Controversies in the
PANDEMIC

Controversies in the PANDEMIC

Editors

Joseph Varon MD FACP FCCP FCCM FRSM
Professor
The University of Houston
College of Medicine
Houston, Texas, United States

Paul E Marik MD MBBS
Chief Medical Officer
Front Line Critical Care Consortium
FLCCC Alliance
Washington, DC, USA

Marc Rendell MD
Medical Director
The Rose Salter Medical Research Foundation
34 Versailles
Newport Coast, California, United States

Jose Iglesias DO FASN
Department of Medicine
Rutgers Health/Community Medical Center
Internal Medicine Residency Program
Community Medical Center
RWJBH, Toms River,
New Jersey, United States

Christopher de Souza
DORL MS DNB FACS(USA) FRCS(England) FRCS(Ireland)
Fellow of the American Neurotology Society
Doctor of Literature (Honoris Causa)
Maharashtra University of Health Sciences
Nashik, Maharashtra, India

Prahlad Prabhudesai
MBBS MD DNB FCCP
Consultant Pulmonary Medicine
Lilavati Hospital and Research Center
Mumbai, Maharashtra, India

Forewords

Randeep Guleria
Ron Johnson and Robert F Kennedy, Jr

JAYPEE

JAYPEE BROTHERS MEDICAL PUBLISHERS
The Health Sciences Publisher
New Delhi | London

Jaypee Brothers Medical Publishers (P) Ltd

Headquarters
EMCA House
23/23-B, Ansari Road, Daryaganj
New Delhi 110 002, India
Landline: +91-11-23272143, +91-11-23272703
+91-11-23282021, +91-11-23245672
E-mail: jaypee@jaypeebrothers.com

Corporate Office
Jaypee Brothers Medical Publishers (P) Ltd.
4838/24, Ansari Road, Daryaganj
New Delhi 110 002, India
Phone: +91-11-43574357
Fax: +91-11-43574314
E-mail: jaypee@jaypeebrothers.com

Overseas Office
JP Medical Ltd.
83, Victoria Street, London
SW1H 0HW (UK)
Phone: +44-20 3170 8910
Fax: +44(0)20 3008 6180
E-mail: info@jpmedpub.com

Website: www.jaypeebrothers.com
Website: www.jaypeedigital.com

Inquiries for bulk sales may be solicited at: jaypee@jaypeebrothers.com

Controversies in the Pandemic / ***Joseph Varon, Paul E Marik, Marc Rendell, Jose Iglesias, Christopher de Souza, Prahlad Prabhudesai***

First Edition: **2024**

ISBN: 978-93-5696-730-4

Printed in India

This book is dedicated to

Mr Ratan N Tata

Who most graciously and generously supported all the healthcare workers during the pandemic. We remain ever grateful to him for his unselfish and generous support.

Contributors

Abha Mahashur MBBS DNB IDCCM
Consultant Pulmonary Medicine
Lilavati Hospital and Research Center
Mumbai, Maharashtra, India

Adriana Luzariaga MD
Department of Medicine
Rutgers Health Community Medical Center Internal Medicine Residency Program, Community Medical Center
Toms River, New Jersey, United States

Aishan Patil MD
Department of Surgery
Borders Hospital
Melrose, Scotland, United Kingdom

Alessandro D Santin MD
Department of Obstetrics, Gynecology and Reproductive Sciences
Yale School of Medicine
New Haven, CT 06520, United States

Allen G Hirsh PhD
CryoBioPhysica Inc.
Chevy Chase, Maryland, United States

Andrew C Berry DO
Private Practic Gastroenterologist
ABIM Board Certified: Internal Medicine and Gastroenterology
Miami, Florida, United States

Anish Patil MB BCh BAO
Royal College of Surgeons (RCSI), Ireland
Masters of Science (MSc), Medical Education, Swansea University
Swansea, Wales, United Kingdom

Anouschka Foltz Dr Phil MA MA
Associate Professor in English Linguistics
Institute of English Studies
University of Graz, Graz, Austria

Arvind Garg MD
Senior Consultant and Head
Department of Pediatrics
Apollo Hospitals
Noida, Uttar Pradesh, India

Bineet Ahluwalia
Clinical Associate
Department of Pulmonary Medicine
Lilavati Hospital and Research Center
Mumbai, Maharashtra, India

Bridgene Bonner
ENT Nurse
Letterkenny University Hospital
Donegal, Ireland

Carlos Valladeres MD
Department of Medicine
Internal Medicine Residency Program
Rutgers Health Community Medical Center
Toms River, New Jersey, United States

Christine Filippone PhD DNP ANP CIC
Director of Nursing/Adult Nurse Practitioner
Ocean County Health Department
Toms River, New Jersey, United States

Christopher de Souza DORL MS DNB FACS(USA) FRCS(England) FRCS(Ireland)
Fellow of the American Neurotology Society
Doctor of Literature (Honoris Causa)
Maharashtra University of Health Sciences
Nashik, Maharashtra, India

Claudia Chaufan MD PhD
Associate Professor
Faculty of Health Profile
School of Health Policy and Global Health
York University
Toronto, Canada

Colleen Aldous PhD
Nelson R Mandela School of Clinical Medicine of the University of KwaZulu-Natal, Durban, South Africa

Dan McDyer MD
Private Consultant in Obstetrics and Gynecology
Jacksonville, Florida, United States

David E Scheim PhD
US Public Health Service
Commissioned Corps, Inactive Reserve
Blacksburg, Virginia, United States

Elaine Cardoso DDS MSc MBA CCRP
Faculty of Dentistry
University of Toronto
Toronto, Ontario, Canada

Eleftherios Gkioulekas PhD
School of Mathematical and Statistical Sciences
University of Texas Rio Grande Valley
Texas, United States

Francesco Salton MD
Department of Pulmonology,
University Hospital of Cattinara, Trieste
Department of Medical, Surgical and Health Sciences, University of Trieste
Trieste, Italy

Francis Johnson PhD
Department of Chemistry and Pharmacological Sciences
School of Medicine
Stony Brook University
Stony Brook, New York, United States

Gianfranco Umberto Meduri MD
Professor of Medicine
Department of Pharmaceutical Sciences
University of Tennessee Health Science Center
Memphis, Tennessee, USA

Howard Tenenbaum DDS Dip Perio PhD FRCD
Faculty of Dentistry
Department of Pathobiology and Laboratory Medicine
Faculty of Medicine
University of Toronto
Toronto, Ontario, Canada

Ivan Fan-Ngai Hung MD
Department of Medicine
The University of Hong Kong
Hong Kong [Special Administrative Region (SAR)], China

Jagan Mohan Rao Vanjarapu MD
Department of Medicine
Rutgers Health Community Medical Center Internal Medicine Residency Program
Community Medical Center, RWJBH
Toms River, New Jersey, USA

Jalil Parkar MD
Consultant Pulmonologist
Department of Pulmonary Medicine
Lilavati Hospital and Research Center
Mumbai, Maharashtra, India

Johannes Scherling Dr Phil
Associate Professor
Department of English Studies
University of Graz, Graz, Austria

Jose Iglesias DO FASN
Department of Medicine
Rutgers Health/Community Medical Center
Internal Medicine Residency Program
Community Medical Center RWJBH,
Toms River, New Jersey, USA

Kavitha Natarajan MD

Konstantinos Giannopolos MD
ENT Specialist
Galatsi Health Center
Athens, Greece

Lorne M Golub DMD MSc MD
Department of Oral Biology and Pathology
School of Dental Medicine
Stony Brook University
Stony Brook, New York, United States

Marco Confalonieri MD
Department of Pulmonology
University Hospital of Cattinara
Trieste, Italy
Department of Medical, Surgical and Health Sciences, University

Marc Rendell MD
Medical Director
The Rose Salter Medical Research Foundation
34 Versailles
Newport Coast, California, United States

Marian P Laderoute PhD(Medical Sciences – Immunology)
Currently Retired
Formerly Laboratory Director
Immune System Management Clinic and Lab
Ottawa, Ontario Canada

Michael Glogauer DDS PhD Dip Perio
Faculty of Dentistry
University of Toronto
Toronto, Ontario, Canada

Michael Goldberg BSc MSc DDS Dip Perio FRCD(C)
Faculty of Dentistry
University of Ontario
Toronto, Ontario, Canada

Nafeesath

Nihal Sriramaneni BS
Garden State Neurology and Neuro-Oncology

Rajesh Mohan MD MBA FACC FSCAI
Department of Medicine Subsection
Department of Cardiology
Rutgers Health Community Medical Center Internal Medicine
Community Medical Center, RWJBH,
Toms River, New Jersey, United States

Ronald Neil Kostoff PhD
Private Consultant
Gainesville, VA, USA

Rosemarie de Souza MD
Head
Department of Internal Medicine
BYL Nair Hospital and TN Medical College
Mumbai, Maharashtra, India

Noah Fine PhD
Faculty of Dentistry
University of Toronto
Toronto, Ontario, Canada

Paola Vottero MA(PhD Candidate)
Department of Biomedical Engineering, University of Alberta,
Edmonton, Alberta, Canada

Patrick Berche MD
Professor Emeritus
Université de Paris
Paris, France

Paul E Marik MD MBBS
Chief Science Officer
Front Line Critical Care Consortium
FLCCC Alliance
Washington, DC, USA

Philip Oldfield DPhil
Scientific and Regulatory Consultant
Rigaud, Quebec, Canada

Prahlad Prabhudesai MBBS MD DNB FCCP
Consultant Pulmonary Medicine
Lilavati Hospital and Research Center
Mumbai, Maharashtra, India

Priyaranjan Kata MD
Department of Medicine
Rutgers Health Community Medical Center Internal Medicine Residency Program
Community Medical Center RWJBH
Toms River, New Jersey, United States

Rajeev Jayadevan MD DNB(Medicine) MRCP ABIM(Medicine) ABIM(Gastroenterology)
Co-Chairman National IMA COVID Task Force
Past President IMA Kochi
Consultant Gastroenterologist
Sunrise Hospital
Kochi, Kerala, India

Ruchi S Raval MPH
MD Candidate
Hackensack Meridian School of Medicine
Research Assistant Garden State Neurology and Neuro-Oncology
Toms River, New Jersey, United States

Shekhar Grover MD
Public Health Consultant
Center for Health Innovation and Policy (CHIP) Foundation
Noida, Uttar Pradesh, India

Sumul N Raval MD DABPN
Neuro-Oncologist
Monmouth Medical Center, RWJBH
Medical Director
David S Zocchi Brain Tumor Center
Leon Hess Cancer Center at Monmouth
Garden State Neurology and Neuro-Oncology
Toms River, New Jersey, United States

Suneela Garg MD
Chair, Program Advisory Committee
National Institute of Health and Family Welfare (NIHFW)
New Delhi, India

Swapnil Chopade MD

Tanu Anand MD
Scientist-E (Medical)
Indian Council of Medical Research
New Delhi, India

Tanvir Hussain MD
Department of ORL-HNS
Sligo University Hospital
Sligo, Ireland

Zahra Sethna BA
Director of Communications
Front Line Critical Care Consortium
FLCCC
Chicago, Illinois

Foreword

Any major outbreak like the COVID-19 pandemic is bound to create controversies. It was a time of uncertainty and fear to some extent. Knowledge and research on how the new virus will interact with the human race was slowly emerging and as the pandemic progressed, it was associated with more and more disruption. As governments, healthcare systems, and individuals struggled to cope with the effects of the virus, several contentious issues arose, leading to intense public discussions and differing opinions.

One of the most significant controversies during the pandemic revolved around government responses and measures implemented to control the spread of the virus. The imposition of lockdowns, mask mandates, and social distancing regulations sparked heated debates about individual freedoms versus public health priorities. Some argued that these measures were necessary to curb the spread of the virus and protect vulnerable populations, while others claimed that they infringed upon personal liberties and had detrimental effects on mental health and the economy. The origin of the virus itself became a contentious issue, with conflicting narratives and conspiracy theories circulating about its source. The debate over whether the virus originated from a natural zoonotic transmission or a laboratory leak fueled geopolitical tensions and added another layer of complexity to the global response to the pandemic. Another controversial topic during the pandemic was the development and distribution of vaccines. As vaccines were developed at an unprecedented pace, concerns about their safety, efficacy, and long-term effects arose. Anti-vaccination movements gained momentum, spreading misinformation and skepticism about the vaccines, leading to hesitancy among certain populations. The debate over vaccine mandates and passports further fueled tensions between those advocating for public health and those emphasizing personal choice. A prominent sport player was not allowed to play an international tournament because he was not vaccinated. Debates about vaccine prioritization, equity, and access have highlighted systemic inequalities and ethical considerations in public health interventions.

In addition to these controversies, COVID-19 has exposed and exacerbated existing societal issues such as healthcare disparities, economic inequality, and racial injustice. The pandemic laid bare the vulnerabilities in our systems and prompted difficult conversations about how to address these underlying issues. Marginalized communities, including low-income populations and people of color, faced disproportionate rates of infection and mortality due to systemic inequalities in healthcare. The lack of equitable vaccine distribution further exacerbated these disparities, highlighting the need for a more inclusive and accessible healthcare system.

The COVID-19 pandemic has been accompanied by a range of controversies that have tested societal norms, values, and systems. As we continue to navigate the challenges posed by the virus, it is essential to engage in constructive dialogue, respect differing viewpoints, and prioritize evidence-based decision-making to address these controversies effectively and unitedly. Several controversies have emerged that have captured public attention and stirred debates across the globe. These controversies range from concerns about government responses and public health measures to issues surrounding misinformation and the development of vaccines.

This well-written book covers all these areas. Chapters have been excellently written by international experts who address these controversies and many more in a balanced and objective manner. The pandemic affected every strata (economy, entertainment, sports, employment, health, etc.) of society and there was an explosion of misinformation in all areas. There is therefore a need to address issues that arose during the pandemic in all sectors and not just in the health sector.

The authors of the book have very skillfully covered all areas that were significantly affected by the pandemic. I would also like to compliment the editors for covering a wide range of topics including telemedicine and censorship of medical literature and highlighting the social work done by many including the art of living volunteers. This book is a great project with support and contributions by so many individuals. A number of chapters have many thought-provoking statements. I am sure the readers will find this an enjoyable and educative experience. Once again, I congratulate the authors and the editors.

Best wishes!

Randeep Guleria
MD DM FAMS DSc(Honoris Causa)
Chairman, Institute of Internal Medicine and Respiratory and Sleep Medicine
Director, Medanta Medical School
Former Director
All India Institute of Medical Sciences
New Delhi, India

Foreword

We are writing this foreword in May of 2024—more than 4 years after the coronavirus pandemic was declared. The changes we have witnessed in the world, the actions taken by governments and global media, and the acquiescence by a majority of the public to those actions are simply breathtaking.

Currently, we would classify the global population into three main categories. The largest group, regardless of the harms they may or may not have suffered or caused, simply wants to move on, trying to forget the pandemic and our response to it.

The next group have had their eyes opened to what the pandemic exposed. They have been awakened to the corruption and ineffectiveness of global government and institutions. They know that they are being lied to, but because the global elite control information, it is exceedingly difficult for them to assess blame and force accountability.

The third group considers themselves to be part of the global elite. They have been preparing for a world-changing pandemic for decades. They quickly sprang into action by stoking fear, covering up their bioweapon research, crushing dissent, and sabotaging any early treatment that might preclude the need for their desired mRNA "vaccine" solution.

They have been depressingly effective because they are in control, and they have no intention of losing control. They will use every tool at their disposal to maintain their power.

Some members of the third group became household names during the pandemic and constitute the ring leaders of the failed response. But in addition to the ring leaders, there are hundreds or thousands of others globally who were all too willing to seize the power made available to them by the pandemic and its ring leaders.

Together, these individuals recommended, implemented, and enforced societal lockdowns, school closures, mask mandates, deadly hospital protocols, emergency use authorizations, and vaccine mandates. They sabotaged early treatment, censored the truth, denied vaccine injuries, and destroyed the careers and reputations of those who questioned their narrative and had the courage and compassion to treat COVID patients with cheap and effective generic drugs. With hindsight, it is hard not to view the actions of some, but not all, as purposeful and malign.

They devised and promoted multiple false media narratives: "safe and effective"; "a pandemic of the unvaccinated"; "no one is safe until everyone is safe"; "vaccinated people do not carry the virus, they don't get sick"; "if you're vaccinated, you're not going to be hospitalized, and you're not going to die"; "the mRNA is likely going to stay right in the arm"; "natural immunity won't protect you"; "side effects of mRNA were mild and short in duration"; and, maybe the most grotesquely hypocritical of all, "follow the science."

Senator Johnson labeled the promoters of our miserably failed response to the coronavirus in the United States the "COVID Cartel"—federal health agencies,

Big Pharma, mainstream media, and social media. This is a powerful and corrupt group of institutions. The evidence of their collusion and corruption continues to grow, but their enormous power allows them to effectively suppress and censor the truth. Unfortunately, the cartel exerted enormous influence around the world, with disastrous consequences for people whose elected officials followed their lead.

A global collection of authors contributed to *"Controversies in the Pandemic."* It is notable the number of contributors from India—a country that supplies much of the active pharmaceutical ingredients (API) for countries around the world. Dr Pierre Kory and others have highlighted the success of the Indian state of Uttar Pradesh in responding to the pandemic, in part through the widespread use of ivermectin. There is much the world can learn and benefit from closer ties to the world's largest democracy. Strengthening our relationship with India should be a major goal of US foreign policy.

The goal, and hopefully the result, of "Controversies in the Pandemic" will be to expose the lies and corruption by providing the truth with science backed by real clinical experience and uncorrupted research. Unlike members of the COVID Cartel, who refuse to provide the public with the data, studies, and analyses that supposedly guided their actions, contributors to this book provide references to back up their conclusions. Readers are free to agree or disagree, propose their own hypotheses, and test them in a process of authentic scientific discovery and debate.

One interesting aspect of the second group, those of us whose eyes have been opened, is its political diversity—the coauthors of this foreword are a prime example. Regardless of past political affiliations, once you have been awakened to the corruption and you see the great harms done as a result, it is impossible to close your eyes. Individuals have put their political differences aside because they are compelled to convey what they have discovered to others. The goal of the second group is to grow our numbers and reduce the size of the first group. This will be the only way we can ensure that those responsible for the harms done to society can be held responsible so their actions will not be repeated.

The pandemic exposed the corruption of science. For the good of us all, it is imperative that scientific integrity be restored. As nonscientists, we are continually amazed at the knowledge mankind has obtained over the millennia, but we would argue that what we do not know vastly exceeds what we do know. As we seek to restore scientific integrity and pursue truth, we must do so with the humility that reality demands.

We have been inspired by the dedication of those in the public eye who have been willing to risk their reputations by speaking the truth. The contributors to this book have made the conscious decision to do just that, and we are truly grateful to them for doing so.

Ron Johnson
US Senator, Wisconsin (2011 to present)
Member of:
- US Senate Committee on the Budget
- US Senate Committee on Finance
- US Senate Committee on Homeland Security and Governmental Affairs (former Committee Chair 2015–2021)
- Permanent Subcommittee on Investigations (current Ranking Member)

Robert F Kennedy, Jr
Candidate for President of the United States

Preface

The title of the textbook "*Controversies in the Pandemic*" may mislead readers to assume that the book itself is contentious. However, the intention of the editors and authors is not to incite but rather to explore the multitude of issues that arose during the pandemic, leading to confusion, uncertainty, and fluctuating opinions. Much of the medical literature published during this time resulted in conflicting claims that caused anxiety and skepticism among both medical professionals and the general public.

Experts contributing to this book present information in an impartial and objective manner, allowing readers to consult the provided references and draw their own conclusions based on credible medical sources. The management of patients during the pandemic highlighted the necessity for collaboration across various medical disciplines to address the health crises, especially in the absence of definitive evidence in the medical literature.

Many healthcare workers devised their own solutions, hoping to alleviate the health problems emerging during the pandemic. Some of these solutions were shared in publications aimed at guiding other healthcare professionals. However, many findings could not be replicated, and in some cases, contradictory results were published, further complicating matters.

To provide clarity amid the confusion, the concept of this book was conceived. Now that the pandemic appears to have eased in the public consciousness, the editors have undertaken a swift review of the myriad dimensions and factors involved in addressing this complex, multidimensional health tragedy.

Some chapters of this book are based on groundbreaking papers such as the one entitled "Sialylated Glycan Bindings from SARS-CoV-2 Spike Protein to Blood and Endothelial Cells Govern the Severe Morbidities of COVID-19," previously published in the *International Journal of Medical Sciences* (IJMS) by Scheim and coauthors, which shed light on the critical interactions between the SARS-CoV-2 spike protein and cellular receptors, providing crucial insights into the mechanisms underlying severe COVID-19 complications. Additionally, Patrick Berche, the great French researcher and historian, in his thought-provoking work "Gain of Function and the Origin of COVID-19", discusses openly the concerns regarding the research aimed at probing enhanced pathogenicity of common viruses. A second contribution by Dr Berche, "The Enigma of the 1889 Russian Flu Pandemic: A Coronavirus?", delves into the historical context of viral pandemics, raising intriguing questions about the potential presence of coronaviruses in past outbreaks, offering valuable perspectives for understanding the current COVID-19 pandemic. We are grateful to Elsevier for allowing us to reprint these classic articles, having first appeared in *La Presse Medicale*, which have contributed significantly to our understanding of viral pathogenesis and the broader implications for public health.

It 'is emphasized by the editors and authors that the pandemic was not solely a medical issue, but also a humanitarian tragedy that profoundly impacted societies worldwide. COVID-19 disrupted the very fabric of communities everywhere, affecting every aspect of daily life. We have secured contributions from thought leaders in many countries throughout the world, in particular from India, the second-most populous nation on Earth, and the leader in the production of many medications and vaccines in use throughout the world.

The editors and authors express profound gratitude to nurses, paramedics, and all frontline workers who selflessly provided care and compassion to those in need. These individuals are the unsung heroes of society, often going above and beyond their human calling to assist others during their most vulnerable moments.

This book is dedicated to these anonymous heroes who exemplify the spirit of selflessness and compassion, embodying the best of humanity in times of crisis. Through their dedication and sacrifice, they have made an indelible impact on the lives of countless individuals, serving as beacons of hope and resilience in the face of adversity.

The Editors
May, 2024

Acknowledgments

The editors would like to acknowledge Elsevier for allowing us to use the following articles by Patrick Berche:

- Berche P. Gain-of-function and origin of Covid19. La Presse Médicale. 2023; 52(1):104167.
- Berche P. The enigma of the 1889 Russian flu pandemic: A coronavirus? Presse Med. 2022;51(3):104111.

The editors and publisher would like to acknowledge MDPI for allowing us to use:

- Scheim DE, Vottero P, Santin AD, Hirsh AG. Sialylated Glycan Bindings from SARS-CoV-2 Spike Protein to Blood and Endothelial Cells Govern the Severe Morbidities of COVID-19. Int J Mol Sci. 2023;24(23):17039.

Contents

SECTION 2: NONPHARMACOLOGIC INTERVENTIONS

SECTION 3: SPECIAL ISSUE OF INTEREST

SECTION 4: THERAPIES

SECTION 5: COMPLICATIONS

1

SECTION

Controversies

CHAPTER 1

Introduction

Jose Iglesias

This January 2023 marks the beginning of the fourth year of the Coronavirus disease 2019 (COVID-19) pandemic. Originating in Wuhan, China, the severe acute respiratory syndrome coronavirus 2 (SARS-CoV-2 virus), the cause of COVID-19 infection, spread throughout the world, overwhelming and stressing healthcare systems to the point of near collapse.[1] During the first year of the pandemic, the capacity of public health authorities, governments, and healthcare systems to properly care for their patients and healthcare workers.[1] In addition to causing millions of deaths, the "state of emergency" generated by the pandemic, the response of governments, politicians, media, public health authorities, and medical research had far-reaching socioeconomic implications that will impact future generations.[2-8] On a translational level, the concept "Bechamp is correct, the microbe is nothing, and the terrain is everything," coined by Pasteur, emphasized and expounded by Antoine Bechamp and by Claude Bernard, can be applied to the interaction of viral infection and societies response to the pandemic.[3,9,10] A pathogen's impact on an individual and socioeconomic level is influenced by various factors.[1,10-12] These include the preexisting health conditions of the population, the response, and robustness of the healthcare system, as well as the role of scientific discovery and information dissemination.[6-8,12] The media plays a crucial role in being a balanced source of information and disseminating information to the public.[6-8] The response of governments and governmental agencies is also critical in determining the severity of a pathogen's impact.[13] In many ways, the nonpathogen factors may have had a more significant impact on the global severity of the pandemic than the pathogen itself. These factors played a crucial role in shaping the pandemic response and mitigating or exacerbating its impact on both an individual and socioeconomic level.[12,14,15]

During these last 3 years, several innumerable controversies have arisen regarding managing the pandemic, early treatment, repurposed medication, and media portrayal of anyone who questions the orthodox view of how the pandemic was managed by institutional medicine and public health authorities. Academic discourse has become toxic, with medical and scientific discourse has become politicized.

THE DEVELOPMENT OF "THE SCIENCE", THE ROLE OF PUBLIC HEALTH AUTHORITIES, INSTITUTIONAL SCIENCE, AND THE MEDIA

From the beginning of the pandemic, there has been a significant amount of mixed messages and controversies. During the COVID-19 pandemic, unclear and inconsistent communication from public health authorities and institutional science has caused confusion and mistrust among the public.[16,17] The media has contributed to this by hyping the pandemic, leading to misinformation.[18] Public attitudes toward governmental actions against COVID-19 varied substantially across the G7 countries due to cultural differences, social norms, and differences in relative positioning on the curve of the pandemic.[19] The disjointed public health response to the pandemic has highlighted the importance of timely and publicly available data, but the lack of open public data standards and sharing has been a significant issue.[20]

Initially, one can attribute this to the lack of knowledge about the novel virus. However, much was known about previous coronavirus outbreaks such as SARS-CoV-1 and Middle East respiratory syndrome (MERS). As time went on, in an attempt to portray the scientific consensus of the narrative, healthcare institutions, institutional science, and scientific bureaucrats working for agencies such as the Center for Disease Control (CDC), National Institute of Health (NIH), and National Health Service (NHS) began to take more control of the scientific debate in order to justify public policy such as employment of nonpharmacological interventions, disease treatment, drug repurposing, and vaccination.[21-25] Thus, institutional science was portrayed by the media and public officials as "the science. Thus, any dissenting views, as Dr Anthony Fauci, head National Institute of Allergy and Infectious Disease (NIAID) stated, "attacks on me are actually attacks on science."[24,26-30]

The advancement of science and scientific inquiry relies on the open exchange of ideas, transparency, and critical evaluation of research, data, and challenges to established knowledge. Regrettably, in recent years, there has been censorship, sometimes even state-sponsored, of dissenting views from reputable scientists and public figures. This may be due to a fear of losing public trust. Instead of fostering transparent and unbiased debate, attempts to silence, disregard, or restrict opposing views can have harmful and long-lasting effects on the fields of public health, science, and medicine.[24,25] It is pertinent to note that the major media and social media began to censor and control public exposure of dissenting views.[22,24,25,31,32] Many dissenting scientists and public figures were deplatformed from social media outlets such as Twitter for spreading misinformation.[24,25,31]

NONPHARMACOLOGIC STRATEGIES AND RESPONSES

China began a "zero COVID strategy" as cases of COVID-19 began appearing. The goals of this public health containment strategy included 5G digital technology to monitor people's movements, large group gatherings, identifying COVID-19 positive cases, and contact tracing. Additionally, entire populations underwent nucleic acid testing with strict quarantine of positive patients and their contacts.[33-35] A long quarantine was enforced on those citizens who traveled abroad.[33-35] Public officials were held accountable with heavy penalties, including imprisonment if policies were not carried out. These rapid containment policies applied to entire cities.[34,36,37] By early March 2020, Italy became the first European country which began to feel the impact of COVID-19.[38,39] Addressing the escalating COVID-19 pandemic in Italy, on 9 March 2020, the Italian government under prime minister Guiseppe Conte instituted restrictions on population movement except for essential needs and by 11 March, Italy was under total lockdown, and only those businesses deemed essential were allowed to operate.[39,40] Following suit, both New Zealand and Australia implemented strict measures to control the spread and elimination of the virus including nationwide lockdowns.[41-43]

From a public health standpoint, as there was no treatment for COVID-19, some epidemiologists, public health authorities, and medical emphasized nonpharmacologic intervention (NPI) strategies, such as Neils Ferguson and the Imperial College of London.[44,45] The Imperial College COVID-19 prediction models had a significant impact on public policy in many developed countries.[44,45] These models were used to analyze the potential impact of various public health measures on slowing and suppressing the spread of coronavirus. The findings were published in a report that predicted dire consequences if countries did not take swift action against the pandemic.[44,45] The updated data from the Imperial team's model indicated that the United Kingdom's health service would soon be overwhelmed with severe cases of COVID-19, and the government might face > 500,000 deaths if no action was taken. This information prompted Prime Minister Boris Johnson to announce stringent new restrictions on people's movements almost immediately.[45,46-50] The same model suggested that the United States might face 2.2 million deaths if no action was taken, and this information was shared with the White House, leading to new guidance on social distancing and escalation of NIP such as "14 days to flatten the curve".[45,46,48,50] The flatten-the-curve policy included NPI strategies such as social distancing, the use of masks, hand washing, and lockdowns eventually led to prolonged lockdowns in many states in the United States.

Michael Levitt and others have criticized the Imperial College predictive models and lockdowns. Levitt, a Nobel laureate in chemistry, has argued that the models were flawed and that the lockdowns were unnecessary and caused more harm than good.[51,52] Other researchers have also questioned the assumptions and projections made by the Imperial College models.

For example, Eubank et al. criticized the models for not taking into account the heterogeneity of the population and the potential for targeted interventions.[44,53,54] Rice et al. replicated the Imperial College model and found that the assumptions made in the model were not supported by the available data at the time.[55] Zala et al. conducted an economic evaluation of the hypothetical suppression policies found in the Imperial College COVID-19 Response Team model and found that the costs of implementing these policies would be substantial.[56] Chin et al. compared the effectiveness of various nonpharmaceutical interventions for COVID-19 using two susceptible groups.[57] Susceptible-infected recovered (SIR) models produced by the Imperial College COVID-19 Response Team and found that the models produced conflicting results.[57] Overall, while the Imperial College predictive models and lockdowns have been widely used and influential, they have also been subject to criticism and debate.[52-54] Although public health measures such as wearing masks, practicing social distancing, and lockdowns attempt to create an environment that lessens the impact of the pandemic, these measures may pose unintended, unforeseen consequences which have significant detrimental effects from a psychological and socioeconomic standpoints.[53,55,56,58,59] In addition, early in the pandemic, it was observed that the majority of morbidity and mortality was found in those > 65 and those with comorbidities, while children and young, healthy adults were minimally impacted or developed the asymptomatic disease.[60-62] This observation and the potential collateral damage that lockdowns could have led some scientists to propose an alternative paradigm to lockdowns.[51,53,55,56] The Great Barrington Declaration (GBD), pioneered by Dr's Jay Bhattacharya, Sunetra Gupta, and Martin Kulldorff, advocated for an approach called "Focused Protection" to address the COVID-19 pandemic. The declaration expresses grave concerns about the damaging physical and mental health impacts of prevailing COVID-19 policies and recommends allowing those who are at minimal risk of death to live their lives normally to build up immunity to the virus through natural infection while better protecting those who are at highest risk.[63,64] The GBD was criticized by Dr Anthony Fauci, director of NAID, and Dr Francis Collins, the then director of the NIH.[24,65,66] The writers of the GBD, all of whom were notable scientists in their respects, were called "fringe epidemiologists" by Francis Collins, and emails between Fauci and Collins released under the Freedom of information act revealed the following comments in regards to the "Barrington Declaration". "There needs to be a quick and devastating published take-down of its premises."[24,65,66] Dr Collins is on public record to have called the declaration "a fringe component of epidemiology. This is not mainstream science. It is dangerous."[24,65,66]

The effectiveness of wearing masks to prevent the spread of COVID-19 has been examined in several studies with mixed results.[67-73] Some studies have shown that masks can prevent the spread of respiratory droplets that may contain the virus. For example, a study by Howard et al. found that masks can be effective in reducing the transmission of COVID-19 when used in combination with other preventive measures.[67] However, other studies have shown that wearing masks alone may not be effective in reducing transmission.[68,70,73] A study by Cardoso[14] found that other preventive measures, such as social distancing, may be more effective in reducing the transmission of COVID-19.[74] A recent Cochrane review conducted by Jefferson et al., which has met much criticism, assessed the effectiveness of physical interventions, including face masks, to interrupt or reduce the spread of acute respiratory viruses.[73] The review found that wearing medical/surgical masks in the community makes little or no difference to the outcome of influenza-like illness (ILI)/COVID-19-like illness compared to not wearing masks.[73] However, the risk of bias for the randomized controlled trials (RCTs) and cluster-RCTs was mostly high or unclear, and adherence with interventions was low in many studies.[73] These findings add to the controversy surrounding mask-wearing during the pandemic, as some studies have shown that masks can reduce transmission while others have found little or no benefit.[67,68,70,72,73] It is important to consider the limitations and context of these studies when interpreting their findings.[67,73] Adding to the confusion Anthony Fauci has recently been quoted in an interview stating, "from a broad public-health standpoint, at the population level, masks work at the margins—may be 10%. But for an individual who religiously wears a mask, a well-fitted KN95, or N95, it is not at the margin. It really does work."[75,76]

As noted above, during the COVID-19 pandemic, many countries implemented stringent public health measures such as lockdowns, quarantines, social distancing, and mask-wearing to slow the progression of the virus. In contrast, Sweden took a unique approach of not implementing strict closures, instead urging personal responsibility.[77,78] The Swedish COVID-19 strategy has thus far yielded a striking result—mild mandates overlaid with voluntary measures can achieve results highly similar to late-onset stringent mandates.[77-81] However, this policy causes more healthcare demand and more deaths than early stringent control and depends on continued public will. Swedish mortality rates are intermediate between rates for European countries that quickly imposed stringent public health controls and those for countries that acted later.[77-81]

MEDICAL THERAPY WITH REPURPOSED DRUGS AND VACCINES

On the clinical front, during the first several months of the pandemic, there was no effective treatment for COVID-19 patients were told to stay home and go to the hospital when they could not breathe and were turning blue, there developed an increased interest in drug repurposing for the treatment of early COVID-19.[82-85] Based on basic science data, molecular docking studies, knowledge of the pathophysiology of disease, and observational empirical evidence some clinicians began employing many repurposed agents in the management of COVID-19.[82,83,85-88] Among these, hydroxychloroquine (HCQ), chloroquine (CQ), ivermectin, fluvoxamine, tocilizumab anticoagulants, and corticosteroids have been the most popular and sometimes most controversial.[89-91] During the first several months of the pandemic, HCQ demonstrated promise as an effective agent in the treatment of early COVID-19.[92-94] Unfortunately, the use of this agent became highly politicized.[95-98] Furthermore, disinformation by the Surgisphere and the somewhat exaggerated concerns about cardiac toxicity studies further hampered its use and approval for early outpatient treatment in high-risk groups.[93,97,99-101] Ivermectin suffered a similar fate.[102-106] What has ensued over the last 2.5 years with drug repurposing has been ridicule, censorship by academics, and public health authorities.[102,105-111] In addition, there are reasonable concerns that many trials on repurposed drugs were inadequately run, had a low incidence of endpoints problems with populations enrolled, questionable endpoints, and issues with timing, dosage, and timing of drug administration.[93,101,112-116] In the case of fluvoxamine and budesonide, despite evidence supporting benefits, they have yet to be approved by health authorities. To date, with the exception of corticosteroids, remdesivir, Paxlovid, and molnupiravir, and for a period of time, monoclonal antibodies have been approved for early treatment of COVID-19 by the Food and Drug Administration (FDA). In some cases, physicians using other agents have been under the threat of losing their licenses and board certification.[117-119]

Since the beginning of the COVID-19 pandemic, institutional medicine and public health institutions have emphasized the importance of developing vaccines and achieving vaccine-induced herd immunity as the only way out of the pandemic.[120-123] Although the initial presumption was that the vaccines would prevent transmission, as time went on, it is important to note that there was a significant amount of breakthrough infections.[124,125]

The focus on vaccines was so intense that there was initially a denial of natural immunity by institutional medicine, and there was a denial or minimization of the protective effect of natural immunity by institutional medicine, with a focus on vaccine development and distribution.[120,121,126-128] As time has progressed, there is evidence that natural immunity provides prolonged immunity.[121,127,128-130] In addition, as the pandemic progressed, the efficacy of vaccines has waxed and waned, with the emergence of new variants leading to breakthrough infections and the need for booster shots.[131,132] Recent evidence suggests that boosters for young adults and teenagers are of questionable benefits.[133,134] Of importance, the vaccine RCTs were not designed to demonstrate prevention of transmission or prevent death.[102,135]

Initially, while the vaccines had been effective in reducing the spread of the virus and preventing severe illness and death, there have also been concerns about vaccine injury.[136,137] The vaccines were developed and approved in record time, and there have been reports of adverse reactions to the vaccines, such as neurologic impairment, thrombotic events, myocarditis, myopericarditis, and death.[136,138-141] It is important to ensure that vaccines are safe and effective, and there should exist transparency and accuracy in reporting serious adverse events.[25,142] Transparency needs to be ensured, and fears that transparency in reporting adverse events will cause vaccine hesitancy should not be a barrier to allowing public knowledge of adverse events. The World Health Organization (WHO) has established the VigiBase system to monitor and report adverse reactions to vaccines.[139] The system allows healthcare professionals and the public to report adverse reactions to vaccines, which are then reviewed by experts to determine if there is a causal relationship between the vaccine and the adverse reaction. This system is critical in ensuring that vaccines are safe and effective and that any adverse reactions are identified and addressed promptly. As of 21 December, there have been >700,000 potential adverse reactions reported to Vigibase.[36,143]

In conclusion, the development of vaccines and achieving vaccine-induced herd immunity has been a major, if not a primary focus of institutional medicine and public health institutions.[122,144-148] To achieve herd immunity by vaccination, a large percentage of the population needs to be vaccinated, and this requires a decrease in vaccine hesitancy and compulsion.[144,149-151]

REFERENCES

1. Connor J, Madhavan S, Mokashi M, Amanuel H, Johnson NR, Pace LE, et al. Health risks and outcomes that disproportionately affect women during the COVID-19 pandemic: A review. Soc Scie Med. 2020;266:113364.
2. Auriemma V, Iannaccone C. COVID-19 pandemic: Socio-economic consequences of social distancing measures in Italy. Front Sociol. 2020;5:575791.
3. Bardosh K, de Figueiredo A, Gur-Arie R, Jamrozik E, Doidge J, Lemmens T, Keshavjee S, et al. The unintended consequences of COVID-19 vaccine policy: Why mandates, passports and restrictions may cause more harm than good. BMJ Global Health. 2022;7(5):e008684.
4. Halperin DT, Hearst N, Hodgins S, Bailey RC, Klausner JD, Jackson H, et al. Revisiting COVID-19 policies: 10 evidence-based recommendations for where to go from here. BMC Public Health. 2021;21(1):2084.
5. Mahase E. COVID-19: Mental Health Consequences of Pandemic Need Urgent Research, Paper Advises. BMJ. 2020;369:m1515.
6. Schabus M, Eigl ES, Widauer SS. The coronavirus pandemic: Psychosocial burden, risk-perception, and attitudes in the Austrian population and its relation to media consumption. Front Public Health. 2022;10:921196.
7. Scherling J, Foltz A. The Use of Certainty in COVID-19 Reporting in Two Austrian Newspapers. Journ Media. 2023;4(2):530-46.
8. Neely SR, Eldredge C, Sanders R. Health Information Seeking Behaviors on Social Media during the COVID-19 Pandemic among American Social Networking Site Users: Survey Study. J Med Internet Res. 2021;23(6):e29802.
9. Rappoport J. Plato's Cave. https://www.platoscave.org/2020_04_19_archive.html
10. Woods TP. Public health policing and the case against vaccine mandates. Thomas L Rev. 2020;33:219.
11. Buck JC, Weinstein SB. The ecological consequences of a pandemic. Biology Letters. 2020;16(11):20200641.

12. Singu S, Acharya A, Challagundla K, Byrareddy SN. Impact of social determinants of health on the emerging COVID-19 pandemic in the United States. Front Public Health. 2020;8:406.
13. Gostin LO, Wiley LF. Governmental public health powers during the COVID-19 pandemic: stay-at-home orders, business closures, and travel restrictions. Jama. 2020;323(21):2137-8.
14. Patterson GE, McIntyre KM, Clough HE, Rushton J. Societal impacts of pandemics: Comparing COVID-19 with history to focus our response. Front Public Health. 2021;9:630449.
15. Pedrosa AL, Bitencourt L, Fróes ACF, Cazumbá MLB, Campos RGB, de Brito SBCS, et al. Emotional, Behavioral, and Psychological Impact of the COVID-19 Pandemic. Frontiers in Psychology. 2020;11:566212.
16. Noar SM, Austin L. (Mis) communicating about COVID-19: Insights from health and crisis communication. Health commun. 2020;35(14):1735-9.
17. Su Z, Zhang H, McDonnell D, Ahmad J, Cheshmehzangi A, Yuan C. Crisis communication strategies for health officials. Front Public Health. 2022;10:796572.
18. Himelein-Wachowiak M, Giorgi S, Devoto A, Rahman M, Ungar L, Schwartz HA, et al. Bots and misinformation spread on social media: Implications for COVID-19. J Med Internet Res. 2021;23(5):e26933.
19. Vardavas C, Odani S, Nikitara K, El Banhawi H, Kyriakos C, Taylor L, et al. Public perspective on the governmental response, communication and trust in the governmental decisions in mitigating COVID-19 early in the pandemic across the G7 countries. Prev Med Rep. 2021;21:101252.
20. Gardner L, Ratcliff J, Dong E, Katz A. A need for open public data standards and sharing in light of COVID-19. Lancet Infect Dis. 2021;21(4):e80.
21. Malhotra A. Curing the pandemic of misinformation on COVID-19 mRNA vaccines through real evidence-based medicine-Part 2. J Insulin Resist. 2022;5(1):10.
22. Niemiec E. COVID-19 and misinformation. EMBO Rep. 2020;21(11):e51420.
23. Woodworth E. (2021). COVID-19 and the Shadowy "Trusted News Initiative." [online] Available from https://www.thelibertybeacon.com/covid-19-the-shadowy-trusted-news-initiative/ [Last accessed November, 2023].
24. Shir-Raz Y, Elisha E, Martin B, Ronel N, Guetzkow J. Censorship and Suppression of COVID-19 Heterodoxy: Tactics and Counter-Tactics. Minerva. 2022:1-27.
25. Elisha E, Guetzkow J, Shir-Raz Y, Ronel N. Suppressing scientific discourse on vaccines? Self-perceptions of researchers and practitioners. HEC Forum. 2022:1-19.
26. Soave R. (2021). Anthony Fauci Says His Critics are Attacking Science Itself. [online] Available from https://reason.com/2021/06/09/anthony-fauci-science-critics-covid-19-chuck-todd/ [Last accessed November, 2023].
27. Dotson T. The Danger of Fact-ist Politics. New Atlantis. 2021;(64):65-74.
28. Graso M, Henwood A, Aquino K, Dolan P, Chen FX. The dark side of belief in COVID-19 scientists and scientific evidence. Pers Individ Dif. 2022;193:111594.
29. March RJ, Yonk RM. (2022). Pandemics and Liberty: An Introduction. [online] Available from https://www.aier.org/article/pandemics-and-liberty-an-introduction/ [Last accessed November, 2023].
30. Ridley M. (2020). What the Pandemic has Taught us about Science. [online] Available from https://www.wsj.com/articles/what-the-pandemic-has-taught-us-about-science-11602255638 [Last accessed November, 2023].
31. Eck K, Hatz S. State surveillance and the COVID-19 crisis. J Hum Rights. 2020;19(5):603-12.
32. Jain A. Restricting Freedom of Speech: An Analysis of Censorship Cases in Relation to Misinformation during the COVID-19 Crisis. Brandeis Univ Law J. 2022;10(1).

33. Li Z, Chen Q, Feng L, Rodewald L, Xia Y, Yu H, et al. Active case finding with case management: the key to tackling the COVID-19 pandemic. Lancet. 2020;396(10243): 63-70.
34. Liu J, Liu M, Liang W. The dynamic COVID-Zero strategy in China. China CDC Weekly. 2022;4(4):74.
35. Wan Z, Lu R, Zhao Y, Zhang C. Diagnostic strategy of SARS-CoV-2 for containment under China's zero-COVID-19 policy. J Infect. 2022;85(1):e7-e9.
36. Yang DL. China's Zero-COVID campaign and the body politic. Curr Hist. 2022;121(836):203-10.
37. Zeng S, Yi C. The impact of accountability on local officials' behavior in the pandemic prevention and control in China based on utility maximization. Glob Health Res Policy. 2022;7(1):1-13.
38. Vaughan A. Italy in lockdown. New Scientist. 2020;245(3273):7.
39. Bull M. The Italian government response to COVID-19 and the making of a prime minister. Contemporary Italian Politics. 2021;13(2):149-65.
40. Young R. Who had their finger on the magic of life-Antoine Bechamp or Louis Pasteur. Int J Vaccines Vaccin. 2016;2(5):00047.
41. Han E, Tan MMJ, Turk E, Sridhar D, Leung GM, Shibuya K, et al. Lessons learnt from easing COVID-19 restrictions: an analysis of countries and regions in Asia Pacific and Europe. The Lancet. 2020;396(10261):1525-34.
42. Bromfield N, McConnell A. Two routes to precarious success: Australia, New Zealand, COVID-19 and the politics of crisis governance. Int Rev Admin Sci. 2021;87(3):518-35.
43. Normile D. 'Zero COVID' countries seek exit strategies. Science. 2021;373(6561):1294-5.
44. Eubank S, Eckstrand I, Lewis B, Venkatramanan S, Marathe M, Barrett CL. Commentary on Ferguson, et al., Impact of Non-pharmaceutical Interventions (NPIs) to Reduce COVID-19 Mortality and Healthcare Demand. Bull Math Biol. 2020;82(4):52.
45. Ferguson N, Laydon D, Nedjati Gilani G, Imai N, Ainslie K, Baguelin M, et al. (2020). Report 9: Impact of non-pharmaceutical interventions (NPIs) to reduce COVID19 mortality and healthcare demand. [online] Available from https://www.imperial.ac.uk/media/imperial-college/medicine/sph/ide/gida-fellowships/Imperial-College-COVID19-NPI-modelling-16-03-2020.pdf [Last accessed November, 2023].
46. Biggs AT, Littlejohn LF. Revisiting the initial COVID-19 pandemic projections. Lancet Microbe. 2021;2(3):e91-2.
47. Enserink M, Kupferschmidt K. With COVID-19, modeling takes on life and death importance. Science. 2020;367(6485):1414-5.
48. Funk S, Abbott S, Atkins BD, Baguelin M, Baillie JK, Birrell P, et al. (2020). Short-term forecasts to inform the response to the COVID-19 epidemic in the UK. [online] Available from https://www.medrxiv.org/content/10.1101/2020.11.11.20220962v2 [Last accessed November, 2023].
49. Adam D. Special report: The simulations driving the world's response to COVID-19. Nature. 2020;580(7802):316-9.
50. Briggs WM. The Most Infamous Coronavirus Forecast. In: Sriboonchitta S, Kreinovich V, Yamaka W (Eds). Credible Asset Allocation, Optimal Transport Methods, and Related Topics. Switzerland: Springer; 2022:39-49.
51. Stringham E; American Institute for Economic Research. (2020). Nobel Laureate Michael Levitt on the lockdowns:" I think it is a huge mistake." [online] Available from https://www.aier.org/article/nobel-laureate-michael-levitt-on-the-lockdowns-i-think-it-is-a-huge-mistake/ [online] [Last accessed November, 2023].
52. Nascimento G. (2020). Multiple Experts, Including Nobel Laureate, Claim Lockdown is More Dangerous Than COVID-19. [online] Available from https://thefreethoughtproject.com/the-state/multiple-experts-including-nobel-laureate-claim-lockdown-is-more-dangerous-than-covid-19 [Last accessed November, 2023].

53. Melnick ER, Ioannidis JP. Should governments continue lockdown to slow the spread of COVID-19? BMJ. 2020;369:m1924.
54. Ioannidis JP, Cripps S, Tanner MA. Forecasting for COVID-19 has failed. Int J Forecast. 2022;38(2):423-38.
55. Rice K, Wynne B, Martin V, Ackland GJ. Effect of school closures on mortality from coronavirus disease 2019: Old and new predictions. BMJ. 2020;371:m3588.
56. Zala D, Mosweu I, Critchlow S, Romeo R, McCrone P. Costing the COVID-19 pandemic: an exploratory economic evaluation of hypothetical suppression policy in the United Kingdom. Value Health. 2020;23(11):1432-7.
57. Chin AW, Chu JT, Perera MR, Hui KPY, Yen HL, Chan MCW, et al. Stability of SARS-CoV-2 in different environmental conditions. Lancet Microbe. 2020;1(1):e10.
58. Joffe AR. COVID-19: Rethinking the Lockdown Groupthink. Front Public Health. 2021;9:625778.
59. Muka T, Li JJ, Farahani SJ, Ioannidis JP. An umbrella review of systematic reviews on the impact of the COVID-19 pandemic on cancer prevention and management, and patient needs. Elife. 2023;12:e85679.
60. Biswas M, Rahaman S, Biswas TK, Haque Z, Ibrahim B. Association of sex, age, and comorbidities with mortality in COVID-19 patients: a systematic review and meta-analysis. Intervirology. 2021;64(1):36-47.
61. Antos A, Kwong ML, Balmorez T, Villanueva A, Murakami S. Unusually high risks of COVID-19 mortality with age-related comorbidities: An adjusted meta-analysis method to improve the risk assessment of mortality using the comorbid mortality data. Infect Dis Rep. 2021;13(3):700-11.
62. Ali AS, Al-Hakami AM, Shati AA, Asseri A, Al-Qahatani SM. Salient Conclusive Remarks on Epidemiology and Clinical Manifestations of Pediatric COVID-19: Narrative Review. Front Pediatr. 2020;8:584694.
63. Kulldorff M, Gupta S, Bhattacharya J. Great Barrington Declaration. Great Barrington Declaration. 2020;4.
64. Ioannidis JP. Citation impact and social media visibility of Great Barrington and John Snow signatories for COVID-19 strategy. BMJ Open. 2022;12(2):e052891.
65. Waldman D. (2022). SARS-CoV-2, the emperor's new clothes and medical tyranny. [online] Available from https://www.oatext.com/sars-cov-2-the-emperors-new-clothes-and-the-return-of-tyranny.php [Last accessed November, 2023].
66. Bertuzzi N, Lagalisse E, Lello E, Gobo G, Sena B. Politics during and after COVID-19: Science, Health and Social Protest. Partecipazione E Conflitto. 2023;15(3):507-29.
67. Howard J, Huang A, Li Z, Tufekci Z, Zdimal V, van der Westhuizen HM, et al. An evidence review of face masks against COVID-19. Proc Natl Acad Sci. 2021;118(4):e2014564118.
68. April MD, Naylor JF, Long B. Analysis of the effects of a texas state-wide mask mandate (Executive Order GA-29) on case load, hospitalizations, and mortality. Southern Med J. 2022;115(3):175.
69. Feng S, Shen C, Xia N, Song W, Fan M, Cowling BJ. Rational Use of Face Masks in the COVID-19 Pandemic. Lancet Resp Med. 2020;8(5):434-6.
70. Kappstein I. Mund-Nasen-Schutz in der Öffentlichkeit: Keine Hinweise für eine Wirksamkeit. Krankenhaushygiene up2date. 2020;15(03):279-95.
71. Klompas M, Morris CA, Sinclair J, Pearson M, Shenoy ES. Universal Masking in Hospitals in the COVID-19 Era. N Engl J Med. 2020;382(21):e63.
72. Lyu W, Wehby GL. Community Use of Face Masks and COVID-19: Evidence From a Natural Experiment of State Mandates in the US. Health Affairs. 2020;39(8):1419-25.
73. Jefferson T, Dooley L, Ferroni E, Al Ansary LA, van Driel ML, Bawazeer GA, et al. Physical interventions to interrupt or reduce the spread of respiratory viruses. Cochrane Databas Syst Rev. 2023;(1):CD006207.

74. de Oliveira Cardoso A, Cardoso RF, Utsumi AG, Sousa NG. (2023). Wearing Masks in COVID-19 pandemic: Mathematical model and simulation for evaluating the impact of non-pharmaceutical intervention strategy associated with social distancing on pandemic behavior in Minas Gerais/Brazil. [online] Available from https://sevenpublicacoes.com.br/index.php/editora/article/view/983 [Last accessed November, 2023].
75. Reason. (2023). Surgeon General Vivek Murthy Refuses to Acknowledge the Government's Misrepresentation of Mask Research. [online] Available from https://reason.com/2023/05/03/surgeon-general-vivek-murthy-refuses-to-acknowledge-the-governments-misrepresentation-of-mask-research/ [Last accessed November, 2023].
76. Wallace-Wells D, The New York Times Magazine. (2023). Dr. Fauci Looks Back: 'Something Clearly Went Wrong.' [online] Available from https://www.nytimes.com/interactive/2023/04/24/magazine/dr-fauci-pandemic.html [Last accessed November, 2023].
77. Ludvigsson JF. How Sweden approached the COVID-19 pandemic: Summary and commentary on the National Commission Inquiry. Acta Paediatrica. 2023;112(1):19-33.
78. Kavaliunas A, Ocaya P, Mumper J, Lindfeldt I, Kyhlstedt M. Swedish policy analysis for COVID-19. Health Policy Technol. 2020;9(4):598-612.
79. Grothe-Hammer M, Roth S. Dying is normal, dying with the coronavirus is not: a sociological analysis of the implicit norms behind the criticism of Swedish 'exceptionalism.' Eur Soc. 2021;23(Sup1):S332-47.
80. Kamerlin SCL, Kasson PM. Managing Coronavirus Disease 2019 Spread with Voluntary Public Health Measures: Sweden as a Case Study for Pandemic Control. Clin Infect Dis. 2020;71(12):3174-81.
81. Renström EA, Bäck H. Anxiety, compassion and pride. How emotions elicited by the government's handling of COVID-19 influences health-promoting behavior. Psychologica Belgica. 2021;61(1):224.
82. Low ZY, Farouk IA, Lal SK. Drug repositioning: New approaches and future prospects for life-debilitating diseases and the COVID-19 pandemic outbreak. Viruses. 2020;12(9):1058.
83. Sultana J, Crisafulli S, Gabbay F, Lynn E, Shakir S, Trifirò G. Challenges for drug repurposing in the COVID-19 pandemic era. Front Pharmacol. 2020;11:588654.
84. Galindez G, Matschinske J, Rose TD, Sadegh S, Salgado-Albarrán M, Späth J, et al. Lessons from the COVID-19 pandemic for advancing computational drug repurposing strategies. Nat Comput Sci. 2021;1(1):33-41.
85. Shah B, Modi P, Sagar SR. In silico studies on therapeutic agents for COVID-19: Drug repurposing approach. Life sciences. 2020;252:117652.
86. Mangione W, Falls Z, Melendy T, Chopra G, Samudrala R. Shotgun drug repurposing biotechnology to tackle epidemics and pandemics. Drug Discov Today. 2020;25(7):1126-8.
87. Baker N, Williams AJ, Tropsha A, Ekins S. Repurposing quaternary ammonium compounds as potential treatments for COVID-19. Pharm Res. 2020;37:1-4.
88. Fadlalla M, Ahmed M, Ali M, Elshiekh AA, Yousef BA. Molecular docking as a potential approach in repurposing drugs against COVID-19: a systematic review and novel pharmacophore models. Curr Pharmacol Rep. 2022;8(3):212-26.
89. Drożdżal S, Rosik J, Lechowicz K, Machaj F, Szostak B, Przybyciński J, et al. An update on drugs with therapeutic potential for SARS-CoV-2 (COVID-19) treatment. Drug Resist Updates. 2021;59:100794.
90. Sultana S. (2022). Medications used for COVID-19 treatment and a comparison of their mechanism of action and therapeutic efficacy. [online] Available from https://dspace.bracu.ac.bd/xmlui/handle/10361/18299 [Last accessed November, 2023].

91. Burkhardt AM, Lu A, Asante I, Louie S. Pharmacologic Therapeutics for COVID-19. In: Gholamrezanezhad A, Dube MP (Eds). Coronavirus Disease 2019 (COVID-19): A Clinical Guide. New York: John Wiley & Sons Ltd; 2023. pp. 290-318
92. Manivannan E, Karthikeyan C, Moorthy NSHN, Chaturvedi SC. The rise and fall of chloroquine/hydroxychloroquine as compassionate therapy of COVID-19. Front Pharmacol. 2021;12:584940.
93. Risch HA. Early outpatient treatment of symptomatic, high-risk COVID-19 patients that should be ramped up immediately as key to the pandemic crisis. Am J Epidemiol. 2020;189(11):1218-26.
94. Million M, Lagier JC, Gautret P, Colson P, Fournier PE, Amrane S, et al. Early treatment of COVID-19 patients with hydroxychloroquine and azithromycin: A retrospective analysis of 1061 cases in Marseille, France. Travel Med Infect Dis. 2020;35:101738.
95. Million M, Raoult D. Re: COVID-19: politicisation,"corruption," and suppression of science.https://www.mediterranee-infection.com/wp-content/uploads/2020/04/Waragainst-Chloroquine.pdf
96. Risch HA. United States Senate Commitee hearing Statement by Harvey A. Risch MD, Phd. https://www.hsgac.senate.gov/wp-content/uploads/imo/media/doc/Testimony-Risch-2020-11-19.pdf Published online November 19, 2020.
97. Piller C. (2020). Former FDA leaders decry emergency authorization of malaria drugs for coronavirus—widespread use of unproven drugs could hurt clinical trials. [online] Available from https://www.science.org/content/article/former-fda-leaders-decry-emergency-authorization-malaria-drugs-coronavirus#:~:text=The%20recent%20Food%20and%20Drug,President%20Donald%20Trump%20and%20former [Last accessed November, 2023].
98. Marcon AR, Caulfield T. (2021). The hydroxychloroquine Twitter war: A case study examining polarization in science communication. [online] Available from https://firstmonday.org/ojs/index.php/fm/article/view/11707 [Last accessed November, 2023].
99. Mehra MR, Desai SS, Kuy S, Henry TD, Patel AN. Retraction: Cardiovascular Disease, Drug Therapy, and Mortality in COVID-19. N Engl J Med. 2020;382(26):2582.
100. Mehra MR, Ruschitzka F, Patel AN. Retraction-hydroxychloroquine or chloroquine with or without a macrolide for treatment of COVID-19: A multinational registry analysis. Lancet. 2020;395(10240):1820.
101. Risch HA. (2021). Hydroxychloroquine in Early Treatment of High-risk COVID-19 Outpatients: Efficacy and Safety Evidence. [online] Available from https://earlycovidcare org/wp-content/uploads/2021/09/Evidence-Brief-Risch-v6 pdf [Last accessed November, 2024].
102. Chaufan C. (2023). "You Are Not a Horse": Medicalization, Social Control, and Academic Discourse in the COVID-19 Era. [online] Available from https://ideas.repec.org/p/osf/socarx/fwvem.html [Last accessed November, 2023].
103. Diaz MI, Hanna JJ, Hughes AE, Lehmann CU, Medford RJ. The politicization of ivermectin tweets during the COVID-19 pandemic. Open Forum Infect Dis. 2022;9(7):ofac263.
104. Tanioka H, Tanioka S, Kaga K. (2021). Shocking conclusions from Africa study expose Big Pharma's suppression of ivermectin data Spread the love. [online] Available from https://climate-science.press/2021/09/04/shocking-conclusions-from-africa-study-expose-big-pharmas-suppression-of-ivermectin-data/# [Last accessed November, 2023].
105. Calello DP, Kazzi Z, Stolbach A. American College of Medical Toxicology (ACMT) cautions against off-label prescribing of ivermectin for the prevention or treatment of COVID-19. J Med Toxicol. 2022;18(1):69-70.
106. Baker SA, Maddox A. From COVID-19 Treatment to Miracle Cure: The Role of Influencers and Public Figures in Amplifying the Hydroxychloroquine and Ivermectin Conspiracy Theories during the Pandemic. M/C J. 2022;25(1):1-13.

107. Bivens M. What About This?: Don't Believe Everything You Read, Ivermectin Edition. Emerg Med News. 2021;43(11B)10.
108. Blaylock RL. COVID UPDATE: What is the truth? Surgical Neurology International. 2022;13:167.
109. Desai AN, Ruidera D, Steinbrink JM, Granwehr B, Lee DH. Misinformation and disinformation: the potential disadvantages of social media in infectious disease and how to combat them. Clin Infect Dis. 2022;74(Supplement_3):e34-9.
110. Gordon JS. A COVID Plea to the CDC: Follow the Science, Respect the People. Integr Med. 2022;21(2):28-9.
111. Gussow L. Toxicology rounds: Ivermectin not the crisis it's claimed to be. Emerg Med News. 2021;43(11):1-33.
112. Marinos A. (2022). TOGETHER Trial Seriously Underdosed its Ivermectin High-BMI Patients. [online] Available from https://doyourownresearch.substack.com/p/together-seriously-underdosed-its [Last accessed November, 2023].
113. Hooper CL, Henderson DR. Ivermeetin and the TOGETHER Trial. Regulation. 2022;45:2.
114. Marinos A. (2022). ACTIV-6 Trial on Ivermectin: NIH Scientists Behaving Badly. [online] Available from https://doyourownresearch.substack.com/p/activ-6-trial-ivermectin-scientists [Last accessed November, 2023].
115. Marinos A. (2022). ACTIV-6 Dosing and Timing: A Fox in the Henhouse. [online] Available from https://doyourownresearch.substack.com/p/activ-6-dosing-and-timing-a-fox-in [Last accessed November, 2023].
116. Hagen K. Misinterpretation of statistical nonsignificance as a sign of potential bias: Hydroxychloroquine as a case study. Account Res. 2022:1-20.
117. DePeau-Wilson M. (2022). Regulators Move Against Two "Misinformation" Doctors. https://www.medpagetoday.com/special-reports/exclusives/101529 [online] Available from https://www.medpagetoday.com/special-reports/exclusives/101529 [Last accessed November, 2023].
118. Clark C. Maine Physician Suspended for COVID Misinformation. [online] Available from https://www.medpagetoday.com/special-reports/exclusives/96652 [Last accessed November, 2023].
119. Saxena V. (2022). Doctor loses license, ordered to have psych eval for Ivermectin scripts, sharing Covid "misinformation. [online] Available from "https://www.bizpacreview.com/2022/01/16/doctor-loses-license-ordered-to-have-psych-eval-for-prescribing-ivermectin-sharing-covid-falsehoods-1189313/ [Last accessed November, 2023].
120. Betsch C, Böhm R, Korn L, Holtmann C. On the benefits of explaining herd immunity in vaccine advocacy. Nat Hum Behav. 2017;1(3):0056.
121. Committee on Oversight and Accountability. (2022). Hearing Wrap Up: Coronaviruses Confer Robust Natural Immunity, Government Officials should have Considered in Policy Decisions. [online] Available from https://oversight.house.gov/release/hearing-wrap-up-coronaviruses-confer-robust-natural-immunity-government-officials-should-have-considered-in-policy-decisions/ [Last accessed November, 2023].
122. Frederiksen LSF, Zhang Y, Foged C, Thakur A. The long road toward COVID-19 herd immunity: vaccine platform technologies and mass immunization strategies. Front Immunol. 2020;11:1817.
123. Pfattheicher S, Petersen MB, Böhm R. Information about herd immunity through vaccination and empathy promote COVID-19 vaccination intentions. Health Psychol. 2022;41:85-93.
124. Singanayagam A, Hakki S, Dunning J, Madon KJ, Crone MA, Koycheva A, et al. Community transmission and viral load kinetics of the SARS-CoV-2 delta (B.1.617.2) variant in vaccinated and unvaccinated individuals in the UK: a prospective, longitudinal, cohort study. Lancet Infect Dis. 2022;22(2):183-95.

125. Stokel-Walker C. What do we know about covid vaccines and preventing transmission? BMJ. 2022;376:o298.
126. Pugh J, Savulescu J, Brown RCH, Wilkinson D. The unnaturalistic fallacy: COVID-19 vaccine mandates should not discriminate against natural immunity. J Med Ethics. 2022;48(6):371.
127. Block J. Vaccinating people who have had COVID-19: Why doesn't natural immunity count in the US? BMJ. 2021;374:n2101.
128. Shenai MB, Rahme R, Noorchashm H. Equivalency of protection from natural immunity in COVID-19 Recovered versus fully vaccinated persons: A systematic review and pooled analysis. Cureus. 2021;13(10):e19102.
129. Lisa Maragakis GDK. (2021). COVID Natural Immunity: What You Need to Know. https://www.hopkinsmedicine.org/health/conditions-and-diseases/coronavirus/covid-natural-immunity-what-you-need-to-know [Last accessed November, 2023].
130. Goldberg Y, Mandel M, Bar-On YM, Bodenheimer O, Freedman LS, Ash N, et al. Protection and Waning of Natural and Hybrid Immunity to SARS-CoV-2. N Engl J Med. 2022;386(23):2201-12.
131. Chemaitelly H, Abu-Raddad LJ. Waning effectiveness of COVID-19 vaccines. Lancet. 2022;399(10327):771-3.
132. Dadras O, SeyedAlinaghi S, Karimi A, Shojaei A, Amiri A, Mahdiabadi S, et al. COVID-19 Vaccines' Protection Over Time and the Need for Booster Doses; a Systematic Review. Arch Acad Emerg Med. 2022;10(1):e53.
133. Bardosh K, Krug A, Jamrozik E, Lemmens T, Keshavjee S, Prasad V, et al. COVID-19 vaccine boosters for young adults: a risk benefit assessment and ethical analysis of mandate policies at universities. J Med Ethics. 2022:medethics-2022-108449.
134. Offit PA. COVID-19 Boosters—Where from Here? N Engl J Med. 2022;386(17):1661-2.
135. Doshi P. Will COVID-19 vaccines save lives? Current trials aren't designed to tell us. BMJ. 2020;371:m4037.
136. Fraiman J, Erviti J, Jones M, Greenland S, Whelan P, Kaplan RM, et al. Serious adverse events of special interest following mRNA COVID-19 vaccination in randomized trials in adults. Vaccine. 2022;40(40):5798-805.
137. Kim MS, Jung SY, Ahn JG, Park SJ, Shoenfeld Y, Kronbichler A, et al. Comparative safety of mRNA COVID-19 vaccines to influenza vaccines: A pharmacovigilance analysis using WHO international database. J Med Virol. 2022;94(3):1085-95.
138. Dutta S, Kaur R, Charan J. Analysis of Neurological Adverse Events Reported in VigiBase From COVID-19 Vaccines. Cureus. 2022;14(1):e21376.
139. Jeet Kaur R, Dutta S, Charan J. Cardiovascular Adverse Events Reported from COVID-19 Vaccines: A Study Based on WHO Database. Int J Gen Med. 2021;14:3909-27.
140. Kant A, Jansen J, van Balveren L, van Hunsel F. Description of Frequencies of Reported Adverse Events Following Immunization among Four Different COVID-19 Vaccine Brands. Drug Saf. 2022;45(4):319-31.
141. Yamoah P, Mensah KB, Attakorah J, Padayachee N, Oosthuizen F, Bangalee V. Adverse events following immunization associated with coronavirus disease 2019 (COVID-19) vaccines: A descriptive analysis from VigiAccess. Hum Vaccin Immunother. 2022;18(6):2109365.
142. Kennedy J, Leask J. Social media platforms have a moral duty to ban misinformation about vaccines: Two leading thinkers on vaccine hesitancy and misinformation debate this crucial question. Index on Censorship. 2020;49(4):76-9.
143. Funke D. (2022). Fact check: 1 million COVID-19 vaccine adverse events are unverified. [online] Available from https://www.usatoday.com/story/news/factcheck/2022/01/05/fact-check-1-million-covid-19-vaccine-adverse-events-unverified/9103381002/ [Last accessed November, 2023].

144. Ahamed F, Ganesan S, James A, Zaher WA. Understanding perception and acceptance of Sinopharm vaccine and vaccination against COVID-19 in the UAE. BMC Public Health. 2021;21(1):1602.

145. Borchering RK, Viboud C, Howerton E, Smith CP, Truelove S, Runge MC, et al. Modeling of Future COVID-19 Cases, Hospitalizations, and Deaths, by Vaccination Rates and Nonpharmaceutical Intervention Scenarios—United States, April–September 2021. MMWR Morb Mortal Wkly Rep. 2021;70(19):719-24.

146. Park H, Kim SH. A Study on Herd Immunity of COVID-19 in South Korea: Using a Stochastic Economic-Epidemiological Model. Environ Resour Econ (Dordr). 2020;76(4):665-70.

147. Fontanet A, Cauchemez S. COVID-19 herd immunity: where are we? Nat Rev Immunol. 2020;20(10):583-4.

148. Rasmussen AL. Vaccination is the only acceptable path to herd immunity. Med (New York, NY). 2020;1:21-3.

149. Graeber D, Schmidt-Petri C, Schroeder CM. Attitudes on voluntary and mandatory vaccination against COVID-19: Evidence from Germany. PLoS ONE. 2020;16:e0248372.

150. Feleszko W, Lewulis P, Czarnecki A, Waszkiewicz P. Flattening the Curve of COVID-19 Vaccine Rejection—An International Overview. Vaccines. 2021;9(1):44.

151. Rozek LS, Jones P, Menon A, Hicken A, Apsley S, King EJ. Understanding Vaccine Hesitancy in the Context of COVID-19: The Role of Trust and Confidence in a Seventeen-Country Survey. Int J Public Health. 2021;66:636255.

CHAPTER 2

The Totality of Evidence

Zahra Sethna, Paul E Marik

INTRODUCTION

Making decisions in medicine can be difficult. The best decisions are based on a combination of:

- The best available evidence
- The clinician's experience, knowledge, and skills
- The patient's individual circumstances, wants, and needs

Evidence can come in many forms such as systematic reviews and meta-analyses (SRMAs), randomized controlled trials (RCTs), observational controlled trials (OCTs), epidemiological analyses, case series, and patient anecdotes.

For a long time, RCTs were considered the "gold standard" of evidence. In this type of clinical trial, participants are randomly assigned to either a treatment group or a control group. You may have heard the term RCT with reference to the various medications being considered as possible coronavirus disease 2019 (COVID-19) treatments.

Another term you may have heard is "meta-analysis" or SRMA. SRMAs involve systematically reviewing the published literature to combine patient data (qualitative and quantitative) from numerous studies of a particular medical intervention to reach a conclusion that has greater statistical power than any single study. Because of the methodology of combining data from multiple studies, SRMAs look at an increased number of subjects, with greater diversity among subjects, and can identify accumulated effects.

However, both RCTs and SRMAs can suffer from the same flaws as other study designs and, unfortunately, these flaws are sometimes intentional due to the financial influences on both researchers and journal editors.

For example, SRMAs can lead to inaccurate results because of biased inclusion or exclusion of study data, flawed analyses, or the exclusion of unpublished studies.

The problems with RCTs are numerous, not least of which is the heavy influence of the pharmaceutical industry in the design and execution of studies, particularly in the larger, well-funded studies published in high-impact medical journals. Studies can be designed to produce a particular set of results, and often are. So much so that often RCTs do not accurately reflect real-world clinical impacts.

"It is simply no longer possible to believe much of the clinical research that is published, or to rely on the judgment of trusted physicians or authoritative medical guidelines," wrote Dr Marcia Angell, in her book *The Truth About Drug Companies: How They Deceive Us and What to Do About It.*[1]

"I take no pleasure in this conclusion, which I reached slowly and reluctantly over my two decades as an editor of the New England Journal of Medicine (NEJM)," she continued.

Angell wrote that medical journals have become "primarily a marketing machine to sell drugs of dubious benefit," and suggested that the pharmaceutical industry has so much wealth and power that it is able to co-opt any institution that might stand in its way. This, she says, includes Congress, the Food and Drug Administration (FDA), academic medical centers, "and the medical profession itself".

Angell and her husband, Arthur Relman, a Harvard professor who also edited NEJM for decades, warned of the undue influence of the pharmaceutical industry for years, as did many other doctors, researchers, and medical ethicists.

"The case against science is straightforward—much of the scientific literature, perhaps half, may simply be untrue. In their quest for telling a compelling story, scientists too often sculpt data to fit their preferred theory of the world. Or they retrofit hypotheses to fit their data," Richard Horton, Editor-in-Chief of The Lancet, wrote in 2015.[2]

In 2005, Stanford Professor John P Ioannidis wrote an article entitled *Why most published research findings are false,*[3] in which he states, "it is more likely for a research claim to be false than true. Moreover, for many current scientific fields, claimed research findings may often be simply accurate measures of the prevailing bias."

In a 2016 paper,[4] Ioannidis analyzed over 9,000 published meta-analyses in biomedicine and found that 20% were flawed beyond repair. Another 33% were redundant and unnecessary, while many others were decent but had "noninformative" evidence. Good and truly informative meta-analyses, he found, were a small minority (3%).

A 2011 analysis of clinical practice guidelines[5] looked at the overall quality of evidence behind 41 guidelines put out by the Infectious Diseases Society of America between 1994 and 2010. Only 14% of the guidelines were based on the supposed "gold standard" of RCTs. Nearly 40% were based on expert opinion alone.

So where, you might ask, does that leave us when it comes to healthcare decision-making?

A NEW MODEL: WEIGHING UP ALL THE EVIDENCE

Just as a jury is asked to review and evaluate all the evidence put forth during a trial, so too must clinicians look at all the best available evidence before them. We propose that researchers rely on the "totality of evidence" and incorporate data from basic science, pharmacology, epidemiology, clinical experience, OCTs, RCTs, and SRMAs. In addition, the intervention should have a sound biological and mechanistic foundation, which is supported by in-vitro and experimental studies.

A common type of observational study is an OCT, where investigators retrospectively assess health outcomes among groups of participants according to a research plan or protocol. The outcomes of study subjects receiving medical interventions (such as drugs, devices, or procedures) are compared to the outcomes of subjects that did not. In these comparisons, the subjects are not randomly assigned to specific interventions by the investigator (as in a prospective RCT). Many people discount the value of findings from OCTs due to an excessive concern that the results can be incorrectly interpreted due to the existence of unmeasured confounders, such as certain characteristics or the behavior of both the patients and the treating physicians.

However, although such concerns are valid when relying on the results of a single OCT, the reality is that findings based on data from groups of OCTs are, on average, identical to the findings from groups of RCTs. Unfortunately, in modern medicine, this fact is rarely taught to or appreciated by physicians and researchers.

Dr William Osler, a Canadian physician often described as the father of modern medicine, is reported to have said that the whole art of medicine is in observation.[6]

A study published in 2014[7] looked at healthcare outcomes assessed with observational study designs compared with those assessed with randomized trials. The researchers reported that— "on average, there is little evidence for significant effect estimate differences between observational studies and RCTs, regardless of specific observational study design, heterogeneity, or inclusion of studies of pharmacological interventions."

In an official 2020 research statement,[8] The American Thoracic Society (ATS) said—"observational studies can provide evidence in representative and diverse patient populations. Quality observational studies should be sought in the development of ATS clinical practice guidelines, and in medical decision making."

THE TOTALITY OF EVIDENCE FOR IVERMECTIN IN COVID-19

Based on the preceding, it is important to look at evidence from all sources when deciding whether to use a particular treatment approach. The Front

Line COVID-19 Critical Care Alliance (FLCCC) used the totality of evidence approach when deciding on whether to recommend ivermectin as a potential treatment for COVID-19.

Some examples of the evidence looked at included the following (not an exhaustive list).

Basic Science

- The FDA-approved drug ivermectin inhibits the replication of severe acute respiratory syndrome coronavirus 2 (SARS-CoV-2) in vitro.[9]
- The broad spectrum antiviral ivermectin targets the host nuclear transport importin-α/β1 heterodimer.[10]
- Ivermectin inhibits DNA polymerase UL42 of pseudorabies virus entrance into the nucleus and proliferation of the virus in vitro and vivo.[11]
- Ivermectin is a potent inhibitor of flavivirus replication specifically targeting NS3 helicase activity—new prospects for an old drug.[12]
- Nuclear localization of dengue virus (DENV) 1–4 nonstructural protein 5; protection against all 4 DENV serotypes by the inhibitor ivermectin.[13]
- Inhibition of human adenovirus replication by the importin-α/β1 nuclear import inhibitor ivermectin.[14]

Pharmacology

- Ivermectin docks to the SARS-CoV-2 spike receptor-binding domain attached to angiotensin-converting enzyme 2 (ACE2)
- Coronavirus (2019-nCoV) deactivation via spike glycoprotein shielding by old drugs, bioinformatic study[15]
- Clinical trial conducted by MedinCell confirms the safety of continuous administration of ivermectin.[16]
- Avermectin exerts anti-inflammatory effect by downregulating the nuclear transcription factor kappa-B and mitogen-activated protein kinase activation pathway.[17]
- Ivermectin inhibits lipopolysaccharide (LPS)-induced production of inflammatory cytokines and improves LPS-induced survival in mice.[18]
- Effect of ivermectin on the cellular and humoral immune responses of rabbits.[19]

Epidemiology

- Uttar Pradesh government says early use of ivermectin helped to keep positivity, deaths low.[20]
- Sharp reductions in COVID-19 case fatalities and excess deaths in Peru in close time conjunction, state-by-state, with ivermectin treatments[21]
- The public health authorities of Missiones released preliminary findings in COVID-19 positive patients receiving Ivermectin. The data suggests that Ivermectin is effective in reducing the symptoms of the disease, with

a considerable record of symptom reduction during the course of the disease. The incidence of hospitalizations and deaths is also shown to be considerably decreased in the population that followed treatment with Ivermectin.[22]

Observational Studies

- Regular use of ivermectin as prophylaxis for COVID-19 led up to a 92% reduction in COVID-19 mortality rate in a dose-response manner: Results of a prospective observational study of a strictly controlled population of 88,012 subjects[23]
- Use of ivermectin is associated with lower mortality in hospitalized patients with COVID-19.[24]
- Ivermectin as preexposure prophylaxis for COVID-19 among healthcare providers in a selected tertiary hospital in Dhaka—an observational study[25]
- Why COVID-19 is not so spread in Africa: How does ivermectin affect it?[26]

Randomized Controlled Trials

- Use of ivermectin as a potential chemoprophylaxis for COVID-19 in Egypt: A RCT[27]
- Role of ivermectin in the prevention of SARS-CoV-2 infection among healthcare workers in India: A matched case-control study.[28]

Systematic Reviews and Meta-analyses

- Review of the emerging evidence demonstrating the efficacy of ivermectin in the prophylaxis and treatment of COVID-19 (this study was what is called a "narrative review.")[29]
- Ivermectin for prevention and treatment of COVID-19 infection: A systematic review, meta-analysis, and trial sequential analysis to inform clinical guidelines.[30]

Case Series

The use of compassionate ivermectin in the management of symptomatic outpatients and hospitalized patients with clinical diagnosis of COVID-19 at the Centro Medico Bournigal and at the Centro Medico Punta Cana, Grupo Rescue, Dominican Republic, from May 1 to August 10, 2020.[31]

Further studies continue to look at the use of ivermectin in COVID-19. A full analysis of all studies is available at c19ivermectin.com,[32] and a real-time meta-analysis is found at ivmmeta.com.[33] You can also read the work of researchers such as Alexandros Marinos (Do Your Own Research)[34] and Phil Harper (The Digger),[35] or follow Dr Pierre Kory's writings about ivermectin and Big Pharma (Pierre Kory's Medical Musings).[36]

REFERENCES

1. Angell M. The Truth About the Drug Companies: How They Deceive us and What to Do About It. New York: Random House; 2004.
2. Horton R. Offline: What is medicine's 5 sigma? Lancet. 2015;385(9976):1380.
3. Ioannidis JP. Why most published research findings are false PLoS Med. 2005;2(8):e124.
4. Ioannidis JP. The mass production of redundant, misleading, and conflicted systematic reviews and meta-analyses. Milbank Q. 2016;94(3):485-514.
5. Lee DH, Vielemeyer O. Analysis of overall level of evidence behind Infectious Diseases Society of America practice guidelines. Arch Intern Med. 2011;171(1):18-22.
6. Silverman ME, Murray TJ, Bryan CS. The Quotable Osler (Vol. 173). Philadelphia: American College of Physicians; 2003.
7. Anglemyer A, Horvath HT, Bero L. Healthcare outcomes assessed with observational study designs compared with those assessed in randomized trials. Cochrane Database Syst Rev. 2014;2014(4):MR000034.
8. Gershon AS, Lindenauer PK, Wilson KC, Rose L, Walkey AJ, Sadatsafavi M, et al. Informing healthcare decisions with observational research assessing causal effect. An Official American Thoracic Society Research Statement. Am J Respir Crit Care Med. 2021;203(1):14-23.
9. Caly L, Druce JD, Catton MG, Jans DA, Wagstaff KM. The FDA-approved drug ivermectin inhibits the replication of SARS-CoV-2 in vitro. Antiviral Res. 2020;178:104787.
10. Yang SNY, Atkinson SC, Wang C, Lee A, Bogoyevitch MA, Borg NA, et al. The broad spectrum antiviral ivermectin targets the host nuclear transport importin α/β1 heterodimer. Antiviral Res. 2020;177:104760.
11. Lv C, Liu W, Wang B, Dang R, Qiu L, Ren J, et al. Ivermectin inhibits DNA polymerase UL42 of pseudorabies virus entrance into the nucleus and proliferation of the virus in vitro and vivo. Antiviral Res. 2018;159:55-62.
12. Mastrangelo E, Pezzullo M, De Burghgraeve T, Kaptein S, Pastorino B, Dallmeier K, et al. Ivermectin is a potent inhibitor of flavivirus replication specifically targeting NS3 helicase activity: new prospects for an old drug. J Antimicrob Chemother. 2012;67(8):1884-94.
13. Tay MY, Fraser JE, Chan WK, Moreland NJ, Rathore AP, Wang C, et al. Nuclear localization of dengue virus (DENV) 1-4 non-structural protein 5; protection against all 4 DENV serotypes by the inhibitor Ivermectin. Antiviral Res. 2013;99(3):301-6.
14. King CR, Tessier TM, Dodge MJ, Weinberg JB, Mymryk JS. Inhibition of human adenovirus replication by the importin α/β1 nuclear import inhibitor ivermectin. J Virol. 2020;94(18):e00710-20.
15. Dayer MR. (2020). Coronavirus (2019-nCoV) deactivation via spike glycoprotein shielding by old drugs, bioinformatic study. [online] Available from https://www.preprints.org/manuscript/202005.0020/v1 [Last accessed November 2023].
16. MedinCell. (2021). Clinical trial conducted by MedinCell confirms the safety of continuous administration of ivermectin. [online] Available from: https://www.medincell.com/en/2021/04/19/clinical-trial-conducted-by-medincell-confirms-the-safety-of-continuous-administration-of-ivermectin/ [Last accessed November 2023].
17. Ci X, Li H, Yu Q, Zhang X, Yu L, Chen N, et al. Avermectin exerts anti-inflammatory effect by downregulating the nuclear transcription factor kappa-B and mitogen-activated protein kinase activation pathway. Fundam Clin Pharmacol. 2009;23(4):449-55.
18. Zhang X, Song Y, Ci X, An N, Ju Y, Li H, et al. Ivermectin inhibits LPS-induced production of inflammatory cytokines and improves LPS-induced survival in mice. Inflamm Res. 2008;57(11):524-9.
19. Sajid MS, Iqbal Z, Muhammad G, Sandhu MA, Khan MN, Saqib M, et al. Effect of ivermectin on the cellular and humoral immune responses of rabbits. Life Sci. 2007;80(21):1966-70.

20. Seth M. (2021). Uttar Pradesh government says early use of Ivermectin helped to keep positivity, deaths low. [online] Available from: https://indianexpress.com/article/cities/lucknow/uttar-pradesh-government-says-ivermectin-helped-to-keep-deaths-low-7311786/ [Last accessed November 2023].
21. Chamie-Quintero J, Hibberd JA, Scheim D. (2022). Sharp reductions in COVID-19 case fatalities and excess deaths in Peru in close time conjunction, state-by-state, with ivermectin treatments. [online] Available from https://osf.io/h7zbg/?utm_medium=email&utm_source=transaction [last accessed November 2023].
22. Página16. (2023) Ivermectina: Brindan resultados parciales de monitoreo en el uso ampliado en pacientes positivos. [online] Available from http://www.pagina16.com.ar/ivermectina-brindan-resultados-parciales-de-monitoreo-en-el-uso-ampliado-en-pacientes-positivos/ [Last accessed November 2023].
23. Kerr L, Baldi F, Lobo R, Assagra WL, Proença FC, Chamie JJ, et al. Regular use of ivermectin as prophylaxis for COVID-19 led up to a 92% reduction in COVID-19 mortality rate in a dose-response manner: Results of a prospective observational study of a strictly controlled population of 88,012 subjects. Cureus. 2022;14(8):e28624.
24. Rajter JC, Sherman MS, Fatteh N, Vogel F, Sacks J, Rajter JJ. Use of ivermectin is associated with lower mortality in hospitalized patients with coronavirus disease 2019: The ivermectin in COVID nineteen study. Chest. 2021;159(1):85-92.
25. Alam MT, Murshed R, Gomes PF, Masud ZM, Saber S, Chaklader M, et al. Ivermectin as Pre-exposure Prophylaxis for COVID-19 among Healthcare Providers in a Selected Tertiary Hospital in Dhaka–An Observational Study. Eur J Med Health Sci. 2020;2(6):1-5.
26. Tanioka H, Tanioka S, Kaga K. (2021). Why COVID-19 is not so spread in Africa: How does Ivermectin affect it? MedRxiv. [online] Available from https://www.medrxiv.org/content/10.1101/2021.03.26.21254377v1 [Last accessed November 2023].
27. Shouman W, Hegazy A, Nafae RM, Ragab M, Anas D, Samra SR, et al. Use of Ivermectin as a potential chemoprophylaxis for COVID-19 in Egypt: A randomised clinical trial. JCDR. 2021;15(2):OC27-OC32.
28. Behera P, Patro BK, Singh AK, Chandanshive PD, S R R, Pradhan SK, et al. Role of ivermectin in the prevention of SARS-CoV-2 infection among healthcare workers in India: A matched case-control study. PLoS One. 2021;16(2):e0247163.
29. Kory P, Meduri GU, Varon J, Iglesias J, Marik PE. Review of the Emerging Evidence Demonstrating the Efficacy of Ivermectin in the Prophylaxis and Treatment of COVID-19. Am J Ther. 2021;28(3):e299-e318.
30. Bryant A, Lawrie TA, Dowswell T, Fordham EJ, Mitchell S, Hill SR, et al. Ivermectin for Prevention and Treatment of COVID-19 Infection: A Systematic Review, Meta-analysis, and Trial Sequential Analysis to Inform Clinical Guidelines. Am J Ther. 2021;28(4):e434-60.
31. Morgenstern J, Redondo JN, De León A, Canela JM, Torres N, Tavares J, et al. The use of compassionate ivermectin in the management of symptomatic outpatients and hospitalized patients with clinical diagnosis of COVID-19 at the Centro Medico Bournigal and at the Centro Medico Punta Cana, Grupo Rescue, Dominican Republic, from May 1 to August 10, 2020. J Clin Trials. 2021;S9:002.
32. COVID Analysis. (2023). Ivermectin for COVID-19: real-time meta analysis of 99 studies. [online] Available from https://c19ivm.org [Last accessed November 2023].
33. COVID Analysis. (2022). Ivermectin for COVID-19: real-time meta analysis of 99 studies. [online] Available from https://c19ivm.org/meta.html [Last accessed November 2023]
34. Marinos A. (2022). Ivermectin: much less than you needed to know. Do Your Own Research. [online] Available from https://doyourownresearch.substack.com [Last accessed November 2023].
35. Harper P. (2022). The 'very unusual paper.' Part 1. The Digger. [online] Available from https://philharper.substack.com/ [Last accessed November 2023].
36. Kory P. (2023). Elon Musk's comments on mechanical ventilation betrayed a stunning amount of ignorance-part 1. Pierre Kory's Medical Musings. [online] Available from https://pierrekory.substack.com [Last accessed November 2023].

CHAPTER 3

COVID-19 Censorship in the European Union: The Example of Austria

Johannes Scherling, Anouschka Foltz

"Of course, all scientists agree when you censor those that don't"

—Author unknown

DECLARING AN INFODEMIC

Coronavirus disease 2019 (COVID-19) was declared a global pandemic by the World Health Organization (WHO) in March 2020.[1] This declaration suddenly and drastically affected the lives of billions of people around the globe—many countries, including most European countries,[2] introduced lockdowns, mask mandates, and social distancing followed in 2021 by mass vaccination programs,[3] vaccination passports[4] and a system of rewards and punishments based on vaccination status.[5-7] Governments presented these measures as inevitable and without alternative,[8-11] a narrative which the mainstream media forcefully echoed.[12,13] From very early on, these media organizations, implicitly but some also explicitly,[14] aligned themselves with governments in the name of public health.

From early on in the pandemic, authorities warned of "fake news" circulating on social media and called on people to only trust "authoritative" information.[15] This was in line with the WHO's assessment in the early days of the pandemic of a so-called "infodemic", defined as "an over-abundance of information, some accurate and some not, that makes it hard for people to find trustworthy sources and reliable guidance when they need it"[15] that was affecting a population hungry for information. Voices that did not conform to the orthodoxy that governments and international authorities, such as the WHO or the CDC, propagated fell silent.[16]

The streamlining of information and sidelining of dissenting views was anything but a coincidence. When the pandemic struck, the European Union (EU) issued several communications attempting to tackle what they saw as a dangerous surge of "disinformation".

EUROPEAN UNION POLICIES ON DISINFORMATION

In a speech on June 4, 2020, Vera Jourová, the vice president of the European Commission, formulated what would later become official EU policy: "I have been saying for a long time that I want (social media) platforms to be more responsible, therefore I support Twitter's action to implement transparent and consistent moderation policy. This is not about censorship (...) But it is about having some limits and taking some responsibility of what is happening in the digital world." She continued that "already on 3 March (2020) I held the first meeting with the social media platforms. We agreed they would promote links to WHO and health authorities [...] They also removed millions of pieces of content that is potentially harmful." She also stressed the importance of journalism in "providing reliable and accurate information". Calling on the health sector specifically to "defend the truth", she concluded her speech by warning that "we must not move into censoring, we must not create ministries of truth."[17] From the beginning, therefore, there was an air of cognitive dissonance in the EU approach toward the "infodemic"—calling to defend "the truth" while refusing to acknowledge that this is the core agenda of any "ministry of truth".

In their Joint Communication from June 10, 2020, termed "Tackling COVID-19 disinformation—getting the facts right",[18] the European Commission identified what they saw as a grave issue: "Given the novelty of the coronavirus, gaps in knowledge have proven to be an ideal breeding ground for false or misleading narratives to spread." They concluded that "this calls for more coordinated action [...] to address the risks for open societies". This strategy was based on an earlier 2018 document called the "Action Plan against Disinformation", which called for combatting disinformation campaigns by foreign state actors.[19] In this updated 2020 action plan, the European commission identified the 'infodemic' as a serious issue as "it can lead people to ignore official health advice and engage in risky behavior, or have a negative impact on our democratic institutions, societies, as well as on our economic and financial situation".[19] It lists various examples on disinformation alongside a proposed course of action, some of which are:

- Dangerous hoaxes and misleading healthcare information including false claims. The suggested response is "to make available and easily visible authoritative health-related content" or "to increase citizens' ability to recognize and react to such disinformation".
- Conspiracy theories that "may endanger human health, harm the cohesion of our societies and may lead to public violence and create social unrest". For such cases, the Commission advises "prompt debunking, demotion, possible removal, or action against accounts".
- Illegal hate speech (the document mentions as an example "a particular ethnic or religious group being blamed for the spread of COVID-19")

which should be subject to removal or "action by competent authorities under the criminal laws of the member states".

- Consumer fraud (the example provided being the sale of "miracle products" against COVID-19), which should trigger legal actions.[19]

The document clarifies that the list is "nonexhaustive", and the examples mentioned (e.g., 5G causes COVID) are sufficiently fringe to make the actions of the commission calls for appear reasonable. However, the problem categories are so vague that they might also be used to censor information that is not actually wrong, but merely unorthodox. For instance, the label "conspiracy theories that harm social cohesion or create social unrest" could be applied to any claim purporting an intentional discrimination of people unvaccinated against COVID-19 as this might lead to social upheaval. Similarly, hate speech could potentially also cover claims that the uniformity of the COVID policies in the West is traceable to an agenda, of whichever shape and form, of the ruling elites and because the commission equates "truth" with "authoritative", the label "false claim" could be attached to any claim that contradicts "authoritative" information at any point in time. All of these, then, would be subject to fact-checks, removal, demoting, or demonetization.

An important distinction that the joint communication attempts to make is between "misinformation", sharing false information without intention to deceive, and 'disinformation' the spread of false information with the intention of harm or deception. In the former case, the commission calls for "rebuttal" and "mythbusting", whereas in the second case they advise "actions taken by governments". This includes "mobilizing the private sector" to tackle accounts that spread disinformation (labeling, demonetizing, and deplatforming) as well as "trainings for media and public opinion shapers in the Union and its neighborhood" and "the creation of teams of multidisciplinary independent fact-checkers, and researchers".[19] A major concern with this distinction is the issue of proving intent. This risks an overly generous interpretation of what constitutes "disinformation", in accordance with the idea of "better safe than sorry".

Another key element of this disinformation policy is the cooperation with international entities, mainly the WHO, the G7, and North Atlantic Treaty Organization (NATO). While cooperation with the WHO seems self-evident in the context of a health crisis, cooperation with the G7 and NATO appears out of place at first sight. However, Vice President Jourová already foreshadowed this in her speech from June 2020, when she called to "beef up our cooperation with international partners, including NATO. Disinformation is part of the hybrid threats, so this is a security issue as well".[17] Furthermore, in the original "action plan against disinformation", disinformation, in the form of "targeted disinformation campaigns", is seen mainly as a threat from foreign state actors, notably Russia and China.[19] Lacking a concrete definition of what "targeted disinformation campaigns" are, this raises the possibility that any information that is pushed by multiple individuals might be summarily seen as a targeted effort to "exacerbate social polarization in the EU".[19] This could thus result in an inflated perception of "disinformation campaigns" and may serve to discredit any information pushing unorthodox views as Russian/Chinese propaganda.

The EU commission's proposed actions to tackle disinformation reflect their dependence on the aforementioned international entities, for example, by:

- Work in partnership with the WHO to enhance its epidemiological surveillance through effective media monitoring and to promote detection and response to misleading and harmful narratives.
- Intensify existing partnerships including with the G7 and NATO.
- Promote the access to reliable information, fight disinformation, work with journalists and media, and support initiatives to address disinformation and misinformation in third countries through EU Delegations and Member States diplomatic missions on the ground.[19]

As a consequence of this identified threat, the 2018 Code of Practice against Disinformation, whose original signatories included Facebook, Google, Twitter, and Mozilla, was expanded to become the Strengthened Code of Practice against Disinformation in 2022,[20] with >40 signatories including big-tech companies, social media giants, and also journalistic networks such as reporters without borders.[21] In this code of practice, the signatories have committed to, among other things:

- Promote authoritative content about COVID-19 from the WHO, national health authorities and media outlets.
- Demote content that is fact-checked as false or misleading.
- Remove content that could harm citizens' health or public safety.[20]

In the context of this code, the commission set up a monitoring system of monthly reports under which online platforms presented their progress in implementing the aforementioned commitments between August 2020 and April 2022. As early as their joint communication from June 2020, the commission commends social media companies for promoting "accurate and authoritative information about COVID-19 from the WHO, national health authorities, and professional media outlets".[19]

In their monthly reports, the social media companies stress their efforts to help people find "reliable information" and "authoritative sources".[22-24] Such content is defined as "expert-voices", such as the WHO, and "government health authorities".[25] Notably absent in this rather vague definition is any mention of medical practitioners in the field or scientific findings, unless they are sanctioned by such authoritative sources. Notably, content is removed if it "contradicts consensus among health authorities".[23] That such consensus can even be established in a fast-changing field like medicine, especially during a pandemic, is, however, disputed.[26,27]

The information stream therefore was strictly top-down and only information that was in-line with the narratives pushed by governments and international health authorities was permitted to go unchecked. Facebook, for instance, in their info text on their COVID-19 policies says that, starting in January 2020, they have been removing information relating to COVID-19 that "according to health authorities, are (1) false, and (2) likely to contribute to imminent physical harm such as increasing the likelihood of exposure to or transmission of the virus or having adverse effects on the public health system's ability to cope with the pandemic".[25] The problematic nature of such a carte blanche for authorities to define what is and is not "disinformation" is revealed later-on in the document, where Facebook explains that it will remove "claims that health authorities do not recommend that healthy people wear masks *where this is not the current public health guidance*" [our emphasis]. This suggests that what is considered to be "disinformation", and as a result what citizens will or will not see, depends on what their governments promote and not on "the science".

In general, social media companies have agreed to take action against "false information" on the following:

- The existence and severity of COVID-19 (including questioning vaccine efficacy or claiming COVID-19 is similar to the flu)
- COVID-19 transmission and immunity
- Guaranteed cures or prevention methods for COVID-19
- Discouraging good health practices (including masking, testing, and vaccinations)

Interestingly, social media companies such as Facebook admit to also remove or otherwise penalize content that "does not violate our COVID-19 or vaccine policies above but that shares potentially or actually true events or facts that raise safety concerns".[25] Similarly, the Twitter Files have revealed that Twitter had a similar policy for "true content which might promote vaccine hesitancy".[28] In short, the EU approach to tackle "disinformation" very likely constitutes an overreach that involved taking down accurate content that ran counter to the orthodox narrative and censoring information, not based on scientific evidence, the much-cited 'the science', but on what the authorities sanctioned as trustworthy. Nevertheless, through the Code of Practice against Disinformation as well as the EU-Rapid Alert System, this practice spread throughout the Union and was adopted not only by social media companies, but also by traditional media outlets, as we will show subsequently with the example of Austria—the only EU member country to later institute a vaccination mandate as well as mandatory lockdowns for unvaccinated people.

AUSTRIAN APPROACH TO COVID DISINFORMATION

On March 19, 2020, the Austrian Government set up a Digital Emergency Task Force ("Digitaler Krisenstab") as well as an "investigative network" ("Aufdecker Netzwerk") to address the issue of the "infodemic". This investigative network also included the major Austrian newspapers and media organizations who committed to identifying and debunking false or misleading information on COVID-19 or measures taken against it and reporting that information to the Digital Emergency Task Force once a day. These news media included the public broadcaster *ORF*, the private broadcaster *PULS 4*, as well as the newspapers *Der Standard, Die Presse, Kleine Zeitung* and *Kronen Zeitung*, amongst others. Members of this network then used this information in their own reporting on the COVID-19 crisis.[29] The Austrian government explicitly mentioned four categories of mis- and disinformation:

1. Conspiracy theories regarding the origins of the virus
2. Trivializing the virus in terms of harm or spread
3. Dangerous recommendations for self-treatment
4. False claims regarding impending measures and restrictions for the public.[30]

In addition, the Austrian government participated in the EU-Rapid Alert System, where member states and EU institutions report cases of perceived mis- and disinformation,[31] with the following intended outcomes:

- Public information and awareness raising
- Flagging serious cases to online platforms
- Empowering researchers, fact-checkers and civil society
- Coordinated responses
- Coordinated attributions[31]

The perpetrators of mis- and disinformation are clearly named in the EU's infodemic approach—they are countries such as Russia or China and, locally, conspiracy platforms and the extreme right.[30] This labeling practice was universally applied to discredit and delegitimize content that went counter to the official narratives at any point during the pandemic.

The potential impact of these measures is palpable—governments and their appointed health authorities decide what is potentially dangerous information. With the help of private companies, social media companies, traditional media via the Code of Practice, networks such as the Austrian "investigative network", and the EU-Rapid Alert System, they target any information that has been labeled as mis- or disinformation. This large and interdependent censorship system may help to explain why government narratives, mainstream media narratives, and published narratives on social media were as monolithic as they turned out to be.

Based on their assessment of the disinformation threat, the EU, its national governments as well as social and traditional media used and promoted a large system of fact-checkers rooted in the so-called International Fact-Checking Network (IFCN) to determine what is and is not permissible information. This widely implemented system was responsible for ensuring that only "authoritative" as well as "authenticated" information got promoted.[32]

FACT-CHECKING IN AUSTRIA

The EU's reliance on fact-checking is clear from the 2022 Strengthened Code of Practice on Disinformation, which contains a total of 121 instances the words *fact, factchecking, factcheckers, factual,* and *factchecked,* but only six instances of the word *scientific* (and no mention of *science*). The European Commission also funds various projects that involve fact-checking, such as the European Digital Media Observatory, which "brings together fact-checkers, media literacy experts, and academic researchers to understand and analyze disinformation, in collaboration with media organizations, online platforms, and media literacy practitioners".[33] Other EU-funded projects addressing disinformation include WeVerify, which states that "The fight is on against fake news"[34] and SocialTruth.[34]

The three main fact-checking organization in Austria are (1) Mimikama,[35] the Austrian Press Agency (APA),[36] and Fakt ist Fakt (fact is fact).[37] Unlike many other fact-checking organizations, which do not disclose how they fact-check information, Mimikama advertises their approach to identify fake news—the FLIP principle.[38] FLIP stands for Fragen, Logik, Interessen, and Plausibilität (questions, logic, interests, and plausibility). The first step, questions, considers whether the source of the information is trustworthy. However, Mimikama does not state which sources they do and do not consider trustworthy. The second step, logic, plays on people's confirmation bias by considering whether the information fits with what we already know or understand. Mimikama gives the following example—"information that claims, for example, that the earth is flat contradicts the generally accepted scientific understanding. Such information should be viewed with scepticism" (our translation).[38] This example implies that there is generally accepted scientific understanding that Mimikama can rely on, which in the case of COVID-19 was and is often not the case. The example can also be seen as a strawman argument in that Mimikama invokes a particularly easily rebukeable example to cast doubt on other claims with more scientific backing. The third step, interests, considers who profits from spreading the information, which, as we will see, they do not apply to information following mainstream narratives. Finally, the fourth step, plausibility, seems to be identical to the second step in that it asks whether the information is in line with what we already know about the world. The approach thus relies heavily on confirming what we think we already know and, as such, risks merely reinforcing those pieces of information that governments and international organizations are pushing via the media. Mimikama also allows people to "report a fake".[35] During the height of the pandemic, Mimikama received around 400 requests for fact-checking daily.[39]

The APA also provides information about their fact-checking approach. Their fact-checks used to consist of three parts—(1) the information to be verified, (2) assessment of the information, and (3) information about the assessment process. Since June 2021, the APA no longer has a paragraph explicitly stating the information to be verified, "so that false assertions are not repeated yet again and thus possibly remain in people's memory" (our translation).[40] In practice, this means that the information to be verified is mentioned differently. Before June 2021, it was given as a declarative statement, as in "according to one study, 13.9% of vaccinated pregnant women suffered a miscarriage and 9.4% a premature birth. This is alarmingly high".[41] Now, the information is typically prefaced by a sentence like "since then, opponents of vaccination have been spreading false and misleading information about it and stirring up fear"[42] in a fact-check about the safety of the COVID-19 vaccines for pregnant women. The APA also does not provide information about how they assess the information. However, they do focus on transparency and provide sources and a rationale to help readers determine how they reached their conclusions. They also acknowledge that not all information can be categorized as completely "true" or completely "false". Fakt ist Fakt focuses on checking statements made by politicians and other public figures. They rate statements as true, half-true, or false, but otherwise provide no information about how they fact-check statements.[43]

Since the media in Austria, via their membership in the "Investigative Network", rely on official "authoritative" information and fact-checking organizations do not provide much information about how they fact-check, we now look at three examples of controversial information in detail—(1) ivermectin, (2) COVID origins, and (3) masks. For media coverage, we use a corpus of the two Austrian broadsheet papers *Der Standard* and *Die Presse* that contain all 2020 and 2021 articles that mentioned "Corona", "COVID-19", and "COVID-19".[27] For our analysis, we consider *collocates*, i.e., words that are up to five words to the left or right of a particular target word. Example fact-checks come from one of the three Austrian fact-checking organizations. In all three cases, the jury is still out, but Austrian media and fact-checkers have prematurely and forcefully come out on one side of the discussion.

AUSTRIAN MEDIA COVERAGE AND FACT-CHECKING OF IVERMECTIN

One of the most controversial topics surrounding COVID-19 has been the use of ivermectin, a broad spectrum antiparasitic that also has antiviral and antibacterial properties,[44] to treat COVID-19. The collocates for "Ivermectin" suggest that the Austrian Media has come down on the anti-ivermectin side. For example, the most common collocates for "ivermectin" include *controversial* (*umstritten*), *deworming agent* (*entwurmungsmittel*), *horse dewormer* (*pferdewurmmittel*), *overdose* (*überdosis*), *intensive care unit* (*invensivstation*), and *FPÖ-circles* (*FPÖ-Kreise*; FPÖ is the far-right party in Austria). The general gist that we get from these collocates is this—ivermectin is horse medication that has been promoted in right-wing circles and has led to people overdosing on the horse medication and ending up in intensive care. The following quotes from these newspapers confirm this picture:

- *It has long been known that ivermectin is dangerous*: Numerous institutes and bodies such as the WHO have already warned against its use, and now the manufacturer itself is doing the same.[45]
- The misbelief that ivermectin helps against COVID is widespread.[46]
- Kickl (the leader of the FPÖ faction) continued his campaign against vaccination with the fake news that there was "rapid spread of infection by the vaccinated," and he recommended the horse worm medication ivermectin, whose ineffectiveness for all but Corona conspiracy theorists has long been proven.[47]
- As is well known, he spreads highly dubious tips for dealing with the coronavirus, for example, that the dangerous worming agent ivermectin or an overdose of vitamin D would help against it. Both substances have already caused severe poisoning in Austria.[48]

Austrian fact-checking websites also position themselves on the anti-ivermectin side. An example comes from Mimikama, which fact-checked the following claim: "After initial reports of an effect against COVID-19, the drug ivermectin, which is used against parasites and worms, was advertised on the internet and triggered hype among opponents of vaccination. These saw in the drug a miracle cure in the pandemic" (our translation).[49] Mimikama's conclusion after fact-checking is "one study concluded that the dewormer, for example, did not reduce the risk of requiring hospitalization after coronavirus infection compared with placebo. Ivermectin thus had no effect on COVID-19 patients and was found to be ineffective" (our translation).[49] As part of their fact-check, they state that a "large study now confirms that the drug ivermectin definitely does not help against COVID-19". However, Mimikama never mentions which study they are referring to. Based on additional information in the text, the study in question turns out to be a 2022 study published in *The New England Journal of Medicine*,[50] which includes authors that have received funding from the Bill and Melinda Gates Foundation, Merck, AstraZeneca, Pfizer, Regeneron Pharmaceuticals, Daiichi Sankyo (the second-largest pharmaceutical company in Japan), and the Australian Government. Here, Mimikama fails to follow their third step, namely considering who profits from spreading the information. If we take into account that there are over 100 studies that look at the effectiveness of ivermectin in the context of COVID-19, basing such a strong conclusion on merely one study is cherry picking.

A look at the scientific literature, specifically at systematic reviews and meta-analyses, suggests that the strong stance against ivermectin is neither factual nor evidence based. Instead, some systematic reviews and meta-analyses conclude that ivermectin shows efficacy against COVID-19,[51-55] whereas others conclude that it does not.[56-58] Despite the ongoing debate about the effectiveness of ivermectin in scientific circles, and a majority of systematic reviews and meta-analyses coming out in favor of ivermectin, many social media sites still censor Ivermectin information in a biased manner, such that an open discussion of the topic on many social media sites is still not possible. As an example, at the time of writing, YouTube still does not allow the following content:[59]

- Content that recommends use of Ivermectin or hydroxychloroquine for the treatment of COVID-19.
- Categorical claims that ivermectin is an effective treatment for COVID-19.
- Claims that ivermectin and hydroxychloroquine are safe to use in the prevention of COVID-19.

AUSTRIAN MEDIA COVERAGE AND FACT-CHECKING OF COVID ORIGINS

Another controversial topic has been the origin of COVID-19, with two main camps—(1) those suggesting that COVID-19 spilled over from animals and (2) those suggesting that COVID-19 was caused by a laboratory leak. The collocates for "origin" ("Ursprung") are not terribly informative, with the most common collocates including *corona virus* (*Coronavirus*), *pandemic* (*Pandemie*), *corona pandemic* (*Coronapandemie*), *Wuhan*, and *China*. What we can see if that the word *origin* occurs near the words related to the pandemic as well as the particular location where the virus originated.

A detailed look at the actual instances on *Ursprung* in the corpus includes many cases of *origin* relating to China not being cooperative in any investigations, references to the WHO investigation into the origins of COVID-19, references to origins of COVID-19 clusters in Austria or of new COVID-19 variants, and statements that the origin of the virus was in Wuhan, China. Of the statements that deal with the search for the origin of COVID-19, the media come down on the side of spill-over proponents. The following statements illustrate this:

- The researchers continue to regard the laboratory hypothesis as "extremely unlikely". All data point in a different direction, namely to wild or farm animals as the origin.[60]
- Two-thirds of all infectious diseases are transmitted from animals to humans including corona. These zoonoses are likely to become even more of a global health risk in the future.[61]
- The draft report of the WHO on the origin of Severe acute respiratory syndrome coronavirus 2 (SARS-CoV-2), which is now available and eagerly awaited, concludes that the pathogen may have been transmitted to humans via an animal. And it does so with a degree of certainty that is cited in the report as "probable to very probable".[62]

The most common suspects are bats,[63,64] but other animals, such as snakes[65] and pangolins,[66] are also mentioned, as is the wet market in Wuhan[67] and Chinese fur farms.[68] The media's bias is most visible in the labels that they choose for proponents of the spill-over theory versus laboratory leak theory. While spill-over theory proponents are called "renowned scientists", laboratory leak proponents are called "conspiracy theorists", as the following quotes illustrate:

- Renowned scientists assume a natural origin, too. "nobody would choose a corona pathogen to make an artificial virus," Stanley Perlman of the University of Iowa said in a recent radio interview. "The coronavirus is difficult to work with."[69]
- In the beginning, mainly conspiracy theorists had pointed to the possible origin of the Corona pandemic in a Chinese biolaboratory.[64]
- The conspiracy theory is mainly based on Fox News. The TV station has never presented any proof or even circumstantial evidence; most scientists still assume an animal origin of the pandemic.[70]

Austrian fact-checking websites also favor the spill-over theory. An example comes again from Mimikama, which fact-checked the theory that the virus came from a laboratory in Wuhan.[71] They conclude that there is no evidence that the coronavirus originated in a biolaboratory in Wuhan: "Contradictory claims are circulating in the media. There is no evidence that the virus originated from a biolaboratory in Wuhan, the natural origin of the virus is almost certain".[57] At the end of the fact-check, Mimikama advertises a related fact-check entitled "Why the new coronavirus cannot come from a laboratory".[72] In this fact-check, they conclude—"even though the new coronavirus resembles the SARS virus, it was determined that it could not have originated from SARS (in a laboratory); instead, it mutated from a lesser-known virus, which would be highly ineffective and complicated for an artificially created virus, but quite common and natural in nature." The article that Mimikama bases this conclusion on is the now infamous and often criticized[73-76] 2020 *Nature* article on, "The proximal origin of SARS-CoV-2".[77]

If we look at the scientific evidence, it is again clear that the jury is still out. As recently as May 2022, researchers published: "A call for an independent inquiry into the origin of the SARS-CoV-2 virus".[78] The authors suggest: "We do not assert that laboratory manipulation was involved in the emergence of SARS-CoV-2, although it is apparent that it could have been. However, we do assert that there has been no independent and transparent scientific scrutiny to date of the full scope of the US-based evidence".[78] Just a few months later, in October 2022, a US Senate Committee on Health Education, Labor and Pensions Minority Oversight Staff report concluded that a laboratory leak is a more likely scenario than spill-over: "Based on the analysis of the publicly available information, it appears reasonable to conclude that the COVID-19 pandemic was, more likely than not, the result of a research-related incident. New information, made publicly available and independently verifiable, could change this assessment. However, the hypothesis of a natural zoonotic origin no longer deserves the benefit of the doubt, or the presumption of accuracy".[79]

AUSTRIAN MEDIA COVERAGE AND FACT-CHECKING OF THE USE OF MASKS

Ever since masks were introduced as a countermeasure to the Corona pandemic, there has been a debate on whether or not, or to what degree, masks were actually a useful tool. In the first few weeks and months, up until approximately mid-April, statements by officials such CDC's Dr Anthony Fauci had been very clear: Healthy people should not be wearing masks.

- *Fauci*: The masks are important for someone who's infected to prevent them from infecting someone else. Right now, in the United States, people should not be walking around with masks.
- *LaPook*: You are sure of it? Because people are listening really closely to this.
- *Fauci*: There's no reason to be walking around with a mask. When you are in the middle of an outbreak, wearing a mask might make people feel a little bit better and it might even block a droplet, but it is not providing the perfect protection that people think that it is. And, often, there are unintended consequences—people keep fiddling with the mask and they keep touching their face.[80]

Even the WHO guidance at the time still affirmed that masks should be prioritized for healthcare workers and that hand hygiene was much more crucial in preventing viral spread.[81] This was even reflected in news coverage at that time, as the following example from the Austrian newspaper *Die Presse* dated January 28, 2020, exemplifies: "Masks can be a health risk—at the moment respiratory masks are out of stock in Austria, even though they don't necessarily prevent transmission. Quite the opposite: They can even provoke an infection" (our translation).[82] This, however, changed about 1 month into the pandemic, with the institution of mandatory masking.

In Austria mask mandates for supermarkets started as early as April 6, 2020 and were gradually escalated to include any public places and buildings.[83] News media supported mask mandates early on, focusing on their perceived effect on the spread of COVID-19 as well as on people who refused to wear them for various reasons.

- The fact that masks, different from what flyers claim, do indeed protect the wearer from the virus is proven.[84]
- New and tightly fitted FFP2-masks are incredibly efficient in protection from infection. Even in case of illness, they are not useless.[85]
- Opponents and proponents fight over the issue of masks, but for most physicians, their medical use is indisputable.[86]
- When medical or FF2-masks are indeed worn to cover mouth and nose, they lower the risk of infection considerably, especially when they have a tight fit.[87]
- A whole range of other studies showed higher numbers (regarding efficiency in blocking infections), but what is indisputable is that masks save lives.[88]

Some more creative articles even praised masks as making their wearers more attractive because they look more competent and healthy.[89]

It does not entirely come as a surprise, then, that people opposed to masking were labeled as "Maskenverweigerer" (mask refuseniks), "Maskenmuffel" (somebody who is too lazy to wear a mask), or "Maskengegner" (anti-maskers), and were pooled together with the likes of "tin foil hat wearers", "COVID deniers" and "antivaxxers".

Collocates to masks do not show anything of interest in particular. Words that collocate the most with "masks" are *tragen* (to wear), *Pflicht* (mandate), *Abstand* (distance), *Ausweitung* (extension), or *Wiedereinführung* (reintroduction). There are no collocates that would show that the media lead a debate on whether or not or to what extent masks are indeed useful in slowing the spread of the virus. Their purpose and efficiency as a physical measure to address the pandemic seems to be presupposed, critical voices remain invisible or are delegitimized via the aforementioned labels.

Fact-checking sites were squarely in the field of the promoted orthodoxy, pleading both for the use of masks and debunking any claims suggesting that they were not effective or perhaps even harmful. For instance, Mimikama responds to criticism of masks by saying: "Indeed masks do not offer their bearer protection from the virus. This needs to be said at this point. In the final analysis, it is not about protecting yourself, but protecting others by wearing a mask and keeping a distance" (our translation).[90] Interestingly, the messaging on who masks protect was contradictory throughout the pandemic. In a fact-check, the Austrian public broadcasting corporation (ORF) wrote: "In particular healthcare workers dealing with COVID-19 patients should wear FFP masks to protect themselves" (our translation).[91] The APA fact-check devotes an entire article to debunking claims that masks do not prevent infection and to promote the wearing of masks.[92] In this context, it is interesting to see that an earlier fact-check by APA was arguing *against* the widespread wearing of masks: "This is why the WHO recommends the wearing of masks "only in particular cases": "If you suffer from coughs and fever and have difficulties breathing, wear a mask and seek out medical attention. If you do not have these symptoms, you also do not need a mask as there is no evidence showing that it protects people who are not sick" and even warning that there might be a "higher risk of infection by wearing a mask" (our translation).[93]

These contradictions and the changing opinions of experts are important because they show the inherent problems with such fact-checks: they are based on developing and fluid information, but at the same time they make dogmatic statements that lead to the stigmatization and censorship of alternative viewpoints. In terms of the actual science on the wearing of masks, it is fair to say that there is no consensus on whether or not mask mandates helped prevent the spread of COVID-19. A recent Cochrane meta-analysis pooling 78 studies on physical interventions to stop people acquiring a respiratory virus infection came to a mixed conclusion on the efficiency and effects of masking, though with low-to-moderate certainty.[94] In their conclusion they write, "The pooled results of RCTs (randomized controlled trials) did not show a clear reduction in respiratory viral infection with the use of medical/surgical masks. There were no clear differences between the use of medical/surgical masks compared with N95/P2 respirators in healthcare workers when used in routine care to reduce respiratory viral infection".[94] This is also in line with the changing recommendations from the likes of the WHO or the CDC during the initial months of the COVID event. Despite all those contradictions, social media giants such as Twitter or YouTube had a policy of censoring "claims that masks do not play a role in preventing the contraction or transmission of COVID-19".[95,96] Facebook still takes down posts containing "claims that wearing a face mask properly does not help prevent the spread of COVID-19".[97] Seeing that the science behind mass masking appears anything but settled, these interventions by social media companies, by fact-checkers and mainstream media, all of whom ascribed definite truth to a medical claim, arguably narrowed the range of possible opinions to a somewhat inconsistent amalgam. In hindsight, the discussion on the usefulness of masks ought to have been led a lot more controversially than it was considering the effects it appears to have had on issues such as mental health and speech and emotional development in children.[98,99]

CONCLUSION

In this chapter, we looked at COVID-19 censorship in the EU, with a focus on the situation in Austria. Censorship occurred both in traditional media and social media. The mainstream media in Austria as well as Austrian fact-checkers mostly followed the official narrative uncritically and merely echoed and amplified official positions, leaving little to no room for dissenting views. This was a result of a centralized system which defined consensus at a very high level through institutions such as the Investigative Network in Austria or the EU Rapid Alert System on a European level. Social media giants as well as traditional media companies as parts of these networks drew their information of what is and is not credible information from the same central pool of information, thus leading to very similar approaches with regard to identifying and then dealing with mis/disinformation.

As we have shown, the claims that the media and fact-checkers made often went far beyond what was warranted by the evidence at the time. As a result, for many of the claims that were portrayed as certain knowledge by both the mainstream media and fact-checkers, often with dubious arguments, we still do not have sufficient evidence to settle the debate. In addition, social media in Europe openly engaged in censorship and even codified censorship into their community rules. Specifically, social media actively removed content that they considered harmful, where, in the case of YouTube, harmful means contradicting local health authorities. Thus, dissenting views were actively suppressed, such that social media essentially functioned as propaganda machines for governments and health authorities.

In the US, there is currently a slow reckoning that the censorship may have gone too far. In a July 4th, 2023 judgment, the US government has been ordered to refrain from "meeting with social-media companies for the purpose of urging, encouraging, pressuring, or inducing in any manner the removal, deletion, suppression, or reduction of content containing protected free speech posted on social media platforms".[100] In the full opinion, Judge Doughty writes: "If the allegations made by Plaintiffs are true, the present case arguably involves the most massive attack against free speech in United States' history".[100] In Austria, the trend seems to go in the opposite direction. The Austrian Directorate for State Protection and Intelligence (DSN) seems to currently consider penalizing the spread of misinformation. Until 2015, spreading false rumors was prohibited in Section 276 of the Austrian Criminal Code. On July 5th, 2023, the DSN proposed that a similar law could prevent the dispersal of unwanted narratives and thus prevent that such narratives influence the population.[101] It seems that stories of the demise of propaganda and censorship in our democracies have been greatly exaggerated; on the contrary, they are alive and well in Austria.

REFERENCES

1. World Health Organization. (2020). Who director-general's opening remarks at the media briefing on COVID-19—11 March 2020. [online] Available from https://www.who.int/director-general/speeches/detail/who-director-general-s-opening-remarks-at-the-media-briefing-on-covid-19---11-march-2020 [Last accessed November, 2023].
2. McClure J, Jones G. (2020). Coronavirus lockdown in Europe. [online] Available from https://www.reuters.com/graphics/HEALTH-CORONAVIRUS-EUROPE/0100B5M347R/index.html [Last accessed November, 2023].
3. France24. (2020). News Wires. Europa rolls out mass vaccinations in bed to beat COVID-19. [online] Available from https://www.france24.com/en/europe/20201228-europe-rolls-out-mass-vaccinations-in-bid-to-beat-covid-19 [Last accessed November, 2023].
4. BBC News. (2021). Covid passports: How do they work around the world? https://www.bbc.com/news/world-europe-56522408 [Last accessed November, 2023].
5. Bor A, Jørgensen F, Petersen MB. Discriminatory attitudes against unvaccinated people during the pandemic. Nature. 2022;613(7945):704-11.
6. Carlo S. (2021). Europe is stripping the unvaccinated of their rights and exploding the EU's claim to be a champion of liberty. [online] Available from https://www.telegraph.co.uk/news/2021/11/19/eu-has-shown-illiberal-double-standards/ [Last accessed November, 2023].
7. BBC News. (2021). Covid: Austria introduces lockdown for unvaccinated. [online] Available from https://www.bbc.com/news/world-europe-59283128 [Last accessed November, 2023].
8. Kupferschmidt K. Europe is locking down a second time. But what is its long-term plan? [online] Available from https://www.science.org/content/article/europe-locking-down-second-time-what-its-long-term-plan [Last accessed November, 2023].

9. Neuman S. Britain's Boris Johnson: "No Alternative" To Strict New Coronavirus Lockdown. [online] Available from https://www.npr.org/sections/coronavirus-live-updates/2020/11/02/930398019/britains-boris-johnson-no-alternative-to-strict-new-coronavirus-lockdown [Last accessed November, 2023].
10. Hubmann D. Diese Mediziner erklären, wie man seltene Thrombosen in zwei Tagen abwendet. [online] Available from https://www.kleinezeitung.at/lebensart/gesundheit/5966492/ImpfNebenwirkung_Diese-Mediziner-erklaeren-wie-man-seltene [Last accessed November, 2023].
11. Zwins K. Die gängigsten Mythen zur Corona-Impfung. [online] Available from https://www.profil.at/faktiv/die-gaengigsten-mythen-zur-corona-impfung-ein-faktencheck/401454709 [Last accessed November, 2023].
12. Palmai J. (2021). Experten leisten Aufklärungsarbeit für Covid-Schutzimpfung. [online] Available from https://www.derstandard.at/story/2000123455134/experten-leisten-aufklaerungsarbeit-fuer-covid-schutzimpfung [Last accessed November, 2023].
13. Fabry C. Anschober: „Bitte stürmen Sie nicht in die Einkaufszentren". [online] Available from https://www.diepresse.com/5908129/anschober-bitte-stuermen-sie-nicht-in-die-einkaufszentren?from=rss [Last accessed November, 2023].
14. Patterer H. Demokratie unter Quarantäne. Kleine Zeitung. https://www.pressreader.com/austria/kleine-zeitung-steiermark/20200322. Published March 22, 2020. Accessed July 7, 2023.
15. World Health Organization. (2020). Novel Coronavirus (2019-nCoV) Situation Report-13. [online] Available from https://www.who.int/docs/default-source/coronaviruse/situation-reports/20200202-sitrep-13-ncov-v3.pdf [Last accessed November, 2023].
16. Shir-Raz Y, Elisha E, Martin B, Ronel N, Guetzkow J. Censorship, and suppression of COVID-19 heterodoxy: Tactics and counter-tactics. Minerva. 2022:1-27.
17. European Commission. (2020). Speech of Vice President Věra Jourová on countering disinformation amid COVID-19 "From pandemic to infodemic." [online] Available from https://ec.europa.eu/commission/presscorner/detail/en/speech_20_1000 [Last accessed November, 2023].
18. European Commission. (2020). JOINT COMMUNICATION TO THE EUROPEAN PARLIAMENT, THE EUROPEAN COUNCIL, THE COUNCIL, THE EUROPEAN ECONOMIC AND SOCIAL COMMITTEE AND THE COMMITTEE OF THE REGIONS Tackling COVID-19 disinformation - Getting the facts right. [online] Available from https://eur-lex.europa.eu/legal-content/EN/TXT/PDF/?uri=CELEX:52020JC0008 [Last accessed November, 2023].
19. European Commission. (2018). JOINT COMMUNICATION TO THE EUROPEAN PARLIAMENT, THE EUROPEAN COUNCIL, THE COUNCIL, THE EUROPEAN ECONOMIC AND SOCIAL COMMITTEE AND THE COMMITTEE OF THE REGIONS Action Plan against Disinformation. [online] Available from https://eur-lex.europa.eu/legal-content/GA/TXT/?uri=CELEX:52018JC0036 [Last accessed November, 2023].
20. Shaping Europe's digital future. (2022). 2018 Code of Practice on Disinformation. [online] Available from https://digital-strategy.ec.europa.eu/en/library/2018-code-practice-disinformation [Last accessed November, 2023].
21. Shaping Europe's digital future. (2022). Signatories of the 2022 Strengthened Code of Practice on Disinformation. [online] Available from https://digital-strategy.ec.europa.eu/en/library/signatories-2022-strengthened-code-practice-disinformation [Last accessed, 2023].
22. Twitter Report: Staying safe and informed on Twitter during Covid-19. Accessed July 7, 2023. https://ec.europa.eu/newsroom/dae/redirection/document/87124
23. European Union. (2022). EU & COVID-19 Disinformation Google Report.[online] Available from https://ec.europa.eu/newsroom/dae/redirection/document/87126 [Last accessed November, 2023].

24. Meta. (2022). March and April 2022 Report: Meta Response to the European Commission Communication on COVID-19 Disinformation.; [online] Available from https://ec.europa.eu/newsroom/dae/redirection/document/87127.
25. Facebook. (2023). COVID-19-Richtlinie–Aktualisierungen und Schutzmaßnahmen. [online] Available from https://www.facebook.com/help/230764881494641 [Last accessed November, 2023].
26. Brownstone Institute. (2023). Scientific Consensus—A Manufactured Construct.[online] Available from https://brownstone.org/articles/scientific-consensus-a-manufactured-construct/ [Last accessed November, 2023].
27. Scherling J, Foltz A. The use of certainty in COVID-19 reporting in two Austrian newspapers. Journ Media. 2023;4(2):530-46.
28. Taibbi M. (2023). Twitter files #19 The Great COVID-19 Lie Machinestanford, the Virality Project, and the Censorship of "True Stories." [online] Available from https://twitter.com/mtaibbi/status/1636729166631432195 [Last accessed November, 2023].
29. 1334/AB. (2020). Österreichisches Parlament. [online] Available from https://www.parlament.gv.at/dokument/XXVII/AB/1334/imfname_799682.pdf [Last accessed November, 2023].
30. Jaklin DC. Desinformation und COVID-19: Österreich und die Europäische Dimension. J Intel, Prop Sec Studies. 2019;13(2):27-44.
31. The Diplomatic Service of the European Union. (2019). Rapid Alert System: Strengthening Coordinated and Joint Responses to Disinformation [online] Available from https://www.eeas.europa.eu/sites/default/files/ras_factsheet_march_2019_0.pdf [Last accessed November, 2023].
32. EU VS DisInfo. (2020). EEAS Special Report: Disinformation on the Coronavirus - Short Assessment of the Information Environment. [online] Available from https://euvsdisinfo.eu/eeas-special-report-disinformation-on-the-coronavirus-short-assessment-of-the-information-environment/ [Last accessed November, 2023].
33. Edmo at a Glance. (2023). European Digital Media Observatory. [online] Available from https://edmo.eu/edmo-at-a-glance/ [Last accessed November, 2023].
34. European Commission. (2023) Digital Solution to Tackle Online Disinformation. [online] Available from https://cordis.europa.eu/project/id/825297 [Last accessed, 2023].
35. Mimikama. (2023). Zuerst Denken—Dann Klicken. [online] Available from https://www.mimikama.org/ [Last accessed November, 2023].
36. APA. (2023). Austria Presse Agentur: Nationale Nachrichtenagentur. [online] Available from https://apa.at/ [Last accessed November, 2023].
37. Fakt ist fakt. (2020). Corona: Warum wir jetzt handeln müssen. [online] Available from https://www.faktistfakt.com/ [Last accessed November, 2023].
38. Mimikama. (2023). FLIP–Ein ausführlicher Blick auf Mimikamas Ansatz zur Identifizierung von Fake News. [online] Available from https://www.mimikama.org/flip-prinzip-mimikama/ [Last accessed November, 2023].
39. Bechtold F. (2020). Coronavirus: Whatsapp ist die größte Fake-News Schleuder. [online] Available from https://futurezone.at/digital-life/coronavirus-whatsapp-ist-die-groesste-fake-news-schleuder/400789952 [Last accessed November, 2023].
40. Austria Presse Agentur. (2023). Die Regeln des APA-Faktenchecks. [online] Available from https://apa.at/faktencheck/regeln/ [Last accessed November, 2023].
41. Schmid V, Shcmidt F. (2021). Fehlgeburten bei Corona Impfstudie im Durchschnitt. [online] Available from https://apa.at/faktencheck/fehlgeburten-bei-corona-impfstudie-im-durchschnitt/ [Last accessed November, 2023].
42. Seidel C. (2022). Corona-Impfung verringert Risiken für Schwangere. [online] Available from https://apa.at/faktencheck/corona-impfung-verringert-risiken-fuer-schwangere/ [Last accessed November, 2023].

43. Fakt ist Fakt. (2023). Faktenchecks. [online] Available from https://www.faktistfakt.com/faktenchecks/ [Last accessed November, 2023].
44. Crump A. Ivermectin: Enigmatic multifaceted "wonder" drug continues to surprise and exceed expectations. J Antibiot. 2017;70(5):495-505.
45. Hagen L, Scherndl G. (2021). Kickls Wurmmittel-Ratschläge bleiben ungestraft. https://www.derstandard.at/story/2000131257806/kickls-wurmmittel-ratschlaege-bleiben-ungestraft [Last accessed November, 2023].
46. Scherndl G. (2021). Wurmmittel für Pferde taugt nicht zur Corona-Bekämpfung. [online] Available from https://www.derstandard.at/story/2000129445304/wurmmittel-fuer-pferde-taugt-nicht-zur-corona-bekaempfung. Published September 7, 2021 [Last accessed November 7, 2023].
47. Rauscher H. (2021). Corona: Die Folgen der Gesundbeterei. [online] Available from https://www.derstandard.at/story/2000130721725/corona-die-folgen-der-gesundbeterei [Last accessed November, 2023].
48. Scherndl G. (2021). Zwei Strafrechtsparagrafen feiern in der Pandemie ihr Comeback. [online] Available from https://www.derstandard.at/story/2000131378169/zwei-strafrechtsparagrafen-feiern-in-der-pandemie-ihr-comeback [Last accessed November, 2023].
49. MIMIKAMA. (2022). Ivermectin Unwirksam Bei COVID-19 (Studie 2022). [online] Available from https://www.mimikama.org/ivermectin-unwirksam-bei-covid-19/ [Last accessed November, 2023].
50. Reis G, Silva EASM, Silva DCM, Thabane L, Milagres AC, Ferreira TS, et al. Effect of early treatment with ivermectin among patients with COVID-19. N Engl J Med. 2022;386(18):1721-31.
51. Bryant A, Lawrie TA, Dowswell T, et al. Ivermectin for prevention and treatment of COVID-19 infection: A Systematic Review, Meta-analysis, and Trial Sequential Analysis to Inform Clinical Guidelines. Am J Ther. 2021;28(4):e434-60.
52. Zein AF, Sulistiyana CS, Raffaelo WM, Pranata R. Ivermectin and mortality in patients with COVID-19: A systematic review, meta-analysis, and meta-regression of randomized controlled trials. Diabetes Metab Syndr. 2021;15(4):102186.
53. Cruciani M, Pati I, Masiello F, Malena M, Pupella S, De Angelis V. Ivermectin for prophylaxis and treatment of COVID-19: A systematic review and meta-analysis. Diagnostics. 2021;11(9):1645.
54. Hariyanto TI, Halim DA, Rosalind J, Gunawan C, Kurniawan A. Ivermectin and outcomes from COVID-19 pneumonia: A systematic review and meta-analysis of Randomized Clinical Trial Studies. Rev Med Virol. 2021;32(2):e2265.
55. Kow CS, Merchant HA, Mustafa ZU, Hasan SS. The association between the use of ivermectin and mortality in patients with COVID-19: A meta-analysis. Pharm Rep. 2021;73(5):1473-9.
56. Roman YM, Burela PA, Pasupuleti V, Piscoya A, Vidal JE, Hernandez AV. Ivermectin for the treatment of coronavirus disease 2019: A systematic review and meta-analysis of randomized controlled trials. Clin Infect Dis. 2021;74(6):1022-9.
57. Deng J, Zhou F, Ali S, Heybati K, Hou W, Huang E, et al. Correction to: Efficacy and safety of ivermectin for the treatment of COVID-19: A systematic review and meta-analysis. QJM. 2022;115(10):706.
58. Marcolino MS, Meira KC, Guimarães NS, Motta PP, Chagas VS, Kelles SMB, et al. Systematic Review and meta-analysis of ivermectin for treatment of COVID-19: Evidence beyond the hype. BMC Infect Dis. 2022;22(1);639.
59. Youtube Help. (2023). COVID-19 Medical Misinformation Policy. [online] Available from https://support.google.com/youtube/answer/9891785?hl=en [Last accessed November, 2023].

60. Oertel F. (2021). Schwierige Suche nach dem Ursprung des Coronavirus. Der Standard. https://www.derstandard.at/story/2000125994064/schwierige-suche-nach-dem-ursprung-des-coronavirus [Last accessed November, 2023].
61. Jansen F. Ludwig S. (2021). Zoonosen–auf der Suche nach dem Ursprung. [online] Available from https://www.derstandard.at/story/2000124261135/zoonosen-auf-der-suche-nach-dem-ursprung [Last accessed November, 2023].
62. Taschwer K, Wallisch G. Weiter Tauziehen um Virus-Ursprung. [online] Available from https://www.pressreader.com/austria/der-standard/20210330/281603833256694 [Last accessed November, 2023].
63. Schmidt V. (2020). Fledermaus als Reservoir für Viren und Wissen. https://www.diepresse.com/5890003/fledermaus-als-reservoir-fuer-viren-und-wissen [Last accessed November, 2023].
64. Escher M, Mattheis P. (2020). Ein Biolabor in Wuhan sorgt für Unruhe. [online] Available from https://www.derstandard.at/story/2000116994821/ein-biolabor-in-wuhan-sorgt-fuer-unruhe [Last accessed November, 2023].
65. Mattheis P. (2020). Coronavirus: Viral ins chinesische Neujahr. https://www.derstandard.at/story/2000113717713/coronavirus-viral-ins-chinesische-neujahr [Last accessed November, 2023].
66. Der Standard. (2020). Schuppentier könnte Überträger des Coronavirus sein. [online] Available from https://www.derstandard.at/story/2000114295301/schuppentier-koennte-uebertraeger-des-coronavirus-sein [Last accessed November, 2023].
67. Mattheis P. (2020). Chinesisches Frühlingsfest im Zeichen des Coronavirus. https://www.derstandard.at/story/2000113575915/chinesisches-fruehlingsfest-im-zeichen-des-coronavirus [Last accessed November, 2023].
68. Kretschmer F. (2021). Der hohe Preis für Pelzkrägen. [online] Available from https://www.diepresse.com/5993036/der-hohe-preis-fuer-pelzkraegen [Last accessed November, 2023].
69. Eder M. (2020). Labor oder Markt: Woher stammt das neue Coronavirus? https://www.diepresse.com/5800883/labor-oder-markt-woher-stammt-das-neue-coronavirus [Last accessed November, 2023].
70. Brändle S. (2020). Frankreichs Frust mit dem Wuhan-Labor. [online] Available from https://www.derstandard.at/story/2000117255496/frankreichs-frust-mit-dem-wuhan-labor [Last accessed November, 2023].
71. Spiess C. (2020). Coronavirous: Spekulationen über Bio-Labor in Wuhan. [online] Available from https://www.mimikama.org/coronavirus-spekulationen-ueber-bio-labor-in-wuhan/ [Last accessed November, 2023].
72. Nowotny R. (2020). Warum das neue Coronavirous nicht aus dem Labor kommen kann. [online] Available from https://www.mimikama.org/warum-das-neue-coronavirus-nicht-aus-einem-labor-kommen-kann/ [Last accessed November, 2023].
73. Hibbett M, Grim R. (2022). House Republicans Release Text of Redacted Fauci Emails on Covid Origins. https://theintercept.com/2022/01/12/covid-origins-fauci-redacted-emails/ [Last accessed November, 2023]
74. Sallard E, Halloy J, Casane D, Decroly E, van Helden J. Tracing the origins of SARS-CoV-2 in coronavirus phylogenies: A Review. Environ Chem Lett. 2021;19(2):769-85.
75. Chaturvedi P, Ramalingam N, Singh A. Is COVID-19 man-made? Cancer Res Stat Treatt. 2020;3(2):284.
76. Segreto R, Deigin Y, McCairn K, Sousa A, Sirotkin D, Sirotkin K, et al. Should we discount the laboratory origin of COVID-19? Environ Chem Lett. 2021;19(4):2743-57.
77. Andersen KG, Rambaut A, Lipkin WI, Holmes EC, Garry RF. The proximal origin of SARS-CoV-2. Nat Med. 2020;26(4):450-2.

78. Harrison NL, Sachs JD. A call for an independent inquiry into the origin of the SARS-CoV-2 virus. Proceed Nat Acad Sci. 2022;119(21):e2202769119.
79. Senate Committee on Homeland Security and Governmental Affairs. An Analysis of the Origins of COVID-19. [online] Available from https://www.help.senate.gov/imo/media/doc/report_an_analysis_of_the_origins_of_covid-19_102722.pdf [Last accessed November, 2023].
80. Farmer BM. (2020). March 2020: Dr. Anthony Fauci talks with Dr Jon LaPook about COVID-19. [online] Available from https://www.cbsnews.com/news/preventing-coronavirus-facemask-60-minutes-2020-03-08/ [Last accessed November, 2023].
81. World Health Organization. (2020). Advice on the use of masks in the context of COVID-19. [Last accessed November, 2023].
82. Winroither E, Schuh K. (2020). Atemschutzmaske kann Gesundheit gefährden. [online] Available from https://www.diepresse.com/5759899/atemschutzmaske-kann-gesundheit-gefaehrden [Last accessed November, 2023].
83. Bizeps. (2023). Nach 3 Jahren endet am Sonntag den 30. April 2023 die letzte Maskenpflicht. [online] Available from https://www.bizeps.or.at/nach-3-jahren-endet-am-sonntag-den-30-april-2023-die-letzte-maskenpflicht/ [Last accessed November, 2023].
84. Scherndl G. (2021). Organisierte Desinformation: Die Flugblätter der Corona-Skeptiker. [online] Available from https://www.derstandard.at/story/2000125203530/organisierte-desinformation-die-flugblattmaschinerie-der-corona-skeptiker [Last accessed, 2023].
85. Baltaci K. (2022). COVID-19: Die immer noch unterschätzte Wirkung der FFP2-Maske. [online] Available from https://www.diepresse.com/6119371/covid-19-die-immer-noch-unterschaetzte-wirkung-der-ffp2-maske [Last accessed November, 2023].
86. Özkan D, Mezler-Andelberg S. (2020). Warum die Gesichtsmaske so aufregt. [online] Available from https://www.diepresse.com/5838133/warum-die-gesichtsmaske-so-aufregt [Last accessed November, 2023].
87. Der Standard. (2021). Gut sitzende FFP2-Maske schützen 75 mal besser als OP-Masken. [online] Available from https://www.derstandard.at/story/2000131772396/gut-sitzende-ffp2-masken-schuetzen-75-mal-besser-als-op [Last accessed November, 2023].
88. Taschwer K. (2020). Alles nur Angstmache? [online] Available from https://www.pressreader.com/austria/der-standard/20201009/282638920048803. [Last accessed November, 2023.
89. Dinnewitzer E. (2022). Menschen mit Maske erscheinen. [online] Available from https://www.diepresse.com/6086940/menschen-mit-maske-erscheinen-attraktiver [Last accessed November, 2023].
90. Wolf A. (2020). Wen schützt denn nun die Maske? [online] Available from https://www.mimikama.org/maske-schutz/ [Last accessed November, 2023].
91. Science ORF. (2021). Desinformation im Urteil des Verwaltungsgerichts. [online] Available from https://science.orf.at/stories/3205811/ [Last accessed November, 2023].
92. Hochrieser G, Schmid V, Schmidt F. (2021). FFP2-Masken schützen vor Corona-Viren. [online] Available from https://apa.at/faktencheck/ffp2-masken-schuetzen-vor-corona-viren/ [Last accessed November, 2023].
93. Schmid V, Schmidt F. Verpflichtendes Maskentragen im Kampf gegen Coronavirus sinnvoll? [online] Available from https://apa.at/faktencheck/verpflichtendes-maskentragen-im-kampf-gegen-coronavirus-sinnvoll/ [Last accessed November, 2023].
94. Jefferson T, Dooley L, Ferroni E, Ferroni E, Al-Ansary LA, Bawazeer GA, et al. Physical interventions to interrupt or reduce the spread of respiratory viruses. Cochrane Database Syst Rev. 2023;2023(4):CD006207.

95. YouTube Policies. (2023). COVID-19 Medical Misinformation Policy. [online] Available from https://web.archive.org/web/20210614011729/https://support.google.com/youtube/answer/9891785?hl=en [Last accessed November, 2023].
96. Twitter. (2023). Richtlinie zu irreführenden Informationen über COVID-19. [online] Available from https://help.twitter.com/de/rules-and-policies/medical-misinformation-policy [Last accessed November, 2023].
97. Facebook help center. (2023). COVID-19 and vaccine policy updates & protections: [online] Available from https://www.facebook.com/help/230764881494641 [Last accessed November, 2023].
98. Wiren Y. (2021). How Lockdown has affected Children's Speech - and what parents can do to help. [online] Available from https://theconversation.com/how-lockdown-has-affected-childrens-speech-and-what-parents-can-do-to-help-160886 [Last accessed November, 2023].
99. Sohn E. (2022). For Some Teens, as Masks Come Off, Anxiety Sets in. [online] Available from https://www.nytimes.com/2022/03/17/well/family/teenage-student-mask-anxiety.html [Last accessed November, 2023].
100. Washington Post. (2023). United States District Court Western District of Louisiana Monroe Division. [online] Available from https://www.washingtonpost.com/documents/0e1edd23-3c69-4bce-ab7c-903370007a3e.pdf [Last accessed November, 2023].
101. ORF.at. (2023). DSN will Strafen für Verbreitung von Desinformation. news.[online] Available from https://orf.at/stories/3322796/ [Last accessed November, 2023].

CHAPTER 4

COVID-19, Hydroxychloroquine, Politics, and Scientific Author Political Party Donation History—What could Possibly Go Wrong?

Andrew C Berry

INTRODUCTION

Imagine spending your relaxing Saturday morning reading an article on a new, emerging scientific breakthrough that may benefit society and people across the world. You become entrenched in the article's convincing rhetoric and even start highlighting sections, download the PDF, and start sharing the link on your array of social media platforms. Remarkably, you even call your spouse in the room to show what you just read. After the pomp and circumstance of sharing it to every pulsating individual you know, your curious mind starts to wonder more about the article's authors. Meanwhile, some of your colleagues start asking you, "How are these authors so confident in their findings? How are they the only ones so passionate and knowledgeable on this breakthrough without any discourse?" One astute colleague calls you up and asks you the question, "What are the financial disclosures of the authors of the study, as it appears they may have some vested financial interest?" You pause, and solemnly realize that there were no financial disclosures listed for the article. You spend the next few days realizing this finding basically invalidated the whole article and feel shameful for propagating such an article. Imagine the public uproar! It is now standard of practice for authors to list any relevant *financial* disclosures. But what about *political* disclosures?

Flash back to March 11, 2020. The World Health Organization declared a pandemic.[1] Society was in peril, a raging new virus was upon us, uncertainty was rampant. Epidemiologic models used early in the disease course instilled a sense of urgency.[2] The scientific and medical community worked together to swiftly learn more about COVID-19 and potential therapeutic regimens. It was all hands-on deck. A promising study by French scientist Didier Raoult et al. showed hydroxychloroquine (HCQ) as a potential therapeutic drug for COVID-19.[3] Thereafter, President Donald Trump and government officials touted the drug, saying it could "have a chance to be one of the biggest game changers in the history of medicine."[4] The ensuing days that followed caused a surge in patient requests and prescriptions across America. On March 28, 2020, the FDA issued Emergency Use Authorization (EUA) for HCQ and chloroquine (CQ) in treatment for hospitalized COVID-19 patients.[5] Amid rampant political strain, the FDA rescinded its EUA for HCQ on June 15, 2020.[6]

Just like that HCQ was exiled in the United States (US). What happened? Why were favorably-appearing non-US scientific studies and positive patient experiences, both inside and outside the US, still piling up? What happened in the US suddenly that made HCQ—used for decades and by millions and even on the list of most impactful global medications—a blacklisted medication carrying negative and spiteful connotation? The American Medical Association (AMA) and the American Pharmacists Association even issued a joint statement calling for a stop to "inappropriate prescribing and ordering" of HCQ and CQ for COVID-19.[7] Some state medical boards and pharmacists were now even blocking doctor-prescribed HCQ prescriptions for COVID-19 from being filled.[8] Never has a physician's clinical judgment been nullified by pharmacists and medical boards, let alone for a longstanding medication with a known safety profile.

As both a scientist and COVID-19 treating clinical physician, I started to ponder why there was such a discordance between the worldwide data and clinical outcomes and the sudden negative connotation for HCQ and CQ. What were we missing or misinterpreting? Was it the shifting political landscape? Was it big pharmaceutical companies and their push of mass vaccination and costly, highly profitable, nongeneric, and not-yet-approved medications?

After numerous nights of hypothesizing, I finally thought I figured it out. Money! Always follow the money! It had to have been big pharma and their push for a highly profitable mass vaccination campaign, along with newly developed, highly profitable, and urgently authorized, but not approved, therapeutic medications. But this was too easy to figure out, there had to be more depth to this. Then it struck, an EUA for vaccinations or medications can only be granted when no adequate, approved, available alternatives exist, and when the known and potential benefits outweigh the potential risks. Big pharma and its constituents would now be willing to do anything to shut down any potential repurposed therapeutic medications, such as HCQ or CQ.

By scientific publishing ethical law, authors are already required to disclose any *financial* interests in their articles. Albeit, embedded inside small-buried print, an informed observer could and should find this information. Even though it may not be a direct link toward the pharmaceutical product in transparent verbiage. For example, a lead author may have disclosures as the "Bill and Melinda Gates Foundation" or the "Chan Zuckerberg Initiative," potentially acting as a surrogate for their vaccine or therapeutic author biases.[9,10] Although this could account for a full-throttle negative campaign by big pharma toward medications such as HCQ or CQ, there was still something missing in this grand scheme.

In the US, public opinion about the COVID-19 pandemic is deeply divided by political affiliation and has shifted toward polarizing political views.[11] I hypothesized that scientific author political viewpoints may have impacted the study design, discussion, and conclusions of numerous COVID-19 research papers relating to HCQ and CQ. Unlike financial disclosures, political party affiliations or voting patterns are not required in published work. In my opinion, this had to be the dagger and the illusive missing piece to this HCQ/CQ dilemma. How could we objectively evaluate this, let alone, quickly and in a manner providing the truest snapshot of any shifting viewpoints? The first thing to mind was to find a way to obtain the political party registrations of each main author on any HCQ/CQ COVID-19 paper. This would theoretically involve manually checking each main author and their author-listed state addresses on their paper correspondence. However, this was not feasible due to various state laws on the availability of obtaining such political party registration data. Some states have open, mixed, or closed voter file information, with some requiring a long wait period for such information, or a high cost to obtain the information.[12] Other states limit the commercial use of such information. In the end, this could not be done practically and to completion.

We had to think smarter and more practical—*FollowTheMoney.org*.[13] And so our study design came to fruition.[14] We utilized publicly available online natural language processing software, Collabovid (*https://www.collabovid*) to electronically search all COVID-19/SARS-CoV-2 preprint and published papers from main preprint servers (medRxiv, BioRxiv, arXiv) and noted peer-reviewed publication servers (Elsevier, PubMed) between January 1, 2020 and July 26, 2020.[15] We then inputted a search using the words "HCQ" or "CQ", and 312 listings were noted. Exclusions and redundant papers were noted per our methods.[14] The detailing of the methods below is imperative to show the transparency and process of this analysis.[14]

Study result favorability was recorded by one author (A.C.B.) by reviewing the abstract and discussion/conclusion sections of the full manuscript. Unfavorable studies coincided with a negative conclusion based on the particular study hypothesis. For example, HCQ/CQ may have provided "no benefit, no decrease in hospitalization, no decrease in mortality, no prophylaxis benefit, harm to the patient in any manner, lack of positive benefit, etc." Favorability coincided with a positive study conclusion based on the particular study hypothesis and the medication in question, HCQ, and/or CQ. Any study with neutral conclusions was noted as neutral. Any study with ambiguous conclusions was noted as neutral. To note, all article favorability extraction was performed before any search into author political party donation history. In order to gauge differences in severity of the favorability findings above, we tested the proportion of studies that concluded HCQ/CQ was medically harmful from US versus non-US based authors.

First and last author demographics were extracted, as these authors represent the lead author and article guarantor for the content of the article, referred to as the main authors throughout this article. Subsequently, any US-based main author was manually searched by one study author (A.C.B.) on publicly available Website FollowTheMoney.org (https: //www.followthemoney.org/).[13] If a search yielded a match for the name and state, further listing description was evaluated for the donor's professional title or workplace. Only then, after all checkpoints for full verification that the author was indeed the match for the listed donor, was it counted as such. Political party of the donation was noted as Democratic, Republican, and Other. If no match was noted or in question, it was deemed no donation was made by the author. To serve as a control subset for COVID-19 publication trends and author characteristics, we randomly selected 68 control studies pertaining to COVID-19 but not involving HCQ/CQ from the same time period. We searched Collabovid with the filter UNITED STATES, yielding 810 studies (from the 27,028 total). A random sampling technique was used, and if the study matched a prior reason for exclusion or if there was only one author, it was not selected. The same study characteristics were recorded and the same process used to assess political party donation history.[14]

Any US citizen with a political party donation is by law required to have it recorded, as such, *FollowTheMoney.org* gave us the perfect public and fully available platform to search all political party donation histories of the study main authors.[13] This was the final piece to the puzzle. Nobody had thought to do such a thing, let alone, real-time in the heat of the COVID-19 political moment mid-2020. This was the best objective way to explore the degree to which political bias in medicine and study authors could explain the stark variation in HCQ/CQ study favorability in the US compared to the rest of the world. We believed the authors' own political motives may have fueled their supposed-objective study design and analysis. Two major questions then remained. What would the results show? And the most difficult question, how could this data get published to the public and past potentially-biased and siphoning journal editors?

There were 267 HCQ/CQ papers extracted, of which, 68 had first or last authors affiliated with a US-based institution **(Table 1)**. Of the 68, 17 total main authors were political donors: 15 (88.2%) Democratic, 2 (11.8%) Republican, and 0 other party. Of the time-matched 68 COVID-19 non-HCQ-CQ COVID-19 only controls, there were 20 total main author donors: 8 (40%) Democratic, 8 (40%) Republican, and 4 (20%) other party **(Table 2)**. This time-match comparison demonstrated there was a predilection toward HCQ/CQ papers having more polarizing authors, toward one political party, the Democratic party, compared to other COVID-19 (but not HCQ/CQ) research at the same snapshot in time **(Table 3)**. US studies having at least one main author donating to the Democratic party were 20.4% more likely to have unfavorable results and 17% less likely to report neutral results. Wow, so much for objectivity in science.

To a keen observer, why did it initially appear that HCQ/CQ studies were more favorable outside the US, and outside the evolving US political climate?

TABLE 1: Study demographics.

	HCQ/CQ studies	COVID-19 controls
	n = 267	*n* = 68
HCQ	153 (57.3)	–
CQ	38 (14.2)	–
Both	76 (28.5)	–
Favorable	76 (28.5)	–
Unfavorable	105 (39.3)	–
Neutral	86 (32.2)	–
Preprint	71 (26.6)	30 (44.1)
Elsevier	63 (23.6)	13 (19.1)
PubMed	133 (49.8)	25 (36.8)
RCT	11 (4.1)	0 (0.0)
Prospective	26 (9.7)	6 (8.8)
Retrospective	45 (16.9)	33 (48.5)
Systematic review	36 (13.5)	0 (0.0)
Basic science	52 (19.5)	0 (0.0)
Review/Editorial	97 (36.3)	29 (42.6)
Impact factor	5.0	3.6
Altimetric score	549.6	41.4
Cardiac	38 (14.2)	–
Patient involvement	146 (54.7)	–
Pharmacy-based	37 (13.9)	–

(CQ: chloroquine; HCQ: hydroxychloroquine; RCT: randomized controlled trial)

TABLE 2: Donation political party for US studies.

	Democratic (%)	Republican (%)	Other (%)	Non-donors	Number of authors
HCQ/CQ	15 (88.2)	2 (11.8)	0 (0.0)	108	125
COVID-19 controls	8 (40.0)	8 (40.0)	4 (20.0)	116	136

Note: Total donors includes unique first and last main authors only.
(CQ: chloroquine; HCQ: hydroxychloroquine)

Our analysis showed non-US studies having a basically even one-third split among unfavorable, favorable, and neutral studies. However, 57.4% of US author studies were unfavorable, with only 10.3% having favorable results **(Table 4)**. How could objective science with a finite identical medication of the same structural chemical component (ex., HCQ) regardless of physical longitude and latitude, have such varying favorability patterns

TABLE 3: HCQ/CQ versus COVID-19 control political party donations.

	HCQ/CQ studies	COVID-19 control	Difference	*p*-value
Democrat	0.120	0.059	0.061	0.041[a]
Republican	0.016	0.059	−0.043	0.036[a]
Nondonors	0.864	0.858	0.011	0.400
Amount ($)	159.496	67.081	92.415	0.100
Number of donations	0.296	0.191	0.105	0.177
Authors[b]	125	136		
Total studies	68	68		

[a] $p < 0.05$.
[b] Authors: Encompasses first and last (main) author totals only.
Note: Difference in means test.
For *p*-values—one-tail test used to determine significance.
(CQ: chloroquine; HCQ: hydroxychloroquine)

TABLE 4: HCQ/CQ study favorability for US versus non-US studies.

	US (%)	Non-US (96)
Unfavorable	39 (57.4)	66 (33.2)
Favorable	7 (10.3)	69 (34.7)
Neutral	22 (32.4)	64 (32.2)
Total	68	199

(CQ: chloroquine; HCQ: hydroxychloroquine)

TABLE 5: Difference in proportion of a conclusion of harm between US and non-US studies.

			p-values	
US (%)	Non-US (96)	Difference (96)		
			t-test	Boschloo
Harmful 41/125 (32.8)	63/409 (15.4)	17.4	0.001[a]	0.001[a]

[a] $p < 0.001$
Note: Out of a total of 534 authors, 63/409 non-US authors and 41/125 US authors were main authors of studies with harmful conclusions.

strictly based on the author country of origin? We even did a subanalysis with study conclusions noting “medical harm”, finding US studies had a significantly higher proportion yielding harmful conclusions than non-US studies **(Table 5)**. Remarkably, US-based authors in general, and those with a federally required, documented, and objective political party donation history, and to the Democratic party, were authors of unfavorable HCQ/CQ studies. The secret was out. Once deemed the most objective ethical scientists, those who publish medical literature, were now propagating the medical-political narrative from ground zero-perceived objective COVID-19 research. This was invisible to the public's eye. Nobody thought to investigate this nor had a manner to objectively do so, nor had a means to publicly explain their results. One could also visually see, as noted in **Figure 1**, a graphical representation of a clear shift away from studies with favorable results toward those of unfavorable results starting around April 2020, reaching a paradigm shift in May-July. HCQ/CQ became politicized right around this time after Donald Trump's tweet in March 2020 and push toward US investigation and use of these medications.[4]

Typically, medical literature takes a few months to successfully publish, after a rigorous peer-review process and edits and delayed print publication. This pandemic was the start of a new publishing era—preprint servers. In fact, within 10 months of the first confirmed COVID-19 case, the scientific community had released over 125,000 COVID-19-related scientific articles, of which, >30,000 were hosted by preprint servers.[16] What does this mean? Quick, nonpeer-reviewed, easily disseminated, news headline-catching "scientific" literature was being propagated en mass to the public eye. Some may argue this was a much-needed revelation of red-tape dissolution in medical publishing, especially during a global health crisis, while others may see a much gloomier scenario playing out—a pathway for corruption and misinformation. What's to say that a group of researchers with a motive

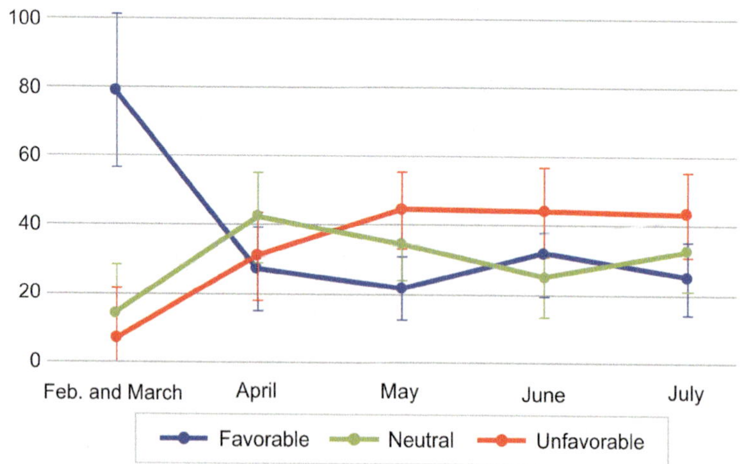

FIGURE 1: HCQ/CQ study release timeline and study favorability. All studies are for year 2020. July is until July 26, 2020 only.
(CQ: chloroquine; HCQ: hydroxychloroquine)

wouldn't "publish" a preprint on a topic they wanted disseminated, without being properly peer-reviewed and vetted. News outlets were salivating for persuasive headline-sparking preprints. Our analysis found 26.6% of the analyzed HCQ/CQ studies were preprint, unpublished studies. Remarkably, just 12.3% of preprints reviewed (of the 26.6%) went from preprint status to eventual publication during our 7-month study period.[14] This just reinforces that there were many preprint studies out there on HCQ/CQ and very few of them ever reached peer-reviewed journal publication status, let alone, in a timely fashion. From a keen eye, this means there was ample avenues to propagate false scientific narratives to the scientific community and general public, unchecked. Another means to rapidly spread "scientific results" or "expert opinions" was via research studies classified as "editorial reviews". These were purely subjective, yet came from what we assumed "experts" on the topic, touting long personal degree suffixes, and fancy institutional professional headings. We knew this was yet another route for demonizing HCQ/CQ and sought to find objective means for our hypothesis testing. We found that HCQ/CQ studies characterized as editorial reviews were 38.6% less likely to yield favorable results.[14] Furthermore, **Table 6** displays US author editorial review totals and author political party donation history. Almost all of the editorial reviews were unfavorable or neutral (21/22, 95.5%), with any listed history of donation all coming from a main author of a Democratic party donation record (7/7, 100%). Wow, yet again, we are objectively not surprised, and the general public was naïve to this all, and still is.

Not only did scientific paper main authors with studies showing unfavorable results for HCQ/CQ have significant propensity for Democratic political party donation histories, but they utilized both preprint servers and editorial "expert reviews" to quickly and exponentially propagate their biased findings. If there was a Hippocratic Oath for scientific research, this last statement would violate every last facet of that sworn-on creed.

As long as your preprint submission was formatted correctly and had valid institutions, your preprint would almost certainly get published online. One of the most remarkable facets of this whole situation was that *we* (with over 125 prior peer-reviewed journal publications between our three physician authors) were rejected from the most popular preprint server at the time of submission in 2020.[17] I think we may have been one of only a few

TABLE 6: US editorial reviews and donation history. Number of editorials that are democratic, republican, other.

	Number of editorials (%)	Democratic (%)	Republican (%)	Other (%)
Unfavorable	11 (50.0)	6 (85.7)	0	0
Favorable	1 (4.5)	0 (0.0)	0	0
Neutral	10 (45.5)	1 (14.3)	0	0
Total	22	7	0	0

authors to ever get rejected from a preprint server, in fact, with personalized commentary in our rejection email stating, "this manuscript was judged to fall into that category. Given the subject is the *motivations* of authors rather than the clinical research per se." The unnamed "affiliate scientist" rejected our submission without review, likely based on the topic of HCQ/CQ and political bias. I even saved the official response, **(Fig. 2)**. I later attempted to obtain the name of the "affiliate scientist" who subjectively rejected our preprint submission, in order to look up their political donation history on *FollowTheMoney.org*, however, the service kept their "affiliated scientists" unnamed and unidentified on the Website or e-mail communication. To further encompass this whole preprint server experience, if you search to the bottom of their Website, you'll see the name of the preprint server financial sponsor—the "Chan Zuckerberg Initiative".[17] The same group vehemently attempting suppression of nonvaccine therapeutics for their own vested vaccine financial interests.[10] "*The irony*"

Our HCQ/CQ author political party donation paper was published in the literature amid numerous editorial board immediate rejections without concrete study design reason.[14] We have been cited a few times, made some news outlets, but with much dismay, there has been no additional research from the scientific community similar to ours since our publication. It has been awkwardly quiet, especially on such a profound, rip-roaring, uproar of scientific ethical principles we helped uncover. Anyone speaking on this medication was shunned going forward, with any research exiled among the scientific community. These medications became the scarlet letter of the medical community. And then came the public health researchers at Harvard University, late to the party, with their April 2022 *JAMA Internal Medicine* brief study report titled "*Association of county-level prescriptions for hydroxychloroquine and ivermectin with county-level political voting patterns in the 2020 US presidential election*."[18] They initially start their publication stating "there is increased prescribing of these treatments despite evidence against their effectiveness."[18] What a blunt finite nonargumentative opening statement to set their study tone. Their study looked at medical claim data to see prescribing patterns of HCQ/CQ [and ivermectin (IVM)] as compared to other drugs over various time intervals, while analyzing these prescribing patterns in various quartiles of county Republican voter share (based on

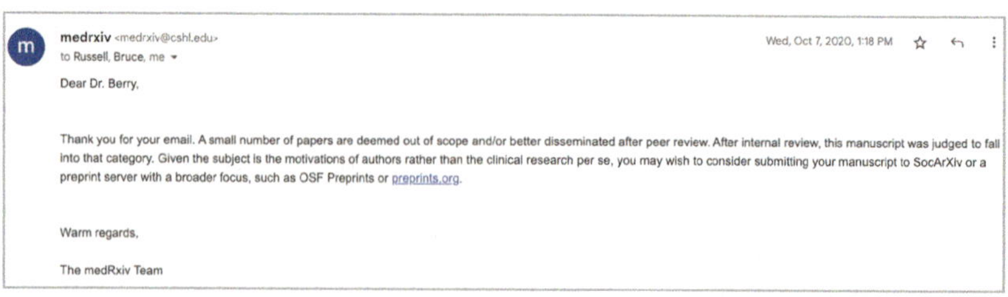
medrxiv <medrxiv@cshl.edu>
to Russell, Bruce, me
Wed, Oct 7, 2020, 1:18 PM

Dear Dr. Berry,

Thank you for your email. A small number of papers are deemed out of scope and/or better disseminated after peer review. After internal review, this manuscript was judged to fall into that category. Given the subject is the motivations of authors rather than the clinical research per se, you may wish to consider submitting your manuscript to SocArXiv or a preprint server with a broader focus, such as OSF Preprints or preprints.org.

Warm regards,

The medRxiv Team

FIGURE 2: Official response.

the 2020 US presential election results). They found that before the FDA's revocation of HCQ/CQ's EUA, the prescribing volume for HCQ was higher in counties with a lower Republican (i.e., higher Democrat) vote share. However, since the EUA revocation, the number of new HCQ and IVM prescriptions was higher in counties with a higher quartile Republican voter share. They concluded that prescribing patterns were influenced by political party affiliation. This study's discussion fails to account for the possibility that Democrats were potentially simply distraught about any mention of HCQ/CQ/IVM, and due to its affiliation with certain leaders and scientists, they would at all costs refuse discussion, advice, and treatment considerations with any of these therapeutics. To be extreme, some would rather gasp for oxygen than discuss with their providers clinical use of such meds. The final concluding line of their scientific report states, "because political affiliation should not be a factor in clinical treatment decisions, our findings raise concerns for public trust in a nonpartisan healthcare system." Their study results were extrapolated to convey their own opinions. And you might know exactly what I did after reading their report, I searched the main authors on *FollowTheMoney.org*, to see their own personal history of political party donations. Both the lead author (ML Barnett) and the final author (A Mehrota), both who have presumably (based on their departmental listings) never treated a single COVID-19 patient clinically, had a documented monetary political donation history listed to one party—the Democratic party.[13] You can't make this up. These partisan academic authors are so motivated to prove and indoctrinate their personal beliefs, that they fail to see their own study design fallacies, which basically invalidates their whole study conclusions. Caught, red-handed. But the public and scientific community has no idea, yet again. And we wonder why trust in the scientific community has waned since the pandemic began.

One of the main reasons why such minimal non-negative research on HCQ/CQ/IVM has been published is because the editors of the journals simply will not entertain any studies on these meds that do not fit their own personal agenda. The editors go out of their way to stress an apolitical manner to scientific research, however, at the same time they make statements signed as a whole editorial board that are purely political. For example, for the first time in their 175-year existence, the *Scientific American* published a scientific article backing a presidential candidate (Joe Biden), saying "we are compelled to do so".[19] Yet in the same issue publishing an article titled, "We can't allow the CDC (Centers for Disease Control and Prevention) to be tainted by politics."[20] *The Lancet* editors published a blatantly political editorial calling for President Trump's ouster.[21] *The New England Journal of Medicine (NEJM)* published an article, signed by the prestigious journal editors, called "*Dying in a leadership vacuum*".[22] This article was strategically published October 8, 2020, <1 month before the next presidential election. This article was downright nasty, partisan, and full of hate and scientifically uncharacteristic personal political opinion, with excerpts shown below.[22]

"The response of our nation's leaders has been consistently inadequate."

"Our current leaders have undercut trust in science and in government, causing damage that will certainly outlast them. Instead of relying on expertise, the administration has turned to uninformed "opinion leaders" and charlatans who obscure the truth and facilitate the promulgation of outright lies."

"Our leaders have largely claimed immunity for their actions. But this election gives us the power to render judgment."

"When it comes to the response to the largest public health crisis of our time, our current political leaders have demonstrated that they are dangerously incompetent. We should not abet them and enable the deaths of thousands more Americans by allowing them to keep their jobs."[22]

These are the same editors that are making objective reviews on your scientific research. HCQ/CQ/IVM never had a chance in the scientific literature in 2020, or ever, under these editorial circumstances. Things even went the other way, with some proactively trying to fabricate negative HCQ/CQ data. *The Lancet* had to retract an unfavorable HCQ/CQ COVID-19 study, because the data could not be verified.[23] Ironically, *The Lancet's* current editor at the time of publication, Richard Horton, in 2015, offered this insightful opinion:

"The case against science is straightforward: much of the scientific literature, perhaps half, may simply be untrue. Afflicted by studies with small sample sizes, tiny effects, invalid exploratory analyses, and flagrant conflicts of interest, together with an obsession for pursuing fashionable trends of dubious importance, science has taken a turn toward darkness."[24]

Large academic institutions trying to objectively research HCQ/CQ for therapeutic purposes succumbed to peer institutional pressures to back down their investigation efforts. The Henry Ford Health System issued the following:

"Unfortunately, the political climate that has persisted has made any objective discussion about this drug impossible, and we are deeply saddened by this turn of events. Our goal as scientists has solely been to report validated findings and allow the science to speak for itself, regardless of political considerations. To that end, we have made the heartfelt decision to have no further comment about this outside the medical community-staying focused on our core mission in the interest of our patients, our community, and our commitment to clinical and academic integrity."[25]

There was simply no avenue to study these medications without personal, institutional, or governmental backlash. It was easy to publish a hit piece, when the editors were seeking such pieces to fit their own narratives. Either to agree en mass with the overarching social mantra at the time, or to propagate their own personal agendas. But how could science advance?

> *"Politically, it is convenient to present an alleged "consensus" and dismiss any contrary findings as inherently illegitimate. But that action overlooks the fact that science often advances the most when presented with contradictory findings that must be resolved. If scientists routinely dismissed research findings just because they differed from previous research, science would make no progress."*[26]

Political bias is a now probable explanation for the unfavorable outcomes of the HCQ/CQ research authored in the US, influencing public and government opinions, and the subsequent nonuse of the drugs here in the US.[14] Many authors were inaccurately propagating false cardiac-related adverse effects of HCQ/CQ used in the COVID-19 patient as a means to assign unfavorability to the medication.[14] The abrupt demarcation of study favorability with timing of political events and social pressures further illustrates the potential infiltration of politics into the once-objective scientific community. Our societal future depends on tested and reproducible scientific advancements, we must continue to objectively evaluate scientific reports in order to succeed as a human race.

We thereby suggest the addition of "*political disclosures*" to the already required "*financial disclosures*" for all scientific research submissions, scientific publications, and journal editorial staff assignments going forth. Let's bring the objectivity back to science.

ACKNOWLEDGMENTS

Russell S Gonnering, Ivan Rodriguez, Qianying Zhang, Bruce B Berry.[14]

REFERENCES

1. World Health Organization. (2020). WHO Director-General's opening remarks at the media briefing on COVID-19. [online] Available from https://www.who.int/dg/speeches/detail/who-director-general-s-opening-remarks-at-the-media-briefing-on-covid-19 [Last accessed November, 2023].
2. Holmdahl I, Buckee C. Wrong but useful-what COVID-19 epidemiologic models can and cannot tell us. N Engl J Med. 2020;383:303-5.
3. Gautret P, Lagier JC, Parola P, Hoang VT, Meddeb L, Mailhe M, et al. Hydroxychloroquine and azithromycin as a treatment of COVID-19: results of an open-label non-randomized clinical trial. Int J Antimicrob Agents. 2020;56(1):105949.
4. @realDonaldTrump. (2020). HYDROXYCHLOROQUINE & AZITHROMYCIN, taken together, have a real chance to be one of the biggest game changers in the history of medicine. The FDA has moved mountain -Thank You! Hopefully they will BOTH (H works better with A, International Journal of Antimicrobial Agents). [online]

Available from //twitter.com/realDonaldTrump/status/1241367239900778501 [Last accessed November, 2023].

5. U.S. Food and Drug Administration. (2020). Letter of authorization-chloroquine phosphate and hydroxychloroquine sulfate. [Last accessed November, 2023] https://www.fda.gov/media/136534/download [Last accessed November, 2023].
6. U.S. Food and Drug Administration. (2020). Coronavirus (COVID19) Update: FDA revokes emergency use authorization for chloroquine and hydroxychloroquine. [online] Available from https://www.fda.gov/news-events/press-announcements/coronavirus-covid-19-update-fda-revokes-emergency-use-authorization-chloroquine-and [Last accessed November, 2023].
7. American Medical Association. (2020). Boards of pharmacy and other actions relating to COVID-19 prescribing. [online] Available from https://www.ama-assn.org/system/files/2020-04/board-of-pharmacy-covid-19-prescribing.pdf [Last accessed November, 2023].
8. State of Ohio Board of Pharmacy. (2020). Requirements for Dispensing or Selling Chloroquine and Hydroxychloroquine in Ohio. [online] Available from https://www.pharmacy.ohio.gov/Documents/Pubs/Special/COVID19Resources/Requirements%20for%20Dispensing%20or%20Selling%20Chloroquine%20and%20Hydroxychloroquine%20in%20Ohio.pdf [Last accessed November, 2023].
9. Bill and Melinda Gates Foundation. (2022). Novo Nordisk Foundation, Open Philanthropy, and Bill & Melinda Gates Foundation Launch Initiative to Support New Antiviral Medicines for Future Pandemics. [online] Available from https://www.gatesfoundation.org/ideas/media-center/press-releases/2022/03/funding-new-antiviral-medicines-and-preventing-future-pandemics [Last accessed November, 2023].
10. Chan Zuckerberg Initiative. (2023). COVID-19 Response. [online]Available from https://chanzuckerberg.com/covid-19/ [Last accessed November, 2023].
11. Geana MV, Rabb N, Sloman S. Walking the party line: the growing role of political ideology in shaping health behavior in the United States. SSM Popul Health. 2021;16:100950.
12. U.S. Election Assistance Commission. (2020). Availability of state voter file and confidential information. [online] Available from https://www.eac.gov/sites/default/files/voters/Available_Voter_File_Information.pdf [Last accessed November, 2023].
13. FollowTheMoney.org. (2020). The National Institute on Money in Politics and the Center for Responsive Politics have joined forces to become OpenSecrets. [online] Available from https://www.followthemoney.org [Last accessed November, 2023].
14. Berry AC, Gonnering RS, Rodriguez I, Zhang Q, Berry BB. Unfavorable hydroxychloroquine COVID-19 research associated with authors having a history of political party donations. Rev Cardiovasc Med. 2021;22(1):191-8.
15. Collabovid. (2020). Explore COVID-19 publications. 2020. [online] Available from https://www.collabovid.org/ [Last accessed November, 2023].
16. Fraser N, Brierley L, Dey G, Polka JK, Pálfy M, Nanni F, et al. The evolving role of preprints in the dissemination of COVID-19 research and their impact on the science communication landscape. PLoS Biol. 2021;19(4):e3000959.
17. MedRxiv. (2023). The preprint server for health sciences. [online] Available from https://www.medrxiv.org/ [Last accessed November, 2023].
18. Barnett ML, Gaye M, Jena AB, Mehrotra A. Association of County-Level Prescriptions for Hydroxychloroquine and Ivermectin with County-Level Political Voting Patterns in the 2020 US Presidential Election. JAMA Intern Med. 2022;182(4):452-4.
19. Scientific American. (2020). Scientific American endorses Joe Biden [online] Available from https://www.scientificamerican.com/article/scientific-american-endorses-joe-biden/ [Last accessed November, 2023].

20. Scientific American. (2020). We can't allow the CDC to be tainted by politics. [online] Available from https://www.scientificamerican.com/article/we-cant-allow-the-cdc-to-be-tainted-by-politics/ [Last accessed November, 2023].
21. Smith K. (2023). Trump derangement syndrome at The Lancet. National Review. [online] Available from https://www.nationalreview.com/2020/06/trump-derangement-syndrome-at-the-lancet/ [Last accessed November, 2023].
22. Editors. Dying in a Leadership Vacuum. N Engl J Med. 2020;383(15):1479-80.
23. Mehra MR, Desai SS, Ruschitzka F, Patel AN. RETRACTED: hydroxychloroquine or chloroquine with or without a macrolide for treatment of COVID-19: a multinational registry analysis. Lancet. 2020;S0140-6736(20)31180-6.
24. Horton R. Offline: what is medicine's 5 sigma? Lancet. 2015;385:1380.
25. Henry Ford Health System. (2020). Hydroxychloroquine: an open letter to our community and beyond. [online] Available from https://www.henryford.com/news/2020/08/hydroxychloroquine-an-open-letter [Last accessed November, 2023].
26. Schumm WR. Navigating treacherous waters-one researcher's 40 years of experience with controversial scientific research. Comprehensive Psychol. 2015;4.

CHAPTER 5

"You are not a Horse": Medicalization, Social Control, and Academic Discourse in the COVID-19 Era

Claudia Chaufan

ABSTRACT

Since early 2020, public figures in government, medicine, public health, and academia have accused critics of official coronavirus disease 2019 (COVID-19) policy of subverting efforts to contain the crisis by spreading "misinformation" leading to concerning levels of "vaccine hesitancy" or to the uptake of unproven, even dangerous, therapeutics. These accusations were compellingly captured in an August 2021 tweet from the US Food and Drug Administration (FDA), "You're not a horse. You are not a cow. Seriously, y'all. Stop it", warning anyone considering or already consuming the antiparasitic drug ivermectin to treat or prevent COVID-19 that the drug could be "dangerous and even lethal" if used outside of the scope of the FDA guidelines. In this study, I examine the role of academic discourse in COVID-19 debates. Drawing from theories and methods that share a concern with how medical language and frames are deployed to control social behavior, I appraise articles from *The Conversation*, an outlet that disseminates academic knowledge to facilitate open exchange and democratic governance. My analysis challenges the outlet's self-presentation, suggesting instead that, in the COVID-19 era, far from contributing to its ostensible goals, *The Conversation*'s stigmatizing and censorious messaging is largely undermining them, with dire implication for the normative academic principles of open inquiry, the free pursuit of knowledge, and the promotion of critical thinking among younger generations. The study is part of a larger project appraising health narratives and social control in times of COVID-19.

Disinformation is the common denominator to many of the problems we are facing in our democratic society. Disinformation is the wicked sister of misinformation: The latter happens when someone spreads false information, the former is a deliberate attempt to deceive by propagating misleading or fabricated facts [...]. Facts matter. Science matters. Expertise matters.

Scott White, Disinformation is an epidemic. We are the vaccine. The Conversation, 2022

> Interactionist theories of deviance [pay] attention to differentials in the power to define. [...] Such research has special sting to it when it allows us to inspect the practice of an institution in the light of its own professed aims and its own preferred description of what it is about [...] by making moral entrepreneurs as objects of study [and questioning] the monopoly on the truth of the "whole story" claimed by those in positions of power and authority. [...] When authorities, political and otherwise, wield power in part by obfuscation and mystification, a science which makes things clearer inevitably attacks the bases of that power.
>
> ***Howard S Becker, Outsiders, 1963***
>
> **Keywords**: COVID-19; medicalization and social control; suppression of dissent in science; stigmatization and deviance; academic discourse.

INTRODUCTION

Since early 2020, academia has aligned with government, public health agencies, medical societies, and the media, to accuse critics of official coronavirus disease 2019 (COVID-19) public health policy of spreading "misinformation", defined by the US Department of Homeland Security as "false information", which becomes "disinformation" when it is "deliberately spread with the intent to deceive or mislead".[1] Researchers with academic affiliations (hereafter "academics") have referred to these critics with negative epithets—"anti-vaxxers" or "conspiracy theorists"—also deployed by leaders in public health, medicine, and the media, and portrayed them as "anti-science", or as *misusing* science to promote "extreme" (meaning usually "far right") political agendas.[2-4] Especially concerning, goes the argument, is that "misinformation" about COVID-19 "vaccines",* produced by a loose, fringe

*I write "vaccine" between quotations (only this first time for the sake of readability), to call attention to two mechanisms of social control through linguistic manipulation triggered by the use of term "vaccine" to refer to messenger ribonucleic acid (mRNA)/ deoxyribonucleic acid (DNA) biologicals: One is *legal*, in that the label "vaccine" affords drug companies that produce these biologicals a full liability protections that they would otherwise not enjoy; the second one is *sociological*, in that calling these biologicals "vaccines" elicits the social trust, warranted or not, afforded to so-called "traditional" vaccines. The response would be very different if these biologicals were referred to as "gene therapy", as per the US Food and Drug Administration (FDA) description that "human gene therapy seeks to modify or manipulate the expression of a gene or to alter the biological properties of living cells for therapeutic use",[5] precisely what the COVID-19 inoculations do by delivering synthetic nucleic acids that instruct our cells to produce a modified form of severe acute respiratory syndrome coronavirus 2 (SARS-CoV-2) spike protein. For a technical discussion of these issues I refer readers to Rose's work on pharmacovigilance[6] and Garner and Hooker's work on health outcomes among vaccinated and unvaccinated populations.[7,8]

but very vocal, alliance of anti-vaccination individuals and groups, promotes "vaccine hesitancy", defined by the Strategic Advisory Group of Experts on Immunization (SAGE) as a complex set of beliefs, attitudes, and behaviors leading to "the reluctance or refusal to vaccinate despite the availability of vaccines".[9] This definition was popularized by the World Health Organization (WHO) in 2019, when it announced that "vaccine hesitancy"—along with droughts, famine, and armed conflict—was "one of 10 major global health threats" that, if left unchecked, could dramatically increase the global burden of disease.[10]

In this study, I examine the role of academic discourse in COVID-19 debates. Drawing from theories and methods that share a concern with how medical language and frames are deployed to control social behavior, I appraise selected articles from *The Conversation*, an outlet that disseminates academic knowledge within and beyond academia with the ostensible goals of facilitating open exchange and democratic governance. I focus on how identified discourses frame the COVID-19 crisis, whether and how they challenge or reproduce orthodox medical/public health dominance, and what are the implications of this framing and discursive strategies for the normative academic principles of open inquiry, the free pursuit of knowledge, and the promotion of critical thinking among younger generations. In the next section, I lay out selected historical and medical landmarks in the COVID-19 crisis to contextualize my study, then describe theories and methods, followed by my findings and analysis, and concluding with a discussion of their potential explanations and implications for human rights and democratic governance. The study is part of a larger project appraising health narratives and social control in the COVID-19 era.

BACKGROUND

Fighting "Disinformation One Click at a Time" or Controlling the Narrative?

On August 21, 2021, the FDA tweeted "You're not a horse. You are not a cow. Seriously, y'all. Stop it", warning anyone considering or already consuming the antiparasitic drug ivermectin to treat or prevent COVID-19 that the drug could be "dangerous and even lethal" if used outside of the scope of FDA guidelines.[11] An earlier press release from the Office of the US Surgeon General upon publication of its report, "*Confronting Health Misinformation: The U.S. Surgeon General's Advisory on Building a Healthy Information Environment*", had already warned against "misinformation about masks and social distancing, treatments, and vaccines" that was undermining the public's trust in COVID-19 policies, importantly, vaccination.[12] The Surgeon General was heeding an earlier call to action by the WHO that, in collaboration with the UK government, was fighting, "one click at a time", misinformation causing "vaccine hesitancy" and leading to unnecessary hospitalizations and deaths worldwide.[13] In a similar spirit, a multiauthor report from the Center for Health Security at the prestigious Johns Hopkins Bloomberg School of Public Health had warned that "health-related misinformation and disinformation" were undermining the response to the COVID-19 crisis and eroding trust in public health institutions, through "contradictory messages" about "false medical cures".[14] The authors called for the establishment of "a multiagency national security response effort that prioritizes management of public health misinformation to prevent disinformation campaigns and educate the public on their use" (ibid).

The summer of 2021 also witnessed the then chief medical advisor to the US president, Dr Anthony Fauci, warning that "attacks on [him] are attacks on science", responding to Republican accusations that Fauci was attempting to "control the [COVID-19] narrative" to impose policies that suppressed civil liberties.[15] Into the fall, major media—the Globe and Mail in Canada,[16] the Guardian in the United Kingdom (UK),[17] and the New York Times in the United States (USA)[18] alerted readers about a "pandemic of the unvaccinated" overwhelming health services, reinforcing messages from the WHO, the FDA, the US Surgeon General, and the Johns Hopkins Bloomberg School of Public Health. Relevant to appraising the role of academia in the COVID-19 saga, warnings about misinformation subverting crucial public health efforts, especially campaigns about the need to embrace "safe and effective" vaccines, would be echoed through the following summer by academics in Canada, the USA, the UK, and beyond.[2-4,19]

Pandemic Politics

No matter how "unprecedented" COVID-19, and how "novel" and "deadly" SARS CoV-2, have been presented to be, the historical record shows that the specter of plague along with fear-producing narratives of diseases and death have long-standing roots. Whether the goal was to distract the public's attention away from deplorable living conditions and exploitative social practices, legitimize colonial domination, or curtail civil and political liberties, the ultimate purpose has always been to manage, and if necessary, suppress, social unrest.[20] Selected examples should illustrate the process. European Jews, blamed for the bubonic plague, were scapegoated to manage class struggles in the late Middle Ages.[21] In the late 19th century, Southern Italians immigrants to the Americas were stigmatized as disease carriers, drawing from arguments provided by medical and public health authorities that scapegoated immigrant communities as sources of societal decay.[22] The history of the collective response to leprosy is revealing. The epitome of a stigmatizing disease eliciting fear due to its physical deformity and perception of high contagiousness, the fear of leprosy, going back to Biblical times, was revived in the late 19th century by Western colonial powers, as they laid territorial claims and signaled "culturally inferior people" for discrimination to meet a variety of political goals—from setting immigration limits, to isolating immigrants from locals, to using taxpayer money to reward public employees with "hazardous duty" pay to reinforce the image of lepers as a public danger even when the risks of contagion were minimal.[23] Religious missions also contributed to the stigmatization of sufferers through exaggerated accounts of deformity and explicit links with ecclesiastic texts.[23] In our times, and despite the fact that the secularization of leprosy largely ended these processes and that the disease is all but nonexistent other than among impoverished, nutritionally deficient communities,[24] leprosy is still officially framed as "caused" by a bacillus, i.e., "infectious", albeit not "contagious" but "chronic", with around 200,000 cases worldwide,[25] and lingering stigma.[26]

Fear-producing disease narratives continued into the 20th century, when the early 1900s witnessed the death of a Chinese immigrant in San Francisco, which was attributed to the bubonic plague and used to legitimize a campaign of forced inoculation of Asians with an experimental drug.[22] They also witnessed "tramps" blamed for smallpox,[27] redirecting popular anger away from the dire living conditions that put workers at risk of disease and death in the first place.[22] Well into the 21st century, these processes have continued, with Western media's framing of China and of COVID-19 as linked existential threats[28-30] deflecting the public anger against the deteriorating living conditions and increasing concentration of wealth that had exploded in 2019,[31] redirecting it toward Asians in the West.[32] As COVID-19 policies soon restructured social, economic, and political relationships, setting boundaries to permissible cognitions, attitudes, and behaviors, groupings of diverse ethnicities, religions, classes, and political affiliations, coalescing around scepticism about, or resistance to, these policies, were blamed for the never-ending crisis and became the object of scapegoating and stigmatizing health narratives.[3,4] What matters for our purpose is that while the object of these narratives has shifted over time, the narratives themselves are similar in that they have unleashed time and again hate and violence toward an "other" that is framed as less than human, an enemy that must be "managed" to "protect" humanity from (always "unprecedented") destruction and death.

Behind the Scenes of "The Science"

As national and international health authorities painted a picture of seemingly uncontrollable disease, spread by unsuspecting healthy people harboring a deadly, "equal opportunity", pathogen manageable only by securing "vaccines in every arm", publicly available health data conveyed a strikingly contrasting message that called into question both official COVID-19 policy—lockdowns, mass masking, and the like—as well as authorities' claims about COVID-19 "misinformation". A few highlights from this message should suffice to make the point. Already early in 2020, frontline physicians were experimenting with generic and inexpensive, repurposed drugs that dramatically reduced hospitalization and death—by over 80%—and even prevented infection among highly exposed (e.g., health workers) or vulnerable (e.g., elderly) populations.[33-36] With 93 clinical trials—43 of them randomized controlled trials (RCTs)—at the time of this writing, ivermectin was merely one of many repurposed drugs that made it into the proposed multidrug therapy approach.[37]

Notably, the *actual* history and properties of ivermectin stand in stark contrast with the image that emerges from the FDA tweet: Ivermectin is no more "dangerous and lethal" than other widely used drugs, like statins or angiotensin-converting enzyme (ACE) inhibitors, and has in addition a few remarkable properties. Upon its discovery and use in the 1970s as a potent drug to treat parasites in animals, ivermectin was adopted for human use in the 1980s, when it was found effective to treat two disabling conditions: Onchocerciasis, commonly known as "river blindness", and a decade later, lymphatic filariasis, commonly known as "elephantiasis", both ravaging poverty-stricken populations.[38] The public health campaign that then delivered thousands of ivermectin doses—millions have since been delivered upon its FDA approval for human use in 1987—was so successful that William C Campbell and Satoshi Ōmura, the scientists that developed it, received the 2015 Nobel Prize in Medicine and Physiology.[39] In addition to its antiparasitic, antiviral, and anti-inflammatory properties that allow many off-label uses,[40] as most experienced general conditions can attest, ivermectin has shown a robust safety profile.[41-43] Further light was shed on the science behind "The Science" when a refereed article in *Nature* indicated no reason to believe that healthy people posed a threat: At the very center of the storm, in Wuhan, China, of 9,899,828 participants in a study, only 300 with no symptoms had been diagnosed positive for SARS CoV-2 as early as June 2020, with *zero* positive tests among 1,174 close contacts.[44] Another highlight was the estimate that in the prevaccine era, the median COVID-19 infection fatality rate (IFR—death rate per individuals infected with SARS-CoV-2) was 0.27%, no higher than the seasonal flu,[45] an IRF that would later be estimated to have been even lower—a median IFR of 0.095% for the 0–69 years old, with a age gradient of 0.0003% at 0–19 years and 0.002% at 20–29 years.[46]

Upon the launch of the global mass vaccination campaign in December of 2020, the website *Our World in Data* soon revealed that as vaccination rates increased, generally in wealthy countries, *so did COVID-19 cases,* whereas in poor countries, notably in Africa, vaccination rates and cases remained flat.[47] In the summer of 2021, a peer-reviewed study in the European Journal of Epidemiology, of 68 countries and 2,947 US counties, showing no correlation between COVID-19 vaccination rates and cases, confirmed this observation.[48] These numbers did not surprise those paying attention to the design of the COVID-19 vaccine original trials, who noted as early as October 2020 that such trials did not include transmission, hospitalizations, or deaths as clinical endpoints.[49] Official claims were also challenged when authorities urged boosters to prepare for the winter, even as public health agencies data showed cases skyrocketing among the boosted.[50] Soon came the realization that at least part of the disease, hospitalization, and death counts may have been overestimated, i.e., not due not to SARS-CoV-2 but to misleading diagnostic criteria for determining them. When on March 11, 2022, Public Health Ontario revised their criteria, 411 deaths were dropped from the total count, and hospitalizations fell by 104 in 1 week—from 821 to 717.[51]

Pertaining to young adults, the main demographic group in academic institutions, not only the *effectiveness* but also the *safety* of COVID-19 vaccines would be called into question, when Canada, following several European countries, suspended the administration of AstraZeneca due to concerns with blood clotting.[52,53] Over time, public health reports and publications by university affiliated medical researchers would also note "safety signals"—in reality, signals of *harm*—such as myopericarditis among young adult males receiving mRNA vaccines, while still *encouraging* vaccination for this demographic group.[54,55] Another "anti-vax" message came no less than from a UK government's Public Assessment Report, in November of 2022, revealing that due to the absence of animal studies' data on the reproductive toxicity of their leading COVID-19 vaccine (AstraZeneca), "sufficient reassurance of the safe use of the vaccine in pregnant [or breast-feeding] women *could not be provided at the present time*" (emphasis added), yet stopped short of *discouraging* vaccination in these demographic groups.[56] This publicly available evidence should provide readers a standard to gauge claims and counterclaims about 'the science of COVID-19'.

THEORETICAL AND METHODOLOGICAL CONSIDERATIONS

I draw from theories and methods that help to appraise social control, such as *medicalization studies,* that seek to explain how medical frames, categories, and discourse can be deployed to achieve political or moral goals concealed by a façade of scientific objectivity.[57,58] Similarly, theories of deviance,[59] including the concept of *stigma,* reveal how social groups identified through contingent features (e.g., physical appearance and behavioral idiosyncrasies) and morally loaded labels operate to prepare the public to accept some form of "management" of the threat those groups allegedly represent.[60] Stigmatization, a process where power differentials are critical, legitimizes the disciplining of "dangerous others" until "public order" is restored.[59] I have chosen academia as an object of study because it sees itself, and is seen by other social institutions and the larger public, as an authoritative producer of knowledge often used to inform public policy.[61] More generally, my study heeds the invitation to *study up,* proposed by anthropologist Laura Nader, who encouraged those willing to understand power to study not only the *effects* of the exercise of power (on the less powerful) but also social actors and institutions that hold power over others such as "the Pentagon or Universities"[62] (p.6). I also consider documents as "social facts", i.e., windows into the social world, and assume that discourses—oral, written, or visual—are a form of social practice that dialectically relates to other forms of social practice and can be deployed to legitimize or challenge relations of power.[63-65]

To represent academic discourse intended to disseminate expert knowledge (hereafter "academic popularizing discourse")—as opposed to the one produced for exchanges within the academy, such as presentations at professional conferences or submissions to peer-reviewed journals—I retrieved articles from *The Conversation*, a web-based outlet that describes itself as "an independent source of news and views from the academic and research community" whose goal is to "unlock [academic] knowledge for use by the wider public" because "access to independent, high-quality, authenticated, and explanatory journalism underpins a functional democracy".[66] I retrieved all articles from the Canadian (English) edition, geared to a Canadian audience but also showcasing the work of academics elsewhere in the English-speaking world (e.g., USA and UK). In contrast to other outlets where academics may share their work (e.g., *Substack*), *The Conversation* is highly respected by influential social institutions, including government funding agencies such as the Social Sciences and Humanities Research Council of Canada.[67] The combination of academic legitimacy and media outreach makes *The Conversation* a unique window into the dynamics of academic power in society.

To compare alignment of the messaging with what has been dubbed the "scientific consensus" on COVID-19,[68] I drew from major documents, including reports such as the SAGE Report on Vaccine Hesitancy,[9] the US Surgeon General report on Misinformation,[12] the WHO initiative communications on "infodemic management",[13] global health public-private partnerships like the Coalition for Epidemic Preparedness Innovations (CEPI alliance), Department of Homeland Security Internal Working Group documents;[1] peer-reviewed articles in leading medical journals such as the New England Journal of Medicine, the British Medical Journal, and The Lancet;[69-71] and definitions from the US National Library of medicine database (PubMed) of Medical Subject Headings (MeSH).

My research questions were: (1) How is dissent with the official COVID-19 narrative represented in academic popularizing discourse? (2) What assumptions about the medical nature of COVID-19 underpin these representations? (3) What are the implications for the role of academia in society of the ideological work performed by these discourses? To identify answers to my questions I selected *The Conversation* articles with the search terms "misinformation", "vaccine hesitancy", and "anti-vaxxer" that following widespread official (FDA, DHS, and PubMed), or dictionary (https://dictionary.cambridge.org/) definitions, denote morally tainted objects or persons, an "other" that elicits distrust or rejection. Therefore, these terms possess the analytic power to illuminate the process of representation that I sought to document, examine, and explain. I limited article selection to July 1, 2021 (ending in June 2022) to capture the point in time when universities announced that vaccine mandates would be adopted by most North American institutions, and academics raised (or not) their voices for or against university policies.

Articles selected for analysis had to include any of the three terms in their title or summary paragraph and be relevant, i.e., not include these terms as one-off comments. I assessed trends through counts per label over time and meanings through thematic and critical discourse analysis.[72,73] I treated articles as "participants" and "asked" all of them similar questions, varying only the search term that identified the article in question [misinformation/vaccine hesitancy/anti-vaxxer]: (1) How do you define/what do you mean by [misinformation/vaccine hesitancy/anti-vaxxer]? (2) Are they a problem and if so, why and for whom? (3) What should be done (and by whom) about the problem assuming it is one? The public nature of the data did not require Institutional Review Board ethics approval.

FINDINGS AND ANALYSIS

I identified 210 articles with the term "vaccine hesitancy", 140 with the term "misinformation", and 65 with the term "anti-vaxxer" **(Appendix 1)** and, upon examining the summaries, selected a purposive sample[74]—most of them from authors with Canadian affiliations—for further analysis, based on their potential to inform my research questions. **Appendix 2** identifies articles by codes used within the analysis. Most months, the most frequent term was "vaccine hesitancy", followed by "misinformation", followed by "anti-vaxxer", a frequency that may reflect the chronology of the appearance of these terms in the medical discourse: the most authoritative document on "vaccine hesitancy" was published in 2014 and the concept was incorporated as a MeSH term in 2022. "Misinformation" was popularized later, by the 2021 report of the US Surgeon General, and was subsequently included as a MeSH term in 2022, whereas no official, certainly no medical, document, has, to this author's knowledge, discussed the figure of the "anti-vaxxer", although a functional equivalent, "anti-vaccination groups", was included as a MeSH term in 2017, preceding the other two. Within the purposive sample, the (predictably) largest group of authors (24; 36%) were affiliated with Canadian institutions, followed by authors affiliated with either UK (13; 19%) or US institutions (13; 19%), Australia (11; 0.16%), South Africa (4; 0.06%), and New Zealand (2; 0.03%). First authors' disciplines varied and included communications, psychology, history, religion, history, accounting, sociology, science studies, and English, with a small number of authors (7; 0.10%) indicating biomedical credentials (e.g., MD; PhD immunology) **(Appendix 3)**.

Regardless of how articles were identified (i.e., through which search term) and characteristics of first authors—country location of institution, departmental affiliation, or disciplinary background—the most salient narrative was about "*misinformation*", a concept that stood at the center of a homogeneous message alerting about a form of speech act dangerous to society because it drove "*vaccine hesitancy*", a major threat to global health, and for this reason, the sources that produced it, the "*anti-vaxxers*", were to be identified, managed, and if needed, silenced, a process described as "more encompassing than censorship, suppression, or peer review rejection [such that heterodox ideas] have little or no impact on what is taught in the classroom, what is published in textbooks and reference books, or what becomes public health policy"[75] (p. 3). Within this homogeneous narrative, the discursive treatment of the three concepts varied, ranging from highly condemnatory to sympathetic. Over the next paragraphs, I present my analysis organized around these concepts and following the order in the message just described.

Misinformation: A Prosecutable Offense?

Across the data set, the meaning of "misinformation" blended seamlessly with the official one of "false information that may be unintentionally spread", to be distinguished from the "more insidious [...] disinformation", i.e., "false information [...] deliberately spread" (M19). These two entities encompassed essentially any claim that contradicted official policy, even when these claims relied on official sources such as signals of harm identified by vaccine adverse events reporting systems, conventional medical advice about the role of lifestyle in disease prevention, or medications with decades of use, billions of doses delivered, and well-established safety profiles,[38] all presented as misleading or potentially threatening:

> *The Vaccine Adverse Event Reporting System (VAERS) relies on unverified self-reports of side effects. Anyone who received a vaccine can submit a report. And because this information is publicly available, misinterpretations of its data has been used to amplify COVID-19 misinformation through dubious social media channels and mass media, including one of the most popular shows on cable news (M05).*

> *No lifestyle approach, including strict adherence to a holistic, nutrient-dense diet—vegan, plant-forward, or otherwise—will confer total protection against COVID-19. The vaccines aren't perfect either; breakthrough infections do occur [...], though vaccines continue to provide robust protection against severe illness and death. I encourage people to do all they can to improve [...] their immune system, naturally. Then, seriously consider what additional protection would be gained from vaccination against COVID-19. When people make decisions based on the latest science—which is always evolving—rather than*

> *on emotions and misinformation, the decision should become much clearer (M08).*
>
> *...health authorities are concerned at the number of people taking ivermectin and warn against it for anyone else who may have COVID symptoms or has been diagnosed with the virus [...] known ivermectin side-effects range from mild to the life-threatening, including seizures and coma (M07).*

In addition to intentionality, authors identified different *types* of misinformation, ranging from "misleading information" to more extreme "conspiracy theories", whose producers "*believe they have discovered the hidden truth that world events result from the deliberate actions of unseen, malevolent actors* (M12). "Malevolent" actors so described were presented as both suffering from a mental health dysfunction—holding implausible cognitions—*and* engaging in immoral behaviors—intentionally "polarizing" society through "manipulating the feelings" of audiences for their own self-serving purposes (M11). Specific "conspiracy theories" included the belief that "*Bill Gates will implant microchips to track people's movement, using the vaccine as the method of delivery"* (M03) or that mask wearing does not stop viral spread, both "polarizing" because, "*...this tension between those who are vaccinated and those who reject vaccines or dispute the science [even if vaccinated] can divide families [...] when loved ones are immersed in conspiracy theories about, for example [...] mask wearing* (M13)."

The accusations are revealing considering scientific and other sources of evidence seemingly unknown to *The Conversation* authors. These include a 91-page 2019 WHO systematic review of the literature concluding that "there is [...] lack of evidence for the use of facemasks in community settings" during influenza pandemics (p. 4), a claim recently confirmed for COVID-19 by a Cochrane review;[76] the Reuters announcement, early in 2022, that Swedish Technology start-up Epicenter was developing "microchip implants [to] store COVID-19 vaccine information" which were already being used by "willing employees";[77] and the well-established understanding that vulnerability to infections strongly depends on the state of the immune system of the host, which varies with age, comorbidities, stress, social determinants of health, and so on.[78,79] If there is any reason to believe that SARS-CoV-2 would behave differently from any past or current microorganism, readers of *The Conversation* were not told. Be that as it may, *The Conversation* authors often presented dissenting physicians and scientists as "misinformation spreaders", untrustworthy due to their heterodox position, "right ring", data-driven albeit "misinterpreting" facts about COVID-19. As noted by one author:

> *One conservative group of doctors [has] actively promote[d] vaccine hesitancy [and] taken legal action to encourage parental noncompliance with childhood vaccine mandates, using misinterpreted data to suggest*

that COVID-19 vaccines are uniquely dangerous compared to other vaccines (M22).

The power of this minority was framed as disproportionate to its size, able to operate unhindered by the power of states or other social institutions, merely thanks to the assistance of a "*well-developed disinformation ecosystem on social media platforms that extends to offline anti-vaccine activism*" (M02, p. 2). The "conspiracy theory" variety of misinformation was perceived as polarizing and contributing to "extremism" and violent behaviors—even a "threat to democracy" and linked to foreign enemies. As two authors compellingly put it:

> *...conspiracy theories have the potential to promote political polarization, extremism, and violence. Some [instances] might seem relatively trivial, such as sticker campaigns disputing the safety of the vaccination program [...]. But there have also been [...] attempts to disrupt the work of vaccination centers and even footage of threats of violence [...] against public figures associated with the pandemic response (M12).*

> *Social media is being manipulated on an industrial scale, including a Russian campaign pushing disinformation about COVID-19 vaccines. Researchers have found that people who rely on Facebook as their primary source of news [...] are less likely to be vaccinated than people who get their coronavirus news from any other source (M02).*

Recommendations on how to handle misinformation followed logically from the nature of the threat: countering it with behavioral techniques—"nudges"—to *"build trust and acceptance of vaccines"* (M02) while forcefully neutralizing the sources appeared as the only way to deal with "aggressive" cases, such as the "disinformation dozen", cited by several authors, and described as a "small but vocal group" of physicians and alternative medicine practitioners identified by the *nonprofit Center for Countering Digital Hate* as misinformation "super-spreaders" (M14):

> *Reports suggest that most of the vaccine disinformation on Facebook and Twitter comes from a dozen users [...] the disinformation dozen [who] engage in coordinated sharing of content, which increases their effectiveness in spreading disinformation and [...] makes it all the more important to block them. Social media platforms need to flag harmful content and remove people known to traffic in vaccine-related disinformation (M02).*

Other proposed policy approaches included employing fact checkers "*to identify and recommend that harmful misinformation be removed from [social media] sites*" (M15), applying "*credibility scores*" to authors and stories on social media to help readers assess the credibility of the information (M24), and implementing media algorithms to detect and counter misinformation and hesitancy (M10). The assumption seemed to be that nothing less than full embrace of vaccination was safe, such that even low levels of "hesitancy" posed a societal threat, as indicated by the *"...15% of adults [in the USA who] refuse to get a COVID vaccine [...] leading to what's been dubbed the pandemic of the unvaccinated"* (M16). Hesitancy was framed as even more troubling when expressed by disadvantaged groups—in low/middle income (M03), racialized groups in North America (M01, M02), and children and parents (M09, M14, M25), especially racialized, perceived as particularly vulnerable to *"anti-vaccine disinformation and propaganda"* (M01), that, as per one author, was *"rife on Spanish-language Facebook [groups]",* and that could lead to *"vaccine inequities'* (M02), messages that I elaborate on in the next section.

Vaccine Hesitancy: A Redeemable Condition?

Authors generally relied on official definitions of "vaccine hesitancy"—most often the SAGE definition mentioned earlier. They also invariably presented "hesitancy" as a "problem" varying "considerably across place, time, and even vaccines" thus in need of "framing" depending on social and cultural contexts (VH12). Vaccine hesitancy populations were described as geographically widespread—to be found in high-income countries such as Canada and the UK (VH18, VH26) as well as in lower middle-income countries like Ghana (VH24)—although sharing certain traits, such as political conservatism (VH10) and low education and income (VH02). Some authors also observed that vaccine hesitancy *"may arise from positions of both privilege and marginalization",* for instance, among parents from ethnic minorities who, regardless of their current social status, for *"historical reasons have cause to distrust [...] public health initiatives that have devalued their children's lives"* (VH01). The widespread presence of vaccine hesitancy was partly explained by the multiple influences shaping vaccination decisions—*"motivations, ideas, intuition, and feelings"* (VH15), or insufficient knowledge of COVID-19 or vaccines leading to insufficient concern with *"the harmful effects of the virus [or with] transmission to others* (VH07). Another explanation was an influenceable disposition and a habit to *"turn to social media platforms [where individuals are] targeted by anti-vaccine activists who are [...] organized and [...] skilled at tailoring their messages"* (VH28).

Whatever the diversity of backgrounds and drivers of vaccine hesitancy, authors overwhelmingly agreed that a salient issue was distrust in authority, in official social institutions, or in science—the latter overlapping a tendency to "anti-intellectualism"—thus one article reporting on a panel of public opinion experts emphasized the importance of building trust with vaccine hesitant loved ones:

> *... when it comes to vaccine hesitancy, trust is really the major factor. I think we are in an era where there's a real sense of anti-intellectualism [...] in certain corners of the internet. [We must engage] people we love*

in that framework of trust, knowing that we [are] approaching them not because we want to be right but because the consequences of them being wrong are so dire for themselves [...] our families and loved ones (VH15).

Of note, "distrust in science" was not presented as rejecting open debates around matters of fact, scientific or otherwise, as the "scientific consensus" left no space for such debate. Rather, scientific claims that contradicted the "consensus" were presented as evidence of *distrust in the scientific enterprise itself.* The idea of "distrust in science" so construed left no room for debating competing scientific claims and evidence, as this option was *ruled out by the very definition of the concept.* Instead, according to the authors what was needed was a whole-of-society approach to *"take the social and political steps required to increase the trustworthiness of science"* (VH16). This was indeed the general thrust of the discourse around vaccine hesitancy, overall sympathetic to the state of mind of persons expressing it, even when this state was seen as driven by misguided perceptions, cognitions, and emotions. Many such emotions were framed as compounded by a declining trust in public institutions, to be expected among marginalized, often indigenous, communities, in their case driven by *"institutional distrust caused by centuries of colonial medical and legislative violence"* (VH14). These concerns, in the eyes of authors, identified *"an urgent need to repair trust and promote vaccine confidence through evidence-based knowledge"* (VH06), insinuating that while *in past times* there may have been evidence-based knowledge for marginalized communities to distrust government authorities, this was no longer the case, as in COVID-19 times what philosophers call "justified true belief",[80] i.e., evidence-based knowledge, always favors vaccination.

Importantly, vaccine hesitant individuals were also presented as "changeable"—"waiting" to make the right—provaccination decision (VH17), as illustrated in one article expressing relief that while vaccine hesitancy was widespread among indigenous Canadians like the Inuit at the launch of the vaccination campaign, upon *"accelerated vaccination campaigns in the North"* this group has now *"experienced one of the biggest changes in the country, with a dramatic increase in their acceptance of COVID-19 vaccines"* (VH02). Diversity of motivations notwithstanding, it was false information, intentional or not, that was framed as leading vaccine hesitancy, whether *indirectly* by sowing unfounded distrust, or *directly* by creating false beliefs. The following extended quotation, from an article by one of the very few authors in the sample with a biomedical background—an academic as well as a practicing physician—captures compellingly the gist of the message conveyed by the overall body of data:

A common response I heard was that [the vaccine] was simply inconvenient. [...] Curiously, they did not consider the myriad

> *"inconveniences" of becoming infected [or dying]—and associated costs for treatment, lost work, dependence on others for basic necessities [...], the risk of infecting family members, the potential for developing long-haul COVID-19 and more. Others expressed a fervid distrust of vaccine-testing methods, stating that people had been "guinea pigs in past vaccine experiments that later caused autism." Yet more than 25 studies in the past 20-odd years have disproved any causal link between vaccines and autism. Some felt that the forceful public messaging to get vaccinated belied true motivations of the authorities, adding: "I mean, why are they pushing this so hard?" Yet few question the strong public health stance on healthy eating practices and exercise or wearing seat belts while driving. Still others feared [...] life-threatening side effects: "Thousands had heart attacks from the vaccine—it's all on the CDC website" they told me. So I took a close look at the CDC website to understand their claims better. Reports of heart inflammation occurred in 699 cases out of 177 million vaccinated people, or 0.0004%, with causal links to the vaccines still being investigated. Development of blood clots causally associated with the Johnson & Johnson vaccine are also extremely rare, occurring in 28 cases out of 8.73 million doses given as of May 7, 2021—a rate of 0.0003%. This extremely low risk of blood clots is still significantly lower than the risk of blood clots from an actual COVID-19 infection (VH04).*

These and similar assertions across the body of data hinged on a range of assumptions about the potential of exposure to SARS-CoV-2 to infect or cause clinical symptoms, about a risk-benefit analysis always favorable to vaccination regardless of demographic group and clinical profile, about the effectiveness and timeliness of public health policies such as mass testing and mass vaccination, and about the ethics of mandatory medical measures. These assumptions, ignored or dismissed facts or interpretations unfavorable to the dominant narrative, were shared across the body of data, and included the beliefs that vaccination stops or significantly reduces viral transmission as well as poor health outcomes, that mass vaccination is critical to achieving herd immunity, and that COVID-19 inoculations are critical to protect the health of children and youth, while decreasing the burden of disease, this theme vividly captured by one author asserting that many "well-educated" parents were undermining the "*self-evident [...] public health intervention [that] protects billions of children from deadly and debilitating infections, like polio or measles*", now worsened by their "hesitancy" about COVID-19 vaccination (VH12).

Calls to action followed reasonably from these assumptions, with articles recommending raising awareness through public education efforts, promoting "media literacy" to assist the public to navigate the COVID-19 "infodemic" (VH28), and offering "culturally sensitive" education to indigenous communities (VH06). Authors also advised members of the public willing to join in the societal effort to approach the hesitant, especially those "persuaded by anti-vaccine conspiracy theories", to draw from "simple psychological techniques", or share "personal stories" as tools of persuasion, trust building, and "demystification" of the "scientific research process":

> *When talking with people who might be persuaded by anti-vaccine conspiracy theories, a practical step could be to highlight that conspiracy beliefs are not as commonplace as people might think [and] that it's far more usual to vaccinate rather than not vaccinate [...]. This simple psychological technique could be an important tool for addressing vaccine hesitancy, and one that many people could easily have a go at trying (VH13).*

> *...include [...] non-scientists in reports on scientific research so that audiences can [...] feel like they are participating in the debate. For example, with the impending approval of COVID-19 vaccines for five- to 11-year-olds, parents of children who have participated in [vaccine] trials [...] could be used to demystify the scientific research process and provide stories that other parents can relate to (VH09, p. 2).*

Physicians were described as especially apt to shape vaccination decisions given the trust placed on them by the public, a task for which they needed to be provided with "evidence-based information" to share with patients (VH11). In fact, physicians were described as not only *able* but also *morally required* to encourage vaccination, as bearers of an *"absolute"* Kantian *"duty"* (VH23, p. 2). Physicians and other healthcare workers were also advised to apply motivational interviewing which relies on a non-judgmental approach and *"empathetic listening"* that does not aim at changing patients' minds (VH15) and instead offers *"space for people to elaborate on their vaccine concerns"* to become at ease with, and finally embrace, vaccination (VH17, p. 2).

While encouragement, persuasion, and even "white lies"—like "juggling" the delivery of information about potential vaccine harms so as not to increase "apprehension" toward them (VH25, p. 3)—were presented as legitimate alternatives, imposing "coercive measures" was generally discouraged, perceived as damaging trust, and when encouraged, calls were qualified as needing to be *"accompanied with explanations [...] that highlight mutual care"* so as to not *"backfire and lead to vaccine resistance"* (VH08). Coercion would however become a legitimate alternative when addressing "anti-vaxxers", whose *"agenda has been hijacked by far-right groups"* (VH05) and to which I now turn.

Anti-vaxxers: From Sickness to Badness?

Perhaps predictably, the "anti-vaxxers" stood on the other extreme of the mental health continuum, as if reversing the traditional process of medicalization running from "badness" to "sickness".[81] Indeed, "anti-vaxxers" were framed as more immoral than sick because they prioritized "misinformed" notions of individual rights and freedoms over the (assumed) societal benefit of vaccination. Importantly, the "anti-vaxxer" was not deemed immoral *for forcing others to reject vaccination against their will,* but rather for not *voluntarily accepting vaccination for themselves for the benefit of others,* due to their (misinformed) notion of freedom to choose or reject a medical intervention. In the words of one author:

> *Based on a significant number of years of studying, reading and teaching the works of the world's most important philosophies, I am of the view that the anti-vaxxer position that being "forced to take the vaccine is an infringement on their liberal rights" is a misinformed stance...Anti-vaxxers against the COVID-19 vaccine may be considered selfish by demanding freedom in an absolute sense (AV06 p. 1).*

Not only were "anti-vaxxers" perceived to be immoral, they were also described as holding the "wrong" political views, i.e., invariably linked to "far-right/white supremacist" thinking. Nevertheless, medicalized notions often colored these moralistic interpretations, for instance, when "anti-vaxxers" were presented not quite as "evil" but rather holding "wrong" cognitions, i.e., beliefs that would be promptly dismissed by rational beings. In the words of another author:

> *Many anti-vaxxers believe they are resisting evil globalist forces who want to corrupt them and their children by means of tracking devices, microchips and other insidious technology allegedly hidden in COVID-19 vaccines (AV09 p. 3).*

Medicalization of dissenting voices also included psychological assessments, with descriptions of "anti-vaxxers" as angry and frustrated, easy victims of "far right" movements. As per one author attempting to explain the links between "unhealthy" emotions, like misplaced anger, and "wrong" ideology, such as libertarianism or "anti-vaccination" views (as defined earlier):

> *Far right nationalists, anti-vaxxers, libertarians and conspiracy theorists have come together over COVID, and capitalized on the anger and uncertainty simmering in some sections of the community (AV02 p. 1).*

Very occasionally, "anti-vaxxers" elicited sympathetic responses, for instance, when the social and economic disruptions caused by policy responses to COVID-19 were presented as driving the coalescence of "fringe" groups, united by anger, resentment, and disconnection with the "truth":

> *The protests against vaccine mandates [...] 5G technology and the rise of QAnon, suggest there are other emotions [...] feelings of anger, grievance, and resentment. Add to this the restrictions and lockdowns imposed by governments over the last 18 months and the effect is like pouring fuel on the fire. Anger makes us want to lash out [and] has a disinhibiting effect on our relationship to the truth (AV07 p. 5).*

In all cases; however, anti-vaxxers were perceived as a threat to public health because they spread "misinformation" by *"sewing seeds of doubt and subsequently hampering the rollout of COVID-19 vaccines across the country (AV03 p. 2),"* and even a *growing* threat, having transitioned from a "*tiny minority*" (AV02) to a major social movement with connections to other "extreme" movements, including "foreign" threats such as from the United States:

> *The contentious politics on display in the truckers' protest ["Freedom Convoy"] are intertwined with a shift toward more extreme political views among some segments of the population, a trend that's spread from south of the border (AV12, p. 4).*

The thread was compounded by anti-vaccine, "far right", protestors "*targeting schools and hospitals*" (AV04) or "grooming" and radicalizing the vaccine hesitant from within Black and Indigenous communities:

> *Researchers have observed members of white supremacist and far right groups recruiting and grooming vaccine hesitant people via Facebook and encrypted messaging groups like Telegram. Anti-vaxxers have also systematically targeted Black and Indigenous communities with misinformation and propaganda (AV09 p. 4).*

Conclusions across all articles followed predictably: A call for action to neutralize the threat. In this task, experts, notably academics, were seen as playing a critical role, helping to "educate" the public, neutralize offenders while respecting "democratic principles" when possible, and suppress misinformation or criminalize its producers if necessary. Put another way, protecting democratic freedoms was presented as *requiring* the suppression of these freedoms, given the "state of exception" brought about by the COVID-19 threat. In the words of two authors:

> *We as a society need to think carefully about social media [...] about regulation [and] media literacy [...] and educate people about social media echo chambers (AV02 p. 4).*

> *There are many debates to be had in an evolving society where freedom of speech and choice will take center stage. But [...] COVID-19 vaccination* ***shouldn't be one of them****. Armed with ideas such as utilitarianism and the harm principle, the application of positive freedom might see many liberal democracies eventually prohibit the anti-vaxxer's spread of misinformation (AV05, p. 3, bolded added).*

Notably, despite the widespread control of social media by state security agencies, as recently revealed by the "Twitter files",[82] some academics perceived that current systems of surveillance of "anti-vaxxers" were insufficient, especially when compared to surveillance of other social groups. For example, one article argued that there has been "disproportionate" police and state surveillance in Canada, of Indigenous and environmental protestors, and that instead the "anti-vaxx, far-right, conspiratorial movements" had "been met with laissez-faire police responses" (AV06), implying that a more "equitable" distribution of non-laissez-faire "police responses" would have been more just. Others recommended punishing dissenters because, since *"the ethical focus is to promote universal immunization and positive freedom for everyone"*, opponents of such "freedom" should *"be reprimanded [...] for not willingly taking the COVID-19 vaccine"* (AV05). While most recommendations on how to deal with "anti-vaxxers" were severe, a few authors expressed more compassionate approaches, such as increasing employment and social opportunities to prevent young people, particularly men, from being pulled into *"extremism"*, which they linked with anti-vaccination beliefs (AV02), or drawing from traditional philosophies, captured in an African phrase *"I am because we are"* translated as *"I am part of my community, where the good I do reflects back onto the society. This can be incredibly significant in the face of vaccine scepticism and anti-vaccination ideas"* (AV05).

DISCUSSION

Across the body of data, the message about the dangers of "misinformation" and the imperative to "counter" it went virtually unchallenged, seamlessly overlapping with establishment discourses from a wide range of institutions, national and international. Much like these discourses, the academic one was reminiscent of the discourse of "moral intrapreneurs" when they are engaged in the process of "othering",[59] i.e., it was delivered in a tone of moral urgency and as a rallying call to protect society from this form of threatening speech. The construction of this deviant "other" was accomplished through a four-step process:[60] The *first* consisted of a "social selection" of differences"—cognitive, attitudinal, behavioral, and ideological—to assist in identifying "deviance", a process that requires "substantial oversimplification" (p. 367) to create groupings from the diversity of the human condition and experience. The *second* step was the task of linking labeled differences (e.g., "anti-vaxxer") to stereotypes, i.e., contextually specific, socially devalued identities (e.g., in academia and conservatives). Stereotypes, an aspect of stigma noted by Goffman half a century ago[83] and central to its conceptualization since, facilitate "cognitive efficiency", meaning they automatically indicate that no further discussion about the identified deviation from the norm is required to "know" that the bearer of the deviance is a moral outcast. The *third* step involved using labels to separate "us" ("our" claims as based on science") from "them" ("their" claims are "mis/disinformation" even when they may be later confirmed to be true). Labels also help to signal who belongs in the human community (those who "care for others") and who does not (those who are "individualistic" and disregard "positive freedoms").

The ideological work of stigmatization was completed in a fourth and last step, when the identified deviances legitimized exclusion and inequitable treatment having experienced status loss and discrimination, those who spread "misinformation", the "anti-vaxxers", and their victims, the "vaccine hesitant", could unproblematically be "nudged" or coerced into "acceptance", or else deregistered from post-secondary institutions, laid off from work, and otherwise deprived from basic rights of citizenship—sharing public spaces, using public transportation, receiving medical care, and so on—without unleashing the moral outrage that these practices would normally produce.

Importantly, these four steps generally do not suffice to complete the process of stigmatization, because this process depends on power—social, economic, and political power. As Link and Phelan noted over 20 years ago (2001), "when people think of mental illness, obesity, deafness, and having one leg instead of two, there is a tendency to focus on the attributes associated with these conditions rather than on the power differences between people who have them and people who do not. But power [...] is essential to the social production of stigma" (p. 375). This power was in display in the academic popularizing discourse and was deployed to locate "deviants" along a mental health continuum ranging from mild psychological troubles ("vaccine hesitant") to overt psychopathology ("anti-vaxxers"). Most critically, both "conditions" hinged on the central concept of "mis/disinformation", which allowed authors to apply medical frames to "secure adherence to social norms: Specifically, by using medical means or authority to minimize, eliminate, or normalize deviant behavior" (p. 1).[57] Underpinning this hegemonic message was the official assumption that the spread of a "deadly virus" can only be stopped by *mass vaccination across age groups and geographical locations (with scant exceptions), with periodic boosters for the foreseeable future, and that anything standing in the way of this goal should be signaled for elimination.* Alternatives to official policy appeared not only irrational, unscientific, or even evil, but simply *unimaginable.*

My analysis indicates that in the COVID-19 era, the dominant message in *The Conversation* stands in stark contrast with the outlet's self-presentation as a source of high-quality information that seeks to "foster academic freedom" to facilitate a "better understanding of current affairs [and allow] for a better quality of public discourse". Instead, its loudest voices not only stigmatize dissenters, but also distort, selectively interpret, or ignore "inconvenient" data—epidemiological, clinical, and immunological—deploying rhetorical strategies that discredit, discipline, and silence any challenge to official narratives. In so doing, these academic popularizing discourses contribute to a "state of exception" in which the suspension of individual rights and freedoms is presented as the only (temporary) road to collective salvation,[84] a state with long historical roots and chilling effects on normative academic principles, such as the pursuit of knowledge, the protection of freedom of expression, and the promotion of critical thinking among younger generations.[85,86]

The question however remains, what explains the hegemonic message, this "social organization of censorship" against anything and anyone challenging the official narrative? Could it be the generous funding of academia by philanthrocapitalists,[87] or the substantial monetary and symbolic incentives to research "vaccine hesitancy",[88] "vaccine confidence",[89] and "misinformation"[90] showering academic centers? Maybe with the rise of the "corporate university"[91] academics have simply given up on the task of due epistemic diligence, i.e., competent and rigorous testing of knowledge claims and disputes,[92] since their prestige and livelihood depends on ignoring this diligence? Perhaps academia is another example of what some scholars have alerted is the rise of "illiberal liberalism", a re-enactment of an old, bourgeois fear of public opinion (i.e., "the crowd") by a liberal, privileged class, overrepresented in academic circles?[93] Maybe academics as a class "whose major function in the social division of labor [is the] reproduction of capitalist culture and class relations"[94] benefit overall from official COVID-19 policy, hence have little motivation to challenge it? Or perhaps what my study has revealed is merely another instance of silencing dissent in scholarly communication, a practice historically pervasive in academic and scientific institutions,[75] notably in vaccination research?[95-97]

While these issues deserve further research, here I can only call attention to the potential implications for human rights and dignity of authoritative discourses that stigmatize and silence dissent, scientific or otherwise. One revealing example is an article published in the Spring of 2022 in the *Journal of the Canadian Medical Association*[98] whose lead author, university professor and medical researcher David N Fisman, "found" that the unvaccinated represent a threat to the vaccinated and concluded that people should be separated out by vaccination status as a matter of public health policy. This open call for discriminating on the basis of *medical* status—unthinkable had the same discrimination been called for on the basis of race/ethnicity, sexual orientation, gender identity, or disability status, even if for "scientific" reasons, never mind for "moral" ones—quickly hit the headlines.[99] The "science" of the study has been discussed elsewhere.[100,101] For my purpose, I note that the "study" was based not on data but on a *model* built on at least one major false, easily identifiable, and assumption that COVID-19 vaccine-induced immunity never wanes. As any lay observer would realize, if this were true, then why insist on endless "boosters"? If the answer is "we need periodic boosters" because vaccine-immunity wanes, and anyway "the virus mutates"—both of which are true—then the claim that vaccination makes people less "dangerous" to others does not have a scientific leg to stand on.

More troubling than the dubious quality of the science was the fact that the study was deployed to persuade people in Canada who are "fully vaccinated" or repeatedly "boosted", therefore presumably protected, that their "unvaccinated" fellow men and women represent a major health, even an existential, threat to them and to the very fabric of Canadian society. It is also being deployed to legitimize policies of discrimination, exclusion, and criminalization that also violate fundamental bioethical principles agreed-upon internationally over half a century ago in the "Doctors' Trial" in Nuremberg.[102] The social and ethical consequences of these policies have been in broad display, in Canada and elsewhere: to mention just a few, students deregistered for not complying with COVID-19 policies,[103] professors disciplined or even fired for similar reasons,[104-106] and a health sector unable to meet staffing needs.[107,108] with authorities never admitting that the intimidation, demonization, and firing of thousands of "dissenting" health workers[109] could explain at least in part this impending public health crisis.

LIMITATIONS

Limitations of my study include a small, purposive sample that may or not be replicable, subjectivity when articulating my research question; and biases, disciplinary, and personal, when interpreting findings, among others—subjectivity that, I note, also colors quantitative approaches, for instance, when crafting indicators to quantify a phenomenon, or even choosing what question to ask.[110] Nor did I strive to reach out to study authors for clarifications or interviewed them to allow them to elaborate on their views, relying instead on the analysis of documents, which nevertheless has a demonstrated track record of allowing researchers to illuminate important features about social interactions and institutions.[111] With that being said, the limitations of qualitative inquiry have not stopped others from conducting it—and they should not—including potential critics of my position who may wish to appraise the same source with different time frames, purposive samples, or interpretive lenses. Bearing in mind these limitations, I have made my inquiry as transparent as possible so that other researchers can reproduce it.[112] Whatever potential shortcomings indicate the need for further research on academia's role in stigmatizing and silencing dissent in the COVID-19 era.

CONCLUDING REMARKS

Still, critics may argue that drawing these conclusions about academia through the subjective interpretation of a small, purposive sample of articles is unwarranted, "unscientific", and outright unfair. Am I not dismissing or obscuring, perhaps "disinforming" about the freedoms afforded by academia, and the good intentions to promote democratic governance held by a not insignificant number of academics, this author included? Critics may also argue that my study is compromised by my disciplinary biases—I am a nonpracticing medical doctor confident in my ability to assess medical research, whatever "The Science" claims, a sociologist of health and medicine trained in bioethics, and a professor of health policy.

My reply to the first objection is that my analysis is structural, by which I mean that while I do not deny the freedoms and good intentions of specific academics qua individuals, my goal is to reveal issues beyond *subjective* dispositions, i.e., what particular social actors claim their intentions to be, to appraise the *objective* consequences of social action,[113] i.e., the functions or dysfunctions that such actions actually perform in the reproduction or disruption of the dominant social order.[114] Moreover, as Howard Becker pointed out 50 years ago, it is my belief that there is value to paying attention to "differentials in the power to define" in that the task allows us to "inspect the practice of an institution in the light of its own professed aims [...] by making moral entrepreneurs as objects of study [and questioning] the monopoly on the truth of the "whole story" claimed by those in positions of power and authority".[59] To the extent that, as suggested by my analysis, academia and academics are deploying medical categories and frames to silence dissent and suppress free and open debate—even if they do so "for our own good"[58]—the hopes that academia will ever live up to its self-expectations and self-appointed societal role are grim.

ADDITIONAL MATERIAL

Appendix 1: Article search.
Appendix 2: Citations of articles selected for qualitative analysis.
Appendix 3: Characteristics of articles selected for qualitative analysis.

ACKNOWLEDGMENTS

I would like to acknowledge the invaluable support of many organizations, especially the Canadian COVID Care Alliance and Canadian Academics for COVID Ethics, my enthusiastic research team of students and mentees, and my life partner and capable editor, Julian Field. Without their continuing emotional encouragement and intellectual insights, and the challenges posed by their questions and critiques this work would have not been possible. I take full responsibility for its content and any errors are my own.

FUNDING

I received no funding to conduct this research.

CONFLICTS OF INTEREST

I have no relevant conflicts of interest to declare. I am member of many academic and professional organizations (available @ my university profile webpage). None of them have influenced my decision to conduct or publish this study.

APPENDIX 1

All Articles Identified through the Conversation Website Search

Label	No time filters	Time filters
Vaccine hesitancy (VH)	$n = 452$	July 1, 2021 to June 30, 2022, $n = 210$
Misinformation (M)	$n = 299$	July 1, 2021 to June 30, 2022, $n = 140$
Anti-vaxxer (AV)	$n = 191$	July 1, 2021 to June 30, 2022, $n = 65$

Comparison of filtered searches within each month

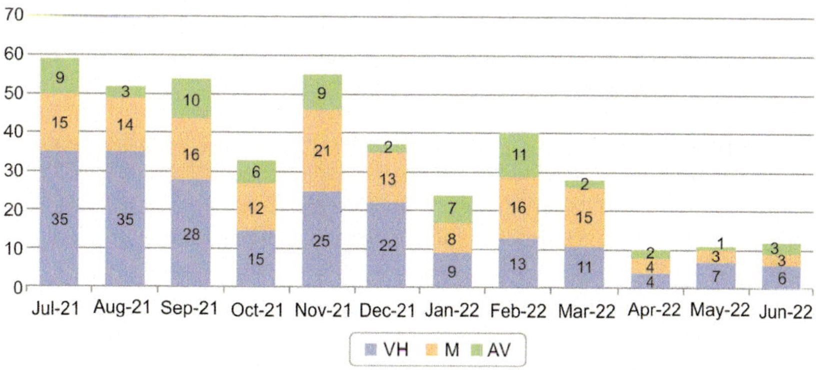

APPENDIX 2

Citations of Articles of Selected for Qualitative Analysis

AV01-Larsson, P. (2021, July 15). *The inherent racism of anti-vaxx movements.* The Conversation. http://theconversation.com/the-inherent-racism-of-anti-vaxx-movements-163456

AV02-Roose, J. (2021, September 21). *"It's almost like grooming": How anti-vaxxers, conspiracy theorists, and the far-right came together over COVID.* The Conversation. http://theconversation.com/its-almost-like-grooming-how-anti-vaxxers-conspiracy-theorists-and-the-far-right-came-together-over-covid-168383

AV03-Chen, S. (2021, September 19). *The anti-vax movement is being radicalized by far-right political extremism.* The Conversation. http://theconversation.com/the-anti-vax-movement-is-being-radicalized-by-far-right-political-extremism-166396

AV04-Fea, J. (2021, October 4). *Cherry-picking the Bible and using verses out of context isn't a practice confined to those opposed to vaccines – it has been done for centuries.* The Conversation. http://theconversation.com/cherry-picking-the-bible-and-using-verses-out-of-context-isnt-a-practice-confined-to-those-opposed-to-vaccines-it-has-been-done-for-centuries-168995

AV05-Poggi, G. (2021, October 6). *Combating COVID-19 anti-vaxxers: Lessons from political philosophy.* The Conversation. http://theconversation.com/combating-covid-19-anti-vaxxers-lessons-from-political-philosophy-168947

AV06-Monaghan, J. (2021, October 27). *Intense police surveillance for Indigenous land defenders contrasts with a laissez-faire stance for anti-vax protesters.* The Conversation. http://theconversation.com/intense-police-surveillance-for-indigenous-land-defenders-contrasts-with-a-laissez-faire-stance-for-anti-vax-protesters-169589

AV07-McKenzie-McHarg, A., & Soyer, F. (2021, November 14). *Anger, grievance, resentment: We need to understand how anti-vaxxers feel to make sense of their actions.* The Conversation. http://theconversation.com/anger-grievance-resentment-we-need-to-understand-how-anti-vaxxers-feel-to-make-sense-of-their-actions-169829

AV08-Parkin, A., & Savoie, J. (2021, November 16). *Who voted for the People's Party of Canada? Anti-vaxxers and those opposed to vaccine mandates.* The Conversation. http://theconversation.com/who-voted-for-the-peoples-party-of-canada-anti-vaxxers-and-those-opposed-to-vaccine-mandates-171575

AV09-Carlson, B., & Day, M. (2021, November 22). *White supremacist and far right ideology underpin anti-vax movements.* The Conversation. http://

theconversation.com/white-supremacist-and-far-right-ideology-underpin-anti-vax-movements-172289

AV10-Ueckermann, V. (2021, December 7). *South Africa must address hesitancy to increase COVID vaccination: Here's how*. The Conversation. http://theconversation.com/south-africa-must-address-hesitancy-to-increase-covid-vaccination-heres-how-173256

AV11-Giubilini, A., & Savulescu, J. (2021, December 16). *Shaming unvaccinated people has to stop. We've turned into an angry mob and it's getting ugly*. The Conversation. http://theconversation.com/shaming-unvaccinated-people-has-to-stop-weve-turned-into-an-angry-mob-and-its-getting-ugly-173137

AV12-Tindall, D. (2022, February 21). *Anti-vax protest or insurrection? Making sense of the "freedom convoy" protest*. The Conversation. http://theconversation.com/anti-vax-protest-or-insurrection-making-sense-of-the-freedom-convoy-protest-176524

AV13-Hannan, J. (2022, May 4). *Why COVID-19 gaslighting by politicians is so dangerous for democracy*. The Conversation. http://theconversation.com/why-covid-19-gaslighting-by-politicians-is-so-dangerous-for-democracy-181103

M01-Larsson, P. (2021, July 15). *The inherent racism of anti-vaxx movements*. The Conversation. http://theconversation.com/the-inherent-racism-of-anti-vaxx-movements-163456

M02-Susarla, A. (2021, July 29). *Big tech has a vaccine misinformation problem – here's what a social media expert recommends*. The Conversation. http://theconversation.com/big-tech-has-a-vaccine-misinformation-problem-heres-what-a-social-media-expert-recommends-164987

M03-Padayachee, N., & Bangalee, V. (2021, July 30). *Reluctant to be vaccinated for COVID-19? Here are six myths you can put to rest*. The Conversation. http://theconversation.com/reluctant-to-be-vaccinated-for-covid-19-here-are-six-myths-you-can-put-to-rest-165027

M04-Whitaker, R. J. (2021, August 4). *"The blood of Jesus is my vaccine": How a fringe group of Christians hijacks faith in a war against science*. The Conversation. http://theconversation.com/the-blood-of-jesus-is-my-vaccine-how-a-fringe-group-of-christians-hijacks-faith-in-a-war-against-science-165236

M05-Stecuła, D., & Motta, M. (2021, August 25). *Unverified reports of vaccine side effects in VAERS aren't the smoking guns portrayed by right-wing media outlets – they can offer insight into vaccine hesitancy*. The Conversation. http://theconversation.com/unverified-reports-of-vaccine-side-effects-in-vaers-arent-the-smoking-guns-portrayed-by-right-wing-media-outlets-they-can-offer-insight-into-vaccine-hesitancy-166401

M06-Woodruff, M. (2021, August 25). *Pregnant or worried about infertility? Get vaccinated against COVID-19.* The Conversation. http://theconversation.com/pregnant-or-worried-about-infertility-get-vaccinated-against-covid-19-166535

M07-Wheate, N., McLachlan, A., & Matthews, S. (n.d.). *Thinking of trying ivermectin for COVID? Here's what can happen with this controversial drug.* Retrieved February 2, 2023, from https://theconversation.com/thinking-of-trying-ivermectin-for-covid-heres-what-can-happen-with-this-controversial-drug-167178

M08-Bloomer, R. (2021, September 28). *Can healthy people who eat right and exercise skip the COVID-19 vaccine? A research scientist and fitness enthusiast explains why the answer is no.* The Conversation. http://theconversation.com/can-healthy-people-who-eat-right-and-exercise-skip-the-covid-19-vaccine-a-research-scientist-and-fitness-enthusiast-explains-why-the-answer-is-no-166393

M09-Head, M. (2021, October 1). *COVID vaccines for teenagers: What UK parents need to know amid a new wave of misinformation.* The Conversation. http://theconversation.com/covid-vaccines-for-teenagers-what-uk-parents-need-to-know-amid-a-new-wave-of-misinformation-169042

M10-Kejriwal, M. (n.d.). *Matching tweets to ZIP codes can spotlight hot spots of COVID-19 vaccine hesitancy.* Retrieved February 2, 2023, from https://theconversation.com/matching-tweets-to-zip-codes-can-spotlight-hot-spots-of-covid-19-vaccine-hesitancy-169596

M11-Harris-Roxas, B., Haire, B., & Seale, H. (2021, November 17). *COVID vaccines don't violate the Nuremberg Code. Here's how to convince the doubters.* The Conversation. http://theconversation.com/covid-vaccines-dont-violate-the-nuremberg-code-heres-how-to-convince-the-doubters-171217

M12-Dacombe, R. (2021, November 24). *Conspiracy theories about the pandemic are spreading offline as well as through social media.* The Conversation. http://theconversation.com/conspiracy-theories-about-the-pandemic-are-spreading-offline-as-well-as-through-social-media-167418

M13-Lewandowsky, S., & Schmid, P. (2021, December 9). *Tackling COVID disinformation with empathy and conversation.* The Conversation. http://theconversation.com/tackling-covid-disinformation-with-empathy-and-conversation-173013

M14-Sidani, J., Hoffman, B., & Ragavan, M. (2021, December 15). *COVID-19 vaccines for children: How parents are influenced by misinformation, and how they can counter it.* The Conversation. http://theconversation.com/covid-19-vaccines-for-children-how-parents-are-influenced-by-misinformation-and-how-they-can-counter-it-173212

M15-Chadwick, A. (2022, January 21). *COVID misinformation is a health risk – tech companies need to remove harmful content not tweak their algorithms.* The Conversation. http://theconversation.com/covid-misinformation-is-a-health-risk-tech-companies-need-to-remove-harmful-content-not-tweak-their-algorithms-175364

M16-Kenny, P. (2022, January 30). *Here's why misinformation is a smaller problem than you think.* The Conversation. http://theconversation.com/heres-why-misinformation-is-a-smaller-problem-than-you-think-172968

M17-Snyder, J. (2022, February 2). *Is GoFundMe violating its own terms of service on the "freedom convoy?"* The Conversation. http://theconversation.com/is-gofundme-violating-its-own-terms-of-service-on-the-freedom-convoy-176147

M18-Sienkiewicz, M., & Marx, N. (2022, February 10). *How Joe Rogan became podcasting's Goliath.* The Conversation. http://theconversation.com/how-joe-rogan-became-podcastings-goliath-176124

M19-Meyers, J. B., Dishart, E., & Morgan, R. (2022, February 18). *Canada's legal disinformation pandemic is exposed by the "freedom convoy."* The Conversation. http://theconversation.com/canadas-legal-disinformation-pandemic-is-exposed-by-the-freedom-convoy-176522

M20-Willett, J. D. S. (2022, March 21). *Research dispels myth that COVID-19 vaccines cause infertility, but misinformation persists.* The Conversation. http://theconversation.com/research-dispels-myth-that-covid-19-vaccines-cause-infertility-but-misinformation-persists-178587

M21-Sutherland, D. (2022, April 4). *With COVID cases still in the thousands, why are some so keen to ditch the things that kept New Zealand safe?* The Conversation. http://theconversation.com/with-covid-cases-still-in-the-thousands-why-are-some-so-keen-to-ditch-the-things-that-kept-new-zealand-safe-180496

M22-Motta, M., & Callaghan, T. (2022, April 5). *The 1 in 10 U.S. doctors with reservations about vaccines could be undermining the fight against COVID-19.* The Conversation. http://theconversation.com/the-1-in-10-u-s-doctors-with-reservations-about-vaccines-could-be-undermining-the-fight-against-covid-19-179929

M23-Jun, J., & Zain, A. (2022, May 10). *Countries with lower-than-expected vaccination rates show unusually negative attitudes to vaccines on Twitter.* The Conversation. http://theconversation.com/countries-with-lower-than-expected-vaccination-rates-show-unusually-negative-attitudes-to-vaccines-on-twitter-178972

M24-Attwell, K., & Harper, T. (2022, June 2). *Social media spreads rumours about COVID vaccine harms ... But it doesn't always start them.* The

Conversation. http://theconversation.com/social-media-spreads-rumours-about-covid-vaccine-harms-but-it-doesnt-always-start-them-184169

M25-Sidani, J., Hoffman, B., & Ragavan, M. (2022, June 24). *Misinformation will be rampant when it comes to COVID-19 shots for young children – here's what you can do to counter it.* The Conversation. http://theconversation.com/misinformation-will-be-rampant-when-it-comes-to-covid-19-shots-for-young-children-heres-what-you-can-do-to-counter-it-185666

Misinformation will be rampant when it comes to COVID-19 shots for young children – here's what you can do to counter it. (n.d.). Retrieved February 15, 2023, from https://theconversation.com/misinformation-will-be-rampant-when-it-comes-to-covid-19-shots-for-young-children-heres-what-you-can-do-to-counter-it-185666

The reasons for science skepticism can be complex and founded on real concerns. (n.d.). Retrieved February 15, 2023, from https://theconversation.com/the-reasons-for-science-skepticism-can-be-complex-and-founded-on-real-concerns-171000

VH01-McGuire, K. (2021, July 5). *Parental COVID-19 vaccine hesitancy may be next challenge for vaccination campaigns.* The Conversation. http://theconversation.com/parental-covid-19-vaccine-hesitancy-may-be-next-challenge-for-vaccination-campaigns-162742

VH02-Parkin, A., Sweetman, A., Rego, V., & Li, Y. (2021, July 28). *Vaccine hesitancy is decreasing in Canada, but it's too soon to celebrate.* The Conversation. http://theconversation.com/vaccine-hesitancy-is-decreasing-in-canada-but-its-too-soon-to-celebrate-165133

VH03-McMurtry, M. (2021, August 17). *Needle fears can cause COVID-19 vaccine hesitancy, but these strategies can manage pain and fear.* The Conversation. http://theconversation.com/needle-fears-can-cause-covid-19-vaccine-hesitancy-but-these-strategies-can-manage-pain-and-fear-165009

VH04-Ramnath, V. (2021, September 7). *Medicine is an imperfect science – but you can still trust its process.* The Conversation. http://theconversation.com/medicine-is-an-imperfect-science-but-you-can-still-trust-its-process-166811

VH05-Chen, S. (2021, September 19). *The anti-vax movement is being radicalized by far-right political extremism.* The Conversation. http://theconversation.com/the-anti-vax-movement-is-being-radicalized-by-far-right-political-extremism-166396

VH06-O'Watch, H., & Sullivan, P. (2021, August 24). *Indigenous children's book 'Little Louis' aims to curb COVID-19 vaccine hesitancy with a culturally relevant story.* The Conversation. http://theconversation.com/indigenous-childrens-book-little-louis-aims-to-curb-covid-19-vaccine-hesitancy-with-a-culturally-relevant-story-165229

VH07-Beaulieu-Pelletier, G. (2021, September 29). *The 9 psychological barriers that lead to COVID-19 vaccine hesitancy and refusal.* The Conversation. http://theconversation.com/the-9-psychological-barriers-that-lead-to-covid-19-vaccine-hesitancy-and-refusal-168643

VH08-Duenas, N., & Mangen, C. (2021, October 7). *Why ensuring trust is important in reducing COVID-19 vaccine hesitancy.* The Conversation. http://theconversation.com/why-ensuring-trust-is-important-in-reducing-covid-19-vaccine-hesitancy-168167

VH09-Basque, J., & Bencherki, N. (2021, October 11). *COVID-19 vaccine hesitancy can be overcome through relatable stories and accessible information.* The Conversation. http://theconversation.com/covid-19-vaccine-hesitancy-can-be-overcome-through-relatable-stories-and-accessible-information-169221

VH10-Maroto, M., Snagovsky, F., & Wesley, J. (2021, October 26). *Financial insecurity and right-wing beliefs drive COVID-19 vaccine hesitancy among Albertans.* The Conversation. http://theconversation.com/financial-insecurity-and-right-wing-beliefs-drive-covid-19-vaccine-hesitancy-among-albertans-170162

VH11-Azarpanah, H., Pilote, L., Farhadloo, M., & Vahidov, R. (2021, November 11). *How cognitive biases and adverse events influence vaccine decisions (maybe even your own).* The Conversation. http://theconversation.com/how-cognitive-biases-and-adverse-events-influence-vaccine-decisions-maybe-even-your-own-170911

VH12-Cooper, S., Swartz, A., Schmidt, B.-M., Wiysonge, C. S., Colvin, C. J., Sambala, E. Z., & Leon, N. (2021, November 16). *Unpacking parents' reasons for not vaccinating their children: Why it matters.* The Conversation. http://theconversation.com/unpacking-parents-reasons-for-not-vaccinating-their-children-why-it-matters-171527

VH13-Cookson, D., Jolley, D., Povey, R., & Dempsey, R. (2021, November 22). *How to dissuade parents from believing in anti-vaxxer conspiracy theories.* The Conversation. http://theconversation.com/how-to-dissuade-parents-from-believing-in-anti-vaxxer-conspiracy-theories-171781

VH14-Day, M., & Carlson, B. (2021, November 22). *White supremacist and far right ideology underpin anti-vax movements.* The Conversation. http://theconversation.com/white-supremacist-and-far-right-ideology-underpin-anti-vax-movements-172289

VH15-White, S. (2021, December 19). *Answers from COVID experts: How do you talk to family members who aren't vaccinated? How can the vaccines be safe if they were developed so quickly? Is natural immunity better than being vaccinated?* The Conversation. http://theconversation.com/answers-from-covid-experts-how-do-you-talk-to-family-members-who-arent-vaccinated-how-can-the-vaccines-be-safe-if-they-were-developed-so-quickly-is-natural-immunity-better-than-being-vaccinated-174032

VH16-Contessa, G. (2022, January 4). *The reasons for science skepticism can be complex and founded on real concerns.* The Conversation. http://theconversation.com/the-reasons-for-science-skepticism-can-be-complex-and-founded-on-real-concerns-171000

VH17-Harbers, V., Kennedy, E. B., & Daoust, J.-F. (2022, January 17). *"Never" or just "not yet?" How timing affects COVID-19 vaccine hesitancy.* The Conversation. http://theconversation.com/never-or-just-not-yet-how-timing-affects-covid-19-vaccine-hesitancy-173127

VH18-Chaudhuri, K., Chakrabarti, A., Chandan, J. S., & Bandyopadhyay, S. (2022, January 18). *Lack of trust in public figures linked to COVID vaccine hesitancy – new research.* The Conversation. http://theconversation.com/lack-of-trust-in-public-figures-linked-to-covid-vaccine-hesitancy-new-research-172323

VH19-Chagla, Z., Kyeremanteng, K., & Baral, S. (2022, February 1). *Politicizing COVID-19 vaccination efforts has fuelled vaccine hesitancy.* The Conversation. http://theconversation.com/politicizing-covid-19-vaccination-efforts-has-fuelled-vaccine-hesitancy-175416

VH20-Goel, V. (2022, February 17). *Vaccine hesitancy: Why 'doing your own research' doesn't work, but reason alone won't change minds.* The Conversation. http://theconversation.com/vaccine-hesitancy-why-doing-your-own-research-doesnt-work-but-reason-alone-wont-change-minds-169814

VH21-Lee, A., Cheng, K. K., Cruickshank, S., & Greenhalgh, T. (2022, March 11). *"We suppressed our scientific imagination": Four experts examine the big successes and failures of the COVID response so far.* The Conversation. http://theconversation.com/we-suppressed-our-scientific-imagination-four-experts-examine-the-big-successes-and-failures-of-the-covid-response-so-far-178705

VH22-Gainty, C., & Arnold-Forster, A. (2022, March 15). *Vaccines are being portrayed as limiting personal freedom – but this can mask the true reasons for hesitancy.* The Conversation. http://theconversation.com/vaccines-are-being-portrayed-as-limiting-personal-freedom-but-this-can-mask-the-true-reasons-for-hesitancy-176813

VH23-Liu, R. (2022, March 24). *Vaccine hesitancy is complicating physicians' obligation to respect patient autonomy during the COVID-19 pandemic.* The Conversation. http://theconversation.com/vaccine-hesitancy-is-complicating-physicians-obligation-to-respect-patient-autonomy-during-the-covid-19-pandemic-176442

VH24-Head, M. (2022, May 23). *What happened to the AstraZeneca vaccine? Now rare in rich countries, it's still saving lives around the world.* The Conversation. http://theconversation.com/what-happened-to-the-astrazeneca-vaccine-now-rare-in-rich-countries-its-still-saving-lives-around-the-world-181791

VH25-Wilson, H. (2022, April 27). *Anticipating a side effect makes it more likely you'll experience it – this could contribute to vaccine hesitancy.* The Conversation. http://theconversation.com/anticipating-a-side-effect-makes-it-more-likely-youll-experience-it-this-could-contribute-to-vaccine-hesitancy-180331

VH26-Williams, S. N. (2022, June 6). *COVID vaccines for children: Uptake in the UK is slow – here's why parents might be hesitant.* The Conversation. http://theconversation.com/covid-vaccines-for-children-uptake-in-the-uk-is-slow-heres-why-parents-might-be-hesitant-183881

VH27-Hitch, D., Yashadhana, A., & Leeuw, E. de. (2022, June 19). *First, COVID hit disadvantaged communities harder. Now, long COVID delivers them a further blow.* The Conversation. http://theconversation.com/first-covid-hit-disadvantaged-communities-harder-now-long-covid-delivers-them-a-further-blow-183908

VH28-Sidani, J., Hoffman, B., & Ragavan, M. (2022, June 24). *Misinformation will be rampant when it comes to COVID-19 shots for young children – here's what you can do to counter it.* The Conversation. http://theconversation.com/misinformation-will-be-rampant-when-it-comes-to-covid-19-shots-for-young-children-heres-what-you-can-do-to-counter-it-185666

APPENDIX 3

Country	Vaccine hesitancy	Misinformation	Anti-Vaxxer	Total
Canada	15	3	6	24
England/UK	6	5	2	13
Australia	2	6	3	11
South Africa	1	1	2	4
United States	3	10	0	13
New Zealand	1	1	0	2
Total	28	26	13	67

Article ID	Authors number	1st author name	Article date	1st author credentials (when available)	1st author academic position	1st author institution	1st author country
AV01	1	Paula Larsson	2021-07-15	Doctoral Student Philosophy	Doctoral Student, Centre for the History of Science, Medicine, and Technology	University of Oxford	UK
AV02	1	Josh Roose	2021-09-21	PhD, Political Science	Political Science Senior Research Fellow	Deakin University	Australia
AV03	1	Sibo Chen	2021-09-21	PhD, Communication	Assistant Professor, School of Professional Communication	Toronto Metropolitan University	Canada
AV04	1	John Fea	2021-10-04	PhD, American History	Professor American History	Messiah College	
AV05	1	Giovanni Poggi	2021-10-06	MA, Political Science	Lecturer Political Science	Nelson Mandela University	South Africa
AV06	1	Jeffrey Monaghan	2021-10-27	Associate Professor Criminology	Associate Professor, Institute of Criminology and Criminal Justice	Carleton University	Canada
AV07	2	Andrew McKenzie-McHarg	2021-11-14	PhD, History	Senior Research Fellow Institute for Religion and Critical Inquiry	Australian Catholic University	Australia
AV08	2	Andrew Parkin	2021-11-16	Post-Doctoral Fellow, Sociology and Social Anthropology	Sessional Lecturer, Munk School of Global Affairs & Public Policy	University of Toronto	Canada
AV09	2	Madi Day	2021-11-16	PhD, Candidate Indigenous Studies	Lecturer, Department of Indigenous Studies	Macquarie University	Australia
AV10	1	Veronica Ueckermann	2021-12-17	MD, Critical Care Specialist and Physician	Adjunct Professor: Department Internal Medicine	University of Pretoria	South Africa

Continued

Continued

Article ID	Authors number	1st author name	Article date	1st author credentials (when available)	1st author academic position	1st author institution	1st author country
AV11	2	Julian Savulescu	2021-12-15	PhD, Practical Ethics	Visiting Professor Biomedical Ethics	University of Oxford	UK
AV12	1	David Tindall	2022-02-21	Professor Sociology	Professor Sociology	University of British Columbia	Canada
AV13	1	Jason Hannan	2021-12-15	Associate Professor Rhetoric and Communications	Associate Professor Rhetoric and Communications	University of Winnipeg	Canada
VH01	1	Kelly McGuire	2021-07-05	Professor Gender and Social Justice	Associate Professor Gender and Social Justice and English	Trent University	Canada
VH02	4	Andrew Parkin	2021-07-28	Post-Doctoral Fellow Sociology and Social Anthropology	Executive Director, Environics Institute/Sessional Lecturer, Munk School of Global Affairs and Public Policy	University of Toronto	Canada
VH03	1	Meghan McMurtry	2021-08-17	Post-Doctoral Fellow Sociology and Social Anthropology; PhD, Peace Studies	Associate Professor Psychology	University of Guelph	Canada
VH04	1	Venktesh Ramnath	2021-07-09	MD, Medicine/Healthcare	Associate Clinical Professor Medicine	University of California	US
VH05	1	Sibo Chen	2021-09-19	PhD, Communication	Assistant Professor, School of Professional Communication	Toronto Metropolitan University	Canada

Continued

Continued

Article ID	Authors number	1st author name	Article date	1st author credentials (when available)	1st author academic position	1st author institution	1st author country
VH06	2	Patrick Sullivan	2021-09-24	Bsc Life Sciences; MPH Indigenous People's Health	Sr. Research Assistant, Morning Star Lodge	University of Saskatchewan	Canada
VH07	1	Geneviève Beaulieu-Pelletier	2021-09-29	PhD, Psychology	Psychologue, conférencière et professeure associée	Université du Québec à Montréal	Canada
VH08	2	Nelson Duenas	2021-10-07	PhD, Candidate Accounting	PhD, Candidate in Accounting	Concordia University	Canada
VH09	2	Joelle Basque	2021-10-11	PhD, Humanities Science	Assistant Professor, Département Sciences humaines, Lettres et Communications	Université TÉLUQ	Canada
VH10	3	Michelle Maroto	2021-10-26	PhD, Sociology	Associate Professor Sociology	University of Alberta	Canada
VH11	4	Hossein Azarpanah	2021-11-11	PhD, Candidate Business Technology Management	PhD, Candidate Business Technology Management	Concordia University	Canada
VH12	7	Sara Cooper	2021-11-16	PhD, Medical Sociology	Senior Scientist, Cochrane South Africa	South African Medical Research Council	South Africa
VH13	4	Darel Cookson	2021-11-21	PhD, (research on Conspiracy Theories); Lecturer Psychology	Lecturer Psychology	Nottingham Trent University	England
VH14	2	Madi Day	2021-11-21	PhD, Candidate Indigenous Studies	Lecturer, Department of Indigenous Studies	Macquarie University	Australia

Continued

Continued

Article ID	Authors number	1st author name	Article date	1st author credentials (when available)	1st author academic position	1st author institution	1st author country
VH15	1	Scott White	2021-12-19	Editor-in-Chief of The Conversation Canada	CEO, Editor-in-Chief	The Conversation Canada	Canada
VH16	1	Gabriele Contessa	2022-01-04	PhD, Philosophy	Associate Professor of Philosophy	Carleton University	Canada
VH17	3	Vivian Harbers	2022-01-17	Master Applied Social Psychology	Project Manager, COVID-19 Canadian Social Impacts Research Study	University of Guelph	Canada
VH18	4	Kausik Chaudhuri	2022-01-18	PhD, Economics	Senior Lecturer in Economics	University of Leeds	England
VH19	3	Zain Chagla	2022-02-01	Fellowship in Infectious Disease	Associate Professor, Infectious Diseases, Department of Medicine	McMaster University	Canada
VH20	1	Vinod Goel	2022-02-17	PhD, Cognitive Science	Professor of Cognitive Neuroscience	York University	Canada
VH21	4	Andrew Lee	2022-03-11	MD, Master Public Health	Professor of Public Health	University of Sheffield	England
VH22	2	Caitjan Gainty	2022-03-15	PhD, History of Medicine	Senior Lecturer, History of Science, Technology and Medicine	King's College London	England
VH23	1	Ryan Liu	2022-03-24	MD	Family Medicine Resident Physician	Penn State	US

Continued

Continued

Article ID	Authors number	1st author name	Article date	1st author credentials (when available)	1st author academic position	1st author institution	1st author country
VH24	1	Michael Head	2022-04-23	PhD, Global Health and Development; Postgraduate Diploma Epidemiology	Senior Research Fellow in Global Health	University of Southampton	US
VH25	1	Hamish Wilson	2022-04-26	Masters General Medical Practice	Associate Professor in General Practice	University of Otago	New Zealand
VH26	3	Simon Nicholas Williams	2022-06-06	PhD, Medical Sociology	Lecturer Psychology	Swansea University	England
VH27	3	Danielle Hitch	2022-06-19	PhD, Occupational Therapy	Senior Lecturer Occupational Therapy	Deakin University	
VH28	3	Jaime Sidani	2022-06-22	PhD, Health Education	Assistant Professor Public Health	University of Pittsburgh	
M01	1	Paula Larsson	2021-07-15	Doctoral Student Philosophy	Doctoral Student, Centre for the History of Science, Medicine, and Technology	University of Oxford	England
M02		Anjana Susarla	2021-07-29	PhD, Information Systems	Omura-Saxena Professor Responsible AI	Michigan State University	US
M03	2	Neelaveni Padayachee	2021-07-30	PhD, Pharmacy and Pharmacology	Senior Lecturer, Department of Pharmacy and Pharmacology	University of the Witwatersrand	South Africa
M04	1	Robyn J. Whitaker	2021-08-04	PhD, Biblical Scholar and Historian	Senior Lecturer in New Testament, Pilgrim Theological College	University of Divinity	Canada
M05	2	Matt Motta	2021-08-25	PhD, Political Science	Assistant Professor Political Science	Oklahoma State University	US

Continued

Continued

Article ID	Authors number	1st author name	Article date	1st author credentials (when available)	1st author academic position	1st author institution	1st author country
M06	1	Matthew Woodruff	2021-08-25	PhD, Immunology and Infectious Disease	Instructor of Human Immunology,	Emory University	US
M07	3	Nial Wheate	2021-09-21	PhD, Medicinal Chemistry	Associate Professor Sydney Pharmacy School	University of Sydney	Australia
M08	1	Richard Bloomer	2021-09-28	PhD, Medicine	Associate Professor Sydney Pharmacy School	University of Sydney	Australia
M09	1	Michael Head	2021-10-01	PhD, Global Health and Development; Postgraduate Diploma Epidemiology	Senior Research Fellow Global Health	University of Southampton	England
M10	1	Mayank Kejriwal	2021-11-05	PhD, Computer Science	Research Assistant Professor Industrial and Systems Engineering	University of Southern California	US
M11	3	Holly Seale	2021-11-17	Associate Professor Social Science	Associate Professor Sydney Pharmacy School	UNSW Sydney	Australia
M12	1	Rod Dacombe	2021-11-24	DPhil Social Policy	Director of the Centre for British Politics and Government	King's College London	England
M13	2	Stephan Lewandowsky	2021-12-09	PhD, Psychology	Chair Cognitive Psychology	University of Bristol	England
M14	3	Jaime Sidani	2021-12-15	PhD, Health Education	Assistant Professor Public Health	University of Pittsburgh	US
M15	1	Andrew Chadwick	2021-01-21	Professor Political Communication	Professor Political Communication	Loughborough University	England

Continued

Continued

Article ID	Authors number	1st author name	Article date	1st author credentials (when available)	1st author academic position	1st author institution	1st author country
M16	1	Paul Kenny	2022-01-30	Doctorate Law	Professor Political Science	Australian Catholic University	England
M17	1	Jeremy Snyder	2022-02-22	Associate Professor Health Sciences	Simon Fraser University	Simon Fraser University	Canada
M18	2	Matt Sienkiewicz	2022-02-10	Associate Professor Communication and International Studies	Associate Professor Communication and International Studies	Boston College	US
M19	3	Jeffrey B. Meyers	2022-02-18	PhD, Political Science	Lecturer, Faculty of Law	Thompson Rivers University	Canada
M20	1	Julian Daniel Sunday Willett	2022-03-21	PhD, Candidate Quantitative Life Science	PhD Candidate, Quantitative Life Sciences	McGill University	Canada
M21	1	Dougal Sutherland	2022-04-04	PhD, Psychology	Clinical Psychologist	Te Herenga Waka—Victoria University of Wellington	New Zealand
M22	2	Matt Motta	2022-04-05	PhD, Political Science	Assistant Professor Political Science	Oklahoma State University	US
M24	2	Jungmi Jun	2022-05-10	PhD, Health Communication Scientist	Associate Professor Information and Communications	University of South Carolina	US
M25	2	Katie Attwell	2022-06-02	PhD, Politics	Associate Professor	The University of Western Australia	Australia
M26	3	Jaime Sidani	2022-06-24	PhD, Health Education	Assistant Professor Public Health	University of Pittsburgh	US

REFERENCES

1. DHS. (2022). Fact Sheet: DHS Internal Working Group Protects Free Speech Other Fundamental Rights When Addressing Disinformation That Threatens the Security of the United States. [online] Available from https://www.dhs.gov/news/2022/05/02/fact-sheet-dhs-internal-working-group-protects-free-speech-other-fundamental-rights. [Last accessed February, 2024].
2. Farhart CE, Douglas-Durham E, Trujillo KL, Vitriol JA. Vax attacks: How conspiracy theory belief undermines vaccine support. Prog Mol Biol Transl Sci. 2022;188:135-69.
3. Lee C, Yang T, Inchoco GD, Jones GM, Satyanarayan A. (2021). Viral Visualizations: How Coronavirus Skeptics Use Orthodox Data Practices to Promote Unorthodox Science Online. [online] Available from https://www.researchgate.net/publication/351420540_Viral_Visualizations_How_Coronavirus_Skeptics_Use_Orthodox_Data_Practices_to_Promote_Unorthodox_Science_Online. [Last accessed February, 2024].
4. van Mulukom V, Pummerer LJ, Alper S, Bai H, Čavojová V, Farias J, et al. Antecedents and consequences of COVID-19 conspiracy beliefs: A systematic review. Soc Sci Med. 2022;301:114912.
5. FDA. (2018). What is Gene Therapy? [online] Available from https://www.fda.gov/vaccines-blood-biologics/cellular-gene-therapy-products/what-gene-therapy. [Last accessed February, 2024].
6. Rose J. Critical Appraisal of VAERS Pharmacovigilance: Is the U.S. Vaccine Adverse Events Reporting System (VAERS) a Functioning Pharmacovigilance System? Sci Pub Health Pol Law. 2021;3:100-29.
7. Garner J. Health versus Disorder, Disease, and Death: Unvaccinated Persons Are Incommensurably Healthier than Vaccinated. Int J Vaccine Theory Pract Res. 2022;2:670-86.
8. Hooker BS. Measles-mumps-rubella vaccination timing and autism among young African American boys: a reanalysis of CDC data. Transl Neurodegener. 2014;3:16.
9. WHO/SAGE. (2014). Report of the SAGE Working Group on Vaccine Hesitancy. [online] https://www.asset-scienceinsociety.eu/sites/default/files/sage_working_group_revised_report_vaccine_hesitancy.pdf. [Last accessed February, 2024].
10. World Health Organization. (2019). Ten threats to global health in 2019. [online] Available from https://www.who.int/news-room/spotlight/ten-threats-to-global-health-in-2019. [Last accessed February, 2024].
11. @US_FDA. (2021). You are not a horse. You are not a cow. Seriously, y'all. Stop it. [online] Available from https://twitter.com/US_FDA/status/1429050070243192839. [Last accessed February, 2024].
12. Primary Care Collaborative. (2021). Surgeon General Issues Advisory during COVID-19 Vaccination Push Warning American Public About Threat of Health Misinformation. [online] Available from https://thepcc.org/it/node/209922. [Last accessed February, 2024].
13. WHO. (2021). Fighting misinformation in the time of COVID-19, one click at a time. [online] Available from https://www.who.int/news-room/feature-stories/detail/fighting-misinformation-in-the-time-of-covid-19-one-click-at-a-time. [Last accessed February, 2024].
14. Sell TK, Hosangadi D, Smith E, Trotochaud M, Vasudevan P, Gronvall GK, et al. (2021). National Priorities to Combat Misinformation and Disinformation for COVID-19 and Future Public Health Threats: A Call for a National Strategy. [online] Available from https://centerforhealthsecurity.org/sites/default/files/2023-02/210322-misinformation.pdf. [Last accessed February, 2024].
15. Kilander G. (2021). 'Attacks on me are attacks on science': Fauci blasts critics in fiery TV appearance. [online] Available from https://www.the-independent.com/news/

world/americas/us-politics/fauci-interview-today-science-covid-b1862899.html. [Last accessed February, 2024].

16. The Globe and Mail. (2021). The pandemic is, more than ever, a pandemic of the unvaccinated. [online] Available from https://www.theglobeandmail.com/opinion/editorials/article-the-pandemic-is-more-than-ever-a-pandemic-of-the-unvaccinated/. [Last accessed February, 2024].
17. The Guardian. (2021). Covid patients in ICU now almost all unvaccinated, says Oxford scientist. [online] Available from https://www.theguardian.com/world/2021/nov/23/covid-patients-in-icu-now-almost-all-unvaccinated-says-oxford-scientist. [Last accessed February, 2024].
18. Anthes E, Petri AE. (2021). C.D.C. Director Warns of a 'Pandemic of the Unvaccinated'. [online] Available from https://www.nytimes.com/2021/07/16/health/covid-delta-cdc-walensky.html. [Last accessed February, 2024].
19. Tang L, Douglas S, Laila A. Among sheeples and antivaxxers: Social media responses to COVID-19 vaccine news posted by Canadian news organizations, and recommendations to counter vaccine hesitancy. Can Commun Dis Rep. 2021;47:524-33.
20. Mullett CF. Politics, Economics and Medicine: Charles Maclean and Anticontagion in England. Osiris. 1952;10:224-51.
21. Cohn SK. The Black Death and the Burning of Jews. Past Present. 2007;196:3-36.
22. Kraut AM. Immigration, Ethnicity, and the Pandemic. Public Health Rep. 2010;125: 123-33.
23. Brandt AM. A Disease and its Specter. Science. 1989;246:679-9.
24. Oktaria S, Hurif NS, Naim W, Thio HB, Nijsten TEC, Richardus JH, et al. Dietary diversity and poverty as risk factors for leprosy in Indonesia: A case-control study. PLoS Negl Trop Dis. 2018;12:e0006317.
25. WHO. (2023). Leprosy. [online] Available from https://www.who.int/news-room/fact-sheets/detail/leprosy. [Last accessed February, 2024].
26. Jarry J. (2021). Leprosy and its Stigma are Both Curable. [online] Available from https://www.mcgill.ca/oss/article/health-and-nutrition-history/leprosy-and-its-stigma-are-both-curable. [Last accessed February, 2024].
27. Lancet. The Spread of Small-pox by Tramps. Lancet. 1904;163:446-7.
28. Kristof N. (2020). Coronavirus Spreads, and the World Pays for China's Dictatorship. [online] Available from https://www.nytimes.com/2020/01/29/opinion/coronavirus-china-government.html. [Last accessed February, 2024].
29. Vanderklippe N. (2020). WHO's early coronavirus response raises awkward questions about Beijing relationship. [online] Available from https://www.theglobeandmail.com/world/article-whos-early-coronavirus-response-raises-awkward-questions-about/. [Last accessed February, 2024].
30. The Guardian. (2020). If China valued free speech, there would be no coronavirus crisis. [online] Available from https://www.theguardian.com/world/2020/feb/08/if-china-valued-free-speech-there-would-be-no-coronavirus-crisis. [Last accessed February, 2024].
31. The Guardian. (2019). 2019: the year in US protests–in pictures. [online] https://www.theguardian.com/world/gallery/2019/dec/29/2019-year-us-protests-in-pictures. [Last accessed February, 2019].
32. Chaufan C. (2021). Geopolitics of anti-Asian racism in times of COVID-19. [online]. Available from https://cancovid.ca/grant/geopolitics-of-anti-asian-racism-in-times-of-covid-19/. [Last accessed February, 2024].
33. Alexander PE, Armstrong R, Fareed G, Lotus J, Oskoui R, Prodromos C. et al. Early multidrug treatment of SARS-CoV-2 infection (COVID-19) and reduced mortality among nursing home (or outpatient/ambulatory) residents. Med Hypotheses. 2021;153:110622.

34. Carvallo H, Hirsch R, Alkis P, Contreras V. Study of the Efficacy and Safety of Topical Ivermectin + Iota-Carrageenan in the Prophylaxis against COVID-19 in Health Personnel. J Biomed Res Clin Investig. 2020;2:1007.
35. Kory P, Meduri GU, Varon J, Iglesias J, Marik PE. Review of the Emerging Evidence Demonstrating the Efficacy of Ivermectin in the Prophylaxis and Treatment of COVID-19. Am J Ther. 2021;28:e299-e318.
36. McCullough PA, Kelly RJ, Ruocco G, Lerma E, Tumlin J, Wheelan KR, et al. Pathophysiological Basis and Rationale for Early Outpatient Treatment of SARS-CoV-2 (COVID-19) Infection. Am J Med. 2021;134:16-22.
37. https://c19ivm.org/. Ivermectin for COVID-19: real-time analysis of all 194 studies. https://c19ivm.org/ [Last accessed March 1, 2023].
38. Crump A. Ivermectin: enigmatic multifaceted 'wonder' drug continues to surprise and exceed expectations. J Antibiot. 2017;70:495-505.
39. The Nobel Prize. (2015). The Nobel Prize in Physiology or Medicine 2015. [online] Available from https://www.nobelprize.org/prizes/medicine/2015/press-release/;[Last accessed February, 2024].
40. Kircik LH, Del Rosso JQ, Layton AM, Schauber J. Over 25 Years of Clinical Experience With Ivermectin: An Overview of Safety for an Increasing Number of Indications. J Drugs Dermatol. 2016;15:325-32.
41. Guzzo CA, Furtek CI, Porras AG, Chen C, Tipping R, Clineschmidt CM, et al. Safety, Tolerability, and Pharmacokinetics of Escalating High Doses of Ivermectin in Healthy Adult Subjects. J Clin Pharmacol. 2002;42:1122-33.
42. Muñoz J, Ballester MR, Antonijoan RM, Gich I, Rodríguez M, Colli E, et al. Safety and pharmacokinetic profile of fixed-dose ivermectin with an innovative 18 mg tablet in healthy adult volunteers. PLoS Negl Trop Dis. 2018;12: e0006020.
43. TrialSite. (2021). France-based MedinCell Safety Study for Ivermectin: Three Decades of Safety. [online] Available from https://www.trialsitenews.com/a/france-based-medincell-safety-study-for-ivermectin-three-decades-of-safety. [Last accessed February, 2024].
44. Cao S, Gan Y, Wang C, Bachmann M, Wei S, Gong J, et al. Post-lockdown SARS-CoV-2 nucleic acid screening in nearly ten million residents of Wuhan, China. Nat Commun. 2020;11:5917.
45. Ioannidis JPA. Infection fatality rate of COVID-19 inferred from seroprevalence data. Bull World Health Organ. 2021;99:19-33F.
46. Pezzullo AM, Axfors C, Contopoulos-Ioannidis DG, Apostolatos A, Ioannidis JPA. Age-stratified infection fatality rate of COVID-19 in the non-elderly population. Environ Res. 2023;216:114655.
47. Our World in Data. (2022). Estimated cumulative excess deaths per 100,000 people during COVID-19. [online] Available from https://ourworldindata.org/explorers/coronavirus-data-explorer. [Last accessed February, 2024].
48. Subramanian SV, Kumar A. Increases in COVID-19 are unrelated to levels of vaccination across 68 countries and 2947 counties in the United States. Eur J Epidemiol. 2021;36(12):1237-40.
49. Doshi P. Will covid-19 vaccines save lives? Current trials aren't designed to tell us. BMJ. 2020;371:m4037.
50. Ontario. (2024). Status of COVID-19 cases in Ontario. [online] Available from https://data.ontario.ca/en/dataset/status-of-covid-19-cases-in-ontario. [Last accessed February, 2024].
51. CBC News. (2022). Ontario removes more than 400 deaths from official COVID-19 count. [online] Available from https://www.cbc.ca/news/canada/toronto/covid19-ontario-march-11-1.6381330. [Last accessed February, 2024].

52. Jordans F. (2021). Major European nations suspend use of AstraZeneca vaccine. [online] Available from https://apnews.com/article/germany-suspends-astrazeneca-vaccine-blood-clotting-0ab2c4fe13370c96c873e896387eb92f. [Last accessed February, 2024].
53. Miller A. (2021). Why Canada is suspending use of AstraZeneca vaccine in people under 55. [online] Available from https://www.cbc.ca/news/health/canada-suspends-astrazeneca-vaccine-covid-19-1.5968657#:~:text=2928-,Canada's%20vaccine%20advisory%20committee%20is%20recommending%20immediately%-20suspending%20the%20use,be%20connected%20to%20the%20shot. [Last accessed February, 2024].
54. Naveed Z, Li J, Spencer M, Wilton J, Naus M, García HAV. Observed versus expected rates of myocarditis after SARS-CoV-2 vaccination: a population-based cohort study. CMAJ. 2022;194:E1529-36.
55. Public Health Agency of Canada. (2021). Statement from the Council of Chief Medical Officers of Health (CCMOH): Update on COVID-19 Vaccines and the Risk of Myocarditis and Pericarditis. [online] Available from https://www.canada.ca/en/public-health/news/2021/10/statement-from-the-council-of-chief-medical-officers-of-health-ccmoh-update-on-covid-19-vaccines-and-the-risk-of-myocarditis-and-pericarditis.html. [Last accessed February, 2024].
56. Gov.UK. (2023). Summary of the Public Assessment Report for COVID-19 Vaccine Pfizer/BioNTech. [online] Available from https://www.gov.uk/government/publications/regulatory-approval-of-pfizer-biontech-vaccine-for-covid-19/summary-public-assessment-report-for-pfizerbiontech-covid-19-vaccine. [Last accessed February, 2024].
57. Conrad P. Types of medical social control. Sociol Health Illn. 1979;1:1-11.
58. Zola IK. In the name of health and illness: On some socio-political consequences of medical influence. Soc Sci Med. 1975;9:83-7.
59. Becker HS. Outsiders: Studies in the Sociology of Deviance. Am J Sociol. 1964;69:417-9.
60. Link BG, Phelan JC. Conceptualizing Stigma. Annu Rev Sociol. 2001;27:363-85.
61. Williams K, Gonzalez Hernando M. Organisations and Policy-Relevant Knowledge Production. Int J Polit Cult Soc. 2018;31:127-9.
62. Nader L. Up the anthropologist: Perspectives gained from studying up. In: Hymes DH (Ed). Reinventing Anthropology. New York: Pantheon Books; 1972. pp. 284-311.
63. Clarke V, Braun V. Teaching thematic analysis: Overcoming challenges and developing strategies for effective learning. Psychologist. 2013;26:120-3.
64. Bowen GA. Document Analysis as a Qualitative Research Method. Qual Res J. 2009;9: 27-40.
65. Fairclough N. Critical discourse analysis and critical policy studies. Crit Policy Stud. 2013;7:177-97.
66. The Conversation. (2024). Who we are. [online] Available from https://theconversation.com/ca/who-we-are. [Last accessed February, 2024].
67. Social Sciences and Humanities Research Council of Canada. (2022). SSHRC and The Conversation Canada launch public talks series featuring award-winning social sciences and humanities scholars. [online] Available from https://www.sshrc-crsh.gc.ca/news_room-salle_de_presse/latest_news-nouvelles_recentes/2022/public_talks_series-serie_entretiens_publics-eng.aspx. [Last accessed February, 2024].
68. Alwan NA, Burgess RA, Ashworth S, Beale R, Bhadelia N, Bogaert D, et al. Scientific consensus on the COVID-19 pandemic: we need to act now. Lancet. 2020;396:e71-e72.
69. Scales D, Gorman J, Jamieson KH. The Covid-19 Infodemic—Applying the Epidemiologic Model to Counter Misinformation. N Engl J Med. 2021;385:678-81.
70. Wardle C, Singerman E. Too little, too late: social media companies' failure to tackle vaccine misinformation poses a real threat. BMJ. 2021;372:n26.

71. Zarocostas J. How to fight an infodemic. Lancet. 2020;395:676.
72. Braun V, Clarke V. Using thematic analysis in psychology. Qual Res Psychol. 2006;3: 77-101.
73. Fairclough N. Language in New Capitalism: Discourse Soc. 2002;13(2):163-6.
74. Creswell J, Poth C. Qualitative Inquiry and Research Design: Choosing among Five Approaches, 4th edition. Thousand Oaks, California: Sage Publications; 2017.
75. Moran G. Silencing Scientists and Scholars in Other Fields: Power, Paradigm Controls, Peer Review, and Scholarly Communication. London: Bloomsbury Publishing; 1998.
76. Jefferson T, Dooley L, Ferroni E, Al-Ansary LA, Driel ML, Bawazeer GA, et al. Physical interventions to interrupt or reduce the spread of respiratory viruses. Cochrane Database Syst Rev. 2023;2023:CD006207.
77. Reuters Fact Check. (2022). Swedish company–not Microsoft–develops microchip implants that can store COVID-19 vaccine information. [online] Available from https://www.reuters.com/article/idUSL1N2U023G/. [Last accessed February, 2024].
78. Cassell J. The contribution of the social environment to host resistance: The fourth Wade Hampton frost lecture. Am J Epidemiol. 1976;104:107-23.
79. Cohen S. Psychological Stress, Immunity, and Upper Respiratory Infections. Curr Dir Psychol Sci. 1996;5:86-90.
80. Ichikawa JJ, Steup M. (2017). The Analysis of Knowledge. [online] Available from https://plato.stanford.edu/entries/knowledge-analysis/. [Last accessed February, 2024].
81. Conrad P, Schneider JW. Deviance and Medicalization: From Badness to Sickness. Philadelphia: Temple University Press; 1992.
82. Weaver MR. (2022). The FBI Colluded with Twitter to Suppress Free Speech. Where's the Outrage? [online] Available from https://www.newsweek.com/fbi-colluded-twitter-suppress-free-speech-where-outrage-opinion-1768801. [Last accessed February, 2024].
83. Goffman E. Stigma: Notes on the Management of Spoiled Identity. London: Penguin Books; 1963.
84. Agamben G. Where are We Now? The Epidemic as Politics. Lanham, Maryland: Rowman & Littlefield Publishers; 2021.
85. American Council on Education. (2022). Open Academic Inquiry and Vigorous Debate are Core Values of Higher Education, Organizations Write. [online] Available from https://www.acenet.edu/News-Room/Pages/Groups-Issue-Statement-on-Open-Academic-Inquiry.aspx. [Last accessed February, 2024].
86. University of Essex. (2016). The importance of critical thinking. [online] Available from https://online.essex.ac.uk/blog/the-importance-of-critical-thinking/. [Last accessed February, 2024].
87. University Philanthropy. (2020). Funding to Universities by the Bill & Melinda Gates Foundation. [online] Available from https://www.universityphilanthropy.com/bill-and-melinda-gates-foundation-funding. [Last accessed February, 2024].
88. Government of Canada. (2023). Immunization Partnership Fund. [online] Available from https://www.canada.ca/en/public-health/services/immunization-vaccine-priorities/immunization-partnership-fund.html. [Last accessed February, 2024].
89. Advancing Health Online. Promoting vaccination confidence and uptake. [online] Available from https://vaccineconfidencefund.org/. [Last accessed February, 2024.
90. Canadian Heritage. (2023). Canadian Heritage funds projects to strengthen Canadians' resilience against harmful online disinformation. [online] Available from https://www.newswire.ca/news-releases/canadian-heritage-funds-projects-to-strengthen-canadians-resilience-against-harmful-online-disinformation-811889904.html. [Last accessed February, 2024].
91. Giroux HA. Democracy's Nemesis: The Rise of the Corporate University. Cult Stud Crit Methodol. 2009;9:669-95.

92. Hayward T. (2022). Counter-Disinformation Fails: Feedback from a Target. [online] Available from https://propagandainfocus.com/counter-disinformation-fails-feedback-from-a-target/. [Last accessed February, 2024].
93. Furedi F. Illiberal Liberalism: A Genealogy. JLS. 2022;2:19-36.
94. Press A. (2019). On the Origins of the Professional-Managerial Class: An Interview with Barbara Ehrenreich. [online] Available from https://www.dissentmagazine.org/online_articles/on-the-origins-of-the-professional-managerial-class-an-interview-with-barbara-ehrenreich/. [Last accessed February, 2024].
95. Elisha E, Guetzkow J, Shir-Raz Y, Ronel N. Suppressing Scientific Discourse on Vaccines? Self-perceptions of researchers and practitioners. HEC Forum. 2022.
96. Elisha E, Guetzkow J, Shir-Raz Y, Ronel N. Retraction of scientific papers: the case of vaccine research. Crit Public Health. 2022;32:533-42.
97. Shir-Raz Y, Elisha E, Martin B, Ronel N, Guetzkow J. Censorship and Suppression of Covid-19 Heterodoxy: Tactics and Counter-Tactics. Minerva. 2022.
98. Fisman DN, Amoako A, Tuite AR. Impact of population mixing between vaccinated and unvaccinated subpopulations on infectious disease dynamics: implications for SARS-CoV-2 transmission. CMAJ. 2022;194:E573-E580.
99. Woo A. (2022). Unvaccinated disproportionately risk safety of those vaccinated against COVID-19, study shows. [online] Available from https://www.theglobeandmail.com/canada/article-unvaccinated-covid-risk-for-vaccinated-canada/. [Last accessed February, 2024].
100. Bridle BW. (2022). Fiction Disguised as Science to Promote Hatred. [online] Available from https://viralimmunologist.substack.com/p/fiction-disguised-as-science-to-promote. [Last accessed February, 2024].
101. Rancourt DG, Hickey J. (2022). OCLA Statement on CMAJ Fisman, et al. Article Claiming Disproportionate Infection Risk from Unvaccinated Population, and on Negligent Media Reporting. [online] Available from https://www.researchgate.net/publication/360227540_OCLA_Statement_on_CMAJ_Fisman_et_al_Article_Claiming_Disproportionate_Infection_Risk_from_Unvaccinated_Population_and_on_Negligent_Media_Reporting. [Last accessed February, 2024].
102. Shuster E. Fifty Years Later: The Significance of the Nuremberg Code. N Engl J Med. 1997;337:1436-40.
103. Gilligan M. (2021). 11 MRU students deregistered for not complying with vaccination policy. [online] Available from https://calgary.ctvnews.ca/11-mru-students-deregistered-for-not-complying-with-vaccination-policy-1.5611963. [Last accessed February, 2024].
104. Caudle D. (2021). Controversial U of G prof criticizes school's vaccine mandate. [online] Available from https://www.guelphtoday.com/local-news/controversial-u-of-g-prof-criticizes-schools-vaccine-mandate-4456348#:~:text=Going%20against%20the%20university's%20mandate,allow%20me%20to%20enter%20buildings. [Last accessed February, 2024].
105. Dawson T. (2021). Ontario professor on paid leave after refusing to get vaccinated or wear a mask. [online] Available from https://nationalpost.com/news/canada/ontario-professor-on-paid-leave-after-refusing-to-get-vaccinated-or-wear-a-mask#:~:text=A%20philosophy%20professor%20at%20a,the%20school's%20COVID%2D19%20policy. [Last accessed February, 2024].
106. Williams R. (2022). University of Waterloo fires professor over vaccine mandate. [online] Available from https://www.therecord.com/news/waterloo-region/university-of-waterloo-fires-professor-over-vaccine-mandate/article_05beda1c-6b47-5a08-907b-00b1c3088f4d.html. [Last accessed February, 2024].
107. Beattie S. (2021). Ontario health-care workers warn of 'brutal' nurse shortage as hospitals brace for 4th wave. [online] Available from https://www.cbc.ca/news/canada/toronto/

ontario-health-care-workers-warn-of-brutal-nurse-shortage-as-hospitals-brace-for-4th-wave-1.6150255. [Last accessed February, 2024].

108. Puri B. (2023). ER doctors at 2 more B.C. hospitals say staffing crisis leaves patients with 'undignified' care. [online] Available from https://www.cbc.ca/news/canada/british-columbia/royal-columbian-hospital-eagle-ridge-hospital-doctors-letter-1.6856310#:~:text=A%20group%20of%20physicians%20from,adequate%2C%20%22dignified%22%20care. [Last accessed February, 2024].

109. United Health Care Workers of Ontario. About Us. [online] Available from https://uhcwo.ca/about-us. [Last accessed February, 2024].

110. Bowker GC, Star SL. Sorting Things Out: Classification and its Consequences. Cambridge: MIT Press; 2000.

111. McCulloch G. Documentary Research: In Education, History and the Social Sciences, 1st edition. London: Routledge; 2004.

112. Tracy SJ. Qualitative Quality: Eight "Big-Tent" Criteria for Excellent Qualitative Research. Qual Inq. 2010;16:837-51.

113. Merton RK. Manifest and Latent Functions. In: Merton RK (Ed). Social Theory and Social Structure. Glencoe, IL: Free Press; 1957. pp. 60-9.

114. Gans HJ. The Positive Functions of Poverty. Am J Sociol. 1972;78:275-89.

CHAPTER 6

Origin of COVID Pandemic: A Natural Calamity or Manmade Adventure

Abha Mahashur, Prahlad Prabhudesai

"The literary depiction of life and its moral dilemmas compel us to use our conscience, to make those infallible distinctions between right and wrong."

—F Sionil Jose

INTRODUCTION

Coronavirus disease (COVID) pandemic has been a historical experience faced by mankind all across the world which paralyzed the population financially, emotionally, and physically. The impact of this journey was seen remarkably on healthcare system in terms of struggle with diagnostic algorithms and devising the treatment. Furthermore, challenges with reducing the transmission of virus due to sudden outburst of cases on one side and poor understanding of epidemiology made the situation even worse. Physicians were caught up with handling alarmingly high patient load day night with their varied expertise in handling something which was for the first time even for the well learned lot. In the early phase, scientists also struggled to establish the origin, transmission, and multifold spread of the virus in community.

Not only scientists and physicians handling the front but also the people who were suffering on large scale were interested to know the origin of such a medical disaster. Unfortunately, the storm of COVID-19 started to inculcate various thought process around, as the experts were not initially in a position to consolidate facts appropriately to come to a single conclusion as to how and why such a huge medical crisis was witnessed. Broadly, the two scenarios put forth were either the novel virus emerged naturally as the previous similar episodes with coronavirus (CoV) outbreaks or it was a manmade weapon which got leaked in the population. Even a slightest thought of this disaster being planned or deliberately executed did create a huge unrest among people who were at loss. To understand the origin of this pandemic, we need to go through the events of pandemic at the source level, how the virus was different than existing CoVs till now and what were the different theories postulated to explain the situation by health authorities.

THE STORY OF PANDEMIC

The first case of this pandemic dates back to around December 8th, 2019, spotted at Wuhan, China. Toward the end of December 2019, health facilities at Wuhan, Hubie province in China, reported clusters of patients with pneumonia of unknown etiology.[1] They had respiratory symptoms such as cough, chest heaviness, and dyspnea rapidly progressing to lung infiltrates along with fever.[2] The pattern of illness somewhat resonated with previous episodes of severe acute respiratory syndrome (SARS) (2002) and Middle Eastern respiratory syndrome (MERS) (2012). As a rapid response, Chinese Center of Disease Control and Prevention (Chinese CDC) deployed a team to conduct an epidemiological and etiological investigations at Hubie province. The first lot of hospitalized patients had a common history of exposure at Huanan Seafood Wholesale Market, a wet market situated at Wuhan, where not only seafood was available but live animals comprising of poultry and wild-life were also sold.[3] Thus, "animal to human transmission" was confirmed at this stage. By January 9th, 2020, the preliminary studies at China found a beta-CoV never identified before as the responsible etiological agent for the emerging disaster. Within no time "human-to-human transmission"[4-6] was established in the community as the virus affected even those people who had not visited the Huanan seafood market. Also, rapid spread was noted in family clusters and healthcare professionals. With the Chinese new year celebrations, remarkable mingling of Chinese people led to a huge number of infected pool in community. By January 23rd, 2020, lockdown was declared in Wuhan city. By the end of January, WHO released 6th situation report of COVID pandemic wherein 29 confirmed cases of COVID were noted in 10 countries other than China.[7] In February 2020, International Committee on Taxonomy of Virus (ICTV) termed this virus as SARS-CoV-2 and WHO termed the disease as COVID-19.[8] In February 2020, China went through a peak of epidemic with COVID-19 illness. Thus, the government curtailed transportation, public gatherings, and any form of intermixing of population which definitely helped them to reduce the daily detected new cases. Unfortunately, toward the end of February, cases in other continents and countries started to rise rapidly.[9] With the alarming number of cases overwhelming the healthcare facilities all across the world, WHO declared COVID-19 illness as a pandemic on March 11th, 2020.[10]

NOVEL CORONAVIRUS (SARS-COV-2)

Coronavirus is a large family of enveloped positive sense single-stranded RNA virus. These viruses can cause illnesses related to not only respiratory system but also enteric, hepatic, and neurological system.[11,12] They can be divided into four genera or subfamilies namely, alpha-, beta-, gamma-, and delta-CoV. Interestingly, human CoV infections are typically caused by alpha- and beta-CoVs. They can cause varied spectrum of respiratory illnesses from mild upper respiratory infection like common flu to a life-threatening state like SARS. The first severe form of respiratory illness caused by CoV was in Foshan, China in November 2002, which was labeled as SARS caused by SARS-CoV. After a decade in 2012, world witnessed yet another deadly outbreak of CoV infection in Saudi Arabia, which was termed as MERS CoV. In both these outbreaks, bats were the reservoirs spreading the disease to humans predominantly through nosocomial transmission.[11,12]

The recently detected CoV was termed as SARS-CoV-2. It is a beta-CoV, an enveloped, nonsegmented RNA virus around 29.9 kb in size. Structurally, it has a nucleocapsid made up of genomic RNA and phosphorylated nucleocapsid protein (N). This is covered by phospholipid bilayers and spike protein (S). The membrane protein (M) hemagglutinin esterase (HE) and the envelope (E) proteins are situated between S proteins in the envelope[11] as depicted in **Figure 1**. Both the CoVs leading to pandemic in past, i.e., SARS-CoV and MERS-CoV, were members of beta-CoV group. This novel virus shares similarities with previous CoV strains but was found to have certain peculiarities which were new. According to the genomic analysis, SARS-CoV-2 shared 79.5% and 50% sequence identity to previously detected SARS-CoV and MERS-CoV, respectively.[1,13]

NOVEL FEATURES OF SARS-COV-2

The SARS-CoV-2 emerged as a tornado and led to massive geographical spread in no time. There were lot a similarities found with other beta-CoVs classifying them as one of the family member. However, certain struggles

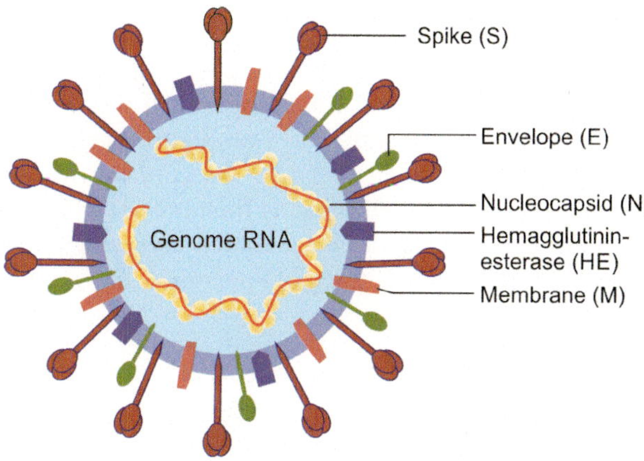

FIGURE 1: SARS-CoV-2 particle.[11]

such as rapid spread, contact transmission, ill understood epidemiology, therapeutic challenges, and postillness symptoms made researches dwell into the peculiar or rather novel virologic features, which could explain the difficulties people faced to curtail this pandemic at the level of epidemic itself.

- *SARS-CoV-2 spike protein*: S protein in SARS-CoV-2 differs from other beta-CoVs in many ways. The amino acid sequence matches up to 76.7–77% with SARS-CoV and 90–92.6% with pangolin CoVs.[13] In the receptor-binding domain (RBD), the similarities are noted only up to 73% with SARS-CoV. There is an insertion of four amino acids residues (PRRA) at the junction of S1 and S2 subunits of S protein.[14] This insertion may reduce the stability of the molecule and allow for easy conformational changes facilitating the binding of RBD to the angiotensin-converting enzyme 2 (ACE2) receptor.[15] Lastly, accessory gene *orf* 8 shows only 40% similarity with that of SARS-CoV. This feature does not trigger intracellular stress pathway as seen in SARS-CoV. It may also indicate a human adaptation after a cross species transmission from an animal host.[16]
- *Contact transmission*: The physicochemical properties showed that SARS-CoV-2 was found to be much more stable on plastic and stainless steel and was viable till 72 hours as compared to previously detected SARS-CoV.[17]
- *Affinity to human receptor*: The biophysical and structural data suggests that SARS-CoV-2 can bind to human ACE2 receptor with 10-20 fold higher affinity than SARS-CoV.[18]
- *Intermediate host*: The intermediate host for SARS-CoV-2 was presumed to be pangolins initially as the sequence identity between pangolin origin CoVs and SARS-CoV-2 was found to be 99%.[19] Eventually, minks CoVs also showed similarities to the novel virus but still the strain was not identical as SARS-CoV-2. Therefore, these presumptions need further validation. Unlike, civets and camels were the intermediate host for SARS-CoV and MERS-CoV in past, intermediate host for SARS-CoV-2 needs further matching of sequence than what we have till now.
- *Transmission*: SARS-CoV-2 was much more infectious and transmissible than SARS-CoV and MERS-CoV. The spread rate was exponential. Several modeling studies postulated that the basic case reproduction (BCR) rate ranges from 2 to 3.6 for SARS-CoV-2 as compared to a value of 2 for SARS-CoV.[20] Transmission of SARS-CoV was noted after beginning of illness and peaked as per the disease severity.[21] In contrast, transmission of SARS-CoV-2 was possible much prior as the viral load in upper airway was highest during first week of illness thereby increasing the maximal risk of viral shedding at the beginning of infection.[22]

ORIGIN OF PANDEMIC

A pandemic is basically a global epidemic affecting lives of people across continents. Impact of COVID-19 illness has been witnessed by every possible sector in the world and every individual on this planet. It is imperative to learn the origin of a pandemic for various reasons. The source identification prevents further reintroduction of virus in the human population. The dynamics of beginning of an outbreak help the public health facilities to devise a plan for not only tackling the current event efficiently but also aid in future preparedness against similar mishaps. Additionally, the course of events in the pandemic also helps in development of therapeutics and vaccines.

With the humongous impact of this deadly pandemic, everyone was warded off in their own houses. There was information floating on social media taking them through several possibilities of origin or cause of such an uncontrollable medical emergency. The biggest controversy has been whether the COVID-19 pandemic was due to a manmade (engineered) virus or it was an unfortunate natural calamity. There were lot of interviews and newspaper articles advocating either sides. Thus, WHO allotted the task to a group of expert scientists from China and other parts of the world to ascertain the facts and an extensive report was released in 2021.

Theories of Origin

As per WHO report released in 2021,[23] several theories were postulated regarding probable origin and transfer of SARS CoV-2 in human population as mentioned below:

- *A natural calamity*: Through a zoonotic transmission
    - Direct (spillover)
    - Through an Intermediate host *with natural selection in animal host or human species*
    - Through food chain (cold chain)
- *A manmade adventure*: Through leak from a laboratory harboring the virus

A Natural Calamity: Through a Zoonotic Transmission

- *Direct zoonotic transmission:* All early cases were found to have a common link to Huanan seafood market. This raised a possibility that if there was an animal infected with SARS-CoV-2 and gave it to human population who were present there. Later, human-to-human transmission facilitated the mass spread. Research showed a definite similarity between bat CoVs and SARS-CoV-2.[13,24] Thus, it was supposed that bats could have served as reservoir host. Although, *Rhinolophus affinis* bat showed 96% similarity with SARS-CoV-2, but spike protein was different and was found to have less affinity toward human ACE2 receptor.[25] Likewise, Malayan Pangolins which were illegally imported in Guangdong province of China had CoVs similar to SARS-CoV-2 even in RBD domain. However, neither of the above CoVs possessed polybasic cleavage site seen in SARS-CoV-2. Interestingly, minks were found to be very susceptible to SARS-CoV-2 as well and more research is warranted to explore if minks were the primary reservoir source of this novel virus. Unfortunately, we are yet to find an identical CoV from any animal species to confirm the direct link. With mutations of different forms, an animal CoV can acquire polybasic cleavage site and spike protein configuration similar to SARS CoV-2 suitable to bind to human ACE2 receptors.[25] These changes can be best explained with a natural evolutionary process. Thus, direct zoonotic transmission is possible but WHO advocated more samples and studies from different animals other than bats to explore the alternate possibility of finding a more suitable reservoir host.

- *Zoonotic transmission through an intermediate host:*
  - *Zoonotic transmission with natural selection in animal host:* This theory postulated that SARS-CoV-2 was first transmitted from the primary reservoir animal to another animal host (intermediate host) and then finally entered into human population. Although, the CoV found in bats and pangolins have shown distinct resemblance to SARS-CoV-2 but to acquire the peculiar genetic mutations some time period should have been required. SARS-CoV-2 was found to show favorable adaptation when introduced to minks, which are also a possible link in transmission. For enzootic transmission, animal must be present in large numbers together to allow to become a potential for transmission. Also, proximity or regular mixing of wildlife with humans is needed for zoonotic transmission to occur swiftly. Thus, many opined that it was much more prudent to look for a farmed animal or domesticated animals as a probable source or carrier to make this happen. To date, sampling from the animals have not shown any promising similarities with SARS-CoV-2. Additionally, after the careful containment and barriers being created at China from the probable animal source, new cases discovered did not show traces of reintroduction of early strains of SARS-CoV-2 derived from animal origin.
  - *Zoonotic transmission with natural selection in humans:* The transfer of progenitor SARS-CoV-2 happened from animal reservoir host and then the virus adapted to above-mentioned state within human. This warranted an undetected human-to-human transmission before the super spreading incident at Huanan seafood market. If the SARS-CoV-2 in Pangolins could show similar RBD region mutation then only the polybasic cleavage site adaptation was pending to occur while human to human transmission. In the timeline of pandemic, this theory makes sense only if this process happened in November 2019 to early December 2019, wherein the virus was circulating in human population in undetected manner before the first confirmed case in Wuhan. In past, a similar situation was seen with MERS-CoV,[26,27] wherein dromedary camels were the intermediate host repeatedly infecting humans. This theory seems to be a bit difficult in view of the timeline of events. However, we need more animal livestock and human genomic sequencing samples from different parts of the world.

- *Food chain /cold chain:* Transmission through a food chain could have happened after a direct spillover event or when an intermediate host transmitted the virus. This theory emphasized on possibility of cold/ food chain products or containers being the carrier for human-to-human transmission. SARS-CoV-2 was found to survive the conditions related to time, temperature, and humidity associated with distribution of frozen products. However, it seems difficult to presume that food chain could have caused the initial outbreak at Huanan seafood market as viral circulation was limited at that time. On the contrary, food chain could have contributed to a certain extent in secondary outbreak in 2020. Also, the genomic sequencing detected human SARS-CoV-2 strains on the cold storage products than the early animal origin SARS-CoV-2. There were isolated incidents of outbreaks due to contaminated frozen food in 2020. There has been evidence of SARS-CoV-2 affecting not only respiratory tract but also gastrointestinal systems. There can be foodborne outbreaks but mostly due to handling of frozen food products by humans harboring SARS-CoV-2 than the animals being the primary problem here.

A Manmade Adventure: Through Leak from a Laboratory Harboring the Virus

This theory surfaced due to innumerable challenges faced by mankind in this battle. The situation of COVID-19 pandemic was way different than previous largescale outbreaks with CoV in terms of virulence, infectiousness, transmissibility, multiorgan involvement, cytokine storm, mortality, and postinfective sequelae with this novel virus. As the expected therapeutics were failing and diagnostic struggles were further allowing the spread of SARS-CoV-2, possibility of an engineered virus was exercised by few. Chinese CDC was found to have a laboratory in Wuhan which was located 300 yards from the Huanan seafood market where the incident happened.[28] As a part of research, bat SARS-CoV like CoVs are being studied in laboratories (biosafety level 2) and there have been documented escape of SARS-CoV accidently in past.[29] Thus, it was theorized that the novel virus was deliberately engineered in the laboratory and was leaked accidently or intentionally to the human population. Most of the information regarding this aspect of origin came from conservative media or political leaders and not from the laboratory researchers.

As per the scientists and researchers, engineering SARS-CoV-2 would have required either a published or otherwise available scientific knowledge about the novel virus which did not exist with us beforehand or evidence of some remnant fingerprints of the engineering. If a leak from laboratory had to happen, the database of laboratory should have revealed the virus or genetic sequence. The novel feature of a polybasic cleavage site which was acclaimed to be engineered was actually found in other bats and human CoVs as well, strengthening the fact that a natural evolution seems to be more possible.[30] Additionally, SARS-CoV-2 shares genetic properties with many other sarbecoviruses, thus a natural evolution with recombination is definitely more possible. Moreover, the laboratories at China were found to be at par with those at United States of America and other developed countries in terms of safety measures, policies, and training.[31]

Thus, COVID-19 pandemic seems to be a natural calamity than any manmade adventure in view of scientific facts favoring natural selection and evolution. The scientific evidences from genomic sequencing definitely dismiss the possibility of an engineered virus as yet but it is currently impossible to approve or disapprove the remaining theories of origin. We definitely need more research to fill in the lacunae in our knowledge to establish the whole sequence of events not only to address this current episode but also to gain information for future preparedness of similar events if any. This calamity has surely taught us a lesson to not disturb the equilibrium between wildlife and human civilization. Human behavior has been responsible for offsetting this balance by direct or indirect intrusion in bat habitats, bat cave tourism, capturing, and eating bats or exposure to animals in wet markets. All these activities breach the thin barrier between the two ecosystem and may encourage future events dangerous zoonotic transmissions taxing human lives. We need protective vaccines and research to preempt the emerging infectious diseases so that public health measures can be taken timely to curtail the spread, effective therapeutics can be devised to fight against such diseases and healthcare system can be supported better.

REFERENCES

1. Zhu N, Zhang D, Wang W, Li X, Yang B, Song J, et al. A Novel Coronavirus from patients with pneumonia in China, 2019. N Engl J Med. 2020;382:727-33.
2. Gralinski LE, Menachery VD. Return of the coronavirus: 2019-nCoV. Viruses. 2020;12:135.
3. Jiang S, Du L, Shi Z. An emerging coronavirus causing pneumonia outbreak in Wuhan, China: calling for developing therapeutic and prophylactic strategies. Emerg Microbes Infect. 2020;9:275-7.
4. Chan JF, Yuan S, Kok KH, To KK, Chu H, Yang J, et al. A familial cluster of pneumonia associated with the 2019 novel coronavirus indicating person-to-person transmission: a study of a family cluster. Lancet. 2020;395:514-23.
5. Chen N, Zhou M, Dong X, Qu J, Gong F, Han Y, et al. Epidemiological and clinical characteristics of 99 cases of 2019 novel coronavirus pneumonia in Wuhan, China: a descriptive study. Lancet. 2020;395:507-13.
6. Wang R, Zhang X, Irwin DM, Shen Y. Emergence of SARS-like coronavirus poses new challenge in China. J Infect. 2020;80:350-71.
7. Muralidar S, Ambi SV, Sekaran S, Krishnan UM. The emergence of COVID-19 as a global pandemic: Understanding the epidemiology, immune response and potential therapeutic targets of SARS-CoV-2. Biochimie. 2020;179:85-100.
8. Coronaviridae Study Group of the International Committee on Taxonomy of Viruses. The species severe acute respiratory syndrome-related coronavirus: Classifying 2019-nCoV and naming it SARS-CoV-2. Nat Microbiol. 2020;5:536-44.
9. Fisher D, Heymann D. Q&A: the novel coronavirus outbreak causing COVID-19. BMC Med. 2020;18:57.

10. World Health Organization. (2020). Coronavirus disease 2019 (COVID-19). Situation report–51. [online] Available from https://www.who.int/docs/default-source/coronaviruse/situation-reports/20200311-sitrep-51-covid-19.pdf [Last accessed November, 2023].
11. Weiss SR, Leibowitz JL. Coronavirus pathogenesis. Adv Virus Res. 2011;81:85-164.
12. De Wilde AH, Snijder EJ, Kikkert M, van Hemert MJ. Host Factors in Coronavirus Replication. In: Tripp RA, Tompkins SM (Eds). Roles of Host Gene and Non-Coding RNA Expression in Virus Infection. Cham, Switzerland: Springer International Publishing; 2018. pp. 1-42.
13. Zhou P, Yang XL, Wang XG, Hu B, Zhang L, Zhang W, et al. A pneumonia outbreak associated with a new coronavirus of probable bat origin. Nature. 2020;579(7798): 270-3.
14. Anderson KG, Rambaut A, Lipkin WI, Holmes EC, Garry RF. The proximal origin of SARS-CoV-2. Nat Med. 2020;26:450-2.
15. Wrobel AG, Benton DJ, Xu P, Roustan C, Martin SR, Rosenthal PB, et al. SARS-CoV-2 and bat RaTG13 spike glycoprotein structures inform on virus evolution and furin-cleavage effects. Nat Struct Mol Biol. 2020;27:763-7.
16. Chan JF, Kok KH, Zhu Z, Chu H, To KK, Yuan S, et al. Genomic characterization of the 2019 novel human-pathogenic coronavirus isolated from a patient with atypical pneumonia after visiting Wuhan. Emerg Microbes Infect. 2020;9:221-36.
17. Van Doremalen N, Bushmaker T, Morris DH, Holbrook MG, Gamble A, Williamson BN, et al. Aerosol and Surface Stability of SARS-CoV-2 as Compared with SARS-CoV-1. N Engl J Med. 2020;382(16):1564-7.
18. Wrapp D, Wang N, Corbett KS, Goldsmith JA, Hsieh CL, Abiona O, et al. Cryo-EM Structure of the 2019-nCoV Spike in the Prefusion Conformation. Science. 2020;367(6483):1260-3.
19. Lam TTY, Shum MHH, Zhu HC, Tong YG, Ni XB, Liao YS, et al. (2020). Identification of 2019-nCoV related coronaviruses in Malayan pangolins in southern China. [online] Available from https://www.biorxiv.org/content/10.1101/2020.02.13.945485v1 [Last accessed November, 2023].
20. Petersen E, Koopmans M, Go U, Hamer DH, Petrosillo N, Castelli F, et al. Comparing SARS-CoV-2 with SARS-CoV and influenza pandemics. Lancet Infect Dis. 2020;20: e238-44.
21. Peiris JS, Chu CM, Cheng VC, Chan KS, Hung IF, Poon LL, et al. Clinical progression and viral load in a community outbreak of coronavirus-associated SARS pneumonia: A prospective study. Lancet. 2003;361:1767-72.
22. Zou L, Ruan F, Huang M, Liang L, Huang H, Hong Z, et al. SARS-CoV-2 viral load in upper respiratory specimens of infected patients. N Engl J Med. 2020;382:1177-9.
23. WHO. (2021). WHO-convened Global Study of Origins of SARS-CoV-2: China Part. Joint WHO-China Study. [online] Available from https://www.who.int/publications/i/item/who-convened-global-study-of-origins-of-sars-cov-2-china-part [Last accessed November, 2023].
24. Wu F, Zhao S, Yu B, Chen YM, Wang W, Song ZG, et al. A new coronavirus associated with human respiratory disease in China. Nature. 2020;579:265-9.
25. Wan Y, Shang J, Graham R, Baric RS, Li F. Receptor recognition by the novel coronavirus from Wuhan: an analysis based on decade-long structural studies of SARS coronavirus. J Virol. 2020;94:e00127-20.
26. Yamada Y, Liu DX. Proteolytic activation of the spike protein at a novel RRRR/S motif is implicated in furin-dependent entry, syncytium formation, and infectivity of coronavirus infectious bronchitis virus in cultured cells. J Virol. 2009;83(17):8744-58.

27. Dudas G, Carvalho LM, Rambaut A, Bedford T. MERS-CoV spillover at the camel-human interface. eLife. 2018;7:e31257.
28. Bolsen T, Palm R, Kingsland JT. Framing the Origins of COVID-19. Sci Commun. 2020;42(5):562-85.
29. Lim PL, Kurup A, Gopalakrishna G, Chan KP, Wong CW, Ng LC, et al. Laboratory-acquired severe acute respiratory syndrome. N Engl J Med. 2004;350:1740-5.
30. Zhou H, Chen X, Hu T, Li J, Song H, Liu Y, et al. (2020). A novel bat coronavirus reveals natural insertions at the S1/S2 cleavage site of the Spike protein and a possible recombinant origin of HCoV-19[online] Available from https://www.biorxiv.org/content/10.1101/2020.03.02.974139v2 [Last accessed November, 2023].
31. Xia H, Huang Y, Ma H, Liu B, Xie W, Song D, et al. Bio-safety level 4 laboratory user training program, China. Emerg Infect Dis. 2019;25:e180220.

CHAPTER 7

Origins of COVID through the Indian Context

Bineet Ahluwalia, Jalil Parkar

INTRODUCTION

The year 2020 brought an unforeseen challenge that the world was evidently unprepared for. It exposed the fragile healthcare system across the globe. Little did anyone imagine the havoc it would bring along, that possibly changed the face of today's world. Physical, mental, emotional, social, and economic, all sectors of life were confronted. Almost all facets of the virus and the disease have been rolled up in various controversies ever since its discovery. We briefly discuss some of the prominent ones which remain points of contention till date and probably for decades to come.

THE ORIGIN OF THE VIRUS

The end of 2019 witnessed the origin of pneumonia of an unknown etiology reported first from the city of Wuhan in China. It was later identified to be caused by a novel coronavirus which was termed as severe acute respiratory syndrome coronavirus 2 (SARS-CoV-2), and the disease was called coronavirus disease-19 (COVID-19).[1,2] It was found to originate from a seafood market in Wuhan. Bats and pangolins were implicated as the primary host and the virus was thought to have jumped the species barrier into humans from an unknown intermediate host.[3] However, there emerged some theories hypothesizing a manmade origin of the pandemic. It was speculated that the virus was manufactured at the Wuhan Institute of Virology from where it accidentally leaked and propagated into a pandemic.[4] While investigations conducted into the same did not yield any concrete findings to support this hypothesis, it still continues to be one of the most controversial theories surrounding the pandemic.

POLITICAL AND SOCIOECONOMIC CONTROVERSIES

The World Health Organization (WHO) declared COVID-19 as a pandemic on March 11, 2020.[5] Its high infectivity led to a rapid and rampant spread across the globe. The statistical data reported by various countries on the prevalence and mortality due to the virus were reported to be severely understated. Epidemiologists claimed a high disparity between the recorded number of fatalities by WHO and the ones reported by the individual nations.[6] One of the most debatable figures came from the Indian subcontinent where a WHO report stated that deaths were nearly 10 times higher than the official report.[7,8] Even though it was vehemently opposed by the government, images of mass cremations and dead bodies found floating in state rivers proved difficult to overlook.[9]

A novel virus with high infectivity required implementation of strict contingent measures to safeguard lives and prevent exhaustion of the healthcare system. Initial reports from China, suggested a massive surge in cases with high fatalities due to lack of effective treatment options. This forced many countries to close their international borders.[10] People were left with limited time to make arrangements for travel back to their native countries. Hence, many were left stranded on foreign lands, looming with insecurities, fear of catching the virus, and the ordeal that would follow. The situation was further aggravated by the stringent local quarantine measures adopted by various countries. Imposition of the nationwide lockdowns allowing for only emergency services further complicated the lives of many. The daily wage workers were suddenly stranded away from their home with no work, money, or roof over their heads. This sparked another debate amongst the policy makers, questioning the lockdown policies which had major socioeconomic repercussions.[11]

Millions of people lost their jobs due to the closure of various professional sectors owing to the pandemic associated policies and lockdown. People were left jobless overnight with pending rents, loans, installments, etc., to be paid, whilst ensuring their families' basic ends meet. The global economic consequences of the same have begun to emerge already and are further expected to unfold in years to come, compounded by the consequences of the ongoing Russia-Ukraine war.

EXHAUSTION OF THE HEALTHCARE SYSTEM

While the bureaucrats were framing policies on ways to contain the spread of the virus, the bigger challenge of facing and treating the infected was combated by the healthcare system. The rapid and unprecedented surge of patients in densely populated countries of Asia and South America overloaded the hospitals, which soon ran short of beds and ventilators.[12,13] Makeshift healthcare facilities were set up overnight to cater to the steeply increasing cases.[14] Reports of oxygen shortage in Delhi, stirred a series of political debates, further complicating an already tensed up situation.[15]

Healthcare workers became the first line of contact with the deadly virus, warranting a skilled team of doctors, nursing staff and support staff, all of whom would together form a robust healthcare system. It was the key weapon in this battle against COVID-19. They worked relentlessly day and night to save lives while risking themselves and their families to the exposure to the deadly virus. Many even succumbed to the disease. However, these extraordinary efforts were met with a harsh and insensitive attitude from the society. Many landlords and housing societies had forbidden the entry of the healthcare workers looking after the infected patients. Instead of being acknowledged for their efforts, courage, compassion, and selflessness, they were socially discriminated against and were asked to search for alternate residence. Even after the government intervened with their set of rules, regulating and preventing the same, it took a very long time for the community to accept the same, adding to their suffering.[16-19]

VARIABLE TREATMENT STRATEGIES

Being a novel virus causing a pandemic, an in depth understanding into its virulence factors and the disease pathophysiology was of utmost importance to explore effective treatment options. However, a high infectivity and mortality gave limited time to doctors to assess the efficacy and response. Tireless efforts were put into searching for the possible treatment options. Lessons learnt from the pandemics in the past offered some treatment modalities but had questionable efficacy.[20] An array of treatment and prophylactic measures were suggested in the beginning months of the pandemic, most of which proved futile eventually. The national guidelines were thus updated frequently as more insight was received into the disease. The repeated changes in guidelines created confusion and panic amongst the common man and hence were also criticized. The fear of getting infected with the virus led many to consume these medications unsupervised, often leading to side effects. Further, irrational consumption of the medication disturbed the demand-supply chain, hence creating their shortage, potentially compromising the treatment for many.[21]

VACCINATION POLICIES

The virus continues to evolve till date with strains showing variable infectivity, disease severity, and effect of different treatment modalities. Lockdowns and travel bans, though bought time to develop effective treatment strategies, already had major socioeconomic repercussions. Hence, the measures to contain the spread of the virus were limited. The situation thus called for building a robust immunity within the community, against the virus. The concept of building a herd immunity, tried by the United States of America, proved futile and backfired with a massive surge in cases, paralyzing their healthcare system. Another effective measure to build immunity is by immunization.[22,23] A vaccine takes decades to develop and reaches out to the public after passing through various phased trials assessing safety and efficacy. However, COVID-19 proved to be an extraordinary situation, calling for an urgent need to develop vaccines to fight against it. This too was surrounded by an intense debate since in no time, multiple pharmaceutical companies came up with vaccines targeting different regions of the virus to build effective immunity in an individual.[24] The trials conducted into the development of vaccines had major limitations. Many severe adverse events were reported following immunization with COVID-19 jabs. Few deaths were also attributed to have occurred due to the vaccines.[25-28]

Further, the distribution and access of vaccines were also controversial with claims that some wealthier countries secured a greater number of vaccine doses per capita compared to poorer countries raising concerns about potential inequalities in health outcomes. The Indian subcontinent, harboring a humongous population with limited healthcare resources, faced the challenge of a uniform, and widespread distribution of the vaccine. On January 16th, 2021, India launched a nationwide vaccination drive, making the vaccines accessible even in remote areas. It was lauded on the international platform as the world's largest COVID-19 vaccination drive.[29]

CONCLUSION

The pandemic has highlighted the need for better global coordination in addressing public health crises. Some critics argued that the lack of a coherent global response allowed the virus to spread more quickly and widely. Nature has its own sets of rules governed by the theory of survival of the fittest. While the microorganisms continue to mutate and evolve, the bigger question stays—have we learnt enough today in order to deal better with a similar tomorrow?

REFERENCES

1. Li J, Lai S, Gao GF, Shi W. The emergence, genomic diversity and global spread of SARS-CoV-2. Nature. 2021;600(7889):408-18.
2. Kumar S, Tao Q, Weaver S, Sanderford M, Caraballo-Ortiz MA, Sharma S, Pond SL, Miura S. An evolutionary portrait of the progenitor SARS-CoV-2 and its dominant offshoots in COVID-19 pandemic. Molecular Biology and Evolution. 2021;38(8):3046-59.
3. World Health Organization. WHO-convened global study of origins of SARS-CoV-2: China Part.
4. Bloom JD, Chan YA, Baric RS, Bjorkman PJ, Cobey S, Deverman BE, et al. Investigate the origins of COVID-19. Science. 2021;372(6543):694.
5. World Health Organization. WHO Director-General's opening remarks at the media briefing on COVID-19. (No Title). 2020.
6. Klobucista C. By how much are countries underreporting COVID-19 cases and deaths. Council on Foreign Relations. 2021 May 10. Available at: https://www.cfr.org/in-brief/how-much-are-countries-underreporting-covid-19-cases-and-deaths
7. Wang H, Paulson KR, Pease SA, Watson S, Comfort H, Zheng P, et al. Estimating excess mortality due to the COVID-19 pandemic: a systematic analysis of COVID-19-related mortality, 2020–21. The Lancet. 2022;399(10334):1513-36.

8. Koshy Jacob. WHO estimates 4.7 million COVID-19 linked deaths in India. The Hindu. 2022 May 5. Available at: https://www.thehindu.com/sci-tech/health/who-estimates-47-million-covid-linked-deaths-in-india-10-times-official-count/article65385669.ece
9. Jaiswal R. Floating bodies spotted at varanasi ghats, more found buried in Unnao, Covid panic spreads. India Today. 2021 May13. Available at https://www.indiatoday.in/india/story/floating-bodies-spotted-in-varanasi-unnao-locals-in-covid-panic-1801978-2021-05-13
10. Koh D. COVID-19 lockdowns throughout the world. Occupational Medicine. 2020;70(5):322.
11. Engage EP. COVID-19: Examining the impact of lockdown in India after one year. Economic and Political Weekly. 2021.
12. Marson FA. COVID-19–The Availability of ICU Beds in Brazil during the Onset of Pandemic. Ann Glob Health. 2020;86(1):100.
13. Ray R. COVID-19 exposes India's weak public healthcare. East Asia Forum. 2020 July 18. Available at: https://eastasiaforum.org/2020/07/18/covid-19-exposes-indias-weak-public-healthcare/
14. Tare K. BMC outsources treatment of coronavirus patients at Mumbai's makeshift hospitals. India Today. 2020 July 8. Available at https://www.indiatoday.in/india/story/bmc-outsources-treatment-of-coronavirus-patients-at-mumbai-s-makeshift-hospitals-1698456-2020-07-08
15. Mishra Ashutosh. Delhi oxygen crisis: All you need to know about oxygen supply, distribution. India Today. 2021 April 5. Available at: https://www.indiatoday.in/coronavirus-outbreak/story/coronavirus-in-india-all-you-need-to-know-about-oxygen-supply-distribution-in-delhi-1794761-2021-04-25
16. Yeung J, Gupta S. Doctors evicted from their homes in India as fear spreads amid coronavirus lockdown. CNN. 2020 March 25. Available at https://edition.cnn.com/2020/03/25/asia/india-coronavirus-doctors-discrimination-intl-hnk/index.html
17. World Health Organization (WHO). Attacks on health care in the context of COVID-19.2020 July 30. Available at https://www.who.int/news-room/feature-stories/detail/attacks-on-health-care-in-the-context-of-covid-19
18. Ulfa M, Azuma M, Steiner A. Burnout status of healthcare workers in the world during the peak period of the COVID-19 pandemic. Frontiers in psychology. 2022;13:952783.
19. Gupta N, Dhamija S, Patil J, Chaudhari B. Impact of COVID-19 pandemic on healthcare workers. Industrial psychiatry journal. 2021;30(Suppl 1):S282.
20. Bartoli A, Gabrielli F, Alicandro T, Nascimbeni F, Andreone P. COVID-19 treatment options: a difficult journey between failed attempts and experimental drugs. Internal and emergency medicine. 2021;16:281-308.
21. Ray I, Bardhan M, Hasan MM, Sahito AM, Khan E, Patel S, Jani I, Bhatt PK, Sp R, Swed S. Over the counter drugs and self-medication: A worldwide paranoia and a troublesome situation in India during the COVID-19 pandemic. Annals of Medicine and Surgery. 2022;78:103797.
22. Morens DM, Folkers GK, Fauci AS. The concept of classical herd immunity may not apply to COVID-19. The Journal of Infectious Diseases. 2022;226(2):195-8.
23. Yamey G. the White House wants to achieve Herd Immunity by letting the Virus Rip, that is dangerous and inhumane. Time. 2020 October 14. Available at https://time.com/5900024/covid-19-herd-immunity-dangerous/
24. Rahman MM, Masum MH, Wajed S, Talukder A. A comprehensive review on COVID-19 vaccines: development, effectiveness, adverse effects, distribution and challenges. Virusdisease. 2022;33(1):1-22.

25. Perappadan B. First death confirmed due to anaphylaxis following COVID-19 vaccination. The Hindu. 2021 June 15. Available at https://www.thehindu.com/sci-tech/health/india-confirms-first-death-following-covid-19-vaccination/article34820939.ece
26. Express News Service. Govt panel confirms first death linked to vaccines. The Indian Express. 2021 june16. Available at https://indianexpress.com/article/india/covid-19-vaccine-death-side-effect-7360141/
27. Liu JY, Chen TJ, Hou MC. Does COVID-19 vaccination cause excess deaths?. Journal of the Chinese Medical Association. 2021;84(9):811-2.
28. Jha D. ICMR studying if Covid shots linked to deaths in young people. The Times of India. 2023 June 21. Available at http://timesofindia.indiatimes.com/articleshow/101147306.cms?from=mdr&utm_source=contentofinterest&utm_medium=text&utm_c
29. Bagcchi S. The world's largest COVID-19 vaccination campaign. The Lancet infectious diseases. 2021;21(3):323

CHAPTER 8

Gain-of-function and Origin of COVID-19

Patrick Berche

ABSTRACT

In nature, wild viruses adapted for transmission circulate in many animal species (bats, birds, primates...). Contamination of other animals, including humans, may occur by crossing of the species barrier. Genetic manipulations have been carried out on wild viruses to favor the species jumping and to increase of viral virulence. The aim was to identify the critical genes for pathogenicity. This has been mainly performed on potentially epidemic pathogens, as *Myxovirus influenzae* of avian flu and coronaviruses of SARS and MERS epidemics. These dangerous experiments were subject to a moratorium in the United States (2014–2017). Three years after the emergence of COVID-19, the origin of SARS-CoV-2 remains a mystery. COVID-19 appeared in Wuhan, officially in December 2019, but probably during the autumn 2019. The virus was identified in January 2020. It belongs to the genus *Betacoronavirus* (subgenus *Sarbecovirus*). It was at once highly contagious. In addition, the primary isolates were genetically very homogeneous, differing only by two nucleotides without evidence for adaptive mutations. In addition, the Spike protein, a major virulence factor, has a furin site, not found in any other known sarbecovirus. Unlike the SARS and MERS epidemics, no intermediate host has been detected so far. Finally, no other outbreaks were reported at the beginning of the pandemic outside of Wuhan, contrary to what happened with the emergence of SARS (2002) and H7N9 avian influenza (2013). Today, there are two scenarios to explain the emergence of SARS-CoV-2. Proponents of the natural origin argue that the bat virus might have directly infected humans, spreading silently at a low level in humans for years, without eliminating the existence

---

This article is an update to the Quarterly Medical Review (QMR) devoted to the history of modern pandemics.

To access this QMR contents, please go here: https://www.sciencedirect.com/journal/la-presse-medicale/vol/ 51/issue/3

of undetected intermediate hosts. This does not explain the origin in Wuhan, far away from the natural virus reservoirs. The furin site would have arisen spontaneously from other coronaviruses. The alternative scenario is that of a laboratory accident after gain-of-function manipulations from a SARS-like virus, or even the occurrence of a human contamination by a natural CoV virus grown on cells in Wuhan.

INTRODUCTION

The virulence of a virus depends on several factors, including the mode of transmission, tissue tropism, escape from the immune system and survival in the environment. Wild viruses highly adapted to the species in which they circulate recognize specific receptors to enter and multiply in cells. Encountering a new animal species, a virus cannot bind with high affinity to heterologous receptors to invade the cells: this is the main species barrier. Crossing this barrier depends in part on the genetic distance between animal species, the plasticity of viral genomes and the frequency of exposure to the virus. Most often, the first contacts with new viruses fail (epidemiological dead ends), resulting in few sporadic clinical or asymptomatic cases,[1-3] as for avian influenza H5N1 in humans. Initial contacts may leave traces in the viral genomes as adaptive mutations, reflecting attempts to cross the species barrier.[3] Serological markers can also be found in contacts. For example, about 80% of living animals sold in 2002 in thc Guangzhou markets had antibodies to the virus SARS-CoV-1.[4] For viruses as *Myxoviruses influenzae*, SARS-CoV-1 and MERS-CoV, the emergence appears as a sequential process requiring progressive adaptation through intermediate hosts in which mutations occur as well as reassortments in case of coinfections **(Fig. 1)**. Thus, intermediate hosts play a crucial role for crossing the species barrier of these viruses, as for other bat viruses as Hendra virus **(Fig. 2)**.[5]

Advances in molecular biology have provided complete genomes for most pathogens that can be genetically manipulated to identify virulence genes. The virulence of infectious agents can be reduced or enhanced by creating mutations, deletions or insertions in certain genes. These genetic approaches might allow to link the phenotype to the genotype of pathogenic viruses. There are researchers who claim that understanding viral virulence is of utmost interest to design vaccines and antiviral drugs. However, the gain-of-function (GoF) manipulations creating hypervirulent viruses are problematic. This is true not only when dealing with emerging potentially pandemic pathogens (PPP), such as influenza viruses or coronaviruses, but also with low pathogenic viruses. The US National Science Advisory Board for Biosecurity (NSABB) has recently recommended going beyond PPPs, to low pathogenic infectious agents.[6] Indeed, the creation of hypervirulent pathogens poses problems of dual research and biosafety, including risks of escape by laboratory accidents. This is why the GoF are designated dual use research of concern (DURC), emphasizing the potential

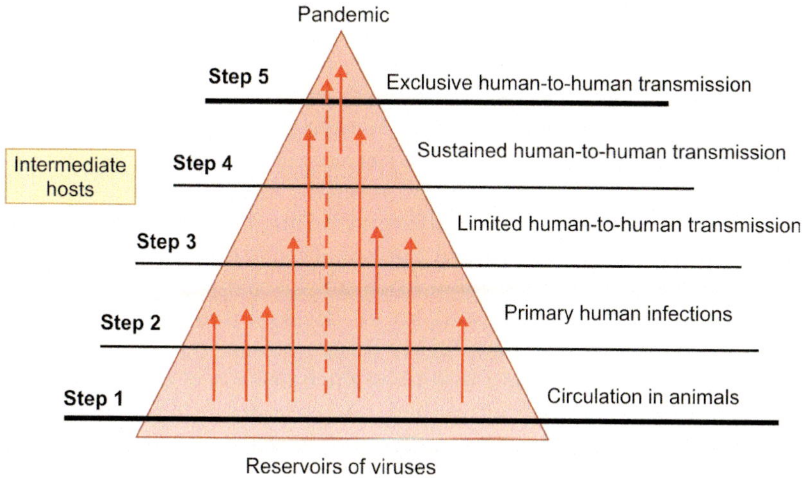

FIGURE 1: Crossing the species barrier.[2]

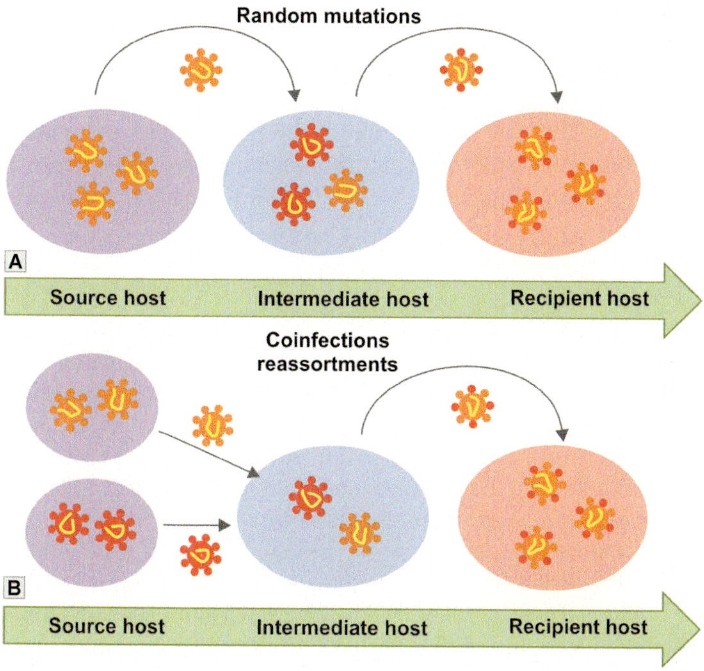

FIGURES 2A AND B: Gain-of-function (GoF) of a virus in nature. (A) Adaptive mutations through an intermediate host; (B) Coinfections of the intermediate host and reassortments.

danger of such experiments.[7] The GoF research must be questioned according to the benefit-risk ratio and must be strictly controlled at several levels, notably before financial funding and before publication of data.

GAIN-OF-FUNCTION EXPERIMENTS

There are several approaches to exacerbate the viral virulence: (1) random mutations by iterative passages on animals or cell cultures; (2) mutations obtained by directed mutagenesis or reverse genetics (cDNA from RNA viruses is transfected into virus-producing cell cultures to generate mutants by genetic reassortment); (3) random insertion of genetic material in the viral genomes (including DNA shuffling by mixing DNA of different alleles of the same gene). Thus, the cellular tropism of a viral mutant can be altered. It may happen that an experiment leads unexpectedly to a GoF. In 2001, Australian researchers who wanted to develop immunocontraceptive viral vaccines, produced a new, highly virulent mouse poxvirus, the agent of ectromelia (mouse variola). By adding the murine *IL-4* gene to the viral genome, the recombinant virus resulted in 100% mortality in all mouse lines, even after vaccination. The novel hypervirulent virus resulted in complete suppression of NK and T responses.[8] Knowing that the Variola virus is closely related to this virus, one may fear that these data become a recipe for a dreadful biological weapon. Was it necessary to publish his results?

Facing the recent repeated pandemic threats, researchers tried to understand the molecular mechanisms of viral pathogenicity of avian flu (H5N1, H7N9, H7N1), SARS (2002) and MERS (2012), studying virulence factors as the hemagglutinin HA of myxoviruses and the Spike(S) protein of coronaviruses. The aim was to monitor the pool of viruses circulating in wild animal reservoirs and to predict the emergence of new viruses better adapted to humans. This includes GoF experiments on influenza and coronaviruses.

Influenza Viruses

The influenza virus (*M. influenzae*) consists of single-stranded RNA (12–15 kb), encoding 8 genes, including two main virulence genes encoding HA and neuraminidase NA, expressed on the surface of the virus envelope. The genes are carried on separate segments of virus, which facilitates reassortment during coinfections of avian viruses in the pig as intermediate host. Several influenza pandemics over the past century (1918, 1957, 1968, 2009) were the result of such reassortments, involving HA and NA. This is the reason why one fears today the emergence of a new influenza pandemic during avian influenza epizootics. This includes the H5N1 virus reported in Hong Kong in 1996–1997 with a few human cases.[9] This virus is highly contagious and lethal in birds. Sporadically, it can infect humans with a mortality of 60%, but it is not contagious. However, a pandemic alert was triggered in 2005 in Hong Kong, following clustered human cases suggesting human-to-human transmission.[10] Between 2005 and 2011, 562 human cases have been reported, including 329 deaths (60% mortality). It is known that the H5N1 virus recognizes avian sialic acids (SA) (SA-a 2.3

galactose), but not human SA (SA a 2.6 galactose) present on the human upper respiratory tract. In contrast, avian receptors are present in human bronchioles, explaining human cases after deep inhalation of avian virus from close contact with poultry. This explains the high mortality and low viral contagiousness to humans. The question was then to identify in H5N1 virus what mutations of HA are required for human SA recognition. In 2012–2013, three teams in Rotterdam (Netherlands), Madison (USA) and Harbin (China) tried to identify crucial mutations of HA gene, conferring human contagiousness.

Yoshihiro Kawaoka's US team first replaced the HA gene of a human H1N1 virus from the 2009 flu pandemic, with the *H5* gene from an avian H5N1 virus.[11] This new virus is not contagious in ferrets, unlike the H1N1 virus. The researchers created random mutations in the *H5* gene by reverse genetics and sieved mutants that bind to avian erythrocytes expressing (after treatment) predominantly human SA. They selected 370 mutants in the 120–259 HA region, 9 of which are located in the H5 receptor binding domain (RBD). Four of these mutants inoculated into ferrets via the nasal route were contagious by saliva and aerosols and weakly pathogenic to the ferret. The species barrier between birds and mammals was crossed with only four HA mutations (N186K, S227N, Q226L, G228S).[11] Ron Fouchier's Dutch team introduced facilitating mutations into a H5N1 virus, two in SA recognition site of HA and one in *PB2* gene coding the RNA polymerase active at >40°C, allowing the H5N1 to replicate at 37°C in mammals. This adapted mutant was then inoculated into ferrets by nasal route. After 10 successive passages, the resulting mutant viruses induced a fatal disease and became contagious by airborne route between ferrets. The researchers were able to identify 5 critical mutations in H5 (N182K, Q222L, G224S, F627K, N154K), required for mammals adaptation.[12,13] A Chinese team from the Harbin Veterinary Institute also used a similarly adapted H5N1 mutant to infect cells that were transfected with cDNA of the 8 genes of a 2009 H1N1 virus. This resulted in 126 hybrid viruses, 35 of which were found to be highly pathogenic to mice and guinea pigs. These mutants are able to bind to human SA receptors and carry mutations in many viral genes (HA, NA, PB1, PB2, M, NS). They identified HA mutations favoring interactions with the human receptor (G224K, Q226L, G228S).[14] Thus, these dangerous experiments show that specific mutations in HA gene from H5N1 virus allow attachment to human SA receptors. Interestingly, these experiments indicate that pathogenicity is a complex multigene phenomenon, not limited to HA.

In October 2022, a major H5N1 epizootic occurred in mink farms in Spain, affecting nearly 52,000 animals, with an increasing mortality switching from 0.7% initially to 4.3% after 3 weeks. Genome analysis of contagious mink-adapted H5N1 viruses has detected mutations in PB2 (T171A) polymerase, which would facilitate replication at 37°C and the genesis of

HA mutations.[15] The HA experimental mutations previously described by experimental GoF were not found. These GoF experiments with potentially pandemic viruses led to a moratorium in the USA in October 2014 on financial funding for this type of research, not on banning it. This moratorium was finally lifted in December 2017.

Coronaviruses

Seven pathogenic coronaviruses are known in humans. Four viruses (designated 229E, NL63, OC43, HKU1) cause mild respiratory infections (rhinitis...), widespread in the infant population. Three are responsible for more severe respiratory infections, as severe acute respiratory syndrome (SARS) in 2002–2003 (8346 cases, 646 deaths, lethality 7.8%), Middle East Respiratory Syndrome (MERS) in 2012 (714 cases, 618 deaths 2012–2015, lethality 35%) in the Middle East with an epidemic in South Korea in 2015 (154 cases, 19 deaths). The MERS pneumonia is not very contagious, but sporadically persists today (> 2000 cases since 2012). Finally, the pandemic COVID-19 emerged in December 2019 in Wuhan, evolving in iterative waves.[16] In January 2023, COVID-19 has taken more than 17 million deaths in the world according to WHO estimates, and more than 660 million infected cases. Overall lethality would be around 0.6% in Western countries, although it may reach 1–2% in poor countries.

Coronaviruses are enveloped viruses bristled with spicules of S protein, hence its name, Spike. Their viral genomes are single-stranded RNA of 26–32 kb. The genome of SARS-CoV-1 responsible for SARS includes 11 genes encoding the proteins S, E (envelope), M (membrane) and N (nucleocapsid) and an additional gene 1a-1b encoding an RNA polymerase consisting of 16 proteins. After proteolysis, the viral genome encodes 33 functional proteins, all of which play an essential role in the penetration and intracellular replication of virus. SARS-CoV-1 and SARS-CoV-2 recognize human ACE-2 receptors (angiotensin-converting enzyme 2). MERS-CoV recognizes the human receptor DPP-4 (human dipeptidyl-peptidase 4).

In Wuhan, the emergence of SARS in 2002 has stimulated intense research on coronaviruses, including the constitution of a sample collection in Wuhan from bats captured in caves of South China and Southeast Asia, from 2004. A stock of nearly 15,000 samples (blood, saliva, urine, etc.) has been built up, allowing identification by RT-PCR and sequencing of about 220 SARS-like coronaviruses. About 100 sequences have been published.

It is well established that bats constitute the wild reservoir of the three pathogenic human coronaviruses. The SARS-CoV-1 virus reservoir was identified in 2005 in bats (*Rhinolophus* species) by Wuhan Institute of Virology (WIV) teams.[17] In a cave in Yunnan province in 2017, these researchers discovered 8 unknown bat viruses closely related to SARS-CoV-1, including two with a functional protein S and 6 with deletions of RBD of protein S. The S protein of virus Rs4874 was identical (99.9%) to that of SARS-CoV-1.[18] Intermediate hosts carrying viruses very similar to SARS-CoV-1 were also identified in the webbed civets, raccoon dogs and badgers. Similarly, the intermediate host of MERS-CoV has been shown to be the dromedary contaminated by bats.

In 2008, a GoF experiment was performed by Ralph Baric's US team at Chapel Hill (North Carolina) on a wild strain of SARS-like coronavirus (Bat-ScoV) that poorly penetrates human cells expressing ACE-2. From the published nucleotide sequence, a cDNA was synthesized and transfected into cultured cells, thereby producing a replicative virus. By replacing the Spike-RBD with that of SARS-CoV-1, the virus very easily invades cell cultures and becomes pathogenic in mice. This demonstrates the importance of the RBD of Spike.[19]

In 2013, Chinese researchers discovered several coronaviruses (RsSHC014, Rs3367, SL-CoV-WIV1) in bat samples from the province of Yunnan, whose S sequences are very similar to that of SARS-CoV-1. These viruses can bind to human, civet and *Rhinolophus* ACE-2 receptors expressed by HeLa cells where they can multiply.[20] Phylogenetic studies showed significant differences in 14 aminoacid residues, which favored Spike binding to these receptors, including 5 critical substitutions for the host spectrum (Y442, L472, N479, D487, Y411).

During the period of the US embargo (2014–2017), US and Chinese teams of Ralph Baric and Zhengli Shi, cooperatively performed GoF experiments in 2015 using the "skeleton" coronavirus M15. This is an avirulent SARS-CoV-1 virus, adapted to humanized transgenic mice expressing the human ACE-2 receptor. This M15 virus is unable to penetrate human cells. The addition to M15 of gene S from a wild-type SARS-like coronavirus (SHCO14-CoV) found in *R. affinis* generated a new virus capable to recognize multiple orthologs of human ACE-2 **(Fig. 3)**. This recombinant virus was serially transmitted in vitro to primary human respiratory epithelial cells, where it reached high titers. Passage in humanized mice showed extensive replication in lungs. This mutant was no longer neutralized by anti-SARS-CoV-1 antibodies neither protected by SARS vaccines.[21]

In 2014 during the moratorium, a US team from the University of Iowa implemented GoF experiments on MERS-CoV, which bears two furin sites in protein S.[22] The wild-type virus was propagated in transgenic mice expressing the human DPP-4 receptor for this virus. Nasal infection of these mice does not result in disease, but after 30 passages the virus causes a lethal infection with a 100-fold increase of growth in lungs, as compared to the parental virus. Genetic analysis of these strains detects 13 to 22 mutations, several affecting the MERS protein S.[23] These mutations make the virus sensitive to cellular proteases. Very recently, in October 2022, a team from the *Boston School of Medicine* constructed from the original Wuhan-Hu-2 virus, a recombinant virus carrying the S protein of an omicron BA.1 variant, known to be more contagious and less virulent than the original virus. This variant carrying

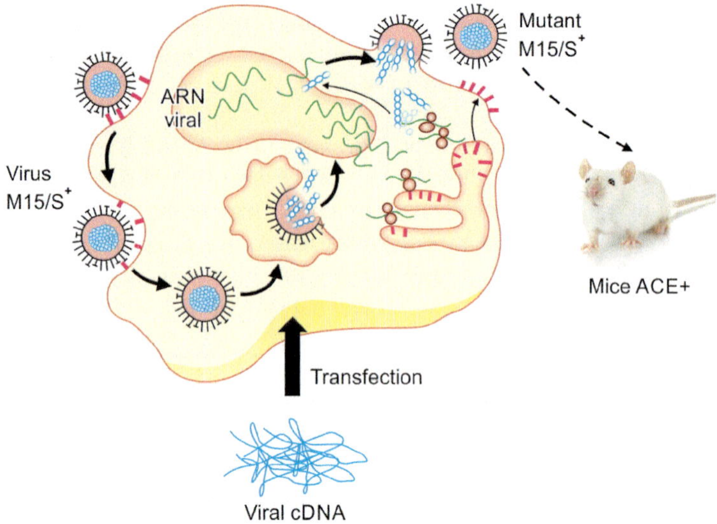

FIGURE 3: Example of GoF experiment: Creation of chimeric coronavirus—cells infected by M15 virus (avirulent mutant SARS-CoV-1) were transfected with cDNA from a wild-type bat coronavirus isolate (SHC014-CoV). Chimeric mutants are produced in culture and used to infect transgenic mice expressing human ACE-2. After serial passages, mutants become highly pathogenic.[21]

numerous mutations in the Spike-RBD escaped humoral vaccine-induced immunity. While the omega virus causes a mild nonlethal infection in humanized K18-hACE mice, the chimeric virus carrying the S gene from omicron virus induces an 80% fatal infection.[24]

EMERGENCE OF SARS-CoV-2

According to Chinese authorities, the first case of severe pneumonia occurred on December 8, 2019, in Wuhan (population 11 million) in Hubei Province.[25] The new virus was quickly identified.[26,27] It is immediately recorded that 33% of initial cases defined by pulmonary symptomatology were associated with a downtown fish market (Huanan Seafood Market).[28] As of February 5, nearly 50% of the first 99 reported cases were reported to have attended this market,[29] where many living animals were sold, kept in unsanitary conditions and possibly shedding viruses.[30] This market was closed on January 1, 2020.

Events then followed one another very quickly. Containment of the city was declared on 23 January 2020, a few days after the Lunar New Year celebrations on 20 January, but nearly 5 million people have left Wuhan to join their families throughout the country, thus dispersing the virus. The first hypothesis was that infection came from live animals sold in the market, a scenario similar to that of SARS in November 2002 in Foshan, near Guangzhou, in the Guangdong province. Chinese authorities have said that they have not detected virus in living animals at the Huanan Seafood Market, nor in the many factory farms that breed minks, foxes and raccoon dogs. Only some environmental samples from the Huanan market were found to contain the virus found by RT-PCR.[25] Therein begins the enigma of the COVID-19 origin and the questions that arise. A recent US Senate report in October 2022 revived the claim that SARS-CoV-2 escaped from a high-security laboratory in Wuhan.[31]

Epidemiology of COVID-19

The occurrence of natural zoonotic infections is determined by the degree of exposure to viruses carried by an intermediate host. The overpopulation of live animals sold in markets, often in poor sanitary conditions, implies close promiscuity favorable to viral spread between animals and humans, as well as during the transit across the country to markets. Therefore, one might expect that many limited human clusters would occur during the emergence throughout various places during transportation. The Chinese epidemiological surveillance network did not report any pneumonia outbreaks outside Wuhan in the last quarter of 2019.[25] For the SARS emergence in 2002, there were at least five human clusters followed by epidemic dissemination of virus. Multiple geographically distant locations were observed in the markets of Foshan, Guangzhou, and Hong Kong, where the virus first emerged **(Fig. 4A)**.[32,33] Intermediate hosts, such as the webbed civet and raccoon dog, were identified in the early months of SARS epidemic. The other example is the H7N9 avian influenza virus that occurred in humans in 2013 in China. This limited human epidemic began with multiple independent viral introductions into humans in multiple locations, although the total number of human cases was less than 500 **(Fig. 4B)**.[34] Furthermore, the intermediate host of SARS-CoV-2 could not be identified, despite more than 80,000 specimens from a wide range of animal species in China **(Fig. 5)**. The only example of animal-to-human transmission of SARS-CoV-2 was reported in factory farms in Denmark where the virus has been transmitted from minks to animal house staff.[35]

Very recently, a Chinese team published the results of the virological survey performed at the Huanan Fish Market after its closure on January 1, 2020. Out of 457 samples collected from 18 animal species (118 individuals) and identified by RT-PCR and direct sequencing, SARS-CoV-2 RNA was not found in any of these samples. In contrast, of 718 environmental samples, 40 were positive by RT-PCR between January 1 and March 2, 2020.[36] The metagenomic DNA sequences of environmental samples were posted on the Gisaid database. A French researcher has identified mitochondrial DNA from various animals in virus-positive samples, including raccoon

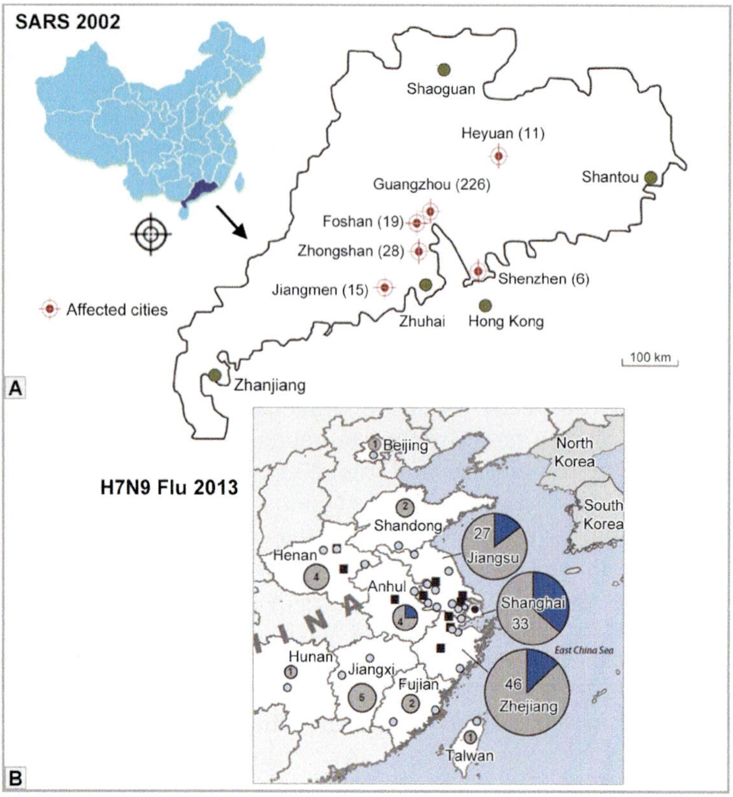

FIGURES 4A AND B: Epidemic outbreaks at the start of SARS and H7N9 influenza epidemic. (A). Outbreaks of SARS in Guangdong province,[32] according to (B) H7N9 avian influenza outbreaks in the Shanghai area.[34]

dog and civet, animals not present in the market according to Chinese authorities. These species are known to be capable of spreading SARS-CoV-like coronaviruses.[37] These results might be in favor of an undeclared intermediate host, but do not establish a causal link, due to natural DNA persistence in the environment.

The Singularities of SARS-CoV-2

SARS-CoV-2 was identified in early January 2020. It is an enveloped single-stranded RNA virus of 29,600 nucleotides. Classified as a β-coronavirus, it belongs to the *sarbecovirus* subgenus (*SARS-like* β-*coronavirus*). Analysis of SARS-CoV-2 genome shows three important features: (1) a very low diversity among initial isolates; (2) a strong affinity of these isolates for the human ACE-2 receptor; (3) the presence of a furin site absent in other known sarbecoviruses.[38,39] The first identified viruses differed by only two nucleotides: Wuhan-Hu-1 (clade B) and Wuhan/ME-WHO/2019 (clade A),

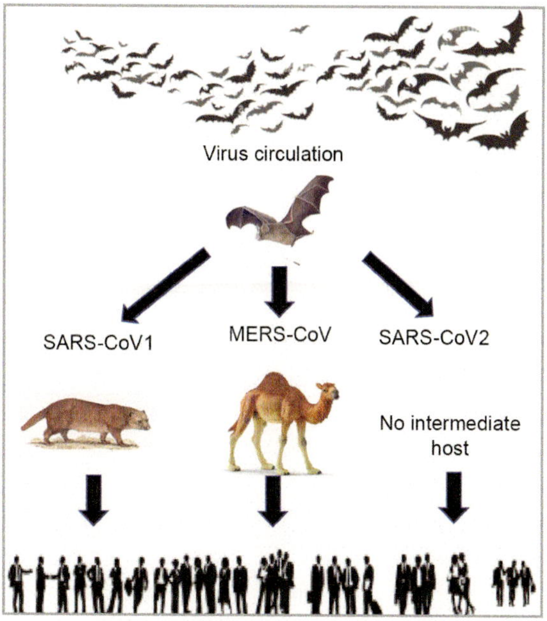

FIGURE 5: Circulation of coronaviruses in *Rhinolophus* species bats, and crossing of the species barrier by intermediate hosts for SARS-CoV-1 (civet), for MERS-CoV (dromedary). So far, no intermediate hosts have been discovered for SARS-CoV-2.

suggesting a very recent origin. This is in contrast with the very rapid diversification of virus by mutations subsequently observed, ultimately resulting in iterative waves of a, b, g, o mutants during the next three years **(Fig. 6)**. This recent origin is also predicted by epidemiological modeling between mid-October and mid-November 2019. Surprisingly, the emerging viruses were at once highly adapted to human-to-human transmission, i.e., they recognized human ACE-2 with a high affinity. It is known that wild bat viruses similar to SARS-CoV-1 are often unable to infect human cells because these viruses are adapted to the bat ACE-2.[40] Moreover, adaptive mutations reflecting prior virus circulation in the hosts are not detected in the SARS-CoV-2 genome, in contrast to observations made on SARS-CoV-1 in 2002.

The discovery of a furin site in SARS-CoV-2 has been much discussed. Furin is a ubiquitous intracellular protease localized to the Golgi apparatus and the nucleoplasm, cleaving the S protein and other proteins from various other viruses. The furin site consists of four amino acids (pro-arg-arg-ala/PRRA), corresponding to an insert of 12 nucleotides (T-CCT-CGG-CGG-GC[A]). It is located at the junction of the two subunits S1 and S2 of S protein **(Fig. 7)**. The cleavage promotes the penetration of virus into cells. Furin sites are present in some β-coronaviruses (other than sarbecoviruses), notably

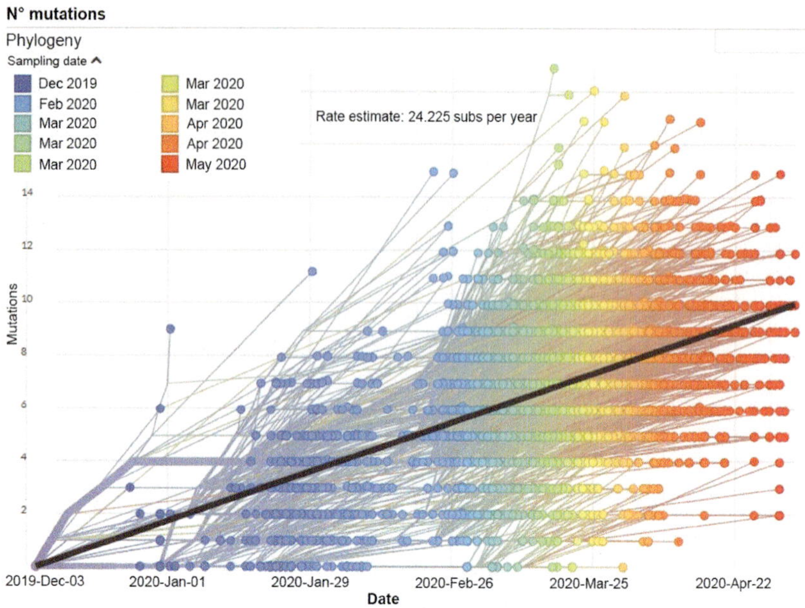

FIGURE 6: Evolution of SARS-CoV-2 mutations from December 2019 to April 2020. It is shown the initial homogeneity of virus that rapidly diversifies with multiple mutations.

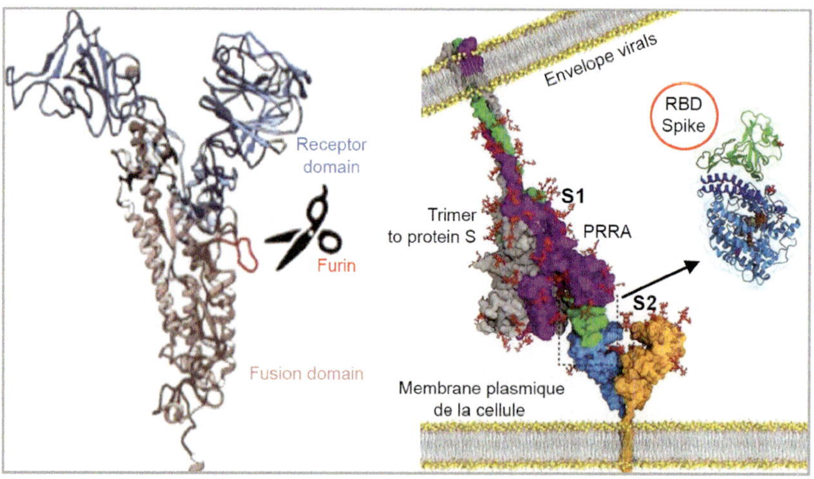

FIGURE 7: Schematic of action of furin—it is a cellular protease that cleaves the S protein between subunits 1 and 2, recognizing a specific PRRA site. This facilitates the virus entry in cells after interaction with ACE2.

in MERS-CoV which presents two furin sites,[23] and also in avian influenza viruses and Ebola virus. No furin sites can be found in the other known sarbecovirus sequences.

Coronavirus Research in Wuhan

Since the deadly SARS epidemic of 2002–2003 and the pandemic threat of H5N1 avian flu in 2005, Chinese authorities have focused on viruses potentially dangerous viruses. For example, in late 2018–2019, a deadly African swine fever epizootic due to a DNA Asfivirus spread throughout China and Southeast Asia, resulting in an economic disaster. The aim of the research was to prevent the emergence of unknown pathogens, to develop vaccines and medical countermeasures. Wuhan has thus become a center of excellence for virus research. Teams from the WIV and Wuhan Chinese CDC were sent to collect samples on the field in South China and Southeast Asia, where bats abound, more than 1600 km from Wuhan **(Fig. 8)**. It is accepted that the SARS-CoV-2 originates from *Rhinolophus* spp, living in South China and Southeast Asia, but absent in Wuhan. Among

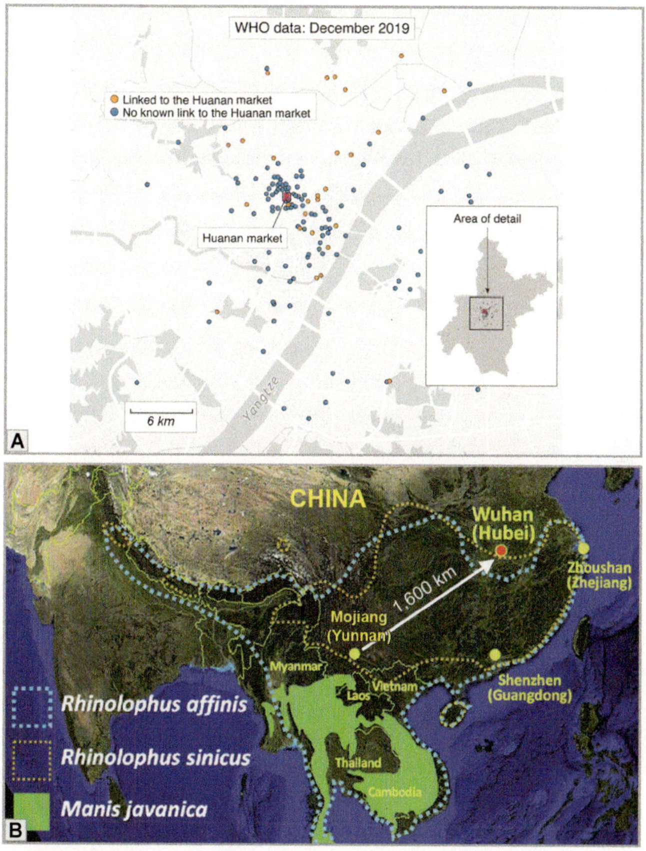

FIGURES 8A AND B: Origin of SARS-CoV-2. (A) The first cases that appeared at Huanan Seafood Market in Wuhan (December 2016)[30] (B) Geographical areas of *Rhinolophus* species bats, reservoirs of coronavirus, 1,600 km from Wuhan.

the coronavirus isolates most closely related to SARS-CoV-2 is RaTG13 (96.1% nucleotide similarity) collected in 2013. The previous year in April 2012, an outbreak occurred in an abandoned copper mine of Tongguan near Mojiang (Yunnan), where miners were cleaning from bat guano. Six workers between 30 and 63 years of age developed severe acute pneumonia and were hospitalized in the provincial capital of Kunming. Three died.[41,42] The Chinese authorities indicated that the patients' samples sent to Wuhan did not reveal the presence of coronavirus. They specified that pneumonia was caused by a fungus.[25] The sequence of RaTG13 was finally published in February 2020.[43] A French team directed by Marc Eloit has collected in Laos several β-coronaviruses very close to SARS-CoV-2 from bats, including BANAL-52 (96.8% nucleotide similarity), BANAL-103 and BANAL-236.[44] Phylogenetic studies show that all these wild-type viruses have diverged for decades **(Fig. 9)**.

In Wuhan, there are eight institutions working on coronaviruses in 2019 with microbiological safety laboratories (BSL2–3–4). This includes the Wuhan Institute of Virology (WIV) located in two places, one at the historic Xiaohongshan site in the heart of the city, and another at the Zhengdian site about 20 km away in the southern suburbs for the BSL-4 laboratory recently opened in 2018. The virus collection is stored next to the BSL-4 laboratory. Security infrastructure in most other institutions, including BSL-3

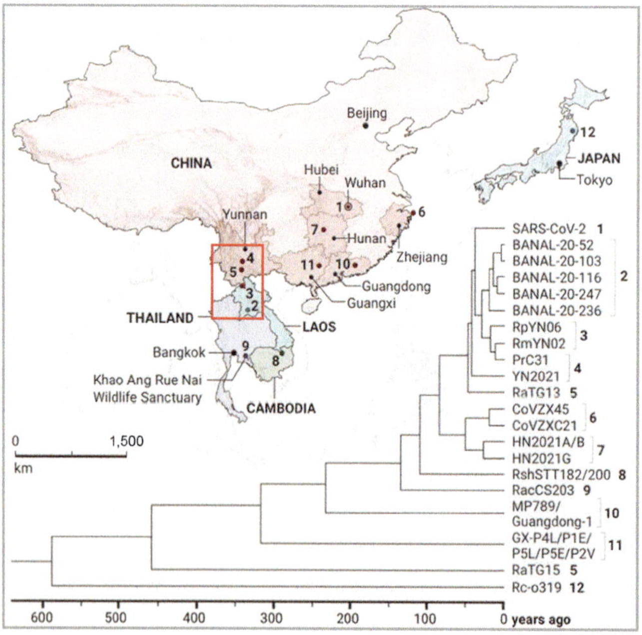

FIGURE 9: Phylogenetic studies showing the areas where the most closely related virus to SARS-CoV-2 were isolated[44]

and animal facilities, were recently established in the last 5 years. These include Wuhan Chinese CDC, Hubei Chinese CDC, Hubei Animal CDC, Wuhan Institute of Biological Products harboring the vaccine production branch of Sinopharm, Wuhan University, Huazhong Agricultural University and Wuhan Entry Exit Inspection. Thus, coronaviruses are handled at 9 different sites, including numerous BSL2 laboratories, six BSL3 laboratories, three ABSL-3 animal facilities, and one BSL4 laboratory (WIV). The Wuhan Chinese CDC is located close to the Huanan Seafood Market.

The WIV has conducted genetic manipulations and chimera construction experiments in BSL-2–3 laboratories. The researchers used humanized transgenic mice expressing human ACE-2 receptors. This allows them to create and selected adaptive mutations by iterative passages in mice and to evaluate the efficacy of vaccines. They also test the virulence of coronaviruses on civets which have an ACE-2 close to the human receptor.[45] The most dangerous experiments are those done in animal houses that produce highly infectious aerosols difficult to detect. A Chinese biosafety expert recommended in May 2019 that all experiments in animals should now be done in BSL3 or BSL 4, no more in BSL2.[46] It must be added that field collection conditions were often not safe in terms of protective equipment and bat handling.

In March 2018, a joint funding application was submitted to DARPA (*Defense Advanced Research Projects Agency*), a US research funding agency. It involved teams from WIV and the US nongovernmental organization *EcoHealth Alliance*. It is proposed to search bat coronavirus samples collected in Yunnan by the WIV team, which are genetically close SARS-CoV-1 and possibly bearing furin cleavage sites. The project stipulates that, in case of failure to find such viruses, researchers intend to manipulate SARS-like coronaviruses to increase binding affinity to human lung tissue and possibly to insert furin sites at the same location as those found in SARS-CoV-2.[47] This project was rejected by DARPA. Addition of furin site has been made in the past in various viruses. For example, researchers at Huazhong Agricultural University in Wuhan in 2015 inserted a furin site into an α-coronavirus responsible for Porcine Epidemic Diarrhea, facilitating entry and replication in cell culture.[48] Similarly in 2019, researchers in Beijing modified a furin site in the coronavirus of the Infectious Poultry Bronchitis, with increased virulence and neurotropism of virus.[49]

THE TWO SCENARIOS FOR THE ORIGIN OF COVID-19

The first scenario is that of a natural origin of SARS-CoV-2.[50-52] The virus would have directly contaminated humans from bats, with a silent, low-level infections not detected by China's epidemiological surveillance system. The alternative is that there was an intermediate host that has not yet been detected. During the adaptation phase, the virus would have naturally acquired the furin site by accumulation of mutations, implying that random has allowed the juxtaposition of 4 amino-acids at the right place at the S1/S2 junction. It is also possible to hypothesize recombination with other coronaviruses carrying furin sites. Scientists holding up this scenario support the idea that a predecessor of SARS-CoV-2 might have circulated silently in human populations for years until acquiring the cleavage site, then triggering the COVID-19 pandemic.

The alternative scenario is that of a laboratory accident after gain-of-function manipulation of SARS-CoV-2. First, there is the absence of identified intermediate hosts after three years of pandemics. Second, why Wuhan? This megapolis where the first cases of COVID-19 were detected is remote from the areas of bat reservoirs. In the early phase of the pandemic, the absence of secondary outbreaks that would have accompanied the trade of living animals is surprising. During the emergence of other recent viral respiratory diseases transmitted by animals on markets, as SARS and H7N9 avian influenza, multiple scattered clusters were observed.[32-34] In Wuhan and elsewhere, researchers have practiced GoF on sarbecoviruses. According to publications, chimeric viruses were created in 2015, followed by 8 more viruses in 2017, two of which were pathogenic to humanized mice. All indications are that the origin of SARS-CoV-2 in December 2019 was very recent, a hypothesis corroborated by epidemiological models. We also observe very low genetic diversity of initial isolates, contrasting with the high diversity that viruses can deploy in a few weeks. Moreover, the SARS-CoV-2 was immediately highly contagious, witnessing a remarkable adaptation of this bat virus to humans. The presence of a furin site in SARS-CoV-2, which is not found in any other known sarbecovirus, is also a singular feature that remains to be explained. Moreover, the hypothesis of a researcher be infected by a nonengineered natural CoV grown on cells in Wuhan cannot be eliminated.

Accidents may occur even in high security microbiology laboratories (BSL3–4). For example for the 2002 SARS-CoV-1, four lab leaks (1 in Singapore, 1 in Taïwan and 2 in Beijing) were reported after manipulations in such laboratories.[53-56] Similarly, the reemergence in 1977 of a H1N1 epidemic virus ("Russian flu"), which was eradicated during the 1957 asiatic pandemic, was a laboratory accident, most probably linked to a vaccine trial in the Soviet Union or China.[57-59] This results in a flu pandemic (1977–1979), then the H1N1 virus persists until the porcine pandemic in 2009. One must also remember the three accidents linked to the handling of smallpox virus in high-security laboratories that occurred in 1972 in London and in 1966 and 1978 in Birmingham, resulting in 80 smallpox cases and three deaths.[60] For respiratory viruses, as coronaviruses, influenza viruses or smallpox, the most dangerous manipulations are those that take place in animal houses and cellular cultures, producing infectious aerosols difficult to detect. We must also mention the risks during field collections, requiring protective equipment and handling of bats. Breaches in the security systems of the WIV have also been suspected, particularly in mid-November 2019.[36] The natural or accidental origin of SARS-CoV-2 remains an unsolved conundrum. But sooner or later, the truth will emerge.

CONCLUSION

The GoF experiments on viruses require strict controls, including an assessment of the benefit-risk and of a possible dual research, and the appropriateness of publishing. Biosafety and biosecurity conditions in laboratories and animal facilities must be at the forefront. Finally, it is important that the scientific community must adhere to this approach through educational actions.

Declaration of Competing Interest.

The author has no conflict of interest and no financial support.

REFERENCES

1. Pike BL, Saylors KE, Fair JN, et al. The origin and prevention of pandemics. Clin Infect Dis. 2010;50(12):1636-40.
2. Plowright RK, Parrish CR, McCallum H, et al. Pathways to zoonotic spillover. Nature Rev Microbiol. 2017;15:502-10.
3. Ye ZW, Yuan S, Yuen KS, et al. Zoonotic origins of human coronaviruses. Int J Bio Sci. 2021;16(10):1686-97.
4. Tu C, Crameri G, Kong X, et al. Antibodies to SARS coronavirus in civets. Emerg Infect Dis. 2004;10:2244-8.
5. Ellwanger JH, Chies JAB. Zoonotic spillover: Understanding basic aspects for better prevention. Genet Mol Biol. 2021;44(S1): e20200355.
6. National Science Advisory Board for Biosecurity, Proposed biosecurity oversight framework for the future of Science, January 2023. Available from: https://osp.od.nih.gov/wp-con- tent/uploads/2023/01/DRAFT-NSABB-WG-Report.pdf
7. Fink Report. Biotechnology research in an age of terrorism. Washington DC: National Research Council of National Academies; 2004.
8. Jackson RJ, Ramsay AJ, Christensen CD, Beaton S, Hall DF, Ramshaw IA. Expression of mouse interleukin-4 by a recombinant ectromelia virus suppresses cytolytic lymphocyte responses and overcomes genetic resistance to mousepox. J Virol. 2001;75(3):1205-2010.
9. Sims LD, Ellis TM, Liu KK, et al. Avian influenza in Hong Kong 1997-2002. Avian Dis. 2003;47(S3):832-8.
10. Ungchusak K, Auewarakul P, Dowell SF, et al. Probable person-to-person transmission of avian influenza A (H5N1). N Engl J Med. 2005;352(4):333-40.
11. Imai M, Watanabe T, Hatta M, et al. Experimental adaptation of an influenza H5 HA confers respiratory droplet transmission to a reassortant H5 HA/H1N1 virus in ferrets. Nature. 2012;486:420-8.
12. Herfst S, Schrauwen EJA, Linster M, et al. Airborne transmission of influenza A/H5N1 virus between ferrets. Science. 2012;336(6088):1534-41.
13. Russell CA, Fonville JM, Brown AEX, et al. The potential for respiratory droplet-transmissible A/H5N1 influenza virus to evolve in a mammalian host. Science. 2012;336(6088):1541-7.

14. Zhang Y, Zhang Q, Kong H, et al. H5N1 hybrid viruses bearing 2009/H1N1 virus genes transmit in guinea pigs by respiratory droplet. Science. 2013;340 (6139):1459-63.
15. Agüero M, Monne I, Sánche A, et al. Highly pathogenic avian influenza A(H5N1) virus infection in farmed minks, Spain, October 2022. Euro Surveill. 2023;28(3):2300001. pp. 1560-79.
16. Buisson Y. Covid-19, an unfinished story. Presse Med (QMR). 2022;51:104131.
17. Li W, Shi Z, Yu M, et al. Bats are natural reservoirs of SARS-like coronaviruses. Science. 2005;310:676-9.
18. Hu B, Zeng LP, Yang XL, et al. Discovery of a rich gene pool of bat SARS-related coronaviruses provides new insights into the origin of SARS coronavirus. PLoS Pathog. 2017;13(11):e1006698.
19. Becker MM, Graham RL, Donaldson EF, et al. Synthetic recombinant bat SARS-like coronavirus is infectious in cultured cells and in mice. Proc Natl Acad Sci USA. 2008;105(50):19944-9.
20. Ge XY, Li JL, Yang XL, et al. Isolation and characterization of a bat SARS-like coronavirus that uses the ACE2 receptor. Nature. 2013;503(7477):535-8.
21. Menachery VD, Yount BL, Debbink K, et al. A SARS-like cluster of circulating bat coronaviruses shows potential for human emergence. Nat Med. 2015;21(12):1508-13.
22. Millet JK, Whittaker GR. Host cell entry of Middle East respiratory syndrome coronavirus after two-step, furin-mediated activation of the spike protein. Proc Natl Acad Sci USA. 2014;111(42):15214-9.
23. Li K, Wohlford-Lenane CL, Channappanavar R, et al. Mouse-adapted MERS coronavirus causes lethal lung disease in human DPP4 knockin mice. Proc Natl Acad Sci USA. 2017;114(15):E3119-28.
24. Chen DY, Kenney D, Chin CV, et al. Role of spike in the pathogenic and anti-genic behavior of SARS-CoV-2 BA.1 Omicron, BioRxiv doi: https://doi.org/ 10.1101/2022.10.13.512134
25. Joint WHO-China Study (14 january-10 february 2021). WHO-convened global study of origins of SARS-CoV-2. Geneva: WHO; 20 March 2021.
26. Zhou P, Yang XL, Wang XG, et al. A pneumonia outbreak associated with a new coronavirus of probable bat origin. Nature. 2020;579(7798):270-3.
27. Huang C, Wang Y, Li X, et al. Clinical features of patients infected with 2019 novel coronavirus in Wuhan, China. Lancet. 2020;395:497-506.
28. Anonymous. The Epidemiological Characteristics of an Outbreak of 2019 Novel Coronavirus Diseases (COVID-19), China 2020. China CDC Weekly. 2020;2(8):113-22.
29. Chen N, Zhou M, Dong X, et al. Epidemiological and clinical characteristics of 99 cases of 2019 novel coronavirus pneumonia in Wuhan, China: a descriptive study. Lancet. 2020;395(10223):507-13.
30. Worobey M, Levy JI, Serrano LM, et al. The Huanan Seafood Wholesale Market in Wuhan was the early epicenter of the COVID-19 pandemic. Science. 2022;377(6609): 951-9.
31. Senate Committee on Health Education, Labor and pensions, An analysis of the origins of Covid-19 pandemic, October 2022. Available from: https://www.help.senate.gov/imo/ media/doc/report an analysis of the origins of covid-19 102722.
32. Zhong N, Zheng BJ, Li YM, et al. Epidemiology and cause of severe acute respiratory syndrome (SARS) in Guangdong, People's Republic of China, in February 2003. Lancet. 2003;362(9393):1353-8.
33. Wang LF, Eaton BT. Bats, civets and the emergence of SARS. Curr Top Microbiol Immunol. 2007;315:325-44.

34. Butler D. Mapping the H7N9 avian flu outbreaks. Nature 2013. doi: 10.1038/ nature.2013.
35. Pomorska-Mo'l M, Włodarek J, Gogulski M, Rybska M. SARS-CoV-2 infection in farmed minks - an overview of current knowledge on occurrence, disease and epidemiology. Animal. 2021;15(7):100272.
36. US Senate Report on the origin of Covid-19, Senator R. Marshall https://www. marshall. senate.gov/wp-content/uploads/MWG-EXECUTIVE-SUMMARY-4.17-Final- Version.pdf.
37. Liu WJ, et al. Surveillance of SARS-CoV-2 at the Huanan Seafood Market. Nature 3 April 2023. doi: 10.1038/s41586-023-06043-2.
38. NG Coutard B, Valle C, X de Lamballerie X, Canard B, Seidah NG, Decroly E. The spike glycoprotein of the new coronavirus 2019-nCoV contains a furin-like cleavage site absent in CoV of the same clade. Antiviral Res. 2020;176:104742.
39. Jaimes JA, Millet JK, Whittaker GR. Proteolytic cleavage of the SARS-CoV-2 spike protein and the role of the novel S1/S2 site. iScience. 2020;23(6):101212.
40. Yan H, Jiao H, Liu Q, et al. ACE2 receptor usage reveals variation in susceptibility to SARS-CoV and SARS-CoV-2 infection among bat species. Nat Ecol Evol. 2021;5: 600-8.
41. Rahalkar MC, Bahulikar RA. Lethal pneumonia cases in Mojiang miners (2012) and the mine shaft could provide important clues to the origin of SARS-CoV-2. Front Public Health. 2020;8. doi: 10.3389/fpubh.2020.581569.
42. Rahalkar MC, Bahulikar RA. Mojiang mine, RaTG13, miners' disease and related samples remain essential clues in the origin SARS-CoV-2. Curr Sci. 2022;122(3):247-50.
43. Zhu N, Zhang D, Wang W, et al. A novel coronavirus from patients with pneumonia in China, 2019. N Engl J Med. 2020;382:727-33.
44. Temmam S, Vongphayloth K, Baquero E, et al. Bat coronaviruses related to SARS- CoV-2 and infectious for human cells. Nature. 2022;604(7905):330-6.
45. Lytras S, Xia W, Hughes J, Jiang X, Robertson DL. The animal origin of SARS-CoV-2 trading of animals susceptible to bat coronaviruses is the likely cause of the COVID-19 pandemic. Science. 2021;373(6558):968-70.
46. Wu G. Laboratory biosafety in China: past, present, and future. Biosaf Heal. 2019;1:56-8.
47. EcoHealth Alliance Project DEFUSE Proposal, https://drasticresearch.files.word- press. com/2021/09/main-document-preempt-volume-1-no-ess-hr00118s0017- ecohealth-alliance.pdf.
48. Li W, Wicht O, van Kuppeveld FJM, He Q, Rottier PJM, Bosch BJ. A single point mutation creating a furin cleavage site in the spike protein renders porcine epidemic diarrhea coronavirus trypsin independent for cell entry and fusion. J Virol. 2015;89(15):80778081.
49. Cheng J, Zhao Y, Hu Y, Zhao J, Xue J, Zhang G. The Furin-S20 site in avian coronavirus plays a key role in central nervous system damage progression. J Virol. 2021;95(11): e02447-520.
50. Holmes EC, et al. The origins of SARS-CoV-2: a critical review. Cell. 2021;184(19): 4848-56.
51. Garry RF. The evidence remains clear: SARS-CoV-2 emerged via the wildlife trade. Proc Natl Acad Sci USA. 2022;119(47):e2214427119.
52. Pekar JE, Magee A, Parker E, et al. The molecular epidemiology of multiple zoonotic origins of SARS-CoV-2. Science. 2022;377(6609):960-6.
53. Senio K. Recent Singapore SARS case a laboratory accident. Lancet Infect Dis. 2003;3(11):679.
54. CIDRAP News. Taiwanese SARS researcher infected. University of Minnesota.; Dec. 17, 2003 https://www.cidrap.umn.edu/SARS/taiwanese-SARS-researcher-infected.

55. Walgate R. SARS escaped Beijing lab twice. Genome Biol. 2004;4 spotlight-20040427-03. doi: 10.1186/gb-spotlight-20040427-0.
56. Lim PL, Kurup A, Gopalakrishna G, et al. Laboratory-acquired severe acute respiratory syndrome. N Engl J Med. 2004;350:1740-5.
57. Rozo M, Gronvall GK. The reemergent 1977 H1N1 strain and the gain-of-function debate. MBio. 2015;6(4):e01013-5.
58. Scholtissek C, von Hoyningen V, Rott R. Genetic relatedness between the new 1977 epidemic strains (H1N1) of influenza and human influenza strains isolated between 1947 and 1957 (H1N1). Virology. 1978;89:613-7.
59. Nakajima K, Desselberger U, Palese P. Recent human influenza A (H1N1) viruses are closely related genetically to strains isolated in 1950. Nature. 1978;274:334-9.
60. Shooter RA, Booth CC, Evans D, McDonald JR, Tyrrell DAJ, Williams R. Report of the investigation into the cause of the 1978 Birmingham smallpox occurrence. London: Her Majesty Stationary Office; 1980.

CHAPTER 9

The Enigma of the 1889 Russian Flu Pandemic: A Coronavirus?

Patrick Berche

ABSTRACT

The "Russian flu", which raged from 1889 to 1894, is considered as the first pandemic of the industrial era for which statistics have been collected. This planetary event started in Turkestan and hit the Russian Empire, before reaching all European countries, the United States of America, and the whole world. Contemporaries were surprised by its high contagiousness as evidenced by attack rates averaging 60% in urban populations, its rapid spread in successive waves circling the globe in a few months by rail and sea, and the tendency of the disease to relapse. Despite its low case-fatality rate (0.10–0.28%), it is estimated to have caused one million deaths worldwide. On serological grounds, it is generally accepted that the causative agent of Russian influenza was *Myxovirus influenzae*, the virus identified for all influenza pandemics since the "Spanish flu" of 1918. In light of the CORONAVIRUS DISEASE 2019 (COVID-19) pandemic, which has underscored the extraordinary epidemic potential of coronaviruses, this assumption has recently been questioned. Coronaviruses come from wild reservoirs (bats, rodents, birds, ...). They induce respiratory symptoms mimicking influenza, possibly leading to respiratory distress with pneumonia. In addition to the COVID-19 pandemic, recent deadly and limited epidemics, such as severe acute respiratory syndrome (SARS) in 2002 and Middle East respiratory syndrome (MERS) in 2012, have occurred. Russian influenza presented as an influenza-like syndrome with clinical peculiarities (multivisceral and neurological involvement, skin rash, early iterative relapses), evoking some particularities of COVID-19. Four other coronaviruses circulating in the human population for decades (HCoV-229E, HCoV-NL63, HCoV-OC43, HCoV-HKU1) have been found to be responsible for 15–30% of seasonal colds. All of these viruses are of animal origin. Recently, phylogenetic studies have revealed the genetic proximity between a bovine coronavirus BCoV and the human virus HCoV-OC43, indicating that the latter emerged around 1890, at the time of the Russian flu, when an epizootic was raging among cattle throughout Europe. Could the current human virus be the attenuated remnant that appeared after the Russian flu in 1894? Was there a coronavirus pandemic before COVID-19?

INTRODUCTION

Since the Renaissance, the world has faced multiple influenza pandemics, punctuated by lulls lasting a few decades. "Influenza" has been defined by the sudden onset of respiratory signs with fever and high contagiousness in the population. In the 19th century, several pandemics originating in the East were reported, including 1831–1833, 1847–1848 and, finally, from 1889 to 1894, the so-called "Russian flu", which spread throughout Europe and then the world. This episode was well-documented in many countries in several official reports, medical sources, and numerous press articles that covered the pandemic on a daily basis.[1-9]

THE RUSSIAN INFLUENZA PANDEMIC

The first cases were reported in May 1889, in the city of Bukhara in Turkestan; curiously, a few cases were also reported in the city of Athabasca in Western Canada and in Greenland. In mid-October 1889, influenza reached the Russian Empire. It was reported in Tomks in western Siberia, Ufa (100 km from the Ural Mountains), Kazan on the Volga River in western Russia (700 km cast of Moscow), Jekatery- noslav on the Dnieper River in Ukraine, and Novgorod near St. Petersburg. Kiev was stricken, as was the entire region of Lake Baikal, and then Siberia up to the island of Sakhalin. The capital of the Empire was severely hit in November 1889, with 20,000 cases. The flu afflicted all levels of society, including Tsar Alexander III himself. By the beginning of December, one third of hospital beds were occupied by flu patients. Economic activity ground to a halt, factories were closed, as were barracks and schools; 25–50% of soldiers and children had fallen ill. The peak of the epidemic occurred on December 1, 1889 in St Petersburg. The first wave lasted five weeks with a total of 180,000 victims in a city of one million inhabitants.[1,3] From St. Petersburg, the Baltic ports were contaminated, notably Stockholm and the rest of Sweden, where the flu infected 60% of the population for eight weeks, and then Copenhagen and Oslo. The German Empire was affected in December, particularly in Poznan, Warsaw and Lodz. The epidemic resulted in 150,000 cases in Berlin for a population of 1.5 million.[5,6] Within a few weeks from December 1889, all of Europe was ablaze. It was mainly an urban pandemic initially striking the capitals: Paris, London, Vienna, Madrid, Rome, Geneva.[1,7,8] At the beginning of 1890, the first wave spread around the Mediterranean, from Constantinople, where half of the population caught the flu, to Egypt.[1,5,9] The spread of flu to major European cities during the first wave is illustrated in **Figure 1**.[1]

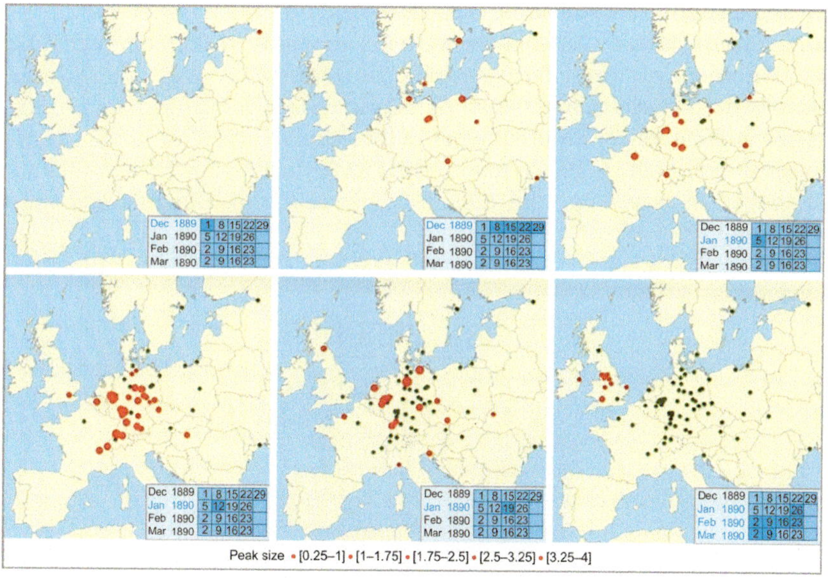

FIGURE 1: Kinetics of the spread of Russian influenza in Europe in 1889–1890 (with the calendar). Red dots: Cities hit by the pandemic (their size corresponds to the magnitude at the peak). Green dots: Extinguished outbreaks (from AJ Valleron).[17]

The pandemic hit Paris in November 1889, afflicting 670 of the 8,000 employees of the *Grands Magasins du louvre*. It was a mild influenza that subsided in about four days. However, it seems to have worsened during the last two weeks of December 1889. Cases of severe pneumonia were reported around December 25–28, with 200 deaths from pneumonia or lung congestion. Patients flocked to hospitals where barracks and emergency tents were set up in the gardens **(Fig. 2)**. Virtually all the doctors of Hôtel-Dieu contracted the disease. The peak occurred on December 28. There were 180,000 symptomatic cases among the 2.5 million inhabitants of Paris. Mortality in the capital was estimated at 62/1,000, a 30% increase compared to the previous winter.[4,9] The epidemic subsided in January 1890, only to return to Paris in late February, after which influenza spread throughout the country, initially affecting regional hubs such as Toulouse, Grenoble, Lyon, Toulon, Montpellier and Angers.[9]

What to do? Almost everywhere the unprepared authorities recommended hygienic measures such as ventilation, disinfection of public places and patients' rooms, prohibition of public gatherings, isolation at home... Needless to say, there was no effective treatment at the time. Quinine was used to treat fever, but without success, as well as treatments such as strychnine, phenol inhalation, carbonic smoke ball that were dangerous or fanciful (castor oil, electric current, brandy, oysters...). Commercial activity likewise collapsed, and schools, colleges, universities, public services, transportation and factories were shut down: a true disaster! Numerous eminent personalities—the President of the Republic, ministers, deputies—were stricken.

From mid-December 1889, the same scenario played out in the United Kingdom. In January 1890, there were 2,258 deaths in London, including 1,070 from pneumonia, far exceeding the seasonal average. The disease spread to other cities, including Edinburgh, Glasgow, Birmingham (50,000 cases) and Dublin.[10-13] Mortality per million due to influenza in the United Kingdom from 1847 to 1905 is reported in **Fig. 3**. The Russian flu was probably prolonged by waves up until 1899–1900, when the so-called flu epidemic occurred.[14,15]

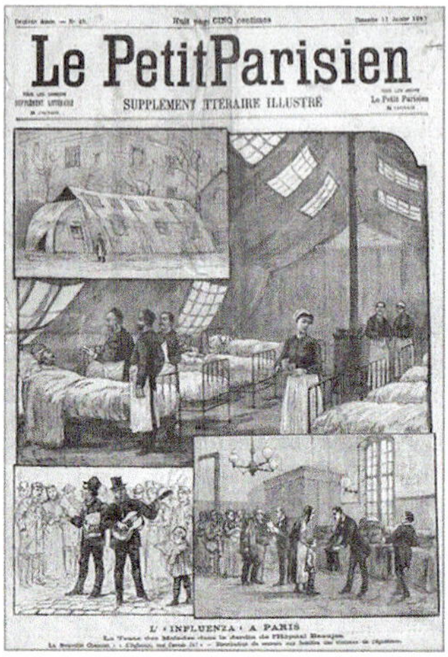

Le PetitParisien

SUPPLEMENT LITTÉRAIRE ILLUSTRÉ

L'INFLUENZA A PARIS

FIGURE 2: "Influenza in Paris". The tent of the sick in the garden of the Beaujon Hospital. Le Petit Parisien (January 12, 1890)—The National Library of Medicine.

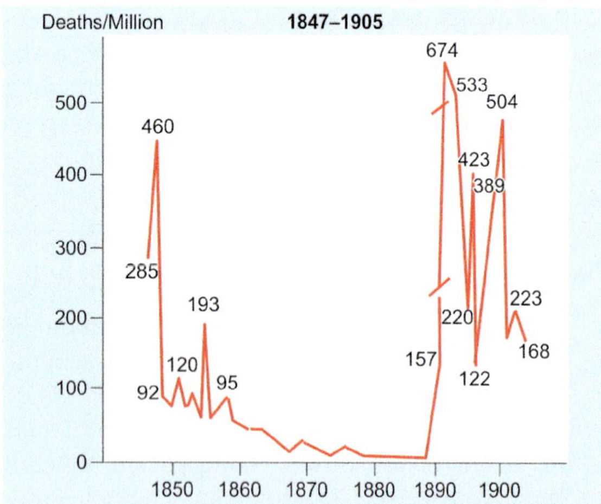

FIGURE 3: Mortality of influenza from 1847 to 1905 in the United-Kingdom. Mortality reached 674/million in 1890, followed by several peaks up until the epidemic of 1900.[14,15]

The epidemic soon crossed the Atlantic, and the first cases in the United States were reported on 18 December 1889. The wave lasted 5 weeks, reaching a peak on 12 January 1890. The epidemic spread along the East Coast before reaching Chicago, Kansas City and San Francisco. Soon afterwards, from Mexico City to Buenos Aires, Latin America was likewise contaminated. In spring 1890, the pandemic spread widely in Africa and Asia. If Africans called it "the white man's disease", it was because they had apparently never previously known influenza. The map of the Russian flu pandemic is shown in **Figure 4**.

The Russian flu pandemic evolved in sequential waves, at least four of them occurring between 1889 and 1894, and rather mysteriously, they varied in severity. In the United Kingdom, the second and third waves were more deadly than the first; the mortality rate (n° deaths/population) was 157 per million in 1890, 574 in 1891 and 534 in 1892.[12] Similar figures were reported in the United States.[2,13] For example, in Indiana (near the Great Lakes), the epidemic began in January 1890, resulting in 3,200 deaths; the waves in that state illustrate the pattern of fatalities during the pandemic **(Fig. 5)**. Case fatality rates (n° deaths/n° symptomatic patients) were 1.56 per 1,000 influenza cases in 1890, 1.64 in 1891 and 2.15 in 1892.[16] Similar rates were recorded in France (1.6/1,000) and Germany (1.3/1,000).[7,9] Mortality was highest among people over 50 years of age, whereas usually influenza affects the oldest and the youngest. A highly detailed study estimated case

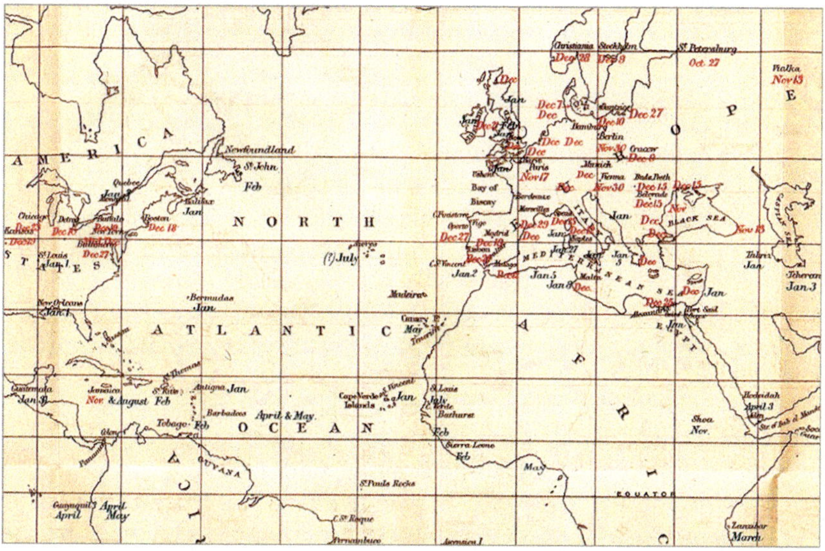

FIGURE 4: Map of the distribution of the Russian influenza pandemic in Europe and the United States of America (from [1] p.65). Outbreaks are shown in red.

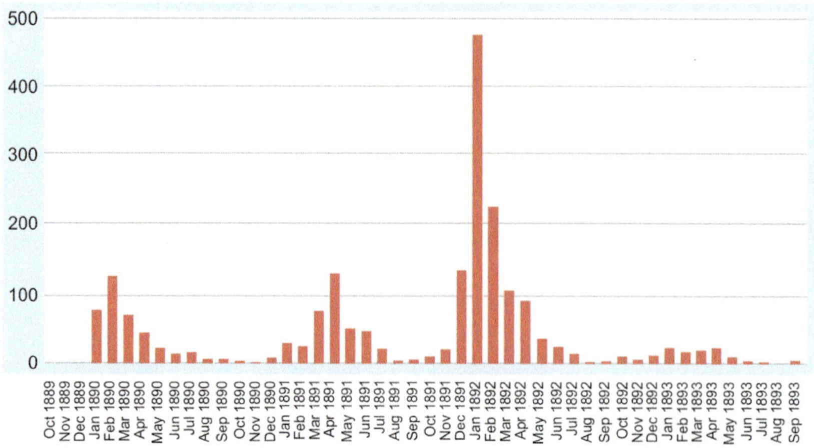

FIGURE 5: Mortality statistics during the Russian influenza in 1890 in Indiana (USA), showing a third wave associated with higher mortality.[16]

fatality rates in Europe as ranging from of 0.10 to 0.28%, proportions similar to those of Asian influenza in 1957 and Hong Kong influenza in 1968.[17] Russian influenza is therefore considered to be fairly mild. However, it resulted in 250,000 deaths in Europe, including 125,000 in England and Wales, 100,000 in the United States, and a total of about one million deaths worldwide, a toll nonetheless in no way comparable with the hecatomb of the Spanish flu of 1918, which killed at least 50 million people worldwide.[18]

THE SINGULARITIES OF THE RUSSIAN FLU

Compared to the previous pandemics of the 19th century, the rapid spread of influenza was surprising. How can it be explained? In 1890, at the outset of the Pastorian era, the proponents of contagion still clashed with those of the miasma theory, which explained the rapid spread by air. In reality, the first wave did not progress steadily from east to west. It first hit successively the major European cities and capitals, which were closely connected by railroads, before disseminating to regions; this explains its predominantly urban impact.

The pandemic also moved upstream, along the rivers; in addition, numerous grouped family cases were reported, indicating that influenza spreads directly through human-to-human contact. There is little doubt that influenza was borne by the European railroads, which were constantly expanding, with 202,887 km of track, and by the ever more rapid steamboats plying the waterways and seas. From May 1889 onwards, influenza was transported from Central Asia to the Russian Empire by the Transcaspian line to Samarkand in August, and then to Tomsk, 3,200 km away, in October. The spread towards the East was slower because the Trans-Siberian Railway did not yet exist. St. Petersburg was afflicted in November 1889 via the Volga River trade routes.[1,3]

The high contagiousness of Russian influenza explains its rapid spread. The average attack rate of symptomatic patients was reported to be 60% of the infected urban population[17]: 50% in Berlin, and 25% in London. The average reproduction rate (R0) was estimated to be 2.15, based on the epidemiological data from 33 European cities collected weekly between November 1889 and February 1890.[17] In some cities, such as St. Petersburg, Amsterdam, and Stuttgart, it was much higher. It bears mentioning that due to their benignity, many cases were not reported.

Russian influenza was more common in men and particularly severe in the elderly[19-21] or in patients with comorbidities, including phthisis, cardiopathies, cerebral diseases and nephritis. In the United Kingdom[1] and in Switzerland,[20] children were attacked much less frequently than adults, in contrast to flu epidemics, which affect the oldest and the very youngest **(Fig. 6)**. That said, young adults were not spared from rare fatal forms; in London, due to pneumonia caused by influenza, the Duke of Clarence died at the age of 28, even though he had no previous medical history.

Physicians of the time distinguished four clinical forms of Russian influenza[22]: a simple, uncomplicated febrile form with mild respiratory symptoms and fever that increased in 48 hours and disappeared in 3 or 4 days; a gastrointestinal form with moderate gastric symptoms, fever, and prostration; an uncommon catarrhal form; and a "nervous" form with intense paroxysmal neuralgic pain. Many people were surprised by the relative rarity of catarrh, which is habitually associated with influenza.[1] For example, around 1780, William Cullen referred to influenza as "catarrhal fever" (*catarrhus a contagio*),[23] leading to further textbook definition of contagious influenza.[24]

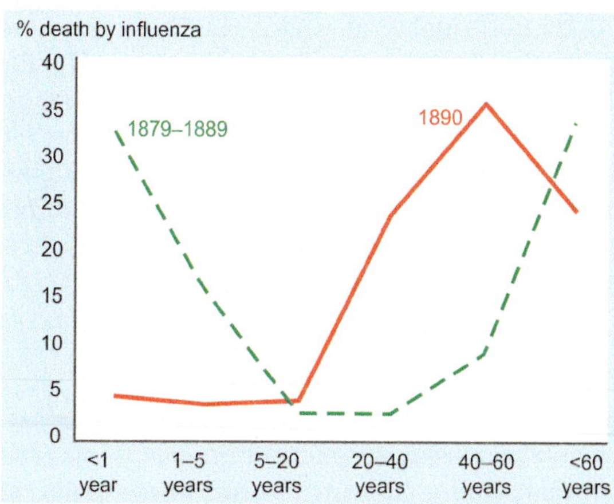

FIGURE 6: Proportion at several ages to 100 deaths from influenza, comparing the period 1847–1889 to 1890 mortality.[1]

At first glance, Russian influenza resembled pandemic episodes having occurred in previous centuries. It begins suddenly with an intense headache, high fever, chills, sweating, sneezing, watery eyes, and dry cough. Some patients suffer from painful bone and muscle, in the back, and in the entire body "up to the hairline". They become prostrate, without appetite, sometimes with slight delirium. Occasionally a loss of smell and photophobia are reported. The illness generally lasts three to five days.[1,9] Rashes of the face and body and unusual swelling of the hands are quite frequent,[1,9] possibly reflecting vasculitis. During SARS-CoV-2, skin lesions, peripheral vascular disease, persistent and painful sudden-onset redness and urticarial lesions with transient vesicles, at times resembling frostbite, have been reported.[25] In severe forms of Russian influenza, patients have difficulty breathing and may experience respiratory distress due to pneumonia, resulting in death.[19] Severe forms with renal, digestive or neurological involvement have also been reported. Dr James Goodhart (1845–1916), who treated numerous patients at Guy's Hospital in London, emphasized the diversity of symptoms and wrote: *"There would appear to be no organ or tissue that has become the subject of attack".*[26] Astonishingly diverse nervous symptoms were observed: Various types of algia, peripheral nerve neuritis with paresis, facial neuralgia, pneumogastric nerve neuritis with alternating tachycardia and bradycardia, occasional loss of smell (anosmia). Frequent psychic manifestations are also known to occur, including a state of prostration in contrast with the apparent benignity of the disease, profound and lasting asthenia, post-influenza depression or melancholy with suicidal tendencies, lethargic, cataleptic, or even psychotic states.

Another peculiarity compared to classical influenza is a tendency to induce short-term recurrences, encountered in about 15% of patients (including the Tsar), the first relapse being the most serious.[1] Due to sequelae, influenza reportedly left thousands of convalescents weakened, depressed, in debt, and unable to work.[11] In London, laborers suffered months of numbness in their limbs, progressing to spinal paralysis after a second bout of influenza in April 1891. Cases of respiratory muscle atrophy, heart failure and tongue paralysis were likewise noteworthy.[11] This atypical symptomatology of Russian influenza combined with splenomegaly, which is generally absent in the course of usual influenza, led the eminent Professor of the Paris Faculty of Medicine, Pierre Potain (1825–1901), to affirm that it was something other than usual influenza.[9]

THE RUSSIAN FLU VIRUS

Which agent was responsible for the pandemic? Needless to say, during the Pastorian revolution search for the germ of Russian flu became a priority, but the search began with a 50-year mistake. In the 1890s, viruses were still unknown. In November 1891, the German Richard Pfeiffer isolated a previously undescribed bacillus, which grew only on blood agar, from patients' nasopharyngeal samples. Terming it *Bacillus influenzae* (now *Haemophilus influenzae*), on January 4, 1892 he announced that he had discovered the agent responsible for influenza.[27] Unfortunately, he was unable to reproduce the disease experimentally in animals and did not fullfill the Koch's postulates, which might have established a causal link. He hypothesized that the agent was a very specific human pathogen, comparable to those of leprosy or cholera. As the bacillus was repeatedly isolated during cases of flu, Pfeiffer's observations seemed to be corroborated. In the years following the discovery, however, the bacillus was also found independently of any epidemic in otitis, mastoiditis, meningitis and pneumopathy. This is in contradiction with the existence of a specific germ at the origin of influenza. During the Spanish flu of 1918, this bacterium was once again incriminated, and many unsuccessful attempts were made to vaccinate against *H. influenzae*. At present, we know that it is a superinfection germ often present in nasopharyngeal samples.

At the end of the First world war, there were serious doubts about the etiology of the Spanish flu. The first major step was taken by Richard Shope, a young physician at the Rockefeller Institute for Medical Research in Princeton. In 1931, he discovered an ultrafiltrable virus that caused swine flu,[28] a disease similar to human flu that was sometimes transmitted to humans. The viral trail led to the discovery in London in 1933 by Wilson Smith, Patrick Laidlaw and Christopher Andrews of the human influenza virus (*Myxovirus influenzae*).[29] It was later shown that influenza viruses originate from birds and pass through an intermediate host, the pig, before infecting humans. Recently, it has become possible to sequence the entire genome of the Spanish flu virus from human remains dating back to 1918,[30] and to show by nucleotide sequence analysis that the H1N1 virus is indeed the agent of the Spanish flu and the ancestor of all subsequent flu pandemics.[31,32] The 1918 virus is believed to be of avian origin and adapted to humans. The H1N1 virus later acquired three new genes by reassortment in pigs, resulting in the H2N2 virus responsible for the Asian influenza of 1957. A new recombination event substituted two new genes, yielding the H3N2 virus of the 1968 influenza pandemic.[32] The same was true for the 2009 swine flu.[33] In 2005, the H1N1 virus of the Spanish flu was resurrected by synthesis and proved to be highly virulent for primates.[34]

After the discovery in 1933 of the influenza virus, it seemed logical to hold it responsible for all the pandemics recorded since the Renaissance, including the 1889 Russian flu. But how can this be proven? There exists a "sero-archeological" approach, which consists in titrating antibodies to strains carrying the H1, H2 or H3 hemagglutinins in the serum of patients born before or after the 1889 pandemic.[35] During the 1957 Asian H2N2 influenza, Dutch researchers found higher levels of anti-H2 antibodies in persons aged 71–94 years born between 1863 and 1886 in the two weeks preceding the epidemic wave in the Netherlands. Could the Russian flu virus be the H2N2 virus? However, the same antibodies were also detected in younger people born after 1910.[36,37] Moreover, the sera were collected just before the pandemic. Other serological studies suggest the H3 virus. During the 1968 H3N2 pandemic, there was less mortality in the elderly, with a higher peak of anti-H3 antibodies, in contrast with a much lower rate of anti-H2 seroprevalence (15–29%), which seems to rule out H2 virus as the cause of Russian influenza. It consequently appears likely that the H1N1 virus may have circulated as seasonal influenza from 1919 to 1957, when it disappeared during the Asian influenza, before reappearing in 1977, probably due to a laboratory accident.[38] The H3N2 virus eliminated the H2N2 from the Asiatic flu and has persisted up until now along with the H1N1 virus. It has been suggested that the agent of the Russian flu and the "mild pandemic" of 1898–1900 was the H3N8 virus,[39] which caused epizootics in horses. During the 1889 pandemic in the United Kingdom, Parsons reported the concomitant occurrence of epidemics of "pink-eye",[1] a form of equine influenza due to endemic H3N8 in horses, birds and dogs. However, the H3 virus hypothesis is based only on sero-epidemiological studies, which provide indirect evidence, and are not free of artifacts related to cross-reactions or serum inhibitors, for example.

THE CORONAVIRUS HYPOTHESIS

While the COVID-19 pandemic resembles the other influenza pandemics, the SARS-CoV-2 coronavirus was identified by sequencing a few weeks after its onset. There are seven coronaviruses pathogenic to humans[1]: Three are highly pathogenic and epidemic: SARS-CoV-1 (9% mortality), MERS-CoV (30% mortality) and the current pandemic virus, SARS-CoV-2 (0.6–2% mortality)[2]; Four are the cause of 15–30% of common colds and have been circulating in populations for decades: HCoV-229E, HCoV-NL63, HCoV-OC43 and HCoV-HKU1. These benign viruses are of animal origin (bats or rodents)[40] and evolve in small seasonal epidemics every 3 to 4 years during the autumn and the winter, conferring short-term immunity.[41,42]

In 2005, Belgian researchers sequenced the entire genome of a laboratory strain of HCoV-OC43 (which had undergone multiple passages in culture), demonstrating its phylogenetic proximity to another betacoronavirus of bovine origin, BCoV, which originated from rodents and yields acute diarrhea in calves.[43] The nucleotide sequence of HCoV-OC43 is almost identical to BCov, from which it was derived in about 1890 **(Fig. 7)**. These investigators confirmed their discovery by comparing different sequences of wild-type HCoV-OC43 strains isolated from patients with acute rhinitis.[44] They also found these viruses to be close to PHEV, a coronavirus causing porcine hemagglutinating encephalomyelitis.[45] In light of the COVID-19 pandemic, these phylogenic observations raise the question of the role of a coronavirus

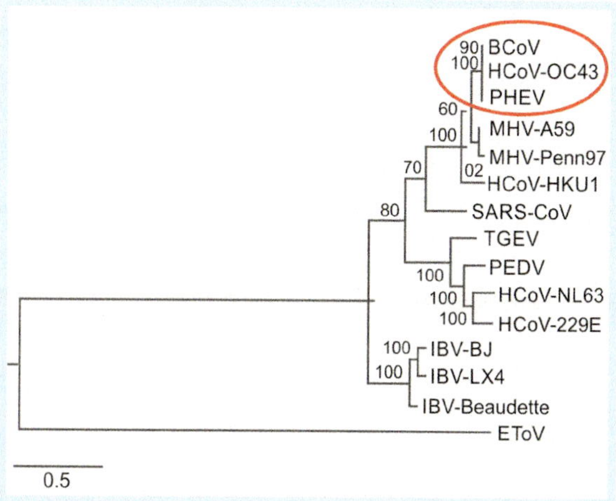

FIGURE 7: The phylogenetic tree of amino acid sequences of HCoV (OC43, NL63, 229E, HKU1) compared to the animal coronavirus (bovine BoCoV, porcine PHEV, PEDV, TGEV, murine MHV, avian IBV). The divergence between HCOV-OC43 occurred around 1890.[44]

in Russian influenza and make HCoV-OC43 an unexpectedly plausible candidate.

Can epidemiological arguments support this hypothesis? It is known that the second half of the 19th century was marked by concerted expansion of the live cattle trade, which was greatly facilitated by railways. Between 1870 and 1890, the world's cattle herd was decimated by a panzootic of contagious peripneumonia attributed to *Mycoplasma mycoides*, a wall-less bacterium. This epidemic necessitated the slaughter of hundreds of thousands of cattle as a means of controlling the disease worldwide. It has been speculated that the operatives performing the stamping out were exposed to bovine respiratory viruses, including BCoV. Such a scenario occurred during the SARS epidemic in 2002, related to the slaughter of civets for human consumption. In 1889, it was noted that cows showed the same symptoms as humans.[1] This led to the hypothesis that an HCoV-OC43 mutant had emerged from a bovine virus, following contamination by people in contact with cattle. Direct transmission of BCoV to humans has been observed in the past, particularly in a 6-year-old child with acute diarrhea.[46] Finally, by comparing the waves of flu pandemics **(Fig. 8)**, the evolution of the Russian pandemic was not similar to the seasonality of the flu pandemics of 1918, 1957 and 1968.[47] Recently, an attempt was made to predict the uncertain evolution of the COVID-19 pandemic using modeling based on the epidemiology of seasonal coronaviruses HCoV-OC43 and HCoV-HKU1. While the R0 transmission rate was shown to be 2.2 during winter and 1.3 during summer,[48] the emergence of highly

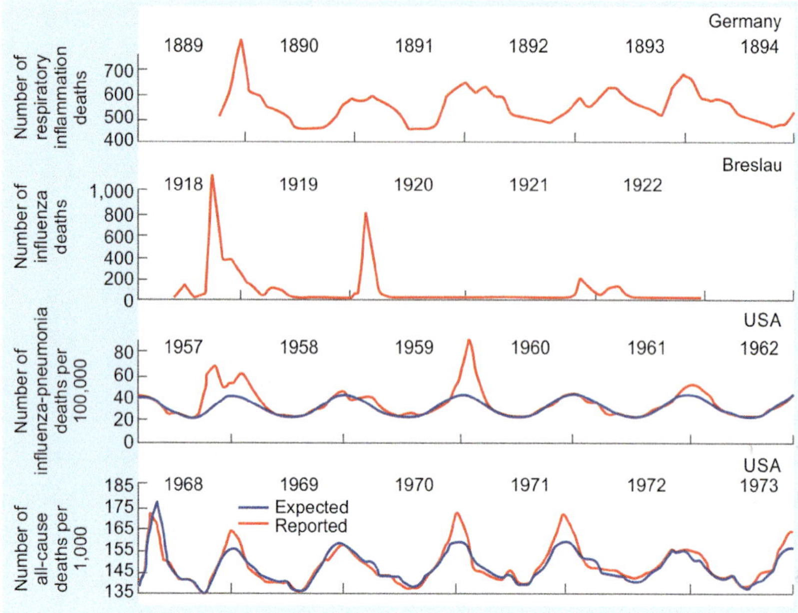

FIGURE 8: Comparison of the waves of the flu pandemics since 1889.[47]

contagious mutants of SARS-CoV-2 call these data into question. The hypothesis of a coronavirus at the origin of the Russian influenza is also corroborated by singular clinical features, e.g., the protean character of its clinical symptomatology, which resembles COVID-19, with multivisceral (pulmonary, digestive, renal, neurological) attacks, as well as prostration and psychiatric disorders.[49-51] The early relapses and sequelae are likewise reminiscent of COVID-19 complications.

While HCoV-OC43 is mostly benign, it appears to have retained some neurotropism (as does HCoV-229E). In 2000, Canadian researchers found traces of HCoV-OC43 RNA (23% of samples) and HCoV-229E RNA (44%) in postmortem brain samples from 90 patients having died of various neurological diseases or due to non-neurological causes. HCoV-OC43 RNA was significantly more frequently found in patients with multiple sclerosis (39% vs. 14% in controls).[52] Respiratory infections are known to trigger relapses of multiple sclerosis. Another Canadian team described a 2003 epidemic of respiratory infections due to HCoV-OC43 in institutionalized residents (95 infected/142) and caregivers (53 infected/160). There were eight deaths among residents.[53] HCoV-OC43 coronavirus is thought by some to be an attenuated mutant of a pandemic virus that triggered Russian influenza.

CONCLUSION

The emergence of the SARS-CoV-2 pandemic prompts a revisiting of the cause of past influenza pandemics. It should be remembered that there exist many wild reservoirs of coronaviruses, including bats, rodents, and birds, in whom the viruses are not (or only weakly) pathogenic.[54] As many as 5,000 types of coronaviruses have been identified, including 500 in bats, which may be the cause of many animal infections and epizootics. Could the loss of virulence be due to the natural evolution of pandemic viruses, an avatar of Darwinian selection of variants well-adapted to the species and persisting in the form of benign diseases or asymptomatic carriage, as in wild reservoirs? Chiropterans that appeared 50 million years ago,[55] most of them asymptomatic carriers of many viruses, may have survived iterative lethal epidemics since the dawn of time. A balance was conceivably found between host-adapted viruses and hosts that developed specific and original defense systems conferring "natural" resistance to viruses.[56]

Clinical, epidemiological and phylogenetic clues point to a coronavirus that caused the Russian influenza pandemic, as occurred in COVID-19, with its flu-like symptoms. Could there exist a historical precedent of a pandemic due to a coronavirus? Could the benign coronaviruses encountered in human populations be the relics of ancient epidemics yielding mild viruses that are perpetuated in the human species? This alternative hypothesis deserves further investigation.

Conflict of interest

None.

Funding

None.

ACKNOWLEDGMENTS

I wish to thank Alain-Jacques Valleron and Francis Barin for helpful discussion.

REFERENCES

1. Parsons H. Report on the influenza epidemic of 1889-90, Londres: HMSO, Eyre & Spottiswoode, 1891, & further report and papers on epidemic influenza 1889-92. Londres: HMSO; 1893.
2. Abbott SW. Twenty-first annual report of the state board of health of massachusetts. Boston: State Board of Health; 1890.
3. Teissier J. L'influenza de 1889-1890 en Russie. Rapport de mission adressé, à M. le Ministre de l'Instruction Publique. Paris: Baillie re JB; 1891.
4. Bertillon J. Annuaire statistique de la ville de Paris pour l'année 1890. Paris. 1892.
5. Friedrich PL. Die Influenza Epidemie 1889-1890. Deutschen Reiche Arbeiten aus dem Kaiserlichen Gesundheitsamte. 1894;9:139-378.

6. Bäumler C. Ueber die Influenza von 1889-90. Ver handl d Cong f innere Med Wiesb. 1890;IX:293-327.
7. Schmid F. Die influenza in der Schweiz in den Jahren 1889-1894. Bern: Schmid, Francke & Co; 1895.
8. Kempinska-Miroslawska B, Wozniak-Kosek A. The influenza epidemic of 1889–90 in selected European cities - a picture based on the reports of two Poznan daily newspapers from the second half of the nineteenth century. Med Sci Monit. 2013;19: 1131-41.
9. André, G. La grippe ou influenza. Paris: Masson; 1908.
10. Creighton C. The history of epidemics in Britain, Vol II, from the extinction of plague to the present time. Cambridge: Cambridge University Press; 1894. pp. 393-400.
11. Smith FB. The Russian Influenza in the United Kingdom, 1889-1894. Soc Hist Med 1995;8(1):55-73.
12. Honigsbaum M. The Russian influenzae in the UK: lessons learned, opportunities missed. Vaccine 2011;295:B11-5.
13. Patterson KD. Pandemic influenza, 1700-1900 : a study in historical epidemiology. New York: Rowan & Littlefield; 1986.
14. Sixty-Third Annual Report of the Registrar General. London: HMSO; 1900 1902, ixvi.
15. Newsholme A. Influenza for the public Health standpoint. Practionner 1907;77:118.
16. Ewing ET. La Grippe or Russian Influenzae: mortality statistics during the 1890 Epidemic in Indiana. Influenza Other Resp Viruses. 2019;13:279-87.
17. Valleron AJ, Cori A, Valtat S, Meurisse S, Carrat F, Boëlle PY. Transmissibility and geographic spread of the 1889 influenza pandemic. Proc Natl Acad Sci USA. 2010;107(19):8778-81.
18. Barry JM. The great influenza, the epic story of the deadliest plague in history. New York: Penguin Books; 2004.
19. Bresalier M. A most protean disease : aligning medical knowledge of modern influenza, 1890-1914. Med Hist. 2012;56(4):481-510.
20. Valtat S, Cori A, Carrat F, Valleron AJ. Age distribution of cases and deaths during the 1889 influenza pandemic. Vaccine. 2011;29(Suppl 2):B6-10.
21. Ramiro D, Garcia S, Casado Y, Cilek L, Chowell G. Age-specific excess mortality patterns and transmissibility during the 1889–1890 influenza pandemic in Madrid, Spain. Ann Epidemiol. 2018;28(5):267-72.
22. West S. The influenza epidemic of 1890. St Bartolomew's Hospital reports. 1890;26: 193-258.
23. Thomson J. The works of William Cullen, vol 1. Edinburgh Londres: William Blackwood & TG Underwood; 1827. p. 290.
24. Peacock TB. On the influenza or epidemic cattharal fever of 1847-1848. Londres: Churchill; 1848.
25. Genovese G, Moltrasio C, Berti E, Marzano AV. Skin manifestations associated with COVID-19: current knowledge and future perspectives. Dermatology. 2021;237:1-12.
26. Goodhart JF. Influenza. In: Talbutt TC, editor. A system of medicine. Londres: Longmans & Co.; 1896. p. 690.
27. Pfeiffer R. Aus dem Institut für Infektionskrankheiten. II. Vorläufige Mittheilungen über die Erreger der Influenza. Dtsch Med Wochenschr. 1892;18:28.
28. Shope R. Swine influenza. I. Experimental transmission and pathology. J Exp Med. 1931;54:349-59.
29. Smith W, Andrewes C, Laidlaw P. A virus obtained from influenza patients. Lancet. 1933;2:66-8.
30. Taubenberger JK, Reid AH, Kraft AE, Bijwaard KE, Fanning TG. Initial genetic characterization of the 1918 "Spanish" influenza virus. Science. 1997;275(5307):1793-6.

31. Taubenberger JK, Reid AH, Janczewski TA, Fanning TG. Integrating historical, clinical and molecular genetic data in order to explain the origin and virulence of the 1918 Spanish influenza virus. Philos Trans R Soc Lond B. 2001;356:1829-39.
32. Taubenberger JK, Morens DM. 1918 Influenza: the mother of all pandemics. Emerg Infect Dis. 2006;12(1):15-22.
33. Garten RJ, Davis CT, Russell CA, Shu B, Lindstrom S, Balish A, et al. Antigenic and genetic characteristics of swine-origin 2009 A(H1N1) influenza viruses circulating in humans. Science. 2009;325(5937):197-201.
34. Tumpey TM, Basler CF, Aguilar PV, Zeng H, Solorzano A, Swayne DE, et al. Characterization of the reconstructed 1918 Spanish influenza pandemic virus. Science. 2005;310: 77-80.
35. Dowdle WR. Influenza A virus recycling revisited. Bull WHO. 1999;77(10):820-8.
36. Mulder J, Masurel N. Pre-epidemic antibody against 1957, strain of asiatic influenza in serum of older people living in the Netherlands. Lancet. 1958;1(7025):810-4.
37. Masurel N. Serological characteristics of a "new" serotype of influenza A virus: the Hong Kong strain. Bull WHO. 1969;41:461-8.
38. Nakajima K, Desselberger U, Palese P. Recent human influenza A (H1N1) viruses are closely related genetically to strains isolated in 1950. Nature. 1978;274:334-9.
39. Taubenberger JK, Morens DM, Fauci AS. The next influenza pandemic: can it be predicted ? JAMA. 2007;297(18):2025-7.
40. Cui J, Li F, Shi ZL. Origin and evolution of pathogenic coronaviruses. Nat Rev Microbiol. 2019;17:181-92.
41. Vabret A, Dina J, Brison E, Brouard J, Freymuth F. Coronavirus humains (HCoV). Pathol Biol. 2009;57(2):149-60.
42. Killerby ME, Biggs HM, Haynes A, Dahl RM, Mustaquim D, Gerber SI, Watson JT. Human coronavirus circulation in the United States 2014–2017. J Clin Virol. 2018;101: 52 6.
43. Vijgen L, Keyaerts E, Moës E, Thoelen I, Wollants E, et al. Complete genomic sequence of human coronavirus OC43: molecular clock analysis suggests a relatively recent zoonotic coronavirus transmission event. J Virol. 2005;79:1595-604.
44. Vijgen L, Keyaerts E, Lemey P, Moës E, Li S, Vandamme A-M, et al. Circulation of genetically distinct contemporary human coronavirus OC43 strains. Virology. 2005; 337(1):85-92.
45. Vijgen L, Keyaerts E, Lemey P, Maes P, Van Reeth K, Nauwynck H, et al. Evolutionary history of the closely related group 2 coronaviruses: porcine hemagglutinating encephalomyelitis virus, bovine coronavirus, and human coronavirus OC43. J Virol. 2006;80(14):7270-4.
46. Zhang M, Herbst W, Kousoulas KG, Storz J. Biological and genetic characterization of a hemagglutinating coronavirus isolated from a diarrhoeic child. J Med Virol. 1994;44: 152-61.
47. Morens DM, Taubenberger JK. Pandemic influenza: certain uncertainties. Rev Med Virol. 2011;21(5):262-84.
48. Kissler SM, Tedijanto C, Goldstein E, Grad YH, Lipsitch M. Projecting the transmission dynamics of SARS-CoV-2 through the postpandemic period. Science. 2020;368: 860-8.
49. Zhou P, Yang XL, Wang XG, Hu B, Zhang L, Zhang W, et al. A pneumonia outbreak associated with a new coronavirus of probable bat origin. Nature. 2020;579:270-3.
50. Zhu N, Zhang D, Wang W, Li X, Yang B, Song J, et al. A novel coronavirus from patients with pneumonia in China, 2019. N Engl J Med. 2020;382:727-33.
51. Zhou F, Yu T, Du R, Fan G, Liu Y, Liu Z, et al. Clinical course and risk factors for mortality of adult inpatients with COVID-19 in Wuhan, China: a retrospective cohort study. Lancet. 2020;395(10229):1054-62.

52. Arbour N, Day R, Newcombe J, Talbot PJ. Neuroinvasion by human respiratory coronaviruses. J Virol. 2000;74(19):8913-21.
53. Patrick DM, Petric M, Skowronski DM, Guasparini R, Booth TF, Krajden M, McGeer P, Bastien N, et al. An outbreak of human coronavirus OC43 infection and serological cross-reactivity with SARS coronavirus. Can J Infect Dis Med Microbiol. 2006;17(6):330-6.
54. Haymans DTS. Bats as viral reservoirs. Ann Rev Virol. 2016;3:77-99.
55. Teeling EC, Springer MS, Madsen O, Bates P, O'Brien SJ, Murphy WJ. A molecular phylogeny for bats illuminates biogeography and the fossil record. Science. 2005;307(5709):580-4.
56. Irving AT, Ahn M, Goh G, Anderson DE, Wang LF. Lessons from the host defences of bats, a unique viral reservoir. Nature. 2021;589:363-70.

2

SECTION

Nonpharmacologic Interventions

CHAPTER 10

The Use of Masks in the Prevention of SARS-CoV-2 Transmission

Christine Filippone

INTRODUCTION

Severe acute respiratory syndrome coronavirus 2 (SARS-CoV-2) is a respiratory virus that is transmitted via contact, droplet, and aerosol.[1] Direct transmission occurs by infectious droplets expelled from coughing or sneezing onto a mucous membrane, or by aerosols generated from a person singing, talking or from mechanical ventilation or other aerosolized generating procedures, and lastly direct contact may occur when touching contaminated parts of a persons' body such as their hands. Indirect transmission may occur when there is contact with the contaminated environment such as surfaces, devices, and equipment.[2]

Masks are one of the major protection measures at the beginning of the COVID-19 pandemic. Controversy regarding the best type of mask to provide protection from transmission of the virus occurred as the science regarding the virus evolved. The effectiveness of different types of masks in preventing the transmission of SARS-CoV-2 has been a topic of discussion in the public health arena and in healthcare settings. Due to the increasing transmission of COVID-19 many different approaches to decrease transmission including nonpharmaceutical interventions including the use of masks have been required. SARS-CoV-2 is primarily transmitted from person to person through close contact with respiratory secretions.

The prevention of the transmission of COVID-19 requires a hierarchy of controls. These controls include early identification and treatment of a suspect or confirm patient with COVID-19. Environmental controls include the use of negative air flow to reduce the concentration of infectious particles in the air, reducing or eliminating direct contact of contaminated surfaces, thorough cleaning surfaces with appropriate agents and physical distancing. Other infection prevention measures include isolation precautions, hand hygiene, respiratory etiquette, and the use of respiratory personal protective equipment (PPE).

When an in infectious person sneezes, coughs, speaks, sings, or breathes their respiratory droplets could be transmitted to others. Viruses can be transmitted through aerosolization, remaining suspended in the air for hours.[3] Masks help decrease the spread of SARS-CoV-2 in two ways—(1) they reduce the number of respiratory droplets in the air and (2) they limit how many droplets the person wearing a mask inhales into their respiratory system. Some masks are more effective than others in the prevention of infectious respiratory particles.

CHOOSING THE RIGHT MASK TYPE

Masks provide different levels of protection depending on the type of mask and how the mask fits the healthcare provider. Choosing the correct type of mask and proper use of the mask assists in the protection against COVID-19. Using a mask to protect against infectious particles is dependents on the type of mask and how well the mask fits and seals to your face. To achieve the best protection, ensure there are no gaps around the side of the mask and the mask fits as close to the face as possible. Do not use masks with exhalation valves, vents or opening through which droplets can be expelled. Wear a mask with a nose piece that can be molded to your face to prevent the penetration of infectious particles. The mask should have at least two layers of protection, completely covers your nose and mouth, fits snugly against your face without gaps, and has a nose wire piece that can be molded to fit the bridge of your nose.[4] The efficacy of filtration of mask depends on many factors from the structural components of each mask to the practice of the person wearing the mask. The masks effectiveness is based on the fit of the mask, the integrity of the mask and the consistency of wearing the mask, and the practices of the person wearing the mask.

TYPES OF MASKS

There are different types of face masks—cloth, surgical, N95, elastomeric, and powered air-purifying respirators (PAPR). Other types of respirators include atmosphere-supplying respirators (ASR), supplied air respirators (SAR), self-contained breathing apparatus (SCBA), and hybrid systems. The later grouping of respirators requires air oxygen to be piped in from an outside source and will not be discussed in this chapter.[5] The types of masks available vary depending on the material, design, and purpose for which they are manufactured.

Because masks are utilized in healthcare settings specific standards are required by the following agencies in the United States Food and Drug Administration (FDA), the National Institute for Occupational Safety and Health (NIOSH), and the Occupational Safety and Health Administration (OSHA). The term facemask is used to describe many types of masks—cloth masks, procedure masks, and surgical masks. A face mask is worn over the wearer's nose and mouth and are used to control the respiratory secretions of the person wearing the mask, this is known as source control. The NIOSH and the FDA have specific definitions for types of face coverings. A "face mask" defined by the FDA and the NIOSH is a loose fitting, disposable device with or without a face shield that creates a physical barrier between the mouth and the nose of the wearer and potential contaminants in the environment. The facemask is not considered respiratory protection.[6]

Cloth Masks

Cloth masks are made from a variety of fabrics and usually have usually have one or two layers of fabric. The primary purpose of cloth facemasks is to contain respiratory droplets that are expelled from the wearer of the mask when they talk, cough, or sneeze. The cloth mask acts as a source control for the wearer more than protecting the wearer from the inhalation of infectious droplet particles.[7] This is an important concept, as it is estimated at least 50% or more of transmission is from persons who never develop symptoms or those who are in the presymptomatic phase of COVID-19. Cloth masks with multiple layers and higher thread counts can improve filtration of small droplets particles from inhaled air.[8] These masks provide the least protection against infectious particles and should not be worn in a hospital setting.

Surgical Masks

Surgical masks also called medical, or procedure masks are loose-fitting, disposable devices. These masks are fluid resistant, flammable, and provide protection from splashes, sprays, and splatter. This mask can be made of a variety of materials and usually has three layers. Some of these masks have a wire nose piece but not all. These masks are a barrier between the mouth and nose of the healthcare provider and potential infectious particles in the immediate environment. If worn properly these masks will prevent large droplets, splashes, and sprays of infectious particles from contact to mucous membranes. Surgical masks prevent infection spreading from the source (the infected person wearing the mask) by reducing the exposure of the wearer's saliva and respiratory secretion from spreading to others. This type of mask is a good option for asymptomatic and symptomatic persons to wear.

The surgical mask will not prevent the transmission of aerosolized or very small infectious particles produced from an infectious person coughs, sneezes, or talks or from certain medical procedures are performed.[9] Data reveals surgical masks with ties had a 71.5% filtration and surgical masks with ear loops only provided 38.1% filtration.[10]

N95 Masks

N95 masks are also called respirators. The N95 respirator is an air-purifying respirator with NIOSH-approved filter or filter material. This respirator is a polyester-based filtering facepiece respirator. The "N" stands for "nonoil," which indicates it protects against solid and nonoil-based particles. The "95" refers to the efficiency rating which indicates this respirator can filter at least 95% of particles.

The NIOSH regulates N95 respirators, therefore ensure all N95 masks are NIOSH approved.

The OSHA mandates safety requirements for the N95 mask which includes fit testing to ensure the proper fit. This mask when fit tested and worn properly is capable to prevent the particles from penetrating the mask. Fit testing should be performed for a specific mask produced by a specific manufacturer, using a specific size mask.

Should another manufacturers N95 mask be utilized, fit testing of that specific mask needs to occur to ensure the safety of the provider.

After donning the N95 mask, the wearer should check for an adequate seal by performing a user seal check every time the respirator is worn. The user seal check is also referred to as the fit check. The seal check or fit check requires the wearer to cup their hands over the facepiece, covering the edges of the mask where there is contact with the face. This check can be either a positive pressure or negative pressure user seal check depending upon the manufacturer's instructions. A positive pressure user seal check includes the wearer to exhale gently while covering the paths for air to exit the facepiece. A seal check is successful when the facepiece is slightly pressurized before increased pressure causes outward leakage of air. A negative pressure user seal check includes the wearer to inhale sharply while covering the paths for air to enter the mask. A seal check is successful when the facepiece collapses slightly under the negative pressure that occurs during the inhalation.[11] The mask forms a seal around the nose and mouth preventing the transmission of airborne infectious particle. The N95 mask is not fluid resistant, the healthcare provider should also wear a face shield if there is a potential for exposure to blood or body fluid.[12]

Persons with chronic respiratory, cardiac, or other medical conditions that may impair breathing should be medically screening prior to use of the N95 mask. Persons with facial hair cannot use an N95 mask, as a tight seal cannot be achieved, thereby allowing infectious particles to be inhaled. Any significant change in body weight requires a repeat fit test to ensure the proper mask size. Fit testing protocols are mandatory and have specific testing procedures.[13]

KN95

KN95 masks are a type of mask that meets certain international standards. This mask filters better than a surgical mask, but in the United States they are not considered a respirator and do not need to meet the same standards as respirators.[14]

ELASTOMERIC RESPIRATORS

Elastomeric respirators provide excellent protection and are a large reusable facemask made of synthetic or natural rubber material. These respirators require specific maintenance including reusable filter and are not fluid resistant. Some concerns regarding the use of this mask in healthcare include the clumsiness of respirator, the expense, distorted verbal communication, and due to the size and the tight fit persons may feel claustrophobic.[15]

Transmission of SARS-CoV-2 and Choosing the Correct Mask

The SARS-CoV-2 virus is approximately 0.1 μm in diameter. Respiratory droplets are produced when an infected person sneezes, sings, or talks, or has certain medical procedures performed that expel respiratory droplets. These respiratory droplets are categorized into two categories based upon their size and evaporation times.

Large droplets, which are particles > 5 μm in diameter are known as spray droplets or droplets. These large droplets fall rapidly to the ground therefore are transmitted over short distances. These large droplets contaminate the immediate surroundings of the patient. Small droplets are particles ≤ 5 μm in diameter and are known as aerosols or droplet nuclei. These smaller droplets can remain suspended in air for significant periods of time. In this suspended form, the droplet nuclei can be transmitted to a person by inhalation.[16] Once the infectious particle is inhaled, infiltration into the pulmonary system occurs. Fine droplets ≤2.5 μm travel into the lungs, droplet particles 2.5–10.0 μm are deposited in the larger tracheal-bronchial airways leaving the larger particles > 10 μm being deposited in the upper respiratory tract.[17]

The N95 masks reach approximately 99.5% filtration efficiency with particles 0.75 μm in diameter.[18] When an infectious person talks, coughs, sneezes, or sings, or has a medical procedure perform that elicits expelling respiratory secretions the droplet or droplet nuclei that is produced can travel up to 27 feet.[19] Persons who experience respiratory symptoms produce aerosols that contain viable SARS-CoV-2 particles that remain suspended in the air. These particles are expelled in the absence of aerosolized generating procedures.[20] Using a Bayesian regression model, it was demonstrated the SARS-CoV-2 particles could remain viable in aerosols for 3 hours.[21]

Not only can infectious particles be transmitted through the respiratory route via droplet and airborne transmission but also may occur through contact of the infectious particle. The transmission of an infectious particle by contact occurs when a person touches a contaminated surface, device, or equipment then touches their mucous membrane. These findings validate droplets can contaminate the environment as they settle onto surfaces. Hence, the need to ensure the environment is cleaned thoroughly by an approved cleaning agent.[22]

CONTROVERSIES IN THE USE OF MASKS IN THE PREVENTION OF COVID-19

Studies have been conducted regarding the effectiveness of masks and the prevention of the transmission of respiratory illnesses.[23,24,26,27] Jefferson et al. reviewed randomized control trials comparing the lack of wearing masks and not wearing masks with healthcare workers and in the community. The outcomes of influenza-like illness (ILI)/COVID-19, as well as laboratory-confirmed influenza/SARS-CoV-2 were utilized. The wearing of masks in the community probably makes little or no difference to the outcome of ILI/COVID-19 illness compared to not wearing masks [RR 0.95, 95% confidence interval (CI) 0.84–1.09]. Wearing masks in the community probably makes little or no difference to the outcome of laboratory-confirmed influenza/SARS-CoV-2 compared to not wearing masks (RR 101. 95% CI 0.72–1.42).[23]

The same review reviewed pooled trials comparing N95 respirators with surgical masks in healthcare and in a household setting. The outcomes of clinical respiratory illness, ILI, and laboratory confirmed influenza infection were utilized. When comparing the use of the N95 respirator with the surgical mask on the outcome of clinical respiratory illness, the results were "uncertain" (RR 0.70, 95% CI 0.45–1.10). The use of the N95 respirator may be effective when compared with the surgical mask on the outcome of ILI (RR 0.82, 95% CI 0.66–1.03). There was little or no difference on the outcome of laboratory-confirmed influenza infection when comparing the N95 respirator to the surgical mask (RR 1.10, 95% CI 0.90–1.34).[23]

Barycka et al. conducted a meta-analysis that evaluated the effect of the N95 respirator compared to the surgical mask and the transmission of acute respiratory infections and concluded, there is insufficient data to definitively determine if N95 respirators are superior to surgical masks in the protection against acute respiratory infections.[24]

Elgersma et al., in a cross-sectional analysis of 3.209 persons, demonstrated that compared to those who seldom or did not wear masks, those who wore masks often had a 33% chance of developing COVID-19. In addition, this risk increased to 40% among persons who consistently almost always or always wore masks.[25]

The use of a mask alone when caring for a person with active COVID-19 infection is not effective against the transmission of infection if other infection prevention measures such as hand hygiene, eye protection, gloves, and gown are not utilized. Adherence to fundamental infection-control measures is required to prevent the transmission of respiratory infections.

General Care of Masks

Proper donning, doffing, and maintenance of the mask will assist with providing the level of protection determine by the mask chosen. A mask should be discarded and replaced as soon as the integrity of the mask is impaired or if the mask becomes wet, soiled, or contaminated.

Donning an N95 Mask

- Choose the same make, model, and size that was utilized to complete a successful fit test.
- Perform hand hygiene.
- Cup the mask in one hand, the headbands will hang below your hand.
- Hold the mask under your chin with one hand, with the other hand place the top headband over your head and place at the top of your head.
- Place the bottom headband around the neck and under the ears.
- Place your fingertips from both hands over the nose piece and slide the fingertips down both sides of the nose piece molding the nose piece around the bridge of your nose.
- Perform positive or negative pressure seal check based upon manufacturers' instructions.

Doffing an N95 Mask

- Without touching the front of the mask, pull the bottom strap over your head letting the strap, and down over your chest.
- Pull the top strap over and discard the mask
- Discard
- Perform hand hygiene[28]

CONCLUSION

Wearing a mask is only one measure in preventing the transmission of SARS-CoV-2. Good hand hygiene, proper donning and doffing of masks, and attention not to contaminate the mask are all important measure to optimize the use of a mask in preventing the transmission of infectious particles. The use of eye protection, gowns and gloves are also recommended PPE when caring for persons with infectious COVID-19 disease.

Most studies reveal N95 masks are superior to surgical masks for front line healthcare providers engaged in high-risk procedures and when caring for COVID-19 infectious patients. Surgical masks can be worn by healthcare providers who are engaged in low-risk procedures and when providing care to noninfectious COVID-19 patients. The main transmission route for SARS-CoV-2 is respiratory droplets and droplet nuclei. These infectious particle are transmitted primarily from person to person by inhaling infectious particles or by contact of contaminated surfaces.

Nonpharmaceutical measures such as isolation, social distancing, hand hygiene, and wearing masks are important in curtailing the spread of infection. Despite the specifications of masks by the manufacturer and regulatory agencies, the mask is only as effective as the person who wears the mask. Individuals need to be educated about the importance of not touching their eyes, nose, or mouth. Proper donning, doffing, and maintenance of the mask is required to reach the full protective properties outlined for each mask.

REFERENCES

1. Kutter JS, Spronken MI, Fraaij PL, Fouchier RAM, Herfst S. Transmission routes of respiratory viruses among humans. Curr Opin Virol. 2018;28:142-51.
2. Sommerstein R, Fux CA, Vuichard-Gysin D, Abbas M, Marschall J, Balmelli C, et al. Risk of SARS-CoV-2 transmission by aerosols, the rational use of masks, and protection of healthcare workers from COVID-19. Antimicrob Resist Infect Control. 2020;9:100.
3. Wang Y, Deng Z, Shi D. How effective is a mask in preventing COVID-19 infection? Med Devices Sens. 2021;4:e10163.
4. University of Maryland Medical System. (2022). Choosing the Right Mask Type. [online] Available from https://www.umms.org/coronavirus/diagnosis-symptoms/mask-types#:~:text=Choosing%20the%20Right%20Mask%20Type,Is%20comfortable%20and%20breathable [Last accessed December, 2023].
5. De Silva AP, Niriella MA, Janaka de Silva H. Masks in COVID-19: Let's unmask the evidence. Expert Rev Respir Med. 2021;15(3):293-99.
6. Quintana-Díaz MA, Aguilar-Salinas CA. Universal Masking during COVID-19 Pandemic–Current Evidence and Controversies. Rev Invest Clin. 2020;72(3):144-50.
7. O'Kelly E, Pirog S, Ward J, Clarkson PJ. Ability of fabric face mask materials to filter ultrafine particles at coughing velocity. BMJ Open. 2020;10:e039424.
8. Brooks JT, Butler JC. Effectiveness of Mask Wearing to Control Community Spread of SARS-CoV-2. JAMA. 2021;325(10):998-9.
9. The Food and Drug Administration. (2022). N95 Respirators, Surgical Masks, Face Masks, and Barrier Face Coverings. [online] Available from https://www.fda.gov/medical-devices/personal-protective-equipment-infection-control/n95-respirators-surgical-masks-face-masks-and-barrier-face-coverings [Last accessed December, 2023].
10. United States Environmental Protection Agency. (2022). EPA Researchers Test Effectiveness of Face Masks, Disinfection Methods Against COVID-19. [online] Available from https://www.epa.gov/sciencematters/epa-researchers-test-effectiveness-face-masks-disinfection-methods-against-covid-19 [Last accessed December, 2023].
11. The Centers for Disease Control and Prevention. (2018). Filtering out Confusion: Frequently Asked Questions about Respiratory Protection. [online] Available from https://www.cdc.gov/niosh/npptl/FilteringOutConfusion.html [Last accessed December, 2023].
12. BencoDental. (2020). Everything You Want to Know about N95 and KN95 Masks but Were Afraid to Ask. [online] Available from https://www.benco.com/benco-dental-u/faq/everything-you-want-to-know-about-n95-and-kn95-masks-but-were-afraid-to-ask/ [Last accessed December, 2023].
13. Occupational Safety and Health Administration. (2023). Appendix A to § 1910.134–Fit Testing Procedures (Mandatory). [online] Available from https://www.osha.gov/laws-regs/regulations/standardnumber/1910/1910.134AppA [Last accessed December, 2023].
14. The Centers for Disease Control and Prevention. (2022). Types of Masks and Respirator. [online] Available from https://www.cdc.gov/coronavirus/2019-ncov/prevent-getting-sick/types-of-masks.html [Last accessed December, 2023].
15. The Centers for Disease Control and Prevention. (2020). Elastomeric Respirators: Strategies during Conventional and Surge Demand Situations. [online] Available from https://www.cdc.gov/coronavirus/2019-ncov/hcp/elastomeric-respirators-strategy/index.html [Last accessed December, 2023].
16. Bar-On YM, Flamholz A, Phillips R, Milo R. SARS-CoV-2 (COVID-19) by the numbers. Elife. 2020;9:e57309.
17. Stern RA, Koutrakis P, Martins MAG, Lemos B, Dowd SE, Sunderland EM, et al. Characterization of hospital airborne SARS-CoV-2. Respir Res. 2021;22:73.

18. Qian Y, Willeke K, Grinshpun SA, Donnelly J, Coffey CC. Performance of N95 respirators: filtration efficiency for airborne microbial and inert particles. Am Ind Hyg Assoc J. 1998;59(2):128-32.
19. Bourouiba L. Turbulent Gas Clouds and Respiratory Pathogen Emissions: Potential Implications for Reducing Transmission of COVID-19. JAMA. 2020;323(18):1837-8.
20. Lednicky JA, Lauzard M, Fan ZH, Jutla A, Tilly TB, Gangwar M, et al. Viable SARS-CoV-2 in the air of a hospital room with COVID-19 patients. Int J Infect Dis. 2020;100:476-82.
21. van Doremalen N, Bushmaker T, Morris DH, Holbrook MG, Gamble A, Williamson BN, et al. Aerosol and Surface Stability of SARS-CoV-2 as compared with SARS-CoV-1. N Engl J Med. 2020;382(16):1564-7.
22. The Centers for Disease Control and Prevention. (2021). Scientific Brief: SARS-CoV-2 Transmission. 2021. [online] Available from https://www.cdc.gov/coronavirus/2019-ncov/science/science-briefs/sars-cov-2-transmission.html [Last accessed December, 2023].
23. Jefferson T, Del Mar CB, Dooley L, Ferroni E, Al-Ansary LA, Bawazeer GA, et al. Physical interventions to interrupt or reduce the spread of respiratory viruses. Cochrane Database Syst Rev. 2011;2011(7):CD006207.
24. Barycka K, Szarpak L, Filipiak KJ, Jaguszewski M, Smereka J, Ladny JR, et al. Comparative effectiveness of N95 respirators and surgical/face masks in preventing airborne infections in the era of SARS-CoV2 pandemic: A meta-analysis of randomized trials. PLoS One. 2020;15(12):e0242901.
25. Elgersma IH, Fretheim A, Elstrøm P, Aavitsland P. Association between face mask use and risk of SARS-CoV-2 infection: Cross-sectional study. Epidemiology and Infection. 2023;151:e194.
26. Xiao J, Shiu E, Gao H, Wong JY, Fong MW, Ryu S, et al. Nonpharmaceutical Measures for Pandemic Influenza in Nonhealthcare Settings—Personal Protective and Environmental Measures. Emerg Infect Dis. 2020;26(5):967-75.
27. Alexander PE. (2021). The CDC's Mask Mandate Study: Debunked. American Institute for Economic Research. https://www.aier.org/article/the-cdc-mask-mandate-study-debunked/ [Last accessed December, 2023]
28. The Center for Disease Control and Prevention. (2023). How to Properly Put on and Take off a Disposable Respirator. [online] Available from https://ehs.msu.edu/_assets/docs/don-doff-n95.pdf [Last accessed December, 2023]

CHAPTER 11

Managing COVID-19 in Hong Kong: Lessons from SARS 2003 and Effective Strategies for Control

Ivan Fan-Ngai Hung

INTRODUCTION

The outbreak of the novel coronavirus disease (COVID-19) in 2019 has posed significant global health challenges. The management of COVID-19 in Hong Kong has been greatly influenced by the lessons learned from the severe acute respiratory syndrome (SARS) outbreak in 2003.[1,2] The SARS outbreak was a significant public health crisis that resulted in 299 deaths in Hong Kong and had a lasting impact on the city's healthcare system. In fact, as early as 2007, 4 years after the SARS 2003 epidemic, our team had already predicted that the SARS-associated coronavirus (SARS-CoV) would return, given the right condition and mutation.[3] Therefore, drawing from the hard-won lessons of SARS, Hong Kong swiftly implemented a range of measures to combat the spread of COVID-19 in January 2020. The management of the COVID-19 pandemic in Hong Kong has been a complex and dynamic process that required the integration of various public health measures, medical interventions, and community engagement. This chapter delves into the multifaceted approach employed by Hong Kong, focusing on early detection through saliva polymerase chain reaction (PCR) testing, early isolation and quarantine which allows early treatment of repurposing antivirals, mass COVID-19 vaccination, universal face masking, treatment with specific antivirals for high-risk patients at the later phase of the pandemic, and the establishment of the Pandemic Research Alliance in the postpandemic era.

EARLY DETECTION AND ISOLATION

One of the key lessons learned from the SARS outbreak was the importance of early detection and isolation. In response to COVID-19, Hong Kong quickly implemented quarantine measures, establishing dedicated facilities with adequate negative pressure isolation capabilities. Environmental studies within the negative pressure facilities have demonstrated minimal contamination.[4] These facilities allowed for the effective isolation of infected individuals, preventing the spread of the virus within the community and hospitals. By isolating and treating infected individuals promptly, Hong Kong was able to contain the spread of the virus and prevent widespread outbreaks.

FACE MASK MANDATES AND PERSONAL PROTECTIVE EQUIPMENT

Another important lesson learned from the SARS 2003 outbreak was the importance of face masking. During the SARS 2003 outbreak, it became evident that wearing face masks could significantly reduce the risk of respiratory droplet transmission.[5] As a result, Hong Kong implemented early and comprehensive face mask mandates during the COVID-19 pandemic. The use of face masks became a social norm, and public education campaigns were launched to promote their importance. This strategy helped to limit the spread of COVID-19 within the community. Adequate supply of the personal protective equipment and stringent infection-control measures have prevented nosocomial COVID-19 infection within the hospitals.

DIAGNOSTIC TESTING

Hong Kong has adopted early and widespread testing measures for COVID-19. The city quickly implemented convenient and noninvasive testing methods, such as saliva SARS-CoV-2 PCR testing,[6] allowing for large-scale screening and early detection of asymptomatic carriers. This proactive approach has helped to identify and isolate infected individuals promptly, preventing community transmission. The adoption of saliva PCR testing had also significantly reduced the need of manpower to perform nasopharyngeal swabs and reduced the risk of viral transmission.

EARLY AND EFFECTIVE ANTIVIRAL TREATMENT

Research from recent epidemics including SARS 2003, Middle East respiratory syndrome, and the 2009 swine-flu pandemic has demonstrated the importance of early treatment among high-risk elderly and patients with chronic illness. Hong Kong has embraced early and effective repurposing antiviral treatment options for COVID-19 before specific antivirals against SARS-CoV-2 became available. Both in vitro studies and randomized controlled trials have demonstrated that the use of interferon beta-1b, lopinavir–ritonavir, and ribavirin triple therapy has shown promising results in viral load suppression, reduced the severity of symptoms, and prevented disease progression.[7] Subsequently, during the 2nd year of the pandemic, specific antivirals including nitrelmavir/ritonavir and molnupiravir became available. Early outpatient treatment with these antivirals among the elderlies and immunocompromised patients has effectively reduced mortality, disease severity, hospitalization, and intensive care units admission.[8] Effective viral-load suppression has also reduced subsequent cytokine activation and inflammatory reaction. This minimizes the use of prolonged steroid treatment and associated adverse effects. The application of monoclonal antibodies against SARS-CoV-2 was also effective in the immunocompromised patients who failed to mount sufficient immunogenicity after multiple doses of COVID-19 vaccination.

VACCINATION CAMPAIGN

Hong Kong recognized the importance of a comprehensive vaccination strategy to achieve population-wide immunity. The government collaborated with global vaccine manufacturers to secure a diverse portfolio of vaccines, including inactivated and messenger ribonucleic acid (mRNA) vaccines. This allowed individuals to choose the vaccine that best suited their needs and preferences, enhancing vaccine uptake and coverage. More than 90% and 85% of the population have received two and three doses of the COVID-19 vaccine, respectively.[9] Studies have demonstrated that the elderly population receiving three doses of either the inactivated or mRNA vaccines would achieve a 95% effectiveness in preventing death and severe diseases.[10] Other studies have demonstrated that heterologous vaccine boosting was highly immunogenic.[11] Hong Kong is also the only city to have a continuous monitoring of adverse events following immunization for the entire vaccinated population.

CONTROL OF COVID-19 AND HYBRID IMMUNITY

Through a combination of early quarantine measures, face masking, early diagnostic testing, effective treatment options, and whole-population vaccination, Hong Kong has achieved significant control over the spread of COVID-19. The concept of hybrid immunity, which involves a combination of natural immunity acquired through previous infection and vaccination-induced immunity, has played a crucial role in reducing the impact of the virus on the population. This hybrid immunity approach has helped Hong Kong transition from pandemic to endemic status, where the virus remains present but with minimal impact on public health.

PANDEMIC RESEARCH ALLIANCE

To enhance and strengthen the management of COVID-19, Hong Kong has recently established the Pandemic Research Alliance in the postpandemic era. Anchored by various renowned global experts, this alliance aimed to pool resources, expertise, and research findings to detect the emergence of novel viruses from animals with the potential of causing pandemics among humans. This allows the development of universal vaccines and antivirals against these emerging viral infections, which threaten to cause another pandemic.[12]

CONCLUSION

Experience learned from the SARS 2003 and COVID-19 have completely changed the strategies for tackling future pandemics. A close surveillance of emerging viral infections, modernization of hospital isolation facilities, rapid diagnostic techniques, and development of a universal vaccine will allow us to prevent future pandemics, with the least interruption to global activities and the economy.

REFERENCES

1. Peiris JS, Lai ST, Poon LL, Guan Y, Yam LY, Lim W, et al; SARS study group. Coronavirus as a possible cause of severe acute respiratory syndrome. Lancet. 2003;361(9366): 1319-25.
2. Peiris JS, Chu CM, Cheng VC, Chan KS, Hung IF, Poon LL, et al; HKU/UCH SARS Study Group. Clinical progression and viral load in a community outbreak of coronavirus-associated SARS pneumonia: A prospective study. Lancet. 2003;361(9371):1767-72.
3. Cheng VC, Lau SK, Woo PC, Yuen KY. Severe acute respiratory syndrome coronavirus as an agent of emerging and reemerging infection. Clin Microbiol Rev. 2007;20(4): 660-94.
4. Cheng VC, Wong SC, Chan VW, So SY, Chen JH, Yip CC, et al. Air and environmental sampling for SARS-CoV-2 around hospitalized patients with coronavirus disease 2019 (COVID-19). Infect Control Hosp Epidemiol. 2020;41(11):1258-65.
5. Cheng VC, Wong SC, Chuang VW, So SY, Chen JH, Sridhar S, et al. The role of community-wide wearing of face mask for control of coronavirus disease 2019 (COVID-19) epidemic due to SARS-CoV-2. J Infect. 2020;81(1):107-14.
6. To KK, Tsang OT, Leung WS, Tam AR, Wu TC, Lung DC, et al. Temporal profiles of viral load in posterior oropharyngeal saliva samples and serum antibody responses during infection by SARS-CoV-2: An observational cohort study. Lancet Infect Dis. 2020;20(5):565-74.
7. Hung IF, Lung KC, Tso EY, Liu R, Chung TW, Chu MY, et al. Triple combination of interferon beta-1b, lopinavir-ritonavir, and ribavirin in the treatment of patients admitted to hospital with COVID-19: An open-label, randomised, phase 2 trial. Lancet. 2020;395(10238):1695-704.
8. Wong CKH, Au ICH, Lau KTK, Lau EHY, Cowling BJ, Leung GM. Real-world effectiveness of molnupiravir and nirmatrelvir plus ritonavir against mortality, hospitalisation, and in-hospital outcomes among community-dwelling, ambulatory patients with confirmed SARS-CoV-2 infection during the omicron wave in Hong Kong: An observational study. Lancet. 2022;400(10359):1213-22.
9. Centre for Health Protection. (2024). Statistics on Government COVID-19 vaccination program. [online] Available from https://www.chp.gov.hk/en/features/106989.html [Last accessed February, 2024].

10. McMenamin ME, Nealon J, Lin Y, Wong JY, Cheung JK, Lau EHY, et al. Vaccine effectiveness of one, two, and three doses of BNT162b2 and CoronaVac against COVID-19 in Hong Kong: A population-based observational study. Lancet Infect Dis. 2022;22(10): 1435-43.
11. Zhang R, Liu D, Leung KY, Fan Y, Lu L, Chan PC, et al. Immunogenicity of a Heterologous Prime-Boost COVID-19 Vaccination with mRNA and Inactivated Virus Vaccines Compared with Homologous Vaccination Strategy against SARS-CoV-2 Variants. Vaccines (Basel). 2022;10(1):72.
12. South China Morning Post. (2023). Pandemic prep: Hong Kong disease expert, global research alliance vow to focus studies on flu and coronaviruses before next major disease emerges. [online] Available from https://www.scmp.com/news/hong-kong/health-environment/article/3243820/hong-kong-disease-expert-global-research-alliance-vow-focus-studies-flu-and-coronaviruses-bid [Last accessed February, 2024].

CHAPTER 12

COVID-19 and Dentistry

Elaine Cardoso, Noah Fine, Michael Glogauer, Francis Johnson, Michael Goldberg, Lorne M Golub, Howard Tenenbaum

SUMMARY

Severe acute respiratory syndrome coronavirus 2 (SARS-CoV-2) is a respiratory virus transmitted rapidly between individuals. In the popular imagination, one cannot conceive of greater viral exposure than the close interpersonal and respiratory contact occurring in dental procedures. Given this belief, it was essential to offer a chapter on dental care and the COVID pandemic. However, the conceptual relationship between COVID-19 and dental treatment goes far beyond these conventional beliefs. In this chapter, we explore a much wider picture connecting dental research with COVID-19.

The pathophysiology of SARS-CoV-2 infection is characterized by rapid virus replication and aggressive inflammatory responses that can lead to acute respiratory distress syndrome (ARDS) within as short a time as a few days after the onset of symptoms. It is suspected that a dysfunctional immune response is the main cause of SARS-CoV-2 infection-induced lung destruction and mortality due to massive infiltration of hyperfunctional neutrophils in these organs. There is an interesting parallel in our dental world. In the oral cavity, neutrophils are recruited constantly to combat microorganisms in the dental biofilm. Hyperfunctional neutrophil phenotypes cause destruction of periodontal tissues leading to chronic periodontitis. Both disease models arise because of elevated host defenses against invading organisms, while concurrently causing host damage/disease when the immune activity becomes excessive. As researchers begin to understand the link between oral and systemic diseases and their potential synergistic impact on general health, we argue that lessons learned from translational periodontology research can suggest therapeutic options potentially effective for the management of both oral and nonoral diseases. In this chapter, we connect concepts from periodontal research on oral inflammation while exploring host modulation therapy (HMT) used for periodontitis as a potential strategy for the prevention of ARDS, a deadly outcome of COVID-19. We suggest that HMT, although developed initially for management of periodontitis could inhibit proteases, cytokines, and the oxidative stress that underlie ARDS, providing safe and effective treatments for COVID-19. We also present potentially useful approaches, evolving from dental research studies for management of transmission of COVID-19/SARS-CoV-2 or any other biopathogens (including nonbiological pathogens) in the setting of dental treatment, approaches that can be adopted readily in any medical facility where similar risks for transmission might exist.

FROM THE RESEARCH BENCH TO THE CHAIRSIDE

The outbreak of viral pneumonia cases from SARS-CoV-2 was first reported by the Chinese government in December 2019.[1] As with other viral diseases SARS-CoV-2 can cause various respiratory infections, including multifocal interstitial pneumonia leading to severe disease and death in infected patients.[2]

Acute respiratory distress syndrome can be caused by many pathogens including influenza and coronavirus. Although its precise pathophysiologic mechanisms are not completely clear, it could be the result of direct damage caused by the viral pathogen and then, more importantly, the triggering of a complex dysregulation of the inflammatory environment.[3,4] Indeed, it has been argued that the host-mediated lung and other tissue damage has more to do with the massive infiltration of polymorphonuclear neutrophils (PMNs) and other cells of the innate immune system in the lungs rather than purely direct viral damage in relation to morbidity and mortality.[4-6]

Immunoinflammatory Pathogenesis of COVID-19

Data from cohorts of critically ill patients with COVID-19-related pneumonia provide evidence of cytokine profiles like those of hyperinflammatory states seen in bacterial and viral pneumonias.[5,7] SARS-CoV-2 invades the host cell by binding of its viral spike glycoprotein to the host's cellular receptor for angiotensin-converting enzyme 2 (ACE2). Once in the cell, the virus may "deceive" the immune system through strategies that prevent pattern recognition receptors (PRRs) such as toll-like receptors (TLRs) from recognizing pathogen-associated molecular patterns (PAMPs) and will start replicating freely using the cells' organelles and other cellular components.[8] In addition, SARS-CoV-2 has also evolved strategies that interfere in the production of type I/III IFN which are essential for the development of effective immunity.[8] As a result of this state of unchecked replication, SARS-CoV-2 can reach high titers shortly after initial infection that leads to an exponential production of PAMPs, with ensuing cell damage and release of damage-associated molecular patterns (DAMPs), all of which trigger hyperactive inflammatory responses.[9]

The attachment of SARS-CoV-2 to ACE2 for host cell entry leads to down-regulation of ACE2 and a subsequent increase of angiotensin II (ANG II)[10-15] which dysregulates the renin-angiotensin system (RAS).[16] In elevated levels, ANG II acts as a proinflammatory mediator that ultimately activates nuclear factor kappa B (NF-κB), disintegrin, and metalloprotease 17 (ADAM17).[17] This activated proinflammatory environment triggers the production of reactive oxygen species (ROS), fibrosis, matrix metalloproteinases (MMPs), and production of cytokines such as interleukin-6 (IL-6) and IL-8 by macrophages and recruitment of PMNs. The virus also activates NF-κB[10,14] that amplifies downstream signaling for cytokine production.[13,14] The release of cytokines rapidly activates pathogenic T helper type 1 (Th1) cells which then secrete additional proinflammatory cytokines.[10,11,18] This is followed by additional infiltration of macrophages and PMNs into alveolar cavities where they begin to contribute to the hyperinflammatory response.[10,13,14] ANG II is also known to trigger the coagulation cascade by activating platelets through surface ANG II receptors binding and inducing platelet shape change[19] both of which are associated with thrombosis.[20] In summary, SARS-CoV-2 binding to ACE2 for cell invasion is likely the first step for activation of the cytokine storm which releases uncontrolled levels of cytokines, including IL-1β, IL-6, IL-8, and IL-10[21] that prime the host for development of hyperactive inflammatory responses. Manifestation of the cytokine storm is extremely complex but in general, in addition to virus-induced infiltration of inflammatory cells to the lungs causing oxidative stress and initial inflammation, it relies on even more PMN infiltration into the lung. The PMNs produce cytokines, MMPs, PMN elastase, ROS, and nitric oxide (NO) which when released into the inflamed tissue[21,22] cause diffuse alveolar damage, pulmonary edema, pulmonary fibrosis, acute lung tissue destruction, multiple organ failure, and death. These developments essentially describe ARDS as seen in patients suffering from COVID-19.[10-15]

The PMNs are the first and most numerous innate immune cells to reach the infection site and therefore play a central role in the resolution of inflammation through specific mechanisms of virus inactivation including the release of MMPs, cytokines, ROS, peroxidases, and PMN neutrophil extracellular traps (NETs).[23] This is of course protective. But PMNs can also become "hyperactive", and when this happens, the PMN contribution to antiviral defense can cause harmful effects to the host including the development of pneumonia and ARDS.[24-26] Paradoxically then, despite the critical roles played by PMN cells insofar as clearance of viral pathogens it is recognized that excessively sensitized/activated PMN responses promote a vicious cycle of inflammatory damage to the very tissues to which they were dispatched as a consequence of a PMN-induced cytokine storm.[23] Notably, MMP-2 and MMP-9 destroy the extracellular matrix in the lungs by degrading collagen found in the basement membrane comprising their parenchymal architecture.[21] The virucidal effects of ROS and the recruitment and activation of even more PMNs through the production of cytokines can perpetuate the hyperinflammatory response thereby leading to lung and other tissue injuries including the development of vasculitides and thrombotic conditions characteristic of ARDS.[23,26] In addition, ROS production increases vascular and epithelial permeability further, allowing for continuous infiltration of PMNs and serosanguinous exudates into the alveolar space.[26] Finally, the formation of NETs aided by activated platelets in response to endothelial damage, ROS and IL-1β production, and virus replication may increase the risk of thromboembolic events in COVID-19 patients by triggering complement activation and further fueling the coagulation cascade **(Flowchart 1)**.[8] A summary of the role of PMNs on the severity of COVID-19 in recent studies is shown in **Table 1**.

To prevent this, we hypothesize that any treatment which could prevent excess PMN infiltration and hyperactivation while also blocking excessive levels of MMP activity, elastase activities, and simultaneously reducing excessive ROS levels or activity might represent a useful approach to the prevention and/or amelioration of the morbidity and mortality associated with the cytokine storm/ARDS in patients with COVID-19.

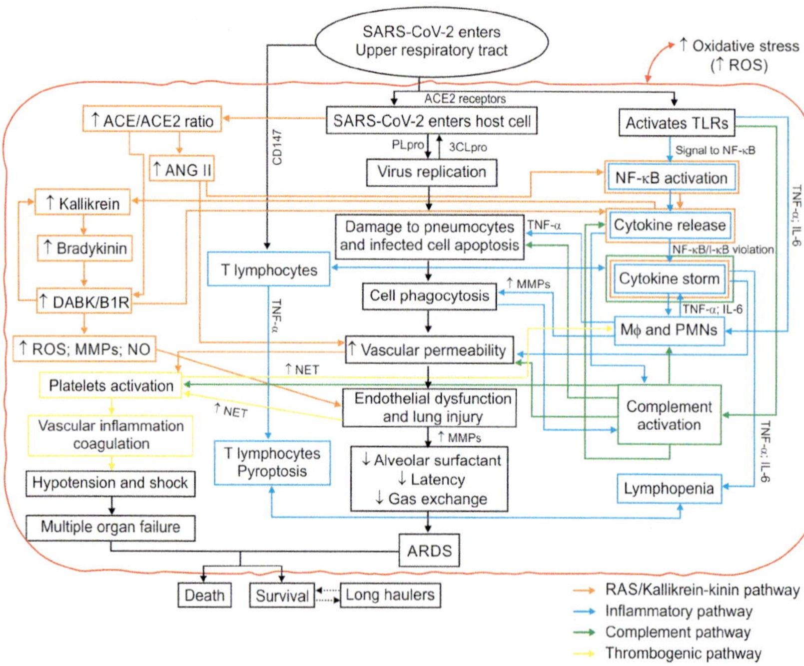

FLOWCHART 1: Schematic representation of the interactions amongst and between four independent pathophysiologic pathways involved in the cytokine storm cascade during COVID-19. Note mechanisms for COVID parallel those also described for periodontal diseases.

(ACE2: angiotensin-converting enzyme 2; ARDS: acute respiratory distress syndrome; DABK: des-Arg[9]-bradykinin; MMPs: matrix metalloproteinases; NF-κB: nuclear factor kappa B; NO: nitric oxide; PMNs: polymorphonuclear neutrophils; ROS: reactive oxygen species; SARS-CoV-2: severe acute respiratory syndrome coronavirus 2)

TABLE 1: Summary of the role of PMNs on the severity of COVID-19 in recent studies.

As predictors of poor outcomes	Higher PMN counts in nonsurvivors than in survivors[5]
	Increased NET formation associated with COVID-19-related ARDS[27]
	Increased NET formation as a potential biomarker for disease severity[27]
	PMN-to-lymphocyte ratio as the most promising predictive factor for critical illness incidence of COVID-19 pneumonia[28]
	Markers of PMN activation amongst the most potent discriminators of critical illness[29]
	PMN activation preceding the onset of critical illness and predicting mortality[29]
	Higher levels of specific markers of NETs in patients receiving mechanical ventilation than in those breathing room air[30]
	Neutrophilia observed In the last 24-h preceding death[31]
	NETs infiltrate in lungs of patients with a fatal outcome[31]
	Dramatic increase of PMNs with COVID-19 severity and ARDS[32]
	Increased number of circulating PMNs as an indicator of worse outcomes[2]
Linked to dysregulated immune response	Blood PMNs produce high levels of NETs; NETs are highly detected in the tracheal aspirate and lung tissue[33]
	SARS-CoV-2–activated PMNs induce lung epithelial cell death through the release of NETs[33]
	PMN activation-associated signatures prominently enriched in severe patient groups[34]
	Dysregulated NET formation in lungs[4]

(ARDS: acute respiratory distress syndrome; NET: neutrophil extracellular trap; PMNs: polymorphonuclear neutrophils; SARS-CoV-2: severe acute respiratory syndrome coronavirus 2)

Links between Oral Inflammation and Systemic Disease

While evidence of associations between periodontal diseases and systemic conditions have long been noted,[35] there has been increased interest in determining the underlying mechanisms that might explain the oral-systemic pathophysiology. We suggest that a causal and indeed bidirectional link may exist between periodontitis and systemic noncommunicable diseases. However, we also have to recognize that they could also be manifestations of common underlying pathophysiological mechanisms. This said, these two concepts are not mutually exclusive, and therefore we must emphasize that both putative mechanisms could be involved in those associations, as demonstrated by studies that show bidirectionality of association. For instance, early epidemiological studies have demonstrated the bidirectional adverse interrelationship between an altered host inflammatory response in

PD and the metabolic imbalance in diabetes[36] while more recently, a causal association was demonstrated between periodontitis and chronic kidney diseases mediated via oxidative stress.[37] We also point out that oxidative stress is a key element of PMN hyperfunctionality related to overproduction of ROS and downregulation of endogenous antioxidants such as NrF2-mediated expression of superoxide dismutase.[38] Inflammation is therefore the common factor amongst periodontitis and the chronic diseases of aging, or simply "the disease".[39] Insofar the individual's susceptibility to systemic diseases, our research supports the hypothesis that PD sensitizes or primes the peripheral innate immune system, and predominantly the PMNs in such a manner as to allow those cells to trigger and/or exacerbate inflammatory diseases in distant organ systems.[40]

Periodontal Disease-induced Immunopathology and COVID-19

The oral cavity is unique in that the teeth are the only structures in the body that de facto protrude through the lining epithelium, in this case the gingival tissues. As such a unique seal exists between the gingiva and tooth surfaces and therefore between the oral cavity and its contents thereby preventing ingress of microbial or other pathogens into the body.[41] This biologic seal, specifically a connective tissue and epithelial attachment to cementum, is not perfect and is permeable even in health but more so in states of inflammation. To enhance protection from pathogens, cells of the innate immune system such as PMNs are recruited constantly to the oral cavity as part of a healthy and self-limiting inflammatory response against the challenges imposed by the oral microorganisms found in the dental biofilm.[42] Interestingly, while bacteria or their byproducts may lead to periodontal tissue damage, it is the host immunoinflammatory response to microorganisms in dental biofilms, when uncontrolled, which is considered the main cause of periodontal pathogenesis,[39,43] something akin to destruction of lung tissues observed in ARDS. In parallel to what is seen in ARDS, the initial host immune response starts when PRRs expressed in the membrane of epithelial cells and gingival fibroblasts interact with PAMPs, including lipopolysaccharide (LPS) found in the cell wall of specific periodontal bacteria.[44] These pathophysiological effects related to periodontitis are similar to the effects of SARS-CoV-2 spike protein produced on host cells that have been transfected with the mRNA provided by the current COVID-19 vaccines. In this regard, there is good evidence that spike protein also activates TLRs.[45] This alone supports the parallelism between the pathophysiological mechanisms of diseases in the mouth to other sites and might also help explain why periodontitis could be a risk factor for the development of severe COVID-19. Other mechanisms might relate to LPS. LPS (in addition to the spike protein) is considered a potent ligand for TLR4[46] and activation of both the TLR2 and TLR4 pathways has been described in studies with *Porphyromonas gingivalis*.[47] PAMP-TLRs binding and MyD88 signaling results in the activation of the downstream signaling pathways associated with inflammation and upregulation of proinflammatory transcription factors, such as NF-κB,[48] leading to the release of inflammatory cytokines and chemokines.[49,50] The most common cytokines involved in this process are tumor necrosis factor-alpha (TNF-α), interleukin-1β (IL-1β), IL-6, and IL-8,[51,52] while chemokines include CXCL8/IL-8, CCL2, CCL3, and CCL5[49,50] and their release causes vasodilation and chemical gradients that facilitate the migration of leukocytes, mostly PMNs from the vasculature to the site of injury.[53] Infiltration of such inflammatory cells leads to release of ROS, MMPs, and NETs, as well as to chemotaxis and phagocytosis as defense mechanisms against infection and inflammation.[54-58] However, as periodontal diseases are not considered as a classic bacterial infection but rather a dysbiotic disease such mechanisms are necessary but possibly not sufficient to cause disease.[59] Periodontal dysbiosis leads to a disturbance of the local homeostasis and immune subversion that increases microbial colonization, virulence, and persistence to disease, and result in persistent recruitment of PMNs[60] with hyperfunctional or hyperactive phenotypes.[42,54-56,61-63] Similar to what happens in patients with COVID-19, these now hyperactivated PMNs pour out high levels of ROS and degradative enzymes along with ever increasing levels of proinflammatory cytokines.[55,56,62] These actions lead to severe destruction of the connective tissues about the affected teeth leading to pain, bleeding, and ultimately tooth loss.[58,64]

This phenotype of hyperinflammatory PMNs has also been observed to play an important role in the pathogenesis of systemic diseases such as diabetes and cardiovascular disease, suggesting an epidemiological association between periodontal diseases and systemic conditions.[65,66] More importantly, these hyperactivated phenotypes have been observed in severe cases of COVID-19,[67,68] as well as in aging-related conditions.[69] Therefore, the presence of periodontitis in patients who are infected with SARS-CoV-2 could represent an as yet unrecognized comorbidity that could contribute to more severe symptoms of COVID-19. While there are now emerging scientific publications that align with this suggestion,[70,71] it still stands in the grounds of scientific inference. Two plausible mechanisms may explain this association—one being related to the periodontitis-induced inflammatory response; a preexisting proinflammatory state. This could act synergistically and therefore amplify the systemic inflammatory response induced by infection with SARS-CoV-2. Another possibility includes the notion there could be a genetic predisposition of the host to develop hyperinflammatory conditions that are favorable to both the development of PD and COVID-19. Regarding the former, our team's previous research has shown that an increase in the level of hyperactivated PMNs in bone marrow and blood can be caused by periodontal inflammation and that this predisposes to an exacerbated PMN response to distant inflammatory conditions. In other words, PD primes the immune system and thus intensifies the overall innate immune response, thus exacerbating general inflammatory disease[40] including COVID-19.

Similarly, in an experimental study of the respiratory mucosa before, during, and after respiratory syncytial virus (RSV) infection in humans, participants who succumbed to infection had more activated PMNs in their airways before exposure to the virus than those who staved off infection. After viral exposure, a reduction in antiviral response in the neutrophilic mucosal environment was observed, more specifically suppression of IL-17, followed by disease onset. The authors hypothesized that primed PMNs, typically associated with immune response to previous bacterial infections might increase the individual's susceptibility to symptomatic viral infections and potentially even COVID-19.[72] A strong hyperactivation phenotype in peripheral PMNs has already been directly associated with severe cases of COVID-19, including increased phagocytosis, degranulation and chemotaxis, and increased expression of genes involved in proinflammatory cytokine release. Within these severe cases, the emergence of an immature PMN population, characteristic of emergency myelopoiesis, was the main difference observed between the immune responses in fatal and nonfatal cases of COVID-19.[73] NET formation in tissue injury and thrombotic complications are additional pathogenic mechanisms whereby circulating PMNs can lead to more severe COVID-19.[4,27,30,31,33] This highlights another potential mechanism linking PD as a potential comorbidity in COVID-19 cases—the prothrombotic state as a result of PD-associated hemodynamic, endothelial, and inflammatory triggers that may lead to an abnormality in the coagulation or fibrinolysis system.[74]

From Bench to Chairside with a Bridge to the Bedside—Host Modulation Therapy

The concept of HMT emerged for the treatment of periodontitis almost 40 years ago, after the identification of host-response mechanisms as the mediators of the destruction of the collagen-rich periodontal tissues and subsequent experiments with systemic drugs that inhibited collagen- and bone-destructive enzymes. Around the same time, HMT was shown to be effective for downregulation of pathologically elevated levels of inflammation in systemic conditions such as arthritis, cancer, lung and cardiovascular diseases, and rosacea.[75] Based on this concept, we have presented evidence, described initially in the periodontal research literature, about the protective properties of a new approach to therapy, HMT, that fits precisely the treatment needs of patients with COVID-19/SARS-CoV-2 infection. And, unlike other medications being investigated for the treatment of COVID-19-mediated lung disease there are virtually no concerns about potential toxicity. Indeed, one might also come to the conclusion that repurposed medications used to control the cytokine storm seen in ARDS and COVID-19 including but not limited to ivermectin and/or hydroxychloroquine could be considered for management of oral inflammatory diseases.

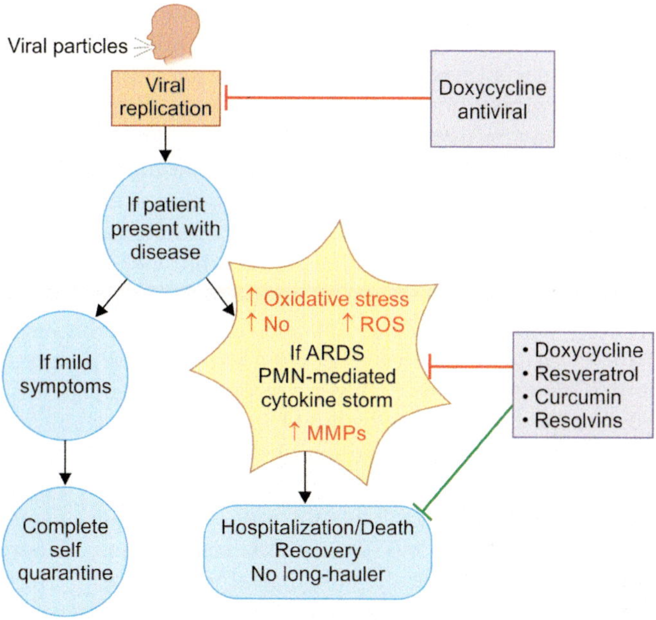

FLOWCHART 2: Proposed multidrug treatment approach, developed in part from therapeutic targets identified for management of periodontal diseases for each phase of COVID-19 presenting both inhibitory (in red) and stimulating or improvement-associated effects (in green). Note also that the use of antivirals (other than doxycycline) is depicted in a slightly faded font to delineate that these other therapeutics were not developed from or based on periodontal research investigations.

(ARDS: acute respiratory distress syndrome; MMPs: matrix metalloproteinases; NO: nitric oxide; ROS: reactive oxygen species)

The rationale for this proposed treatment approach is based on the use of some or all the compounds identified above to inhibit the cytokine storm/ARDS, including PMN-mediated hyperinflammatory responses and tissue destruction and including the development of thromboembolic disorders. This approach could reduce hospitalization, intensive care unit (ICU) admissions, and death associated with COVID-19 markedly as suggested in **Flowchart 2**. We suggest that the SARS-CoV-2 pandemic has highlighted the need for a greater understanding of the role of PMNs in combating viral infections, as COVID-19-related PMN-mediated inflammation in the lungs can be life-threatening.[4] While supporting the potential role of PD-related innate immune response in systemic inflammatory conditions, our team proposes the use of HMT, as designed initially for treatment of PD for treatment of systemic inflammatory diseases that interact with PD,[41] as well as in the prevention and treatment of ARDS, given the similarity of the underlying inflammatory mechanisms. Hereunder we describe the tenets of HMT.

The HMT has been established in periodontology as a successful therapeutic approach for management of chronic periodontal and refractory periodontal diseases, all of which are PMN-mediated disorders. This therapy, pioneered by our group (notably Dr Golub's group), was a paradigm shift in periodontal therapy for using tetracycline-based molecules and not reliant on their antimicrobial properties, to downregulate the activities of PMN-derived MMPs, suppression of inflammatory cytokines, and for quenching of ROS.[76-79] In relation to periodontitis, work has focused on the use of subantimicrobial dose doxycycline (Periostat®), but higher dose use over a short term is certainly feasible when treating extreme cases of inflammation as in the acute stage of COVID-19. This has also led to the development of effective treatment for rosacea using subantimicrobial-dose doxycycline slow release form (Oracea®/Aprillon®).[80] More recently, this concept was boosted by Serhan's studies on proresolving lipid mediators in which he argues that a failure in resolution of inflammation rather than its hyperactivation leads to chronic inflammation.[81,82] Preclinical studies have shown that treatment with lipid mediators after experimentally induced periodontitis in animals was associated with bone loss prevention, regeneration of periodontal tissues, and bacterial shifts in the subgingival microbiota.[83-85] In humans, differences in proresolving lipid mediator profiles were observed between periodontally healthy and periodontitis participants and thus associated with the state of periodontal inflammation.[86] These targets are important factors contributing to the breakdown of periodontal tissues, but also to other tissues being attacked by dysregulated inflammation-mediated destruction observed in periodontitis and ARDS (including stimulation of the vasculitides). Along similar lines, our group has shown that the flavonoids, resveratrol, and curcumin, downregulate ROS-mediated oxidative stress, inhibit ROS production/activity, and inhibit proinflammatory cytokine formation in animal model studies of periodontitis, which should protect tissues under inflammatory attack.[87,88] In animals subjected to cigarette smoke inhalation, we showed that resveratrol effectively blocks the harmful effects of aryl hydrocarbons found in cigarette smoke and the environment, which could be very important inasmuch as smoking represents a significant comorbidity for COVID-19 and is also a major risk factor for periodontitis and favor healing.[89,90] There is also evidence animal model data showing that by using HMT, the development of ARDS can be blocked.[91,92]

We suggest that the effectiveness of HMT could be independent of the type of infectious virus because it targets the host's cellular mechanisms that propagate ARDS (and of course PD) and not only the virus itself. Therefore, we suggest that mutations of the virus should be equally less material insofar as the putative effectiveness of HMT in prevention and treatment of ARDS. Recent evidence showed that tetracyclines have in vitro activity in postentry stages of the infection with SARS-CoV-2[93] and resveratrol blocks replication of coronavirus and other respiratory viruses.[94,95] We propose that the use of drug/nutraceutical HMT described initially for periodontitis could reduce morbidity, mortality, and possibly longer-term sequelae of COVID-19. Another potentially important role related to the use of HMT, and doxycycline in particular, is that it attenuates TLR-induced inflammatory pathways which as discussed above play a critically important role in manifestation of the pathologically elevated inflammatory response to SARS-CoV-2.[96]

Aerosols in dentistry and SARS-CoV-2—what do scientific enquiries tell us about their management and the promotion of a safe working environment?

COVID AND IMPLICATIONS FOR THE CLINICAL MILIEU IN DENTISTRY; ELEVATED UNIVERSAL PRECAUTIONS

In addition to overlapping principles within the biomedical realm, other concepts and procedures developed in relation to the practice of dentistry and pertaining to the SARS-CoV-2 pandemic including COVID-19 (the disease) have arisen which might be useful in other medical settings as we shall describe below. Concepts and measures adopted during the COVID pandemic might prove useful not only for other medical settings as noted above but also can be used should other, possibly even more pathogenic, virulent, or contagious respiratory pathogens emerge, bacterial or vial. This said, we must also point out that within the context of the COVID pandemic there have been no reported incidences of viral contagion being spread to patients even when not all of the measures described below are implemented and this was demonstrated well in another publication that assessed over 2,800 patients over an 6 months period.[97] But to reiterate, other pathogens, for example drug-resistant tuberculosis could emerge at any time and could be managed by way of the approaches described in the following section.

Aerosols Contain Virus/Viral RNA

According to research published recently, aerosols contain virus (in particular SARS-CoV-1 and -2) which can remain viable for 3 hours.[98] This study also demonstrated that viral survival is highly dependent on the surface upon which it finally comes to rest. Although the findings in this paper are reliable insofar as scientific methodology is concerned (albeit with missing methodological information), they might not be wholly comparable to conditions experienced under something we will refer to as "real-world situations". In this investigation, aerosols containing SARS-CoV-2 were manufactured in a laboratory nebulizer and fed into a Goldberg drum.[98] The drum is a 2 by 6 feet chamber that rotates around its axis and in which an internal wedge aids the contained air to move in synchrony with the drum.[99] Due to the compact nature of the drum, the virus cannot dissipate, and it might be anticipated that this favors high aerosol retention and a low settling rate over time.[100] But how closely does this represent the "real-world situations" where air movement, convection, and other factors that could dissipate a naturally occurring aerosol would be present, with or without viral particles that themselves would not alter aerosol behavior?

The investigators then tested for the presence of viral RNA by using reverse transcription polymerase chain reaction (RT-PCR) methods that were not described in detail. Depending on the degree of stringency among other things, this testing method is highly sensitive. It can also have high specificity but in the end, it can only report the presence or absence of viral RNA, and not necessarily the presence of viable virus. However, the investigators also tested for viral viability by inoculating their samples (from aerosol, viral particles placed on cardboard, plastic, stainless steel, and copper) into Vero E6 cells and demonstrated viral replication/cytopathological changes in the cells (data not shown).[98] These findings confirm that, at least for our purposes, viable viral particles remain in artificially generated aerosols for several hours and that aerosols within a Goldberg drum do not settle for about 3 hours. If these findings fastidiously replicate conditions in "real-world situations", then theoretically they could be used to inform us about the presence and dangers of aerosols in a dental operatory. This could mean that rather extraordinary measures might be needed in dental practices in order to remove traces of aerosol following the use of an aerosol-generating procedure (AGP). However, it is unclear as to how closely this laboratory-generated aerosol model represents the actual characteristics of human-exhaled and virally loaded aerosols created by use of ultrasonic or highspeed handpieces and in particular the viability of putative viral particles under "real-world situations" as will be discussed below.

We must also realize that viruses or other microorganisms found in aerosols created by ultrasonic cavitation as well as highspeed handpieces could be destroyed under these conditions thereby actually reducing the viral load. Moreover, the use of oral rinses containing, for example, hydrogen peroxide (1.1–2%) can be used prior to treatment which should also reduce the viral load in aerosols generated in dental practices as will be discussed below (more on this below).[101,102]

Other investigations have also demonstrated the presence of SARS-CoV-2 RNA in aerosols in and other surfaces but in this case under "real-world situations". A study conducted in two hospitals in Wuhan China demonstrated the presence of very low concentrations of viral RNA in aerosols from isolation wards and ventilated patient rooms while elevated concentrations were observed in areas prone to crowding such as a patient's toilet.[103] Similarly, high concentrations of SARS-CoV-2 genes were also found in the air and on object surfaces in ICU and general wards in another hospital in Wuhan.[104] However, neither study tested the amount or presence of viable virus in any of the samples. Therefore, it can be concluded at most that viral particles containing viral RNA had been present at some point, but absent testing of viability it cannot be concluded that the whole virus was present or that even any intact viral particles that might have actually been present retained their ability to replicate and cause infection (in animal or cell culture models). Indeed, it has already been recognized that the mere detection of viral RNA in an aerosol cannot in and of itself be used as a surrogate indicator for the presence of biologically active virus.[105] We suggest that this is a critical issue. We also suggest that it is extremely important to identify whether or not viable viruses in the aerosol, should they be detected represent an actual biothreat. In this regard, only viable viruses are infectious but at the same time we also understand that there is an infectious threshold for the number of viral particles required to cause an actual infection in a human. And it is entirely conceivable that the mere presence of "live" virus within an aerosol or on a surface might not indicate that there is actually enough of the virus to cause infection.[105]

Aerosols come in many mixed forms and can contain anything from particles of dust or soil to microbes including bacteria and viruses. When an aerosol is created in a person infected with a microorganism (viral/bacterial) by coughing, sneezing or even speaking among other things, microbe-containing aerosol droplets, or 'bioaerosols' are formed. These aerosols can be comprised of droplets to actual bioaerosols, whose components measure in the range of 1–5 mm to more representative aerosol components in the range of 0.3–100 μm. Notably, aerosols can travel further (hundreds of meters or more) than droplets (1–2 m) before falling to surfaces.[106,107]

Do Aerosols Contain Virus that is Capable of Transmitting Infection?

Airborne transmission, under certain circumstances based on historical experience related to SARS-CoV-2, can lead to outbreaks of disease.[107] As noted above, there is reliable evidence that one can detect both viral RNA and viable virus in laboratory-generated aerosols. But can the same be said for virus particles within naturally occurring aerosols? And in this regard are such viral particles actually infective?

Of great interest in relation to the question posed here is a study (in press/prepublication) that investigated various characteristics of viral particles and/or residua that had been detected and harvested from various sites within the rooms of SARS-CoV-2-infected patients as opposed to the use of a laboratory model that was referred to above. In this study, samples were taken from the air (i.e., aerosol), the floor, air grates, and several other sites. As demonstrated using RT-PCR, RNA for SARS-CoV-2 was found in all sites tested and even under beds. But in this case, when the samples were tested for infectivity/viability using the Vero E6 cell culture model, almost no viral growth/replication could be demonstrated according to the authors. There was minimal evidence for the cytopathological changes expected in the presence of viral replication and only in a small number of samples. Investigators followed up with additional testing, given the negative cell culture results, and sought to identify viral protein, an indicator of the presence of viral coat proteins that would suggest that some intact viral particles might still be present in the samples, or that at least there are remnants of previously intact virus. The results paralleled those found in cell culture but were even clearer cut. Viral protein could not be identified using either western blot or immunofluorescence tests in any of the samples. While it is possible that the levels of viral protein were below the detection thresholds of these two immunoassays, this is unlikely particularly in light of the mainly negative results found in the cultures.

These data suggest that viral particles from SARS-CoV-2 are either not intact and/or lose infectivity in naturally occurring aerosols (and on other surfaces, replication of virus in some samples was considered to be minimal, while viral protein could not be identified in any of the samples taken as noted above). We suggest then that it is probable that viral particles are degraded under "real-world situations". In light of this, one could conclude that under "real-world situations", the most germane to this topic, survival of virus with the ability to infect to any degree is extremely low and possibly nonexistent. In the end, if neither viral proteins nor clear evidence for viral replication in vitro can be shown, then we could conclude that the ability of SARS-CoV-2 derived from aerosols in a clinical setting cannot cause infection of either patients or staff. As noted above, this supports the notion that the mere presence of viral RNA cannot be used as the sole indicator of the presence of infectious virus. And to reiterate, this would mean that upon entering this environment, the risk for becoming infected from an aerosol is extremely low, if not absent altogether. To make this point more emphatically, it should be pointed out that if significant viral replication cannot even be demonstrated in cell culture (where immunity is not a factor), then the ability to infect patients/staff (who have immune systems; albeit SARS-CoV-2 naïve) cannot occur in all probability.

Why Reduce Aerosol/Viral RNA/Virus in a Dental Operatory?

Based on the above, it could be argued that there is no need to manage aerosols in dental offices. Yet, it must also be recognized that we are in the early stages of research as regard SARS-CoV-2, meaning that newer studies might well demonstrate not only the presence of viable virus within aerosols but that the number of particles present is sufficient to cause infection. Moreover, we can anticipate mutations in SARS-CoV-2 as well as the emergence of new and potentially heartier viruses in the future that could retain infectious capacity for far longer. And in this regard, we need to understand that although the evidence suggests that remaining aerosols might not be highly infective, this is certainly not necessarily the public perception.[108] Similarly, health boards and dental regulatory authorities are likely to proceed with an abundance of caution leading to recommendations for management of the environments in dental offices so as to reduce, as much as possible, the risks for infection of staff or patients who might enter rooms in which an AGP has been performed. Therefore, we present here some strategies that could be used to provide the best possible conditions which aim to reduce/eliminate aerosol related issues, while at the same time allowing for practitioners to work as efficiently as possible in the delivery of oral healthcare to their patients. We will not be addressing issues pertaining to the waiting room, or changes to patient booking schedules although there might be additional changes that can be made to these which would have a positive impact on safety in the dental clinic and operatory.

Do Aerosols Remain Suspended for up to 3 Hours?

Concentrations of microbial aerosols were measured in different dental offices with routine use of high-volume aspirators. Although peak levels were over 10 times higher than those from ventilated rooms in hospitals, aerosols tended to dissipate and return to background levels within 10 and 30 minutes.[109]

- Is there anything we can do to reduce the risk further?
  From an operational point of view, it is easiest to prevent as much airborne contamination as possible by reducing saliva's microbial load and/or using physical barriers before it escapes the treatment site. Then a layering of protective procedures to reduce aerosol generation, such as suction systems, followed by air cleaners will mitigate the remaining risk.
- *Pretreatment rinses*: It is argued that incorporation of a preprocedural mouth rinse with 0.12% chlorhexidine can lead to a reduction in the bacterial loads in saliva, and ergo decreases the levels of aerosolized bacteria during dental procedures.[110,111] Similarly, 0.2% chlorhexidine had yielded a significant reduction in airborne bacteria count after a 1-minute rinse.[112] In addition, it has been suggested that a 2% chlorhexidine concentration in oral rinses is bactericidal for a wide number of different bacteria, fungi, and selected viruses in saliva, targeting the oral biofilm as well.[113] Combinations of hydrogen peroxide and chlorhexidine rinses have also been proposed. It was demonstrated that the use of 1.5% hydrogen peroxide rinse prior to the use of a 0.2% chlorhexidine oral rinse significantly decreased bacterial colony-forming units (CFUs) on a patient's chest, on the operator's side, and on the assistant's side in groups that underwent both oral rinses prior to an operation when compared to groups that used just saline or 0.2% chlorhexidine.[101] Despite this, studies on SARS-CoV-2 disregard chlorhexidine as an effective ingredient to eliminate the virus.[102,113,114] But models developed for reducing bacterial loads in aerosols can be interpreted to mean that the use of rinses that have antiviral activity should yield similar results as regards reductions in the viral load within aerosols that might be formed during dental treatment.

Certain flavonoid groups (specifically rhoifolin, herbacetin, and pectolinarin) demonstrate anticoronaviral properties by inhibition of 3C protease, and others (isobavachalcone, herbacitin, helichrysetin, quercetin, 3-beta-d-glucoside, and Torreya nucifera) by inhibition of Middle East respiratory syndrome (MERS)-CoV/3CLpro enzymatic activity.[113] Citrox®, made from natural soluble bioflavonoids found in citrus fruits, demonstrates various antimicrobial activities on oral microbiota including viral particles due to its oxidizing nature, and should be included as pretreatment oral rinses to reduce viral loads.[113]

Methylated beta-cyclodextrin's ability to reduce infectivity of influenza A virus and coronavirus by eliminating cholesterol access has also been studied and its use along with Citrox® has been encouraged for oral rinses/nasal applications.[113] The foregoing notwithstanding, there is currently no direct scientific evidence regarding the effects of preprocedural mouth rinses to reduce SARS-CoV-2 load within aerosols following an AGP such as performing a dental restoration (AGP). Nevertheless, a logical extension of other studies suggests that a 30-second rinse with a 1–1.5% hydrogen peroxide solution, 0.2% povidone iodine, or the use of Citrox® should reduce viral loads within aerosols due to the vulnerability of the virus to oxidation.[102,114] Given that there's no significant downside to the use of pre-procedural rinses, and only potential gains, we argue in favor of ongoing use of the aforementioned. We also point out that whilst there were numerous online references regarding personal protective equipment (PPE), and nonpharmaceutical interventions (NPIs) in dentistry to which we have referred in many cases tangentially, that were sponsored by various dental professional organizations, these are no longer available at the time of this writing when there was no longer a COVID emergency.

- *Rubber dam use:* It has been demonstrated that the use of a rubber dam for dry-field procedures leads to a reduction in the levels of bacteria-laden aerosols[115] while also reducing the levels of saliva- and blood-contaminated aerosols when high-speed handpieces and dental ultrasonic devices are used along with extra high-volume suction.[102,110,116] Given the use of a rubber dam then, it might be argued that the tooth or teeth under treatment might still be contaminated with viral particles (although possibly not if preprocedural rinses are used). Consequently, even with a rubber dam in place, it is possible that a tooth or teeth undergoing treatment could be sources of aerosols containing various particulates, biopathogens including virus particles.[117] Therefore, we propose that the teeth or tooth surfaces can be decontaminated even more by disinfecting surfaces of teeth about to undergo treatment (with an AGP) with 2.5% sodium hypochlorite (NaOCl) in order to minimize the production of aerosols containing live virus.[118]
- *Using a high-volume Evacuation (HVE) Suction can Reduce > 96% of all bacterial aerosols:* Quantitative data suggest a reduction by three orders of magnitude in the release of bacterial aerosol when including an HVE tip or modified suction tip, the latter of which can be used without an assistant (very important for dental hygienist who often work without an assistant). The effectiveness of aerosol filtration is contingent on limited obstruction to the suction tip throughout the procedure and does not eliminate any larger particles or splatter that aerosolize (due to the high kinetic energy of the particle, allowing it to travel against the air current in the suction).[117] We recognize and appreciate the fact that in this case we

have relied on studies focused on the reduction of bacteria-laden aerosols for evidence, it is worth repeating that aerosol behavior is unaffected by the precise nature of the microbes contained therein and there is no reason to believe that the use of HVE would not have similar effects in relation to spread of aerosols containing SARS-CoV-2.

- *Extraoral suction to reduce aerosols*: The use of extraoral suction devices such as extra-oral vacuum aspirators (EOVA) can produce statistically significant reductions in specific bacteria-containing aerosols compared to a control group. The device's ability to "filter" aerosolized *E. coli* was tested using various common dental procedures to generate aerosols. There were statistically significant reductions in the production of aerosols containing bacteria in comparison to control.[119] Similar efficacy in reducing the quantity of airborne droplets and aerosols was observed when extraoral evacuation devices were used along with special aerosol reduction devices (ARD) in conjunction with ultrasonic scalers.[110]
- *Use of high-efficacy particulate air (HEPA) filters*: The building's general heating, ventilation, and air conditioning (HVAC) system works to prevent the spread of microorganisms in the air by diluting and removing contaminated air from a room, controlling the direction of air flow and airflow patterns in a building.[120] This is important because the presence of high air exchange within treatment rooms will reduce the content of aerosols within the treatment-room environment. When renovation of the general ventilation system is not possible, the use of an in-room HEPA cleaner is a good alternative to reduce the concentration of microorganisms in the air and prevent the spread of infectious diseases.[120] Its effectiveness depends on the airflow rate through the unit's filter and airflow patterns in the room; the greater the number of air changes per hour, the faster the airborne pathogens and particulates are removed from the ambient air.[121] It has been demonstrated that HEPA filters remove 99.97% of airborne particles at 0.3 μm[110] and 99.99% of airborne particles < 0.01 μm[122] **(Table 1)** with an appropriate number of air exchanges per hour **(Table 2)**.[121]
- *Ultraviolet germicidal irradiation (UGVI)*: Along with filtration of airborne microorganisms, air disinfection can be carried out by UGVI. Ultraviolet radiation is produced using mercury vapor lamps within the UVC bandwidth of the electromagnetic spectrum[110] and its effectiveness has already been demonstrated against RNA viruses like MERS-CoV and SARS-CoV.[123] Its effect on viral DNA depends on the intensity of UVGI energy and the duration of the exposure. For instance, a single 17-watt UVGI lamp installed through upper room fixtures added the equivalent of 10 air changes per hour (ACH) to the ambient ventilation of 2 ACH, while 2 lamps producing 46 watts added the equivalent of 33 ACH to the ambient ventilation of 4 ACH.[124] Alternatively, portable UVGI modules are designed to be mounted directly on the clean air outlet of a HEPA filter unit, so they can be moved easily from room to room. They are an

TABLE 2: Summary description of PD-900DW according to manufacturer's specifications.

What	3-in-1 clean air machine [HEPA, UVC germicidal light (nonozone producing) and photocatalytic oxidation]
	Offers the ultimate in air filtration and sterilization
Indications	Residential and light commercial applications
	For those suffering from allergies or asthma
	New construction odors, smokers, pets, cooking odors, mold, water, and sewer damage
Installation	On the return air duct of the heating/cooling system
	A portion of this returned air is by-passed through an opening on the rear of the unit and passes through a 5-stage filtration system to discharge clean air back into the return duct
	Can also be mounted on a wall as a stand-alone unit

(HEPA: high-efficacy particulate air; UVC: ultraviolet C)

Source: CDC Guidelines for Environmental Infection Control in Health Facilities, 2003. Available from https://www.cdc.gov/infectioncontrol/pdf/guidelines/environmental-guidelines-P.pdf.

excellent option for disinfecting air between patients but in this case, the UV source is only disinfecting the actual filter but not the air or other operatory surfaces.[121] In recent years, the use of conventional UVC light sources in public settings has been limited due to carcinogenic and cataractogenic concerns.

Currently, studies exploring low dose-rate far-UVC light (207–222 nm) have shown that it can inactivate airborne aerosolized viruses efficiently, and has become a promising and safe alternative to reduce the spread of airborne-mediated infections.[125] It should be emphasized that these methods apply to a wide array of biopathogens including the ability to kill bacterial spores meaning that absent a coronavirus pandemic, such measures would reduce the overall burden of biopathogens that might arise during any period of time when one contagious disease or another (e.g., TB) is trending. However, at this time, we must rely on UVC irradiation and based on current knowledge, it would take no > 1–2 minutes to kill all viral particles in the air and on most surfaces (except those in shadow, say, on the floor under the dental chair). And even with the use of UVC irradiation, it is still good practice to still clean/disinfect surfaces in the usual manner after irradiation is complete. Finally in this regard, it cannot be overstated that when irradiating an operatory/clinic, the areas should be unoccupied by either patients or staff. This is of particular importance where the use of UVC or other UV light might lead to unavoidable chronic/long-term exposure of staff in the workplace. Therefore, alternate approaches that rely perhaps more heavily upon air exchange/filtration rates and routine surface disinfection would be needed.

- *Masks and other PPEs*: A surgical mask has been recommended in all instances in which there is contact between patients and other people for longer than 15 minutes, as well as a surgical mask with a face shield in the event FFP2/FFP3 masks are unavailable.[114] FFP2 masks are equivalent to N95 masks, and N99 along with its equivalent FFP3's offer even stronger filtration (for aerosols and particulates, most of which are considerably larger than viral particles). Either has been deemed acceptable during procedures that risk aerosol droplet production. This said, the evidence currently shows that surgical grade paper masks (grade 3) are noninferior to N95 masks in reducing infection rates in nurses regardless of the measured efficiency and particulate filtering.[126] It must be stressed though, that in all cases one cannot be considered to be completely protected against viral spread when using masks or other PPEs which at best night mitigate some spread, particularly as relates to aerosols but not necessarily to airborne viral particles. And in reality, FFP or "face filtering face piece 2", the European designation, really only filters the same or less aerosol with some claims that it also filters out viral particles. But since these masks filter approximately 94% of *aerosol/droplets* versus the 95% claimed for N95 masks claims that the former also filters out viral particles like SARS-CoV-2 are tenuous at best (to search NIOSH for PPE and other NPI requirements, check: https://search.cdc.gov/search/index.html?query=ffp2%20vs%20n95&siteLimit=NIOSH&dpage=1&strict=true). Moreover, given that neither system provides leak-free protection even when fit perfectly, protection against airborne viral particles should not be taken as proof that protection against spread of COVID-19 is being provided apart from times when there is some barrier protection that can be taken advantage of when AGPs are being done and when some degree of protection might be anticipated. To reiterate, under office conditions where no aerosols or large numbers of droplets are being generated (e.g., the business office), neither N95s nor FFP2s could provide protection against the spread of an airborne virus (SARS-CoV-2, influenza, or otherwise) the operative term here is droplets, which are large versus microscopically sized airborne viral particles which generally evade PPE protection measures. And again, even the most optimally fitted and constructed masks are still leaky.[127]

The use of long sleeve uniforms is also recommended, single-use surgical gowns on top of the uniform, and disinfecting the uniform with chlorine before washing it.[114] We suggest that the use of multiuse gowns is also effective, as long as they are laundered appropriately. With respect to the above, it cannot be overemphasized that the masking PPE approach could be protective against larger aerosolized droplets found commonly in a dental setting but cannot be relied upon to prevent transmission of virus which is airborne as shown in various studies.[128] Indeed, even N95 masks, often touted as a gold standard form of masking-PPE do not prevent viral contagion and were designed in any case to filter out larger particles created in construction sites. The pore sizes on N95 masks are simply inadequate for prevention of the spread of airborne viral particles.[129] Nevertheless, the use of at most, surgical face masks is a worthy approach for the reduction of viral spread insofar as contaminated droplet contamination might be concerned within a dental office or other clinical setting where aerosols might be generated. And of course, there are other nonbiopathogen-related protections in relation to other particulates that are produced as a consequence of dental treatments.

CONCLUSION

Taken together, the experimental evidence discussed suggests that viral RNA from COVID-19 can be detected readily and is spread easily. Under artificial conditions, it might take up to 3 hours for a virally laden (or any) aerosol to settle but this is not the case under "real-world situations". Moreover, the virtual inability to detect either intact virus, or virus that retains its ability to grow in cell culture suggests that even if an aerosol is present, it is unlikely that anyone entering this environment is going to develop an infection.

These conclusions lead us to suggest that the need to close down dental treatment rooms following the generation of a virus (following an AGP) for any significant amount of time is unnecessary. When combined with readily available methods for reducing aerosol levels in the atmosphere of a dental treatment room (air filtration/exchange units), as well as post-treatment irradiation of the operatory with UV(C) light, we can ensure drastic reduction and probably elimination of infectious viral particles that might be left behind after an AGP has been done. In addition, the practice of intratreatment measures including the use of antiviral rinses prior to treatment as well as the use of high-volume suction, we suggest that there is no need to shut down treatment rooms in between patient appointments for 3 hours or even 15 minutes. By following the protocols suggested above, the dental operatory and overall environment of the dental office can be rendered as safe as possible and could even yield general benefits insofar as the quality of air (and safety of surfaces) is concerned even without concerns relating to SARS-CoV-2 or other viral pathogens and this can be done efficiently. Of course, these measures also apply to bacterial pathogens (including their spores) as well as to the reduction of other potentially harmful particulates that are thrown into the air during an AGP.

In general, then, we suggest that we have demonstrated how research focused initially on oral inflammatory diseases has illuminated therapeutic targets that can be attacked by relatively simple and safe compounds, thereby reducing hospitalization, morbidity, and mortality associated with COVID-19. We also discuss potential impact of oral inflammatory diseases and the pathogenesis of COVID-19. In addition to the biomedical parallels that have become evident in the fields of Medicine and Dentistry, we have also discussed some practical or operational matters that have been developed within a dental clinic setting which could prove useful in other clinical settings (e.g., a medical office). And just as importantly the procedures developed for protection from SARS-CoV-2 infection and COVID-19 are just as important in relation to other biopathogens as well as potentially pathogenic particulates that might be found in a clinical setting and in the air. These concepts and their implementation will lead to overall improvements in the atmosphere of active dental clinical centers even under nonpandemic situations and these benefits would apply to any medical center where AGPs might be produced. It cannot be overstated that with implementation of the regimens alluded to above, dental offices will be prepared for any and all respiratory pathogens that might arise so that much needed oral healthcare can proceed even in the midst of a pandemic and without considering the shutting down of this important healthcare service. Yet, we cannot end our discussions in this way alone. To do so would be to implicate dental offices as important and potentially primary sources of contagion, and at this moment in time we refer specifically to SARS-CoV-2 and COVID-19, the disease induced by the former. But this is not the case. There has been absolutely no evidence to show, even before recognition of the presence of SARS-CoV-2 (although it was clearly present prior to recognition!) that dental offices acted as significant sources of contagion. Moreover, and as noted above, the PPE approaches described above are certainly not perfect but even then, with the reintroduction of dental care (and the related aerosols created along with the close contact required between clinicians and patients with open mouths), there have still been no reports showing that attending or working in a dental office poses a greater health risk than attending any other venue. Moreover, the generation of large but inhalable particulates as a result of the performance of dental hard and soft tissue surgical interventions can still contribute to respiratory tract issues which can be mitigated significantly by the use of the NPI and PPE approaches alluded to above.[130] Hence, we also suggest that the responsible approach to these issues might appear to be overcautious but, in the end, will still support improved health and safety needs in the dental clinical setting.

REFERENCES

1. Zhu N, Zhang D, Wang W, Li X, Yang B, Song J, et al. A Novel Coronavirus from Patients with Pneumonia in China, 2019. N Engl J Med. 2020;382:727-33.
2. Huang C, Wang Y, Li X, Ren L, Zhao J, Hu Y, et al. Clinical features of patients infected with 2019 novel coronavirus in Wuhan, China. Lancet. 2020;395:497-506.
3. Wang QW, Su Y, Sheng JT, Gu LM, Zhao Y, Chen XX, et al. Anti-influenza A virus activity of rhein through regulating oxidative stress, TLR4, Akt, MAPK, and NF-κB signal pathways. PLoS One. 2018;13:e0191793.
4. Barnes BJ, Adrover JM, Baxter-Stoltzfus A, Borczuk A, Cools-Lartigue J, Crawford JM, et al. Targeting potential drivers of COVID-19: Neutrophil extracellular traps. J Exp Med. 2020;217:e20200652.
5. Wang D, Hu B, Hu C, Zhu F, Liu X, Zhang J, et al. Clinical characteristics of 138 Hospitalized patients with 2019 Novel coronavirus-infected pneumonia in Wuhan, China. JAMA. 2020;323(11):1061-9.

6. Teijaro JR, Walsh KB, Rice S, Rosen H, Oldstone MB. Mapping the innate signaling cascade essential for cytokine storm during influenza virus infection. Proc Natl Acad Sci U S A. 2014;111:3799-804.
7. Qin C, Zhou L, Hu Z, Zhang S, Yang S, Tao Y, et al. Dysregulation of Immune Response in Patients With Coronavirus 2019 (COVID-19) in Wuhan, China. Clin Infect Dis. 2020;71:762-8.
8. Amor S, Fernández Blanco L, Baker D. Innate immunity during SARS-CoV-2: evasion strategies and activation trigger hypoxia and vascular damage. Clin Exp Immunol. 2020;202:193-209.
9. Domingo P, Mur I, Pomar V, Corominas H, Casademont J, de Benito N. The four horsemen of a viral Apocalypse: The pathogenesis of SARS-CoV-2 infection (COVID-19). EBioMedicine. 2020;58:102887.
10. Hu B, Huang S, Yin L. The cytokine storm and COVID-19. J Med Virol 2020;93(1):250-6.
11. Ragab D, Salah Eldin H, Taeimah M, Khattab R, Salem R. The COVID-19 Cytokine Storm; What We Know So Far. Front Immunol. 2020;11:1446.
12. Sun X, Wang T, Cai D, Hu Z, Chen J, Liao H, et al. Cytokine storm intervention in the early stages of COVID-19 pneumonia. Cytokine Growth Factor Rev. 2020;53:38-42.
13. Hussman JP. Cellular and molecular pathways of COVID-19 and potential points of therapeutic intervention. Front Pharmacol. 2020;11:1169.
14. Mahmudpour M, Roozbeh J, Keshavarz M, Farrokhi S, Nabipour I. COVID-19 cytokine storm: The anger of inflammation. Cytokine. 2020;133:155151.
15. Soy M, Keser G, Atagündüz P, Tabak F, Atagündüz I, Kayhan S. Cytokine storm in COVID-19: pathogenesis and overview of anti-inflammatory agents used in treatment. Clin Rheumatol. 2020;39:2085-94.
16. Ingraham NE, Barakat AG, Reilkoff R, Bezdicek T, Schacker T, Chipman JG, et al. Understanding the renin-angiotensin-aldosterone-SARS-CoV axis: a comprehensive review. Eur Respir J. 2020;56:2000912.
17. Devaux CA, Rolain JM, Raoult D. ACE2 receptor polymorphism: Susceptibility to SARS-CoV-2, hypertension, multi-organ failure, and COVID-19 disease outcome. J Microbiol Immunol Infect. 2020;53:425-35.
18. Ye Q, Wang B, Mao J. The pathogenesis and treatment of the 'Cytokine Storm' in COVID-19. J Infect. 2020;80:607-13.
19. Jagroop IA, Mikhailidis DP. Angiotensin II can induce and potentiate shape change in human platelets: effect of losartan. J Hum Hypertens. 2000;14:581-5.
20. Nachman RL, Rafii S. Platelets, petechiae, and preservation of the vascular wall. N Engl J Med. 2008;359:1261-70.
21. Roy SK, Kendrick D, Sadowitz BD, Gatto L, Snyder K, Satalin JM, et al. Jack of all trades: pleiotropy and the application of chemically modified tetracycline-3 in sepsis and the acute respiratory distress syndrome (ARDS). Pharmacol Res. 2011;64:580-9.
22. Zhou X, Wang D, Ballard-Croft CK, Simon SR, Lee HM, Zwischenberger JB. A tetracycline analog improves acute respiratory distress syndrome survival in an ovine model. Ann Thorac Surg. 2010;90:419-26.
23. Galani IE, Andreakos E. Neutrophils in viral infections: Current concepts and caveats. J Leukoc Biol. 2015;98:557-64.
24. Abraham E. Neutrophils and acute lung injury. Crit Care Med. 2003;31:S195-9.
25. Sideras P, Apostolou E, Stavropoulos A, et al. Activin, neutrophils, and inflammation: just coincidence? Semin Immunopathol. 2013;35:481-99.
26. Potey PM, Rossi AG, Lucas CD, Dorward DA. Neutrophils in the initiation and resolution of acute pulmonary inflammation: understanding biological function and therapeutic potential. J Pathol. 2019;247:672-85.

27. Middleton EA, He XY, Denorme F, Campbell RA, Ng D, Salvatore SP, et al. Neutrophil extracellular traps contribute to immunothrombosis in COVID-19 acute respiratory distress syndrome. Blood. 2020;136:1169-79.
28. Liu J, Liu Y, Xiang P, Pu L, Xiong H, Li C, et al. Neutrophil-to-lymphocyte ratio predicts critical illness patients with 2019 coronavirus disease in the early stage. J Transl Med. 2020;18:206.
29. Meizlish ML, Pine AB, Bishai JD, Goshua G, Nadelmann ER, Simonov M, et al. A neutrophil activation signature predicts critical illness and mortality in COVID-19. Blood Advances. 2021;5:1164-77.
30. Zuo Y, Yalavarthi S, Shi H, Gockman K, Zuo M, Madison JA, et al. Neutrophil extracellular traps in COVID-19. JCI Insight. 2020;5(11):e138999.
31. Radermecker C, Detrembleur N, Guiot J, Cavalier E, Henket M, d'Emal C, et al. Neutrophil extracellular traps infiltrate the lung airway, interstitial, and vascular compartments in severe COVID-19. J Exp Med. 2020;217(12):e20201012.
32. Gong J, Dong H, Xia QS, Huang ZY, Wang DK, Zhao Y, et al. Correlation analysis between disease severity and inflammation-related parameters in patients with COVID-19: a retrospective study. BMC Infect Dis. 2020;20:963.
33. Veras FP, Pontelli MC, Silva CM, Toller-Kawahisa JE, de Lima M, Nascimento DC, et al. SARS-CoV-2-triggered neutrophil extracellular traps mediate COVID-19 pathology. J Exp Med. 2020;217(12):e20201129.
34. Aschenbrenner AC, Mouktaroudi M, Krämer B, Oestreich M, Antonakos N, Nuesch-Germano M, et al. Disease severity-specific neutrophil signatures in blood transcriptomes stratify COVID-19 patients. Genome Med. 2021;13:7.
35. U.S. Department of Health and Human Services. Oral Health in America: A Report of the Surgeon General. United States: National Institute of Dental and Craniofacial Research, National Institutes of Health; 2000.
36. Taylor GW. Bidirectional interrelationships between diabetes and periodontal diseases: an epidemiologic perspective. Ann Periodontol. 2001;6:99-112.
37. Sharma P, Fenton A, Dias IHK, Heaton B, Brown CLR, Sidhu A, et al. Oxidative stress links periodontal inflammation and renal function. J Clin Periodontol. 2021;48:357-67.
38. Chiu AV, Saigh MA, McCulloch CA, Glogauer M. The Role of NrF2 in the regulation of periodontal health and disease. J Dent Res. 2017;96:975-83.
39. Van Dyke TE. Inflammation and periodontal diseases: A reappraisal. J Periodontol. 2008;79:1501-2.
40. Fine N, Chadwick JW, Sun C, Parbhakar KK, Khoury N, Barbour A, et al. Periodontal Inflammation Primes the Systemic Innate Immune Response. J Dent Res. 2021;100: 318-25.
41. Nanci A. Ten Cate's Oral Histology: Development, Structure, and Function. Philadelphia, United States: Elsevier; 2017.
42. Fine N, Hassanpour S, Borenstein A, Sima C, Oveisi M, Scholey J, et al. Distinct Oral Neutrophil Subsets Define Health and Periodontal Disease States. J Dent Res. 2016;95:931-8.
43. Van Dyke TE. The management of inflammation in periodontal disease. J Periodontol. 2008;79:1601-8.
44. Hanada T, Yoshimura A. Regulation of cytokine signaling and inflammation. Cytokine Growth Factor Rev. 2002;13:413-21.
45. Fontes-Dantas FL, Fernandes GG, Gutman EG, De Lima EV, Antonio LS, Hammerle MB, et al. SARS-CoV-2 Spike protein induces TLR4-mediated long-term cognitive dysfunction recapitulating post-COVID-19 syndrome in mice. Cell Rep. 2023;42:112189.
46. Zeng XZ, Zhang YY, Yang Q, Wang S, Zou BH, Tan YH, et al. Artesunate attenuates LPS-induced osteoclastogenesis by suppressing TLR4/TRAF6 and PLCγ1-Ca. Acta Pharmacol Sin. 2020;41:229-36.

47. Hajishengallis G, Sojar H, Genco RJ, DeNardin E. Intracellular signaling and cytokine induction upon interactions of Porphyromonas gingivalis fimbriae with pattern-recognition receptors. Immunol Invest. 2004;33:157-72.
48. Song B, Zhang YL, Chen LJ, T Zhou, WK Huang, X Zhou et al. The role of Toll-like receptors in periodontitis. Oral Dis. 2017;23:168-80.
49. Cavalla F, Araujo-Pires AC, Biguetti CC, Garlet GP. Cytokine Networks Regulating Inflammation and Immune Defense in the Oral Cavity. Curr Oral Health Rep. 2014;1: 104-13.
50. Souto GR, Queiroz CM, Costa FO, Mesquita RA. Relationship between chemokines and dendritic cells in human chronic periodontitis. J Periodontol. 2014;85:1416-23.
51. Garlet GP. Destructive and protective roles of cytokines in periodontitis: a re-appraisal from host defense and tissue destruction viewpoints. J Dent Res. 2010;89:1349-63.
52. Han X, Lin X, Seliger AR, Eastcott J, Kawai T, Taubman MA. Expression of receptor activator of nuclear factor-kappa B ligand by B cells in response to oral bacteria. Oral Microbiol Immunol. 2009;24:190-6.
53. Kolaczkowska E, Kubes P. Neutrophil recruitment and function in health and inflammation. Nat Rev Immunol. 2013;13:159-75.
54. Fredriksson M, Gustafsson A, Asman B, Bergström K. Periodontitis increases chemiluminescence of the peripheral neutrophils independently of priming by the preparation method. Oral Dis. 1999;5:229-33.
55. Matthews JB, Wright HJ, Roberts A, Cooper PR, Chapple IL. Hyperactivity and reactivity of peripheral blood neutrophils in chronic periodontitis. Clin Exp Immunol. 2007;147:255-64.
56. Matthews JB, Wright HJ, Roberts A, Ling-Mountford N, Cooper PR, Chapple IL. Neutrophil hyper-responsiveness in periodontitis. J Dent Res. 2007;86:718-22.
57. Gustafsson A, Asman B. Increased release of free oxygen radicals from peripheral neutrophils in adult periodontitis after Fc delta-receptor stimulation. J Clin Periodontol. 1996;23:38-44.
58. Chapple IL, Matthews JB. The role of reactive oxygen and antioxidant species in periodontal tissue destruction. Periodontol 2000. 2007;43:160-232.
59. Hajishengallis G, Lamont RJ. Beyond the red complex and into more complexity: the polymicrobial synergy and dysbiosis (PSD) model of periodontal disease etiology. Mol Oral Microbiol. 2012;27:409-19.
60. Lamont RJ, Hajishengallis G. Polymicrobial synergy and dysbiosis in inflammatory disease. Trends Mol Med. 2015;21:172-83.
61. Fredriksson M, Gustafsson A, Asman B, Bergström K. Hyper-reactive peripheral neutrophils in adult periodontitis: generation of chemiluminescence and intracellular hydrogen peroxide after in vitro priming and FcgammaR-stimulation. J Clin Periodontol. 1998;25:394-8.
62. Ling MR, Chapple IL, Matthews JB. Peripheral blood neutrophil cytokine hyper-reactivity in chronic periodontitis. Innate Immun. 2015;21:714-25.
63. Wright HJ, Matthews JB, Chapple IL, Ling-Mountford N, Cooper PR. Periodontitis associates with a type 1 IFN signature in peripheral blood neutrophils. J Immunol. 2008;181:5775-84.
64. Figueredo CM, Fischer RG, Gustafsson A. Aberrant neutrophil reactions in periodontitis. J Periodontol. 2005;76:951-55.
65. Hatanaka E, Monteagudo PT, Marrocos MS, Campa A. Neutrophils and monocytes as potentially important sources of proinflammatory cytokines in diabetes. Clin Exp Immunol. 2006;146:443-7.
66. Yasunari K, Watanabe T, Nakamura M. Reactive oxygen species formation by polymorphonuclear cells and mononuclear cells as a risk factor of cardiovascular diseases. Curr Pharm Biotechnol. 2006;7:73-80.

67. Reyes L, A Sanchez-Garcia M, Morrison T, Howden AJM, Watts ER, Arienti S, et al. A type I IFN, prothrombotic hyperinflammatory neutrophil signature is distinct for COVID-19 ARDS. Wellcome Open Res. 2021;6:38.
68. Morrissey SM, Geller AE, Hu X, Tieri D, Ding C, Klaes CK, et al. A specific low-density neutrophil population correlates with hypercoagulation and disease severity in hospitalized COVID-19 patients. JCI Insight. 2021;6:e148435.
69. Tseng CW, Liu GY. Expanding roles of neutrophils in aging hosts. Curr Opin Immunol. 2014;29:43-8.
70. Aquino-Martinez R, Hernández-Vigueras S. Severe COVID-19 lung infection in older people and periodontitis. J Clin Med. 2021;10:279.
71. Marouf N, Cai W, Said KN, Daas H, Diab H, Chinta VR, et al. Association between periodontitis and severity of COVID-19 infection: A case-control study. J Clin Periodontol. 2021;48(4):483-91.
72. Habibi MS, Thwaites RS, Chang M, Jozwik A, Paras A, Kirsebom F, et al. Neutrophilic inflammation in the respiratory mucosa predisposes to RSV infection. Science. 2020;370:eaba9301.
73. Wilk AJ, Lee MJ, Wei B, Parks B, Pi R, Martínez-Colón GJ, et al. Multi-omic profiling reveals widespread dysregulation of innate immunity and hematopoiesis in COVID-19. J Exp Med. 2021;218(8):e20210582.
74. Bizzarro S, van der Velden U, ten Heggeler JM, Leivadaros E, Hoek FJ, Gerdes VE, et al. Periodontitis is characterized by elevated PAI-1 activity. J Clin Periodontol. 2007;34: 574-80.
75. Golub LM, Lee HM. Periodontal therapeutics: Current host-modulation agents and future directions. Periodontol 2000. 2020;82:186-204.
76. Golub LM, McNamara TF, D'Angelo G, Greenwald RA, Ramamurthy NS. A non-antibacterial chemically-modified tetracycline inhibits mammalian collagenase activity. J Dent Res. 1987;66:1310-4.
77. Golub LM, Ramamurthy NS, McNamara TF, Greenwald RA, Rifkin BR. Tetracyclines inhibit connective tissue breakdown: new therapeutic implications for an old family of drugs. Crit Rev Oral Biol Med. 1991;2:297-321.
78. Golub LM, Suomalainen K, Sorsa T. Host modulation with tetracyclines and their chemically modified analogues. Curr Opin Dent. 1992;2:80-90.
79. Golub LM, Wolff M, Roberts S, Lee HM, Leung M, Payonk GS. Treating periodontal diseases by blocking tissue-destructive enzymes. J Am Dent Assoc. 1994;125:163-9.
80. Monk E, Shalita A, Siegel DM. Clinical applications of non-antimicrobial tetracyclines in dermatology. Pharmacol Res. 2011;63:130-45.
81. Serhan CN. Controlling the resolution of acute inflammation: a new genus of dual anti-inflammatory and proresolving mediators. J Periodontol. 2008;79:1520-6.
82. Serhan CN, Chiang N, Van Dyke TE. Resolving inflammation: dual anti-inflammatory and pro-resolution lipid mediators. Nat Rev Immunol. 2008;8:349-61.
83. Lee CT, Teles R, Kantarci A, Chen T, McCafferty J, Starr JR, et al. Resolvin E1 Reverses Experimental Periodontitis and Dysbiosis. J Immunol. 2016;197:2796-806.
84. Van Dyke TE, Hasturk H, Kantarci A, Freire MO, Nguyen D, Dalli J, et al. Proresolving nanomedicines activate bone regeneration in periodontitis. J Dent Res. 2015;94: 148-56.
85. Hasturk H, Kantarci A, Goguet-Surmenian E, Blackwood A, Andry C, Serhan CN, et al. Resolvin E1 regulates inflammation at the cellular and tissue level and restores tissue homeostasis in vivo. J Immunol. 2007;179:7021-9.
86. Ferguson B, Bokka NR, Maddipati KR, Ayilavarapu S, Weltman R, Zhu L, et al. Distinct profiles of specialized pro-resolving lipid mediators and corresponding receptor gene expression in periodontal inflammation. Front Immunol. 2020;11:1307.

87. Corrêa MG, Pires PR, Ribeiro FV, Pimentel SZ, Casarin RC, Cirano FR, et al. Systemic treatment with resveratrol and/or curcumin reduces the progression of experimental periodontitis in rats. J Periodontal Res. 2017;52:201-9.
88. Ikeda E, Ikeda Y, Wang Y, Fine N, Sheikh Z, Viniegra A, et al. Resveratrol derivative-rich melinjo seed extract induces healing in a murine model of established periodontitis. J Periodontol. 2018;89:586-95.
89. Ribeiro FV, Pino DS, Franck FC, Benatti BB, Tenenbaum H, Davies JE, et al. Resveratrol Inhibits Periodontitis-Related Bone Loss in Rats Subjected to Cigarette Smoke Inhalation. J Periodontol. 2017;88:788-98.
90. Corrêa MG, Absy S, Tenenbaum H, Ribeiro FV, Cirano FR, Casati MZ, et al. Resveratrol attenuates oxidative stress during experimental periodontitis in rats exposed to cigarette smoke inhalation. J Periodontal Res. 2019;54:225-32.
91. Steinberg J, Halter J, Schiller H, Gatto L, Carney D, Lee HM, et al. Chemically modified tetracycline prevents the development of septic shock and acute respiratory distress syndrome in a clinically applicable porcine model. Shock. 2005;24:348-56.
92. Steinberg J, Halter J, Schiller HJ, Dasilva M, Landas S, Gatto LA, et al. Metalloproteinase inhibition reduces lung injury and improves survival after cecal ligation and puncture in rats. J Surg Res. 2003;111:185-95.
93. Gendrot M, Andreani J, Jardot P, Hutter S, Delandre O, Boxberger M, et al. In vitro antiviral activity of doxycycline against SARS-CoV-2. Molecules. 2020;25:5064.
94. Campagna M, Rivas C. Antiviral activity of resveratrol. Biochem Soc Trans. 2010;38:50-3.
95. Lin SC, Ho CT, Chuo WH, Li S, Wang TT, Lin CC. Effective inhibition of MERS-CoV infection by resveratrol. BMC Infect Dis. 2017;17:144.
96. Silva Lagos L, Luu TV, De Haan B, Faas M, De Vos P. TLR2 and TLR4 activity in monocytes and macrophages after exposure to amoxicillin, ciprofloxacin, doxycycline and erythromycin. J Antimicrob Chemother. 2022;77:2972-83.
97. Froum SH, Froum SJ. Incidence of COVID-19 Virus Transmission in Three Dental Offices: A 6-Month Retrospective Study. Int J Periodontics Restorative Dent. 2020;40:853-9.
98. van Doremalen N, Bushmaker T, Morris DH, et al. Aerosol and Surface Stability of SARS-CoV-2 as Compared with SARS-CoV-1. N Engl J Med. 2020;382:1564-7.
99. Goldberg LJ, Watkins HM, Boerke EE, Chatigny MA. The use of a rotating drum for the study of aerosols over extended periods of time. Am J Hyg. 1958;68:85-93.
100. Fischer RJ, Bushmaker T, Judson S, Munster VJ. Comparison of the Aerosol Stability of 2 Strains of Zaire ebolavirus From the 1976 and 2013 Outbreaks. J Infect Dis. 2016;214:S290-3.
101. Asha R, Julie Toby T, Muralidharan NP, Sheeja SV. Efficacy of adjunctive usage of hydrogen peroxide with chlorhexidine as preprocedural mouthrinse on dental aerosol. Natl J Physiol Pharm Pharmacol. 2015;5:431.
102. Peng X, Xu X, Li Y, Cheng L, Zhou X, Ren B. Transmission routes of 2019-nCoV and controls in dental practice. Int J Oral Sci. 2020;12:9.
103. Liu Y, Ning Z, Chen Y, Guo M, Liu Y, Gali NK, et al. Aerodynamic analysis of SARS-CoV-2 in two Wuhan hospitals. Nature. 2020;582(7813):557-60.
104. Guo ZD, Wang ZY, Zhang SF, Li X, Li L, Li C, et al. Aerosol and Surface Distribution of Severe Acute Respiratory Syndrome Coronavirus 2 in Hospital Wards, Wuhan, China, 2020. Emerg Infect Dis. 2020;26:1583-91.
105. Pan M, Lednicky JA, Wu CY. Collection, particle sizing and detection of airborne viruses. J Appl Microbiol. 2019;127:1596-611.
106. Kulkarni H, Smith CM, Lee DoH, Hirst RA, Easton AJ, O'Callaghan C. Evidence of Respiratory Syncytial Virus Spread by Aerosol. Time to Revisit Infection Control Strategies? Am J Respir Crit Care Med. 2016;194:308-16.
107. Yu IT, Li Y, Wong TW, Tam W, Chan AT, Lee JH, et al. Evidence of airborne transmission of the severe acute respiratory syndrome virus. N Engl J Med. 2004;350:1731-9.

108. Lloyd M. (2020). COVID-19 concerns could affect your visit to the doctor or dentist. [online] Available from https://vancouver.citynews.ca/2020/03/10/covid-19-visit-doctor-dentist/ [Last accessed February, 2024].
109. Bennett AM, Fulford MR, Walker JT, Bradshaw DJ, Martin MV, Marsh PD. Microbial aerosols in general dental practice. Br Dent J. 2000;189:664-7.
110. Li RW, Leung KW, Sun FC, Samaranayake LP. Severe acute respiratory syndrome (SARS) and the GDP. Part II: implications for GDPs. Br Dent J. 2004;197:130-4.
111. Logothetis DD, Martinez-Welles JM. Reducing bacterial aerosol contamination with a chlorhexidine gluconate pre-rinse. J Am Dent Assoc. 1995;126:1634-9.
112. Ammu A, Varma S, Suragimath G, Zope S, Pisal A, Gangavati R. Evaluation And Comparison Of Two Commercially Available Mouthrinses In Reducing Aerolised Bacteria During Ultrasonic Scaling When Used As A Preprocedural Rinse. Cumhuriyet Dent J. 2019;22:235-40.
113. Carrouel F, Conte MP, Fisher J, Gonçalves LS, Dussart C, Llodra JC, et al. COVID-19: A Recommendation to Examine the Effect of Mouthrinses with β-Cyclodextrin Combined with Citrox in Preventing Infection and Progression. J Clin Med. 2020;9:1126.
114. Lo Giudice R. The Severe Acute Respiratory Syndrome Coronavirus-2 (SARS CoV-2) in Dentistry. Management of Biological Risk in Dental Practice. Int J Environ Res Public Health 2020;17:3067.
115. Micik RE, Miller RL, Mazzarella MA, Ryge G. Studies on dental aerobiology. I. Bacterial aerosols generated during dental procedures. J Dent Res. 1969;48:49-56.
116. Samaranayake LP, Peiris M. Severe acute respiratory syndrome and dentistry: A retrospective view. J Am Dent Assoc. 2004;135:1292-302.
117. Harrel SK, Molinari J. Aerosols and splatter in dentistry: a brief review of the literature and infection control implications. J Am Dent Assoc. 2004;135:429-37.
118. Siqueira JF, Rôças IN, Riche FN, Provenzano JC. Clinical outcome of the endodontic treatment of teeth with apical periodontitis using an antimicrobial protocol. Oral Surg Oral Med Oral Pathol Oral Radiol Endod. 2008;106:757-62.
119. Teanpaisan R, Taeporamaysamai M, Rattanachone P, Poldoung N, Srisintorn S. The usefulness of the modified extra-oral vacuum aspirator (EOVA) from household vacuum cleaner in reducing bacteria in dental aerosols. Int Dent J. 2001;51:413-6.
120. Medical Advisory Secretariat. Air cleaning technologies: an evidence-based analysis. Ont Health Technol Assess Ser. 2005;5:1-52.
121. Sehulster L, Chinn RY; CDC, HICPAC. Guidelines for environmental infection control in health-care facilities. Recommendations of CDC and the Healthcare Infection Control Practices Advisory Committee (HICPAC). MMWR Recomm Rep. 2003;52:1-42.
122. National Aeronautics and Space Administration, Marshall Space Flight Center. (2016). Submicron and Nanoparticulate Matter Removal by HEPA-Rated Media Filters and Packed Beds of Granular Materials. [online] Available from https://ntrs.nasa.gov/citations/20170005166 [Last accessed February, 2024].
123. Bedell K, Buchaklian AH, Perlman S. Efficacy of an Automated Multiple Emitter Whole-Room Ultraviolet-C Disinfection System Against Coronaviruses MHV and MERS-CoV. Infect Control Hosp Epidemiol. 2016;37:598-99.
124. Brickner PW, Vincent RL, First M, Nardell E, Murray M, Kaufman W. The application of ultraviolet germicidal irradiation to control transmission of airborne disease: bioterrorism countermeasure. Public Health Rep. 2003;118:99-114.
125. Welch D, Buonanno M, Grilj V, Shuryak I, Crickmore C, Bigelow AW, et al. Far-UVC light: A new tool to control the spread of airborne-mediated microbial diseases. Sci Rep. 2018;8:2752.
126. Loeb M, Dafoe N, Mahony J, John M, Sarabia A, Glavin V, et al. Surgical mask vs N95 respirator for preventing influenza among health care workers: A randomized trial. JAMA. 2009;302:1865-71.

127. Centers for Disease Control and Prevention & National Institute for Occupational Safety and Health. (2019). Understanding the difference. Available from https://www.cdc.gov/niosh/npptl/pdfs/UnderstandDifferenceInfographic-508.pdf [Last accessed February, 2024].
128. Bundgaard H, Bundgaard JS, Raaschou-Pedersen DET, von Buchwald C, Todsen T, Norsk JB, et al. Effectiveness of Adding a Mask Recommendation to Other Public Health Measures to Prevent SARS-CoV-2 Infection in Danish Mask Wearers : A Randomized Controlled Trial. Ann Intern Med. 2021;174:335-43.
129. Loeb M, Bartholomew A, Hashmi M, Tarhuni W, Hassany M, Youngster I, et al. Medical Masks Versus N95 Respirators for Preventing COVID-19 Among Health Care Workers: A Randomized Trial. Ann Intern Med. 2022;175:1629-38.
130. Ding J, Li J, Qi J, Fu L. Characterization of dental dust particles and their pathogenicity to respiratory system: a narrative review. Clin Oral Investig. 2023;27:1815-29.

CHAPTER 13

The Evolving Role of Simulation in Surgical Training

Tanvir Hussain, Aishan Patil

INTRODUCTION

Simulation is a pedagogical training approach that is applied in various specialties. As a training technique, simulation replaces or amplifies real experiences with immersive guided experiences that evoke and replicate the real-world through an interactive approach. Simulation is a concept that has been introduced previously in medical training.[1] Over recent years, simulation has been widely applied in enhancing healthcare training, promoting quality of care, and promoting patient safety. Even before the coronavirus disease-2019 (COVID-19) outbreak, surgical experts have used simulation to assess patients' operative risks and plan complicated surgical procedures.[2] Nevertheless, the exponential increase in the utilization of simulation for surgical skills training is attributable to the COVID-19 pandemic. The pandemic resulted in reduced elective procedures, rearranged conferences, and canceled examinations.[3,4] These unprecedented changes in surgical training and healthcare at large necessitated resourceful and innovative ways to promote learning and career progression in surgery despite the pandemic-related restrictions regarding in-person training.[5,6] This chapter explores how simulation surgical training was an innovative, adaptive, and alternative approach to surgical training during the COVID-19 pandemic and how such approaches optimize healthcare now and in the future.

NEED FOR SIMULATION SURGICAL TRAINING

The COVID-19 pandemic brought a constant flux to the medical and surgical trainers and trainees within the global healthcare system. Amid the ravaging COVID-19 wave, organizations such as the American College of Surgeons (ACS) recommended the minimization, postponement, or cancelation of elective procedures to reserve hospital space for critically ill

COVID-19 patients and protect healthcare workers.[7-9] Thus, most invasive and endoscopic procedures were deferred "until further notice". Although these recommendations aimed at enhancing patient safety and promoting health outcomes for the critically ill, they left surgical trainees and residents in precarious positions. The reduced operative exposure made it challenging for surgical trainees to retain intraoperative knowledge and maintain surgical skills.[10,11] Fortunately, most healthcare training institutions capitalized on preexisting technological advancements to promote the retention of surgical knowledge and skills beyond the confines of an actual hospital setting. As such, surgical trainees and residents had access to an interactive phone- and computer-based technological platforms for enhanced learning. Surgical education governing bodies such as the ACS approved using these platforms to supplement and satisfy surgical trainees' learning needs. Surgical simulation training increases surgical trainees' technical proficiency, decreases operative time, and decreases intraoperative errors.[12,13]

Despite canceling elective operations due to the spike in COVID-19 cases, the surgical workforce invested in simulation training and other innovative modalities to train surgical residents and trainees and protect surgical services.[3,14] Digital simulation, virtual reality software, and simulation box trainers enabled surgical trainees to develop clinical and procedural skills. Therefore, simulation surgical training was one of the ways that surgical training institutions maximized learning opportunities to enhance learners' career progression against the backdrop of COVID-19 setbacks. This objective was achieved through multidisciplinary team participation for optimal learning outcomes.[15,16]

During the peak of the COVID-19 pandemic, most surgical cases, especially those that did not require emergency intervention, were managed conservatively.[17] For instance, patients with acute appendicitis were treated using antibiotics and anti-inflammatory agents instead of appendectomy. This approach aimed at tapering the spread of infection and protecting medical personnel. As such, surgeons running surgical clinics during the pandemic limited their care to urgent cases that were impossible to handle through the various virtual platforms. Despite reducing the risk of virus transmission, this strategy had counter effects in depriving surgical trainees, such as fellows and residents, of the quality time required to hone their clinical and operative skills through surgical and clinical exposure.[18,19] Surgical simulation redeemed the lost training time by enhancing trainees' access to surgical exposure through level-appropriate learning opportunities. Converting lectures to diverse online learning platforms promoted social distancing and a safe teaching and learning environment. Surgical simulation training also promotes access to various educational resources, surgical techniques, and perspectives with clearly demonstrable benefits.[20-22]

IMPLEMENTING SIMULATION SURGICAL TRAINING

Implementing alternative surgical training modalities replaced the traditional face-to-face surgical training approach as a coping mechanism against the COVID-19 pandemic that had caused significant changes in educational and healthcare operational policies.[23] In addition to surgical skills simulation training, alternative curricular components included virtual rounding, online learning modules, research education, scenario-based multiple choice questions writing exercises, medical education learning, reflection assignments, and video-based interactive learning.[24] The educational value of these alternative curricular components was analyzed in terms of learning effectiveness/knowledge gain, feasibility, feedback, facilitation, and evaluation. The available alternative learning resources were crucial in maximizing learning outcomes in the context of the challenging surgical training during the pandemic.[25]

Various surgical training institutions applied simulation modalities, including virtual reality task trainers, web-based simulations, virtual patients, and high-fidelity mannequins to promote learning during the COVID-19 pandemic.[26] As an evolving specialty, simulation surgical training creates a safe, stress-free, and reproducible learning environment that allows surgical trainers to tailor their training with objective performance evaluation. Simulation can be used to teach four learning domains, i.e., cognitive capabilities, teaching and research skills, psychomotor skills, and professional affect.[27] The specific modality used in simulation training determines the need and extent of supervision.

SIMULATION TRAINING IN HEAD AND NECK SURGERY

The pandemic also significantly affected surgical training in head and neck surgery, as noted by the American Head and Neck Society (AHNS). Despite the unprecedented challenges to healthcare due to the pandemic, there was a need to find the right balance between providing clinical care and continuing high-quality and evidence-based head and neck surgical training through a comprehensive approach aimed at promoting the efficiency of graduates.[28,29] In the context of head and neck surgery, surgical simulation promotes the acquisition and practice of technical skills within settings that permit reflection and discussion while limiting risks to both surgical trainees and patients.[30] Virtual reality simulators, as well as animal or cadaveric models, provided realistic platforms to promote surgical skills training. Virtual reality and physical simulators accurately replicate the complex human anatomy, mimic emergency situations, and introduce practical pathology.[31] Some of the widely used virtual reality simulators in head and neck surgery include virtual reality temporal bone drilling and endoscopic sinus surgery simulations.

Khan et al. (2020) explored the impact of the COVID-19 pandemic on core surgical training. It was essential to continue providing appropriate and evidence-based surgical skills training during the pandemic by using online platforms.[32] Alternative teaching modalities included face-to-face conference calling, modules, lectures, and laparoscopic simulators. Surgical simulators provided a platform for ongoing practical skills development in the absence of real-time operating. Surgical simulation training mitigated the effects of the pandemic on healthcare training by ensuring the continuity of learning and preventing the disruption of practice.[33,34] Technology-based simulations promoted knowledge acquisition through structured teaching sessions and other learning opportunities, thus reducing the learning curve. Simulation surgical training enhances the mastery of surgical skills, promotes patient safety, and improves clinical outcomes.

An ideal simulation training approach provides access to learning and assessment outside the confines of an operating theater.[35,36] Expanded simulation training during the pandemic compensated for the reduced surgical exposure time due to postponed hands-on training and reduced surgical trainees' presence in the theater. Most simulation models involved robotic-assisted and laparoscopic surgical training with task recording and real-time feedback for improved educational outcomes.[37,38] Constructive feedback after simulations allowed surgical trainees to sharpen their surgical skills and practice on increasingly difficult levels. Social distancing hindered onsite simulation training, although some surgical training centers implemented onsite simulated surgical training consoles.[39]

SIMULATION TRAINING IN SURGICAL ONCOLOGY

Computer-based surgical platforms, such as open-access video-based platforms and intraoperative surgical oncology videos, provided valuable learning resources for instructing surgical trainees on surgical indications, operative anatomy, preoperative workup, and surgical techniques within the context of surgical oncology.[40-42] These simulation platforms offered detailed aspects and steps in critical operations in surgical oncology through illustration. In addition to enhancing learning through virtual modalities, simulation surgical training introduced new structured training pathways that conferred geographical flexibility and provided a larger pool of surgical trainers.[43,44]

Although simulation training is not ideal for surgical oncology and other surgical specialties, it temporarily solved the crisis by ensuring the continuity of learning and career progression. Regular training using surgical simulators enhances basic skills and mastery of complex surgeries.[45] Technical skills of operating surgeons influence patients' postoperative outcomes. Approaches to address variations in learning and clinical outcomes and improve surgical trainees' technical skills include consistent debriefing, surgical coaching, feedback, and video reviews.[46,47] In surgical oncology, oncological and theoretical knowledge and experience augment surgical training to optimize learning outcomes.

SIMULATION SURGICAL TRAINING IN CARDIOTHORACIC SURGERY

In the United Kingdom (UK), simulation surgical training was used to bridge the knowledge and practice gaps following changes by the European Working Time Directive due to the COVID-19 pandemic.[48] Simulation surgical training was applied in cardiothoracic surgery to progressively increase basic and advanced surgical skills. The pandemic inadvertently highlighted various areas of weakness within the current surgical training curriculum and necessitated simulation training to meet the increased need for evidence-based practical training.[49] Incorporating simulation training in cardiothoracic surgical training mitigates the challenges brought about by the pandemic while ensuring the continuity of care, learning, and practice.[50]

In addition to reduced elective operations and surgical clinic cancellations, the redeployment of healthcare professionals to medical wards at the peak of COVID-19 limited learning opportunities for learners, including surgical residents.[51] Although surgical education through virtual learning promotes valuable experience and skills, the relevance of in-person simulation must be considered.[52]

Simulation sessions improved doctors' and nurses' confidence in assessing and managing patients with surgical emergencies. Thus, simulation surgical training through diverse learning opportunities maintains the integrity of surgical training.[53] Simulation surgical training was a timely solution to education continuity. The reduced surgical case load and unforeseeable end of the pandemic hindered surgical residents' training and development of surgical skills.[54] With the cessation of various other learning opportunities, such as surgical conferences, cadaveric dissection, and surgical symposiums, training centers considered running these programs virtually. High-fidelity 3D surgical simulators, such as the take-home simulation kits, enabled surgical trainees to acquire and maintain surgical skills even in remote settings.[55] Overall, 3D-printed simulators promote higher degrees of training across various surgical specialties. Developing such simulators requires an effective partnership between academic centers and the open-source community, thus enhancing accessibility to diverse surgical training opportunities.[56] Simulation surgical training during the pandemic also involved designing the curriculum in compliance with the principles of social distancing.[57,58]

SIMULATION SURGICAL TRAINING FOR THE FUTURE

As an emerging surgical training modality, simulation-based education promoted surgical training by enhancing the acquisition of procedural skills while minimizing residents' exposure to contagion.[59] Simulation centers sought to replicate or evoke the real surgical world through evidence-based simulation platforms, constructive feedback, and social distancing protocols.[60,61] Although simulation surgical training was mainly deployed as a mitigating measure against the effects of the COVID-19 pandemic, its benefits render it a valuable entity that could inform evidence-based surgical training even beyond the COVID-19 era.[62] Various surgical simulators can be incorporated into the surgical education program to catalyze knowledge sharing, surgical skills development and maintenance, and career progression.[63] Simulation surgical training effectively diversifies the educational opportunities available to surgical residents and other trainees.

CONCLUSION

The COVID-19 pandemic opened up the surgical world to a wide array of educational opportunities. At the peak of the pandemic, when surgical procedures, conferences, clinics, and symposiums were deferred or canceled with a resultant decline in the surgical caseload, surgical trainees, including residents, were deprived of essential training time needed to hone their clinical and surgical skills. This crisis necessitated innovative and alternative approaches to teaching and learning to optimize learning and clinical outcomes. Despite not matching up to in-person training in the actual surgical environment, simulation surgical training enhances the continuity of learning by promoting learners' ability to acquire and retain surgical knowledge, skills, and experience. The approach promoted surgical training and minimized infection spread by complying with the social distancing principles. Simulation surgical training continues to be relevant, feasible, and practical for evidence-based surgical education beyond COVID-19.

REFERENCES

1. Agha RA, Fowler AJ. The role and validity of surgical simulation. Int Surg. 2015;100(2): 350-7.
2. Alanazi AA, Nicholson N, Thomas S. The use of simulation training to improve knowledge, skills, and confidence among healthcare students: a systematic review. Int J Allied Health Sci Practice. 2017;15(3):2.
3. Ellis R, Scrimgeour DS, Brennan PA. Surgical training during the COVID-19 pandemic: preparing for future uncertainty. Br J Oral Maxillofac Surg. 2022;60(1):42-5.
4. Bhojwani D, McNutt A. 374 Simulation and the Surgeon during COVID-19: The Double 2s Surgical Emergencies Course. Br J Surg. 2021;108(Suppl-2):znab134-132.
5. Doulias T, Gallo G, Rubio-Perez I, Breukink SO, Hahnloser D. Doing more with less: surgical training in the COVID-19 era. J Invest Surg. 2022;35(1):171-9.
6. McKechnie T, Levin M, Zhou K, Freedman B, Palter VN, Grantcharov TP. Virtual surgical training during COVID-19: operating room simulation platforms accessible from home. Ann Surg. 2020;272(2):e153-4.
7. Wady H, Restle D, Park J, Pryor A, Talamini M, Abdel-Misih S. The role of surgeons during the COVID-19 pandemic: impact on training and lessons learned from a surgical resident's perspective. Surg Endosc. 2021;35:3430-6.

8. White EM, Shaughnessy MP, Esposito AC, Slade MD, Korah M, Yoo PS. Surgical education in the time of COVID: understanding the early response of surgical training programs to the novel coronavirus pandemic. J Surg Educ. 2021;78(2):412-21.
9. Hau HM, Weitz J, Bork U. Impact of the COVID-19 pandemic on student and resident teaching and training in surgical oncology. J Clin Med. 2020;9(11):3431.
10. Michaels R, Witsberger CA, Powell AR, Koka K, Cohen K, Nourmohammadi Z, et al. 3D printing in surgical simulation: emphasized importance in the COVID-19 pandemic era. J 3D Print Med. 2021;5(1):5-9.
11. Higham H, Baxendale B. To err is human: use of simulation to enhance training and patient safety in anaesthesia. Br J Anaesth. 2017;119(Suppl-1):i106-14.
12. Adesoye T, Davis CH, Del Calvo H, Shaikh AF, Chegireddy V, Chan EY, et al. Optimization of surgical resident safety and education during the COVID-19 pandemic–lessons learned. J Surg Educ. 2021;78(1):315-20.
13. Sutzko DC, Martin CA, Chu DI. Development and implementation of virtual grand rounds in surgery. Am J Surg. 2021;221(1):46-8.
14. Thomson JE, Poudrier G, Stranix JT, Motosko CC, Hazen A. Current status of simulation training in plastic surgery residency programs: A review. Arch Plast Surg. 2018;45(5): 395-402.
15. Abdelsattar JM, Coleman JR, Nagler A, Shabahang M, Ellison EC, Baker Y, et al. Lived experiences of surgical residents during the COVID-19 pandemic: a qualitative assessment. J Surg Educ. 2021;78(6):1851-62.
16. Agrawal V, Sharma D. Surgical training "Before COVID-19 (BC)" to "After COVID-19 (AC)": Needs-driven approach for the Global South. Br J Surg. 2020;107(12):e585-6.
17. ElHawary H, Salimi A, Alam P, Gilardino MS. Educational alternatives for the maintenance of educational competencies in surgical training programs affected by the COVID-19 pandemic. J Med Educ Curric Dev. 2020;7:2382120520951806.
18. Hourston GJ. The impact of despecialisation and redeployment on surgical training in the midst of the COVID-19 pandemic. Int J Surg. 2020;78:1-2.
19. Arolfo S, Velluti F, Romagnoli R, Lo Secco G, Allaix ME, Morino M. COVID-19 outbreak and the practice of surgery: do we need to change? Br J Surg. 2020;107(9):e307-8.
20. Azadi S, Green IC, Arnold A, Truong M, Potts J, Martino MA. Robotic surgery: the impact of simulation and other innovative platforms on performance and training. J Minim Invasive Gynecol. 2021;28(3):490-5.
21. Feins RH, Burkhart HM, Conte JV, Coore DN, Fann JI, Hicks Jr GL, et al. Simulation-based training in cardiac surgery. Ann Thorac Surg. 2017;103(1):312-21.
22. Fuller S, Vaporciyan A, Dearani JA, Stulak JM, Romano JC. COVID-19 disruption in cardiothoracic surgical training: an opportunity to enhance education. Ann Thorac Surg. 2020;110(5):1443-6.
23. Tuma F, Kamel MK, Shebrain S, Ghanem M, Blebea J. Alternative surgical training approaches during COVID-19 pandemic. Ann Med Surg. 2021;62:253-7.
24. Buléon C, Caton J, Park YS, Eller S, Buyck M, Kardong-Edgren S, et al. The state of distance healthcare simulation during the COVID-19 pandemic: results of an international survey. Adv Simul (Lond). 2022;7(1):10.
25. Chao TN, Frost AS, Newman JG. Interactive virtual surgical education during COVID-19 and beyond. Acad Med. 2020;95(11):e9.
26. Grady ZJ, Gallo LK, Lin HK, Magod BL, Coulthard SL, Flink BJ, et al. From the operating room to online: medical student surgery education in the time of COVID-19. J Surg Res. 2022;270:145-50.
27. Hedman LR, Felländer-Tsai L. Simulation-based skills training in non-performing orthopedic surgeons: skills acquisition, motivation, and flow during the COVID-19 pandemic. Acta Orthopaedica. 2020;91(5):520-2.

28. Givi B, Moore MG, Bewley AF, Coffey CS, Cohen MA, Hessel AC, et al. Advanced head and neck surgery training during the COVID-19 pandemic. Head Neck. 2020;42(7):1411-7.
29. Arezzo A, Vignali A, Ammirati CA, Brodie R, Mintz Y. Is it possible to continue academic teaching in surgery during the COVID pandemic era? Minim Invasive Ther Allied Technol. 2022;31(4):487-95.
30. Coe TM, Jogerst KM, Sell NM, Cassidy DJ, Eurboonyanun C, Gee D, et al. Practical techniques to adapt surgical resident education to the COVID-19 era. Ann Surg. 2020;272(2):e139-41.
31. Daodu O, Panda N, Lopushinsky S, Varghese Jr TK, Brindle M. COVID-19–considerations and implications for surgical learners. Ann Surg. 2020;272(1):e22-3.
32. Khan KS, Keay R, McLellan M, Mahmud S. Impact of the COVID-19 pandemic on core surgical training. Scott Med J. 2020;65(4):133-7.
33. Beaubien JM, Baker DP. The use of simulation for training teamwork skills in health care: how low can you go? Qual Saf Health Care. 2004;13 (Suppl 1):i51-6.
34. Blanco-Colino R, Soares AS, Kuiper SZ, Zaffaroni G, Pata F, Pellino G. Surgical training during and after COVID-19: a joint trainee and trainers manifesto. Ann Surg. 2020;272(1):e24-6.
35. Davis CE, Hayes L, Dent N, Jennings I, Arumugasamy M, Walsh TN. Impact of COVID-19 on surgical training. Br J Surg. 2021;108(5):e199-200.
36. English W, Vulliamy P, Banerjee S, Arya S. Surgical training during the COVID-19 pandemic–the cloud with a silver lining? Br J Surg. 2020;107(9):e343-4.
37. Lungu AJ, Swinkels W, Claesen L, Tu P, Egger J, Chen X. A review on the applications of virtual reality, augmented reality and mixed reality in surgical simulation: an extension to different kinds of surgery. Expert Rev Med Devices. 2021;18(1):47-62.
38. McCarthy CJ, Uppot RN. Advances in virtual and augmented reality—exploring the role in health-care education. J Radiol Nurs. 2019;38(2):104-5.
39. Kapila AK, Farid Y, Kapila V, Schettino M, Vanhoeij M, Hamdi M. The perspective of surgical residents on current and future training in light of the COVID-19 pandemic. Br J Surg. 2020;107(9):e305.
40. Khan S, Mian A. Medical education: COVID-19 and surgery. Br J Surg. 2020;107(8):e269.
41. Goolsarran N, Hamo CE, Lane S, Frawley S, Lu WH. Effectiveness of an interprofessional patient safety team-based learning simulation experience on healthcare professional trainees. BMC Med Educ. 2018;18(1):1-8.
42. Johnston S, Coyer FM, Nash R. Kirkpatrick's evaluation of simulation and debriefing in health care education: a systematic review. J Nurs Educ. 2018;57(7):393-8.
43. Clements JM, Burke JR, Hope C, Nally DM, Doleman B, Giwa L, et al. The quantitative impact of COVID-19 on surgical training in the United Kingdom. BJS Open. 2021;5(3):zrab051.
44. Joyce DP, Ryan D, Kavanagh DO, Traynor O, Tierney S. Impact of COVID-19 on operative experience of junior surgical trainees. Br J Surg. 2021;108(1):e33-4.
45. Liaw SY, Carpio GA, Lau Y, Tan SC, Lim WS, Goh PS. Multiuser virtual worlds in healthcare education: A systematic review. Nurse Educ Today. 2018;65:136-49.
46. Loh CY, Wang AY, Tiong VT, Athanassopoulos T, Loh M, Lim P, et al. Animal models in plastic and reconstructive surgery simulation—a review. J Surg Res. 2018;221:232-45.
47. Kurup V, Matei V, Ray J. Role of in-situ simulation for training in healthcare: opportunities and challenges. Curr Opin Anaesthesiol. 2017;30(6):755-60.
48. Shafi AM, Sheikh AM, Awad WI. Comparison of cardiothoracic surgical training before and during the COVID-19 pandemic in the United Kingdom. JTCVS Open. 2021;7:394-410.
49. McGrath JL, Taekman JM, Dev P, Danforth DR, Mohan D, Kman N, et al. Using virtual reality simulation environments to assess competence for emergency medicine learners. Acad Emerg Med. 2018;25(2):186-95.

50. Metchik A, Boyd S, Kons Z, Vilchez V, Villano AM, Lazar JF, et al. How we do it: implementing a virtual, multi-institutional collaborative education model for the COVID-19 pandemic and beyond. J Surg Educ. 2021;78(4):1041-5.
51. LoSavio PS, Eggerstedt M, Tajudeen BA, Papagiannopoulos P, Revenaugh PC, Batra PS, et al. Rapid implementation of COVID-19 tracheostomy simulation training to increase surgeon safety and confidence. Am J Otolaryngol. 2020;41(5):102574.
52. Lund J, Sadler P, McLarty E. The effect of COVID-19 on surgical training. Surgery (Oxf). 2021;39(12):829-33.
53. Oliveira L, Figueiredo E. Simulation training methods in neurological surgery. Asian J Neurosurg. 2019;14(2):364-70.
54. Oriot D, Alinier G, Alinier G. Pocket Book for Simulation Debriefing in Healthcare, 1st edition. Gewerbestrasse: Springer International Publishing; 2018.
55. So HY, Chen PP, Wong GK, Chan TT. Simulation in medical education. JR Coll Physicians Edinb. 2019;49(1):52-7.
56. Staropoli PC, Gregori NZ, Junk AK, Galor A, Goldhardt R, Goldhagen BE, et al. Surgical simulation training reduces intraoperative cataract surgery complications among residents. Simul Healthc. 2018;13(1):11-5.
57. Muret-Wagstaff SL, Collins JS, Mashman DL, Patel SG, Pettorini K, Rosen SA, Shaffer VO, et al. In situ simulation enables operating room agility in the COVID-19 pandemic. Ann Surg. 2020;272(2):e148.
58. Norman GR, Grierson LE, Sherbino J, Hamstra SJ, Schmidt HG, Mamede S. Expertise in medicine and surgery. In: Ericsson KA, Hoffman RR, Kozbelt A, Williams AM (Eds). The Cambridge Handbook of Expertise and Expert Performance, 2nd edition. Cambridge: Cambridge University Press; 2018. pp. 331-55.
59. Jarry Trujillo C, Achurra Tirado P, Escalona Vivas G, Crovari Eulufi F, Varas Cohen J. Surgical training during COVID-19: a validated solution to keep on practicing. Br J Surg. 2020;107(11):e468-9.
60. Kantar RS, Alfonso AR, Ramly EP, Cohen O, Rifkin WJ, Maliha SG, et al. Knowledge and skills acquisition by plastic surgery residents through digital simulation training: a prospective, randomized, blinded trial. Plast Reconstr Surg. 2020;145(1):184e-92e.
61. Savage N, Jain A, Ng SC. Impacts of the COVID-19 pandemic on medical students in Australia. ANZ J Surg. 2020;90(7-8):1244-5.
62. Shah AP, Falconer R, Watson AJ, Walker KG. Teaching surgical residents in the COVID-19 era: The value of a simulation strategy. J Surg Educ. 2021;78(3):751-2.
63. Okland TS, Pepper JP, Valdez TA. How do we teach surgical residents in the COVID-19 era? J Surg Educ. 2020;77(5):1005-7.

CHAPTER 14

The Impact of the COVID-19 Pandemic on Nursing

Bridgene Bonner

In March of 2020, the world as we knew it underwent a sudden and unwelcome change. The rapid spread of the seemingly unstoppable coronavirus disease 2019 (COVID-19) pandemic ravaged country after country, throwing society into a state of near panic. Very little remained unaffected by this global disaster; from the outright cancellation of long-distance travel and the disruption of supply chains to the overwhelming of services and much more, all that we had become accustomed to had, almost overnight, become unstable and insecure. Few areas felt this impact as deeply as the health services sector. While many businesses closed their doors or shut down operations, those in all facets of healthcare were called upon to come to the front line and aid in the fight against this new and formidable enemy. With limited information and understanding of exactly what they were dealing with, and a hugely increased number of patients to deal with, doctors and nurses stepped into the breach and stood at the forefront of the global response. 3 years have passed since that time, and though the pandemic has been brought somewhat under control, this event brought many changes in the way healthcare is administered. In this chapter, I will be addressing the impact, and changes, for better or worse, that this phenomenon had on the nursing profession.

According to the World Health Organization (WHO), there are an estimated 20.7 million nurses practicing worldwide,[1] accounting for almost 50% of the entire global healthcare workforce (estimated at 43.5 million). This being the case, it is clear to see that nurses were, and continue to be, relied upon heavily from the early days of the pandemic onward. In the initial stages of the outbreak many services, including all but nonelective surgery and outpatients department appointments, ceased operating in an attempt to stem the potential spread of COVID-19 by reducing the exposure for both staff and patients. The nurses who worked in these fields were redeployed to departments and areas that required additional staff to assist with the massive and sudden increase of patients that the pandemic had brought about. As a result of this, the vast majority of nurses were now being put in direct contact with infectious patients at a time when the healthcare industry, along with the rest of the world, was still learning and adapting to new information regarding best practices when it came to minimizing personal risk of contracting the virus. This sudden disruption, combined with an initial shortage of adequate personal protective equipment (PPE) and the insecurity of the situation, resulted in a negative effect on the mental well-being of many nurses. A systematic review conducted in 2020 by Pappa et al.,[3] in which a combined analysis of 13 other studies was taken into consideration, found that out of the combined total of 33,062 participants, 23.2% reported suffering from anxiety, 22.8% reported symptoms of depression, and 38.9% reported problems with insomnia, all directly related to the effects of the pandemic. Indeed, in a study conducted toward the end of 2021,[4] 11% of 5,000 respondents intended to leave their positions, and a further 20% remained undecided, with the pandemic rating high amongst these results as the reason, particularly in those nurses with more than 25 years of experience. In fact, a recent study by the Royal College of Nurses in Britain[5] has found that 43,000 nurses and midwives have left the National Health Service (NHS) in the last 5 years with the pandemic and its aftereffects being cited as one of the predominant reasons. With the WHO reporting a global shortage of healthcare workers,[1] 50% of which is made up of nurses and midwives, this may yet end up being one of the biggest long-term impacts of COVID-19.

Another negative impact on nursing came with the resumption of services and reopening of departments, particularly those such as outpatients, where the general public attend appointments on a continuous basis. For the safety of both staff and patients, guidelines had to be put in place to both minimize risk and maximize output. Documents, such as "Resumption of OPD in HSE Hospital Groups",[6] laid out a specific set of regulations and standard practices that should be followed to achieve this, placing a special emphasis on social distancing, hand hygiene, and the wearing of masks as a primary deterrent to the spread of COVID-19. While these requirements were understood and adhered to by the majority of those attending clinics, they also came with their own set of challenges.

Social media has proved, more than any other source of information, invaluable for the most up-to-date and relevant information during this pandemic. While lockdowns and work-from-home orders were implemented, many people found themselves out of the societal loop and as such turned to social media for news regarding the developing situation. Vengas-Vera et al., in their paper "Positive and negative impact of social media in the COVID-19 era",[7] found that while social media was essential for sharing of news and medical information amongst healthcare workers, it also put responsibility on these same workers to act in the best interests of public health by attempting to curb the rapid spread of huge amounts of misinformation. Unfortunately, with the best will in the world, and due to the speed at which this information spreads, this would have been a Sisyphean task even in prepandemic times. So, as misinformation spread, those healthcare workers, hailed as heroes by some, found themselves on the receiving end of vitriol and accusations of conspiracy and collusion with nefarious entities. Particularly controversial among public health measures was the mask mandate. Research by the Pew Research Centre[8] found that a number of factors affected the likelihood of wearing a mask such as age, political affiliation, education levels, and digital literacy, with older conservatives being the least likely to adhere to these rules. Nurses being the first point of contact in many of these departments and clinics, the task of dealing with patients who refused to comply with these regulations fell mainly to them, often resulting in at a minimum verbal abuse and in some cases physical attack.[9-11] Although we have much more information and a better understanding of COVID-19 since the early days of 2020, the feelings of those against vaccines and public safety measures have only grown,[12] meaning that this is a problem that will likely persist and as such must be taken into account when measuring the impact on nursing.

Relatedly, the increased use of necessary PPE by nurses, particularly that of a face mask, has brought to light another hereto unforeseen issue; the effect of face coverings on the ability to satisfactorily communicate with both colleagues and patients. In the book Nonverbal Communication, Albert Mehrabian asserts through his studies that up to 93% of our communication is nonverbal, with 55% of that relating to the face and facial expressions.[13] These effectively being removed by the use of face coverings has forced a more direct form of communication, meaning heavier reliance on solely verbal instruction, which in Mehrabian's model accounts for only 7% of what is being transmitted. This, obviously, creates more of a challenge in an environment where communication is vital and has required adaptation on the part of both nurse and patient to ensure that each one's needs are understood clearly. Where this has proven particularly problematic is in dealing with those who are hearing impaired. Two studies carried out by Hussain et al.,[14,15] one focused on children and the other on adults, found that the use of face masks had a significant impact on their ability to communicate, removing the ability to lip read and to follow visible facial cues. They found that this was likely to increase the risk of patient dissatisfaction and felt that the use of an advocate by the patient was necessary to ensure clear communication. Regarding children in particular, they found that they displayed a decrease in interest in play or social interaction. As a large part of providing a quality health service is effective communication between providers and users, it is clear to see how this can impact the ability of both nurses and doctors to ensure that this level of service is achieved, particularly in fields, such as ear, nose, and throat (ENT), where these factors are more likely to arise.

Naturally, with an event of this scale and severity there would be, as illustrated above, many negative consequences for nursing and for healthcare in general. However, not all of the outcomes are quite as bleak. With the sudden necessity to approach healthcare in new ways came advances and opportunities that previously were not considered the standard procedure. Chief amongst these was the evolution of the use of telemedicine. As lack of contact was regarded as the best form of prevention regarding infection by COVID-19, telemedicine became an essential tool in continuing to provide a healthcare, to both new and returning patients, as well as being able to safely monitor those with chronic conditions.

Telemedicine is of course not a new concept, its origins stretching back to a time when the telegraph was the main means of long-distance communication. Of course, as technology progressed, so too did the abilities of the medical field to utilize this as a tool for the provision of healthcare.[16] Now, with many people having regular access to mobile communication tools, like phones or tablets, telemedicine has become a more viable option, particularly in a case like the COVID-19 pandemic when safety of patients and staff was critical. While access to these devices has been the norm for a relatively long time, the necessity or will to use such a system was, for the most part, just not there for healthcare providers or users of their services. Certainly, clinicians harbored concerns that the personal connection could be diminished through the use of telemedicine as opposed to in-person visits[17] It was when health services started to be affected, or outright shut down, as a result of the pandemic that the use of these methods really came into play in a serious manner, requiring the apprehensions of both practitioner and patient to be put aside in order to facilitate the provision of care. In the post-shutdown era, when services are largely back to normal levels of accessibility, studies have shown that patients express a higher level of satisfaction with "virtual" services than the prepandemic era.[18] One survey, for example, by Penn Medicine found that 67% of 800 respondents classed a video or telephone "visit" as good or better than an in-person one.[19]

Although the above is positive, on the whole, it predominantly addresses the use of this system between physicians and patients. So, how does the rise of telemedicine impact nursing? For those operating in the field of emergency medicine, a number of benefits have been reported when working in conjunction with doctors.[20] Triaging of patients can be done remotely, with decisions on what level of treatment will be necessary on their presenting at hospital, or indeed if they require emergency medical treatment at all. [21] Obviously, these are beneficial from a point of view of time and resource management, as well as potentially keeping the department less congested, and thereby more able to focus on actual emergencies. Remote appraisal of conditions is also beneficial in that should the patient, currently, be at a distant hospital or medical facility, it can be decided whether it is necessary for them to have to be transported to another facility, both potentially reducing further stress to the patient and aiding with more efficient resource management and cost-effectiveness.[22] The telemedicine approach also allows for a reduced time between first contact and treatment[23] and for decisions on required treatment to be made prior to physical contact with the patient.[24] Given that emergency departments, by their nature, are very often the most overcrowded in a hospital, telemedicine used in this fashion has the potential to reduce the number of patients presenting with minor or nonemergency conditions, allowing for more efficient use of staff and resources as well as efficient running of the department overall.

For a nurse practitioner or a clinical nurse specialist, telemedicine can also be a beneficial tool, particularly when dealing with the patient suffering from a chronic condition or illness.[25] The use of telemedicine in this way allows the nurse to have ready access to the patient and the ability to more frequently monitor and assess them, all without the patient having to constantly travel or attend clinics in person. Naturally, this takes some of the strain off the patient also, as well as allowing the nurse to work more efficiently and make the best use of his/her time. Additionally, telemedicine can be used as a means to further expand and educate on conditions or newly prescribed medications to patients should they feel it necessary.[26] Conversely, the patients have the ability to contact the nurse should they have any questions or concerns, which normally they would have to keep note of until the next time they attend an appointment in person, making for a more efficient and reliable system.[27] In this respect, telemedicine also removes the aforementioned issue concerning the wearing of face coverings and facial cues, allowing for freer and more satisfactory communication, particularly for those who are hearing impaired. Another benefit from this system is the fact that neither nurse nor patient is exposed to potential infection, from COVID or any other infectious conditions. As with the use of telemedicine in emergency care, as mentioned above, the use of these systems, when properly implemented, can allow for a better and more efficient use of time, potentially cutting waiting times and allowing for quicker access to doctors for those in need of more urgent care.[28]

One thing that this pandemic has laid bare to all is the importance of nurses to a fully functioning healthcare system, and as such the post-COVID environment is now primed for nurses to take more of a leadership role and to carry the profession into the future. In an article for the British Medical Journal,[29] Howard Catton, chief executive officer of the International Council of Nurses, makes a number of recommendations for his vision of the future of nursing. Included in these is that nurses, instead of just providing healthcare, should be at the forefront of its design and also that senior nurses should be included at the levels of government responsible for policy making. Though these proposals will undoubtedly take time to come to fruition, there is no doubt that the pandemic has brought about many opportunities for nurses to move ahead in their careers and positions, predominantly through further access to education.[30]

As the emergence of COVID forced us all into a world where virtual communication was necessary, so did it require education providers to adapt. This has opened up a groundswell of educational opportunities for nurses. Previously, where provision of courses for career advancement required planning around an already busy work, and in some cases home, schedule as they were solely available through only physical attendance, the movement of many of these online has allowed more nurses to benefit from the career advancement that these can provide. There are, as with any new system, concerns that perhaps the standard of online learning will be of a lesser value than that provided in person; however, studies have found this not to be the case. In their systematic review,[2] Pei et al.[31] found that online learning, while not more effective, was no less effective than that provided in a traditional way. Additionally, a study by Sarli et al.[32] in the journal "Creative Education", relating to those nurses whose educational path was interrupted and subsequently shifted online due to COVID, concluded that, although initial adaptation was necessary, a high level of educational quality was maintained. As such, the provision of further education in a more accessible manner is likely to encourage more nurses to take the steps necessary for taking on of roles with more responsibility and to train for positions that allow them to provide advanced levels of treatment and care. The benefits of nurses taking on these new roles are twofold; not only will they make it unnecessary for doctors to be responsible for certain procedures, thereby freeing them up to concentrate on more specialized areas, but the ease of access to education and opportunities for advanced nursing positions may help to stem the current flow of nurses away from the healthcare system. Of course, at the base of all healthcare is the benefit of the patient, and with these shifting of roles there is potential for a more-efficient and less-congested system, making changes in this manner advantageous for both providers and end users.

The COVID-19 pandemic has been somewhat of a double-edged sword when it comes to the nursing profession. While it has undoubtedly exposed the inadequacies of healthcare systems and has had a negative effect, mentally and physically, on those practicing at the time of its peak, it has also opened up a number of new doors that, while perhaps previously available, were underutilized and somewhat less accessible. There are those who having experienced the full force of the pandemic, particularly those on the frontline, who will likely never return to the profession. It was, however, through these unfortunate circumstances that the importance of nurses to multiple facets of a functioning and fit-for-purpose system has been exposed. Resultantly, issues that have long needed addressing have come to the forefront, and with the resolution of these comes a better overall situation, not alone for nurses, but also for the patients. Moving into a post-COVID era, nursing is finally being viewed in an entirely new light, and with that importance being acknowledged comes a new era of opportunity for nurses to fill new roles and step up to levels previously unexplored. COVID has undeniably been a disaster on many fronts, and will not quickly be forgotten, but if there is a light at the end of the tunnel, it is certain that the nursing profession may now grow and flourish more than it has in a long time.

REFERENCES

1. World Health Organization. (2022). Health workforce nursing and midwifery. [online] Available from https://www.who.int/news-room/fact-sheets/detail/nursing-and-midwifery [Last accessed February, 2024].
2. World Health Organization. (2021). The impact of COVID-19 on health and care workers: A closer look at deaths. [online] https://www.who.int/publications/i/item/WHO-HWF-WorkingPaper-2021.1 [Last accessed February, 2024].
3. Pappa S, Ntella V, Giannakas T, Giannakoulis VG, Papoutsi E, Katsaounou P. Prevalence of depression, anxiety, and insomnia among healthcare workers during the Covid-19 pandemic: A systematic review and meta-analysis. Brain Behav Immun. 2020;88:97.
4. Raso R, Fitzpatrick JJ, Masick K. Nurses' intent to leave their position and the profession during the COVID-19 pandemic. J Nurs Adm. 2021;51(10):488-94.
5. Royal College of Nursing. (2023). Valuing Nursing in the UK Staffing for safe and effective care in the UK: Interventions to mitigate risks to nursing retention. [online] Available from https://www.rcn.org.uk/-/media/Royal-College-Of-Nursing/Documents/Publications/2023/February/010-695.pdf [Last accessed February, 2024].
6. Patil N, Walsh M (2020). Resumption of OPD Activity in HSE Hospital Groups. Otolaryngology-Head and Neck Surgery. [online] Available from http://iiohns.org/assets/files/covid19/RESUMPTION%20OF%20OPD%20(00000002).pdf [Last accessed February, 2024].
7. Venegas-Vera AV, Colbert GB, Lerma EV. Positive and negative impact of social media in the COVID-19 era. Rev Cardiovasc Med. 2020;21(4):561-4.
8. Ruth Igielnik. (2020). Pew Research Center. Most Americans say they regularly wore a mask in stores in past month; fewer see others doing it. [online] Available from https://www.pewresearch.org/short-reads/2020/06/23/most-americans-say-they-regularly-wore-a-mask-in-stores-in-the-past-month-fewer-see-others-doing-it/ [Last accessed February, 2024].
9. Johnson S, Baloch SM, Nuño A. (2021). The Guardian. 'They stormed the ICU and beat the doctor': Health workers under attack. [online] Available from https://www.theguardian.com/global-development/2021/jun/07/they-stormed-the-icu-and-beat-the-doctor-health-workers-under-attack [Last accessed February, 2024].
10. BBC News. (2021). Guatemala: Anti-vaccine villagers attack and hold nurses with Covid jabs. [online] Available from https://www.bbc.com/news/world-latin-america-58801096 [Last accessed February, 2024].
11. The Guardian. (2021). The Guardian view on attacks on NHS staff: A grim and growing problem. [online] Available from https://www.theguardian.com/commentisfree/2021/aug/29/the-guardian-view-on-attacks-on-nhs-staff-a-grim-and-growing-problem [Last accessed February, 2024].
12. Gallegos M, de Castro Pecanha V, Caycho-Rodríguez T. Anti-vax: the history of a scientific problem. J Public Health (Oxf). 2022:fdac048.
13. Mehrabian A. Nonverbal Communication. Chicago, IL: Aldine Atherton;1972.
14. Hussain T, Munir K, Patil A, Munir J. The use of protective facemasks in hearing-impaired children during the severe acute respiratory syndrome coronavirus 2 pandemic: A new consideration. Int J Contemp Pediatr. 2022;9(4):333-6.

15. Hussain T, Patil A, Munir K, Choo M. Effect of face mask use on hearing impaired adult patients. Int J Community Med Public Health. 2022;9(3):1170-7.
16. Jagarapu J, Savani RC. A brief history of telemedicine and the evolution of teleneonatology. Semin Perinatol. 2021;45(5):151416.
17. Donelan K, Barreto EA, Sossong S, Michael C, Estrada JJ, Cohen AB, et al. Patient and clinician experiences with telehealth for patient follow up care. Am J Manag Care. 2019;25(1):40-4.
18. Nunes F, Ahmad N, Roberts D, Metz DC. (2020). Research Shows Patients and Clinicians Rated Telemedicine Care Positively During COVID-19 Pandemic. Penn Medicine News. [online] Available from https://www.pennmedicine.org/news/news-releases/2020/june/patients-and-clinicians-rated-telemedicine-care-positively-during-covid [Last accessed February, 2024].
19. Doximity. (2020). 2020 State of Telemedicine Report. Examining patient perspectives and physician adoption of telemedicine since the COVID-19 pandemic. [online]. Available from https://press.doximity.com/reports/state-of-telemedicine-report-2020.pdf [Last accessed February, 2024].
20. Sharifi Kia A, Rafizadeh M, Shahmoradi L. Telemedicine in the emergency department: An overview of systematic reviews. Z Gesundh Wiss. 2022:1-15.
21. Ward MM, Jaana M, Natafgi N. Systematic review of telemedicine applications in emergency rooms. Int J Med Inform. 2015;84(9):601-16.
22. du Toit M, Malau-Aduli B, Vangaveti V, Sabesan S, Ray RA. Use of telehealth in the management of non-critical emergencies in rural or remote emergency departments: A systematic review. J Telemed Telecare. 2019;25(1):3-16.
23. Rogers H, Madathil KC, Agnisarman S, Narasimha S, Ashok A, Nair A, et al. A systematic review of the implementation challenges of telemedicine systems in ambulances. Telemed JE Health. 2017;23:707-17.
24. Culmer N, Smith T, Stager C, Meyer H, Quick S, Grimm K. Evaluation of the triple aim of medicine in prehospital telemedicine: A systematic literature review. J Telemed Telecare. 2020;26(10):571-80.
25. Ma Y, Zhao C, Zhao Y, Lu J, Jiang H, Cao Y, Xu Y. Telemedicine application in patients with chronic disease: A systematic review and meta-analysis. BMC Med Inform Decis Mak. 2022;22(1):105.
26. O'Shea J, Berger R, Samra C, Van Durme D. Telemedicine in education: Bridging the gap. Educ Health (Abingdon). 2015;28(1):64-7.
27. Vicente MA, Fernández C, Guilabert M, Carrillo I, Martín-Delgado J, Mira JJ; Prometeo Working Group. Patient Engagement Using Telemedicine in Primary Care during COVID-19 Pandemic: A Trial Study. Int J Environ Res Public Health. 2022;19(22):14682.
28. Caffery LJ, Farjian M, Smith AC. Telehealth interventions for reducing waiting lists and waiting times for specialist outpatient services: A scoping review. J Telemed Telecare. 2016;22(8):504-12.
29. Catton H. How to reposition the nursing profession for a post-covid age. BMJ. 2021;373.
30. Saputri E, Pasinringi S, Ake J. The relationship between career ladder and nurses job satisfaction at a hospital. 2021;9(1):55-66.
31. Pei L, Wu H. Does online learning work better than offline learning in undergraduate medical education? A systematic review and meta-analysis. Med Educ Online. 2019;24(1):1666538.
32. Sarli L, Artioli G, De Luca E, Moretti C, Camacho VC, Di Niro V, et al. Nurses' perceived quality of educational life during the COVID-19 induced rapid transition to online learning in post-graduate courses: A qualitative study. Creative Educ. 2021;12(6):1247-61.

CHAPTER 15

Immunology in COVID-19

Rajeev Jayadevan

BASICS OF IMMUNOLOGY

The human body has the ability to defend itself from the attack of pathogens. These defense systems work in layers. The first line of defense is our innate immunity, which is broad and nonspecific as is the case with lower animals. The next line of defense is adaptive immunity, an advanced feature observed in more evolved species like vertebrates. Adaptive immunity is absent in invertebrates, such as insects, molluscs and worms, which rely on innate immunity as their primary defense mechanism.

Innate Immunity

Innate immunity consists of physical barriers, chemical defenses, and cellular responses.[1] The skin and mucous membrane are almost impenetrable for most pathogens to physically break through. On their own, they serve to keep the body safe, just like the walls of a fortress. Chemical barriers include enzymes found in natural body secretions such as saliva and tears, which destroy pathogens. Hydrochloric acid secreted in the stomach gets rid of many invading bacteria.

Innate cellular responses include phagocytes, such as macrophages and neutrophils, which engulf and destroy pathogens. Natural killer (NK) cells are specialized immune cells that can recognize and kill cells that are already infected or are cancerous. Unlike the adaptive immune system, NK cells do not require external permission to kill based on prior immune memory. This saves time and allows early removal of threats.

Natural killer cells have the ability to detect abnormal cells by assessing the presence or absence of certain molecules on the cell surface. They use a balance of activating and inhibitory receptors to distinguish healthy cells from infected or abnormal cells. Thus, when a patrolling NK cell encounters a sick-appearing cell that lacks proper inhibitory signals or displays activating signals, they can initiate a response to kill the target cell. This helps eliminate the threat early, before it spreads further.

Every day, the innate immune system diligently protects the body by warding off numerous potential pathogens.

Adaptive Immunity

Adaptive immunity refers to more specific and targeted response to pathogens. Also called acquired immunity, this involves the coordinated action of several components of the immune system.

When a new antigen is encountered, specialized antigen-presenting cells (APCs), such as dendritic cells, capture and process fragments of the antigen. These dendritic cells then migrate to the nearest lymph node, where they present the antigen fragments to T cells and B cells, initiating a tailored immune response. These fragments are called epitopes, and can be likened to a barcode of a specific product on the supermarket shelf. While scanning the barcode, the computer at the check-out is able to identify the product without the need to take a photograph of it. Different infectious agents have different barcodes. T cells and B cells located in the lymph node get trained based on these new barcodes (epitopes), and learn to recognize it.

There are several types of T cells, designated to perform different tasks. The CD4 helper T cells help coordinate and modulate the immune response, while CD8 cytotoxic cells scout the area and detect cells that are already infected by the specific pathogen. These T cells are armed with the specific bar-code of the offending agent; thus, their response is precise and targeted.

B cells manufacture antibodies, which are Y-shaped molecules that attack viruses and bacteria. When a B cell, already primed to recognize a specific virus, encounters the virus, the B cell receptors located on its surface recognize the barcode on the body of the virus. This activates the B cell to produce antibodies tailored to attack that virus. Once these antibodies attach to the virus, it can either be neutralized directly or swallowed by other immune cells. Thus, the attachment of antibodies to a virus is a crucial step in the immune response against viral infections.[2] They help eliminate the threat by directly neutralizing it, promoting phagocytosis, activating the complement system, and engaging other immune cells such as NK cells to attack and clear the virus from the body.

Antibody-dependent cellular cytotoxicity (ADCC) involves the coordinated action of various immune components against pathogens such as viruses. Cells that are infected by viruses are able to send distress signals to summon the immune system. One such signal is to display a fragment (epitope) of the virus on its surface, this almost like waving a flag to attract the attention of a passing soldier. Antibodies made specifically for the virus circulate throughout the body. They attach to these bits of virus found on the surface of infected cells. This process highlights the infected cells, making it easy for circulating immune cells to find and destroy them. The Fc ends of these antibodies are recognized by circulating NK cells, which secrete chemicals that destroy the infected cell.

CD8 T cells, also called cytotoxic T cells, also destroy infected cells, through a process that does not require prior flagging by antibodies. Having been trained within the lymph nodes as described earlier, these cells are already armed with specific barcodes (epitopes) of the virus. They can identify infected cells on their own, followed by targeted destruction. CD8 T cells directly identify fragments of the virus displayed on the surface of the infected cell on specialized molecular complexes called major histocompatibility complex-I (MHC-I). Once activated, they secrete cytotoxic chemicals such as perforin and granzymes, which destroy the infected cell along with the viruses contained within it.

Once the immediate threat is eliminated, there is immune contraction. This is essentially a winding down of the immune response, so that normal bodily function can resume. The immune system has its own built-in brakes, which help reduce the activity of the activated immune cells. For instance, regulatory T cells, also called Treg cells play a role in this process. These cells prevent excessive immune responses that could lead to harmful inflammation. By regulating the activity of T helper cells, Treg cells indirectly influence the activity of B cells, thus reducing antibody production.[3]

An outcome of immune contraction is that antibody production slows to a low baseline; this is the reason why circulating levels of antibodies decline after a few months of infection or vaccination.[4]

Along with immune contraction, there is development of immune memory, which means storing of essential identifying information of the virus for future use. Such immune memory exists in both the B cell and T cell compartments, and is long-term. This means that the immune system can readily recognize and respond if ever the same infection occurred again in the future. A prompt immune response helps keep tissue damage to a minimum, and this is the reason why people who have had vaccination have better outcomes following repeat infection.

These immune memory cells are located in different areas of the body. Some memory cells take up permanent residence in the bone marrow, while others live in tissues. A few remain in constant circulation, looking for any signal of the virus entering the body again. The advantage of immune memory is that it jump-starts the immune response, without having to go through the elaborate initial process of identifying and training immune cells.

Mucosal Immunity

In the context of coronavirus disease 2019 (COVID-19), mucosal immunity plays a crucial role, providing protection at the surfaces lining the respiratory tract, gastrointestinal tract, and eye, which serve as the points of entry for the severe acute respiratory syndrome coronavirus 2 (SARS-CoV-2) virus. The protection it provides is both innate and adaptive in nature.

The first line of defense is the physical barrier provided by the mucosal surfaces themselves. These include the mucus layer and epithelial cells. These barriers serve to trap and prevent the entry of the SARS-CoV-2 virus.

Additionally, the mucosal immune system comprises various immune cells and molecules that actively combat viral infections. When a pathogen breaches the mucosal barrier, specialized mucosal cells called APCs capture and process antigens. This sets adaptive immunity in motion, eventually resulting in mucosal immune memory. Virus-specific memory T cells and B cells are found in vaccinated people and among those who have recovered from COVID-19.

Following activation in the mucosa-associated lymphoid tissue (MALT), some B cells differentiate into plasma cells, producing immunoglobulin A (IgA) antibodies. They are specifically designed to neutralize pathogens at the mucosal surfaces. In the case of COVID-19, IgA antibodies can recognize and bind to the spike protein of the SARS-CoV-2 virus, preventing its attachment and entry into host cells.

Mucosal immunity in COVID-19 helps not only in preventing initial infection but also for limiting the spread of the virus from the respiratory and gastrointestinal tracts to other parts of the body. In addition, nonpharmacological interventions such as N95 masks, social distancing, and improving room ventilation help reduce the load of virus entering the respiratory tract, further decreasing the chance of getting infected.

HISTORY OF COVID-19 FROM AN IMMUNOLOGY PERSPECTIVE

When the SARS-CoV-2 virus started spreading in humans, a unique situation arose. This was an all-new virus which had never been encountered by man earlier. Therefore, there was no question of relying on baseline protection from prior immune memory. This meant that immune memory had to be built from zero. Two ways to build immune memory are through natural infection and through vaccination. Unfortunately, the initial death rate from COVID-19 was relatively high, implying that allowing the virus to circulate freely through the community would result in millions of deaths. This would be too high a price to pay for acquiring immune memory, especially for older adults in whom mortality rate was substantially higher than in younger people.

Hence, the world placed its collective hope in vaccines. They were developed on multiple platforms, some of which were new. Several ventures failed; others succeeded. Until vaccines arrived, time-tested mitigation measures kept the virus from spreading uncontrollably. Once vaccines were rolled out, mitigation measures were gradually eased.

Unfortunately, over the course of 3 years, millions of people lost their lives to COVID. Deaths occurred directly from complications of COVID such as pneumonia and cardiovascular events. Deaths also occurred indirectly from overwhelmed healthcare systems failing to deliver the recommended care for other health conditions such as cardiac and respiratory disease. In addition, many people lost their lives following initial recovery from COVID, either from destabilization of their baseline health conditions, or due to delayed vascular complications.

IMMUNOLOGY LESSONS FROM THE PANDEMIC

As the pandemic unfolded, unlike the case of other communicable diseases, no textbook existed for the world to turn to. Knowledge was primarily based on observations on a forward timeline; some events such as the Diamond Princess Cruise ship outbreak and the Seattle fishing boat experience gave the world valuable information.[5] Numerous unknowns existed, particularly about the type of immune response that is elicited by the SARS-CoV-2 virus. Foremost was whether prior exposure to virus antigen would provide any protection from future infection. Experience with circulating common cold coronaviruses suggested that long-term immunity would be unlikely, as these viruses are known to cause repeated infections in the same individual. However, there was an early narrative that for the new virus, achieving immunity could be a realistic goal.

The Diamond Princess Cruise ship outbreak proved that the virus could spread efficiently between people in confined settings. The secondary attack rate was 19%, after 700 people became infected out of 3,700 passengers.

The Seattle fishing boat experience revealed that crew members who had significant levels of antibodies from surviving a prior infection were protected from getting infected during an outbreak that occurred while at sea. While this was encouraging, what the study did not reveal was the duration of such protection.[6]

The early clinical trials of COVID vaccines promised a high percentage of protection from infection.[7] Unfortunately, these percentages referred to the immediate postvaccination period, and did not reflect long-term outcomes.

The Centers for Disease Control and Prevention (CDC) report on 60% of a group of fully vaccinated miners suffering a COVID outbreak in French Guyana by May 2021 was one of the landmark papers revealing the inability of COVID vaccines to provide long-term protection from infection.[8]

Similar stories started getting reported from other parts of the world, including India. An outbreak of COVID occurred among a batch of vaccinated MBBS students in Government Medical College Trissur in July 2021.[9]

It became clear that the SARS-CoV-2 virus was continuously evolving to achieve immune escape, and repeatedly infect the same individual.

Although infections occurred among those who had prior vaccination or natural infection, disease severity and mortality were consistently lower than among immune-naïve individuals.

THE ARRIVAL OF OMICRON

After multiple variants circulated in various parts of the globe, a landmark event occurred on November 2021. A new variant, vastly different from any prior version was reported by scientists in South Africa.[10] This was faster spreading, immune evasive, but apparently causing less severe disease. The speed of spread was unprecedented; within 6 weeks, it spread throughout the globe. Test positivity rate (TPR) in parts of India reached 50%, indicating that one out of every two people tested were carrying the virus, either with or without symptoms.

The COVID-19 outbreak in the Faroe Islands affected 21 out of 33 healthcare workers who had recently received a booster dose and attended a private gathering in December 2021. This event highlighted that under specific circumstances, such as close contact in a social setting, Omicron could still infect individuals who had received a messenger ribonucleic acid (mRNA) booster dose.

The origin of Omicron is not clear. It is believed that such a large number of mutations would have taken considerable time to accumulate, and therefore it could have risen during the course of a chronic infection in a person who was immunosuppressed. The alternative hypothesis is that it might have evolved in an animal as a case of reverse zoonosis, created the new mutations, and then jumped back to man.

There is uncertainty about whether Omicron's lower severity is due to the large number of mutations, or because the world had been already exposed to prior versions of the virus by virtue of vaccination or by surviving natural infection. Hong Kong's experience suggests the latter.[11] As part of zero COVID strategy, Hong Kong was one of the few places in the world that had remained free from natural infection. In addition, there was considerable vaccine hesitancy, especially among older citizens. As a result, when Omicron arrived in Hong Kong, it spread rapidly through the population, and caused substantial mortality among the immune naïve, primarily the unvaccinated elderly. This suggests that the apparent low severity of Omicron is chiefly the result of protection offered by prior immune memory.[12]

NEWER VERSIONS OF OMICRON

The world continued to see newer versions of Omicron, each one capable of causing infection in people who had infection with prior sublineages. XBB is the currently dominant version, being a product of recombination of BM.1.1.1 and BJ.1 sublineages. Various downstream descendants of XBB are circulating in different countries, immune evasiveness being their hallmark.

India recently went through a wave lasting approximately 2 months, from March till May 2023. Although the number of people infected was substantial, the number of patients admitted to hospital was relatively low. Severe outcomes were restricted to those who were elderly or with comorbidity. The lower severity of the wave in India is believed to be the result of preexisting long-term immune memory from vaccination as well as prior bouts of COVID.

The number of reported cases in the most recent wave in India will be an underestimate due to widespread reluctance to undergo SARS-CoV-2 testing. Wastewater surveillance from Tata Institute for Genetics and Society (TIGS) Bengaluru shows that the viral load measured in copies/mL in April 2023 was higher than the first Omicron wave in January 2022. This is an indirect indicator of the amount of virus circulating in the community.

This observation is proof that existing immunity against the SARS-CoV-2 virus is not effective in reducing the number of infections in the community during subsequent waves.

VACCINATION AND IMMUNE IMPRINTING

The ability of newer versions of the SARS-CoV-2 virus to repeatedly infect people who had prior vaccination has been the subject of study. It was observed that XBB sublineages were poorly neutralized by antibodies from convalescent plasma or from prior vaccinated people. This means that current vaccination strategy is not enough to stop repeat infections from occurring, and that any additional protection from infection from extra doses of vaccine will be short-lived.

While studying the reasons for failure of vaccines to stop infection by newer sublineages of Omicron, it was found that each additional dose of vaccine was generating antibodies directed against the older version of the virus, which the vaccines were based on.[13] This phenomenon is called immune imprinting, and was earlier known as "original antigenic sin". It means that when the body is exposed to a new antigen, the immune response generated will primarily target the specific version of the antigen that was encountered earlier.

Consequently, even infections from newer versions of the virus generated antibodies that were directed against the original strain. However, recent evidence suggests it can be overcome by repeated infection with newer versions of Omicron.[14]

In order to counter immune imprinting, updated vaccines were launched in the US since 2022. Also known as bivalent vaccines, they contained the spike protein of the omicron in addition to that of the original strain. Unfortunately, immune imprinting persisted; the antibodies generated were overwhelmingly biased toward older rather than newer versions of the virus. The real-world protection offered against infection was not markedly higher than older monovalent vaccines, according to studies from Cleveland clinic.[15]

A recent study conducted in Qatar compared people who received the bivalent booster vaccine with individuals who had not received recent vaccination. The study revealed that the frequency of COVID-19 cases in the bivalent group was similar to that in the control group. Specifically, the bivalent group had a frequency of 36 cases out of 10,886 individuals, which translates to 0.33%. In comparison, the control group had a frequency of 211 cases out of 53,901 individuals, which corresponds to 0.39%.[16]

The World health Organization (WHO) has recently recommended that any new vaccine be made based only on the latest version of the virus, and that the older spike no longer be used.[17] This was based on observations that immune imprinting can be overcome by repeated exposures to newer versions of the virus.[18]

The updated XBB.1.5 monovalent mRNA vaccine was made available in 2023, but found low acceptance of only 17% among US adults. While data of clinical effectiveness is not yet available at the time of writing, research from Sato Lab Japan indicates that the new variant JN.1 is potentially capable of escaping the antibodies following this vaccine.[19] Its immune evasiveness is greater than the recently circulating XBB sub-lineages. This suggests that the virus is continuously evolving to escape human immune response. This explains the cyclical tendency of the virus infection to a large degree.

LONG CORONAVIRUS DISEASE

Although the mortality rate of COVID-19 has reduced with the arrival of Omicron sublineages, the threat of long COVID looms large. This is defined by the WHO as the persistence of symptoms for at least 3 months following recovery from an acute bout of COVID. The chief symptoms include fatigue, shortness of breath, "brain fog", and myalgia. The estimated incidence is 5%, which implies that one out of twenty infections go on to have long-term symptoms. The recent National Institutes of Health (NIH) Researching COVID to Enhance Recovery (RECOVER) study of 9,764 participants showed that 10% of Omicron infections go on to develop long COVID, the risk increasing with reinfection.[27]

With no approved medications, long COVID remains a challenge, particularly given the cyclical nature of the infection. Immunology of long COVID has been the subject of much study. Initially it was believed to be autoimmune in nature, but more recent research has suggested otherwise. Persistence of virus in remote parts of the body such as the gut has been implicated. Reactivation of latent viruses like Epstein–Barr virus is yet another proposed mechanism. Persistent immune dysfunction is the common theme.[20]

MULTISYSTEM INFLAMMATORY SYNDROME IN CHILDREN

During the earlier waves of the pandemic, a rare yet severe multisystem illness was observed among children following recovery from COVID.[21] Mortality was significant, especially among untreated cases. Multisystem inflammatory syndrome in children (MIS-C) is characterized by immune dysregulation, activation of innate immunity, T cell activation, excessive antibody response, and endothelial dysfunction. Outcomes are better among children who receive multidisciplinary care in hospitals, and favorable results have been achieved with intravenous immunoglobulin and steroids. Fortunately, MIS-C has become uncommon following the arrival of Omicron.

NATURAL IMMUNITY

Much has been discussed about the role of natural immunity in COVID. Unfortunately, it is seldom recognized that to achieve natural immunity, one must first survive natural infection. In an immune naive population, to survive natural infection involves considerable risk. Those who have acquired natural immunity are therefore more aptly called survivors, a term particularly relevant in the prevaccination era. In the early part of the pandemic, nations such as Sweden and Britain believed that allowing the virus to circulate in the community would result in what they called herd immunity. Unfortunately, nations that followed this principle suffered high mortality rates, specifically in the first part of the pandemic.

The concept of herd immunity was borrowed from other infectious diseases, such as measles and polio, where immunity is considered long-lasting or lifelong. In such situations, the presence of a high percentage of people with immunity in a population could arrest the spread of the virus further. However, this concept was found to be invalid in COVID because of the ability of this virus to cause repeated infections even among those with prior immune memory.[22]

Instead, what was observed was a cyclical pattern of infections, where repeated waves occurred in the same geographical region, spread several months apart—with no predilection to seasons. Each wave correlates with several factors coinciding, including a collective drop in level of immunity in the community, increase in travel, drop in pandemic precautions, arrival of new variants, and weather conditions that facilitate spread of the virus.

Studies have shown that those who survived natural infection experienced significant protection from severe disease during future encounters with the virus. However, such protection is relatively less effective among older age groups.

MECHANISMS OF PROTECTION

Following vaccination, two types of protection are obtained. The first is protection from infection and the second is protection from severe disease and death in the event of an infection. The two must be seen separately from an immunological perspective.

Protection from Infection

A correlate of protection refers to a measurable immune response or biomarker that is predictive of protection against a particular infectious disease. It serves as an indirect indicator or surrogate endpoint for vaccine efficacy or the likelihood of immune protection. Unfortunately, there is no clear correlate of protection for COVID-19 despite extensive research. A recent paper has shown that the presence of a high titer of neutralizing antibodies immediately prior to exposure is protective against infection.[23] However, a gradual drop in antibody titers is the norm, and therefore it is unrealistic to expect long-term protection as a result of vaccination or a bout of infection.

As neutralizing antibody levels drop, it becomes easier for the virus to infect the individual. There is some evidence that those who have survived natural infection have more robust mucosal immunity along the airways compared to those who had been vaccinated. This is believed to offer temporary protection against infection.[24,25]

A recent study of reinfections by the CDC has shown that one out of seven reinfections occurred under 2 months.[26] This indicates that multiple infections are the norm, looking forward.

A large study from Washington University has shown that while reinfections are not individually more serious, the collective outcomes are worse among those who had more bouts of infection.[28] This highlights the need for continuing mitigation measures, especially during times of a regional surge.

Protection from Severe Disease

Although the subject of debate, it is increasingly recognized that T cell-mediated adaptive immunity plays a crucial role in providing protection against severe disease. As discussed earlier, T cells from various genres coordinate the adaptive immune response following infection. Although neutralizing antibodies are effective in preventing the virus from infecting a cell, they are of little use after a virus has already entered the cell. In such a scenario, T cells that have been primed through prior exposure, either by natural infection or vaccination, play a significant role.

T cells recognize and eliminate these infected cells, preventing the virus from spreading further and causing organ damage. Continuous evolution has enabled the virus to escape neutralizing antibody protection. However, the smaller and limited epitope repertoire recognized by T cells has made it more challenging for the virus to evade T cell-mediated protection. In other words, the accumulated mutations have primarily aided the virus in evading detection by antibodies, while T cells remain effective in recognizing and responding to even newer versions of the virus.

The absence of a clear correlate of protection remains a challenge in COVID-19. In other words, unlike hepatitis B, where a specific antibody titer signifies protection from infection, no such test is available commercially for COVID-19 outside of laboratory research. In other words, checking the antibody panel in a commercial laboratory will not predict the magnitude or duration of protection from infection or severe disease. The reason is that commercial antibody tests estimate binding antibodies.

Binding antibodies are involved in recognizing and binding to specific viral proteins, while neutralizing antibodies are responsible for blocking the infectivity of the virus. Both types of antibodies contribute to the overall immune response against the virus. However, neutralizing antibodies attach to specific regions of the virus, preventing it from entering cells and causing infection. Their presence can effectively abort an infection before it takes hold.

Currently, measurement of neutralizing antibodies in blood is not widely available through standard commercial laboratory kits. This presents a challenge in accurately assessing the level of protection against infection. Additionally, the progressive decline in antibody levels over time further complicates the ability to provide assurance of long-term protection from infection in real-life scenarios.

HYBRID IMMUNITY

The term hybrid immunity is often used to denote the combination of immunity derived not only from vaccination, but also from natural infection. Studies have suggested that those who have hybrid immunity have more robust protection from infection. This stems from the observation that vaccination in a person who has had prior natural infection, generates a more robust antibody response because of preexisting long-term immune memory. However, some authors have reported more frequent adverse outcomes such as chronic arthralgia among people who have been vaccinated following recovery from natural infection.[29]

SEROPREVALENCE

Multiple studies have assessed the antibody positivity among the general population during the early days of the pandemic. In urban areas, seropositivity has been documented. For example, a study in Delhi showed that 97% of people already had antibodies to COVID—even before the arrival of Omicron.[30] A study from Karnataka had shown that 75% of COVID infections in the pre-Omicron era occurred without noticeable symptoms.[31] This implies that a large part of the world's population has been subjected to repeated bouts of infection over the past 3 years, generating a substantial amount of community immunity. Although this is implicated in the relatively mild recent XBB.1.16 wave in India, whether this translates into long-term protection against severe outcomes from future variants remains unknown.

REFERENCES

1. Paludan SR, Mogensen TH. Innate immunological pathways in COVID-19 pathogenesis. Sci Immunol. 2022;7(67):eabm5505.
2. Tso FY, Lidenge SJ, Poppe LK, Peña PB, Privatt SR, Bennett SJ, et al. Presence of antibody-dependent cellular cytotoxicity (ADCC) against SARS-CoV-2 in COVID-19 plasma. PLoS One. 2021;16(3):e0247640.
3. Marrack P, Scott-Browne J, MacLeod MKL. Terminating the immune response. Immunol Rev. 2010;236(1):5-10.
4. Rickards CG, Kilpatrick AM. Age-specific SARS-CoV-2 infection fatality rates derived from serological data vary with income and income inequality. PloS One. 2023;18(5): e0285612.
5. Gu Y, Chen Y, Wang X, Chen Z. Impact of COVID-19 Epidemic on Port Operations: Evidence from Asian Ports. Case Stud Transp Policy. 2023;12:101014.
6. Bradley BT, Bryan A, Fink SL, Goecker EA, Roychoudhury P, Huang ML, et al. Anti-SARS-CoV-2 Antibody Levels Measured by the AdviseDx SARS-CoV-2 Assay are Concordant with Previously Available Serologic Assays but are Not Fully Predictive of Sterilizing Immunity. J Clin Microbiol. 2021;59(9):e0098921.
7. Polack FP, Thomas SJ, Kitchin N, Absalon J, Gurtman A, Lockhart S, et al. Safety and Efficacy of the BNT162b2 mRNA Covid-19 Vaccine. N Engl J Med. 2020;383(27): 2603-15.
8. Vignier N, Bérot V, Bonnave N, Peugny S, Ballet M, Jacoud E, et al. Breakthrough Infections of SARS-CoV-2 Gamma Variant in Fully Vaccinated Gold Miners, French Guiana, 2021. Emerg Infect Dis. 2021;27(10):2673-76.
9. India Today. (2021). Kerala: 39 fully vaccinated students of govt medical college hospital test positive for COVID. [online] Available from https://www.indiatoday.in/coronavirus-outbreak/story/kerala-39-fully-vaccinated-students-of-govt-medical-college-hospital-test-positive-for-covid-1830177-2021-07-19. [Last accessed February, 2024].
10. Helmsdal G, Hansen OK, Møller LF, Christiansen DH, Petersen MS, Kristiansen MF. Omicron Outbreak at a Private Gathering in the Faroe Islands, Infecting 21 of 33 Triple-Vaccinated Healthcare Workers. Clin Infect Dis. 2022;75(5):893-6.
11. Tegally H, Moir M, Everatt J, Giovanetti M, Scheepers C, Wilkinson E, et al. Emergence of SARS-CoV-2 Omicron lineages BA.4 and BA.5 in South Africa. Nat Med. 28(9): 1785-90.
12. Centre of Health Protection. Statistics on 5th Wave of COVID-19 in Hong Kong. [online] Available from https://www.covidvaccine.gov.hk/pdf/5th_wave_statistics.pdf. [Last accessed February, 2024].
13. Mykytyn AZ, Rosu ME, Kok A, Rissmann M, van Amerongen G, Geurtsvankessel C, et al. Antigenic mapping of emerging SARS-CoV-2 omicron variants BM.1.1.1, BQ.1.1, and XBB.1. Lancet Microbe. 2023;4(5):e294-5.
14. Aydillo T, Rombauts A, Stadlbauer D, Aslam S, Abelenda-Alonso G, Escalera A, et al. Immunological imprinting of the antibody response in COVID-19 patients. Nat Commun. [online]. 2021;12(1):3781.
15. Yisimayi A, Song W, Wang J, Jian F, Yu Y, Chen X, et al. Repeated Omicron infection alleviates SARS-CoV-2 immune imprinting. Nature. 2024;625(7993):148-56.
16. Shrestha NK, Burke PC, Nowacki AS, Simon JF, Hagen A, Gordon SM. Effectiveness of the Coronavirus Disease 2019 Bivalent Vaccine. Open Forum Infect Dis. 2023;10(6): ofad209.
17. Chemaitelly H, Ayoub HH, AlMukdad S, Faust JS, Tang P, Coyle P, et al. Bivalent mRNA-1273.214 vaccine effectiveness against SARS-CoV-2 omicron XBB* infections. J Travel Med. 2023;30(5):taad106.

18. World Health Organization. (2023). Statement on the antigen composition of COVID-19 vaccines. [online] Available from https://www.who.int/news/item/18-05-2023-statement-on-the-antigen-composition-of-covid-19-vaccines. [Last accessed February, 2024].
19. Thaweethai T, Jolley SE, Karlson EW, Levitan EB, Levy B, McComsey GA, et al. Development of a Definition of Postacute Sequelae of SARS-CoV-2 Infection. JAMA. 2023;329(22):1934-46.
20. Gold JE, Okyay RA, Licht WE, Hurley DJ. Investigation of Long COVID Prevalence and its Relationship to Epstein-Barr Virus Reactivation. Pathogens. 2021;10(6):763.
21. Gupta V, Singh A, Ganju S, Singh R, Thiruvengadam R, Natchu UCM, et al. Severity and mortality associated with COVID-19 among children hospitalised in tertiary care centres in India: a cohort study. Lancet Reg Health Southeast Asia. 2023;13:100203.
22. Yewdell JW. Individuals cannot rely on COVID-19 herd immunity: Durable immunity to viral disease is limited to viruses with obligate viremic spread. PLoS Pathog. 2021;17(4):e1009509.
23. Atti A, Insalata F, Carr EJ, Otter A, Foulkes S, Wu MY, et al. Antibody Correlates of Protection Against Delta Infection after Vaccination: A Nested Case-Control within the UK-Based Siren Study. J Infect. 2023;87:420-7.
24. Malato J, Ribeiro RM, Leite PP, Casaca P, Fernandes E, Antunes C, et al. Risk of BA.5 Infection among Persons Exposed to Previous SARS-CoV-2 Variants. N Engl J Med. 2022;387(10):953-4.
25. Tang J, Zeng C, Cox TM, Li C, Son YM, Cheon IS, et al. Respiratory mucosal immunity against SARS-CoV-2 after mRNA vaccination. Sci Immunol. 2022;7:eadd4853.
26. Nguyen NN, Houhamdi L, Delorme L, Colson P, Gautret P. Reinfections with Different SARS-CoV-2 Omicron Subvariants, France. Emerg Infecti Dis. 2022;28(11):2341-3.
27. De Bruijn S, van Hoek AJ, Mutubuki EN, Knoop H, Slootweg J, Tulen AD, et al. Lower prevalence of Post-Covid-19 Condition following Omicron SARS-CoV-2 infection. Medrxiv. 2023.
28. Bowe B, Xie Y, Al-Aly Z. Acute and postacute sequelae associated with SARS-CoV-2 reinfection. Nat Med. 2022;28(11):2398-405.
29. Kaur U, Fatima Z, Maheshwari K, Sahni V, Dehade A, Kl A, et al. Long-term Safety Analysis of the ChAdOx1-nCoV-19 Corona Virus Vaccine: Results from a Prospective Observational Study in Priority Vaccinated Groups in North India. Drug Saf. 2023;46: 553-63.
30. Hindustan Times. (2021). 8 of 10 kids in Delhi have COVID antibodies. [online] Available from https://www.hindustantimes.com/cities/delhi-news/8-of-10-kids-in-delhi-have-covid-antibodies-101635471193829.html. [Last accessed February, 2024].
31. George CE, Inbaraj LR, Rajukutty S, Joan RF, Suseeladevi AK, Muthuraj S, et al. Seroprevalence of COVID-19 infection among vaccine naïve population after the second surge (June 2020) in a rural district of South India: A community-based cross-sectional study. PLoS One. 2022;17(3):e0265236.

CHAPTER 16

The Experience in the Making of COVID-19 Vaccines

Carlos Valladeres, Jose Iglesias

INTRODUCTION

Coronavirus disease 2019 (COVID-19) was first detected in Wuhan, Hubei Province, China, in December 2019.[1] As a result of the emergence of severe acute respiratory syndrome coronavirus 2 (SARS-CoV-2), the virus causing COVID-19, a global pandemic affected individuals and communities in a dramatic manner.[2] By September 2022, there were >95 million cases and >1 million deaths associated with COVID-19 in the United States.[3] People of all ages are at risk for infection and severe disease from COVID-19. However, people with chronic medical conditions, those residing in long-term care facilities, and those over 65 years of age are at greater risk of severe illness. Moreover, racial and ethnic minority communities suffer disproportionately from COVID-19 infections and deaths. Blacks, Hispanics/Latinos (Hispanics), and American Indians/American natives have higher rates of disease, hospitalization, and death than non-Hispanic Whites. As a result of inequities in social determinants of health, racial and ethnic minorities are likely to be more vulnerable to COVID-19. These include overrepresentation in essential workers who are at an increased risk of exposure to COVID-19, have lower incomes, have less access to healthcare, or have higher rates of comorbid conditions.[2]

HOW WAS THE VACCINE DEVELOPED SO QUICKLY?

The researchers at the National Institute of Allergy and Infectious Diseases's (NIAID's) Vaccine Research Center (VRC) and Moderna were able to quickly develop messenger ribonucleic acid-1273 (mRNA-1273) as a result of prior studies on coronaviruses that cause severe acute respiratory syndrome (SARS) and Middle East respiratory syndrome (MERS), which are related coronaviruses. There is a spike on the surface of coronavirus particles, which gives it a crown-like appearance **(Fig. 1)**. This spike binds to human cells,

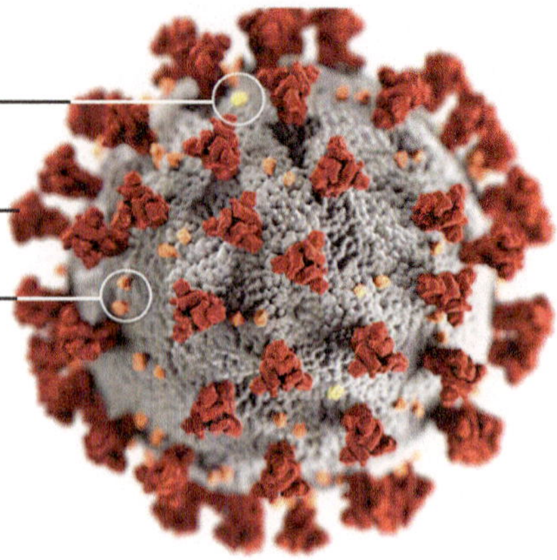

FIGURE 1: This illustration, created at the Centers for Disease Control and Prevention (CDC), reveals ultrastructural morphology exhibited by coronaviruses. Note the spikes that adorn the outer surface of the virus, which impart the look of a corona surrounding the virion, when viewed electron microscopically. A novel coronavirus, named severe acute respiratory syndrome coronavirus 2 (SARS-CoV-2), was identified as the cause of an outbreak of respiratory illness first detected in Wuhan, China in 2019. The illness caused by this virus has been named coronavirus disease 2019 (COVID-19).[11]

Courtesy: Alissa Eckert, MSMI; Dan Higgins, MAMS.

which allows the virus to enter. A vaccine candidate for protection against COVID-19 was already being developed by VRC and Moderna scientists, who were already developing an investigational MERS vaccine targeting the spike. Scientists selected a sequence to express the stabilized spike protein of the virus on the existing mRNA platform immediately after the genetic information for SARS-CoV-2 became available.[1] It is pertinent to note that although the vaccine platforms are different, there have vaccines developed against coronavirus in veterinary medicine for over three decades and have been employed with variable success.[4-7] In addition the development of a successful vaccine against SARS and MERS was met with failure.[8-10]

CLINICAL TRIALS STARTED–RACE FOR A VACCINE

In response to the obvious need for a vaccine against COVID-19, pharmaceutical companies began competing to develop such a vaccine. As different clinical trials were initiated around the world, some relied on well-known vaccine methods and others tested novel technologies to combat this viral infection.

Kaiser Permanente Washington Health Research Institute (KPWHRI) in Seattle conducted the first phase 1 clinical trial evaluating an investigational vaccine designed to protect against COVID-19. During the open-label trial, 45 healthy adult volunteers aged 18–55 years were enrolled, and the investigational vaccine was administered to the first participant on March 16, 2020.[1]

The NIAID scientists and collaborators at the Cambridge, Massachusetts-based biotechnology company Moderna, Inc. developed a vaccine called mRNA-1273. Various doses of the experimental vaccine were evaluated for their safety and their ability to induce an immune response in participants. As part of the clinical trial process, this was the first of several steps evaluating the vaccine's potential benefits.[1]

Based on the genetic platform of mRNA, the investigational vaccine was designed to induce a robust immune response by directing cells to express a virus protein. In animal models, mRNA-1273 had shown promise, but this was the first human trial to test it.[1]

Two doses of the vaccine were administered intramuscularly in the upper arm approximately 28 days apart. Each participant received either 25 μg, 100 μg, or 250 μg dose at both vaccinations, with 15 people in each dose cohort. Four of the participants received a low dose injection, followed by four participants receiving a 100 μg injection. After reviewing safety data, investigators vaccinated the remaining participants in the 25 μg dose group and vaccinated them again before receiving their second vaccination.

After the second vaccination, participants were requested to return to the clinic for follow-up visits and for additional visits over the next year. Clinical staff will monitor participants for symptoms common to vaccination, such as soreness at the injection site, fever, and any other medical problems. Safety data were reviewed regularly by a protocol team, and a safety monitoring committee advised the NIAID on trial safety data on a periodic basis. As part of the study, participants provided blood samples at certain time points, which investigators analyzed in the laboratory to detect and assess the immune response to the experimental vaccine.[1]

It should be noted, however, that this was not the only clinical trial being conducted. The race has also been entered by a number of other well-known companies. A press release issued by Pfizer Inc. and BioNTech SE on May 5, 2020 announced that doses had been administered to the first participants in the Phase 1/2 clinical trial of BNT162 against COVID-19 in the United States. As part of a worldwide development program, the first cohort of patients was dosed in Germany 1 week prior to the start of this study.[12]

During Phase 1/2, four mRNA vaccine candidates were evaluated in a single continuous study to determine safety, immunogenicity, and optimal dose level. It was reported that up to 360 healthy subjects were enrolled into two age cohorts (18–55 and 65–85 years of age) during the dose level escalation phase (Stage 1) of the Phase 1/2 trial in the United States. As part of Stage 1 of the study, healthy adults 18–55 years of age were immunized. Participating sites included NYU Grossman School of Medicine and the University of Maryland School of Medicine.[12]

On June 10th 2020, Johnson & Johnson announced that the early-stage human trials of a potential coronavirus vaccine would begin in the second half of the following month, much earlier than anticipated. Earlier that year, the company began developing a vaccine for COVID-19 using the same technology used to manufacture an experimental Ebola vaccine that was delivered to people in the Democratic Republic of Congo at the end of 2019. A modified adenovirus that causes common colds in humans was combined with genetic material from the coronavirus.[13]

By April 2021, Johnson & Johnson expects to produce 600–900 million doses of the vaccine if it works well and is proven to be safe. In its early-stage clinical trial, Johnson & Johnson planned to test its vaccine on 1,045 healthy adults between the ages of 18 and 55 years, as well as those between the ages of 65 and 74 years. The trial was conducted in the United States and Belgium.[13]

THE FIRST RESULTS

Following the positive results of Phase 1/2 studies, pharmaceutical companies moved on to Phase 3 clinical trials. Over 40,000 people were enrolled in these studies, and the vaccine was tested for safety and adverse reactions were reported. A number of trials were conducted in different parts of the world and the race to develop the first vaccine became increasingly competitive.

The results of Pfizer's Phase 3 clinical trials were announced in November, 2020. Trials for the potential vaccine BNT162b2 commenced on July 27, 2020, and 43,661 participants have been enrolled to date. Nearly 42% of global participants and 30% of US participants are of diverse racial and ethnic backgrounds, and 41% of global participants and 45% of US participants are between the ages of 56 and 85 years.[15]

The results of the study indicate that the vaccine has an efficacy rate of 95% ($p < 0.0001$) in participants without prior SARS-CoV-2 infection, as well as in participants who have had prior SARS-CoV-2 infection, both measured 7 days following the second dose. According to the study protocol, there were 170 cases of COVID-19, of which 162 cases were observed in the placebo group and eight cases in the BNT162b2 group. In terms of effectiveness, there was no difference in effectiveness across age groups, genders, races, and ethnicities. Over 94% of the efficacy defined as relative risk reduction (RRR) was observed in adults over 65 years of age. During the trial, 10 severe cases of COVID-19 were observed, nine of which occurred in the placebo group and one in the BNT162b2 vaccinated group.[15]

There were no serious safety concerns reported in the study. In the final analysis of unblinded reactogenicity data, it was demonstrated that the vaccine was well-tolerated with the majority of solicited adverse events resolved shortly after vaccination. Following doses 1 and 2, fatigue at 3.8%

and headache at 2.0% were the only Grade 3 (severe) solicited adverse reactions ≥2%. Vaccine-related adverse events in older adults were fewer and milder than in younger adults, according to earlier shared results.[15]

Pfizer announced that these results had met the safety milestone required for the Emergency Use Authorization (EUA) by the US Food and Drug Administration (FDA). In November 2020, Pfizer and BioNTech submitted a request for an EUA in response to the totality of safety and efficacy data collected to date, as well as manufacturing data regarding vaccine quality and consistency to the FDA. Additionally, these data would be submitted to other regulatory agencies worldwide.[15]

During that same month, Moderna shared interim results from its Phase 3 trial of mRNA-1273 (COVE), an investigational COVID-19 vaccine. According to this interim review, the vaccine was safe and effective at preventing symptomatic COVID-19 in adults. Among volunteers, 95 cases of symptomatic COVID-19 were included in the interim analysis. It was reported by the data and safety monitoring board that the candidate vaccine was safe and well-tolerated, and that the efficacy rate of the vaccine was 94.5% (RRR), statistically significant. A total of 90 cases occurred in the placebo group, while five cases occurred in the vaccinated group. In the placebo group, 11 cases of severe COVID-19 were reported out of 95 cases.[16]

Based on the interim analyses described above, ModernaTX submitted an EUA application to FDA on November 30, 2020, seeking approval to use mRNA-1273 to prevent COVID-19 related to SARS-CoV-2 infection in individuals 18 years of age and older.[16]

Of note, the primary endpoint in most trials included a small number of events defined as symptomatic disease regardless of severity and a positive polymerase chain reaction (PCR) test.[17-19] The endpoint to determine efficacy of these trials can be summarized as symptomatic disease regardless of the severity of symptoms and a positive PCR test. Efficacy analysis occurred generally with <200 events.[17-19] All test subjects were not PCR tested, only those that displayed symptoms. Therefore, these trials were not designed to demonstrate prevention of transmission.[17-19]

THE FIRST VACCINE APPROVED FOR EMERGENCY USE AUTHORIZATION

It should be noted that an EUA is different from an FDA approval (licensure) of a vaccine. If a benefit-risk assessment indicates that a product can be made available during an emergency, the FDA will issue an EUA by evaluating the available evidence and assessing any known or potential risks and benefits. Manufacturers who submit EUA requests for COVID-19 vaccines to the FDA must first evaluate the request and determine if all of the relevant statutory criteria are met, taking into account the complete scientific evidence available to the FDA regarding this vaccine.[20]

In December 2020, the US FDA granted the first EUA for a vaccine to prevent COVID-19, caused by SARS-CoV-2. Pfizer-BioNTech was granted an EUA for the distribution of the COVID-19 vaccine in the United States.[20] It is necessary to administer two doses of the Pfizer-BioNTech COVID-19 vaccine intramuscularly, 3 weeks apart, over the course of 3 weeks.[21] In the 10 days following the EUA, >1 million people had received their first dose of COVID-19 vaccine.[22]

This achievement will help protect those on the frontlines—our healthcare providers treating patients with COVID-19—and our most vulnerable—seniors living in nursing homes and assisted living facilities—at a critical time as COVID-19 cases continue to increase nationwide.[22]

A second vaccine for the prevention of COVID-19 was issued by the US FDA on December 18, 2020, which permitted the distribution of the Moderna COVID-19 vaccine in the US for individuals aged 18 years and older.[23]

As a result of the EUA, the FDA also expected manufacturers that had been authorized to manufacture COVID-19 vaccines to continue their clinical trials in order to obtain additional safety and effectiveness information and to pursue approval (licensure).[20]

WHAT DID THE CDC SAY ABOUT THIS VACCINE APPROVALS?

Upon authorization by the FDA for the use of an emergency vaccine, an independent panel of medical and health experts referred to as the Advisory Committee on Immunization Practices (ACIP) makes recommendations and provides guidance about the use of the vaccine to the Director of the Centers for Disease Control and Prevention (CDC).[24]

In addition to being voting members, ACIP is composed of 15 experts who are responsible for making vaccine recommendations. Following an application and nomination process, these members are selected by the Secretary of the US Department of Health and Human Services (DHHS). A total of 14 of these members possess expertise in vaccinology, immunology, pediatrics, internal medicine, nursing, family medicine, virology, public health, infectious diseases, or preventive medicine. A consumer representative serves as a member of the committee and provides perspectives on the social and community aspects of vaccination.[24]

One day after the FDA approved the Pfizer vaccines, on December 12, 2020, the ACIP issued an interim recommendation recommending the use of the Pfizer-BioNTech COVID-19 vaccine in persons aged 16 years for the prevention of COVID-19. The recommendation was made public on December 13, 2020.[21]

Among the topics covered in these recommendations were who should be vaccinated, the process of obtaining the vaccine, and possible side effects. They stated that COVID-19 is a major public health issue at the present

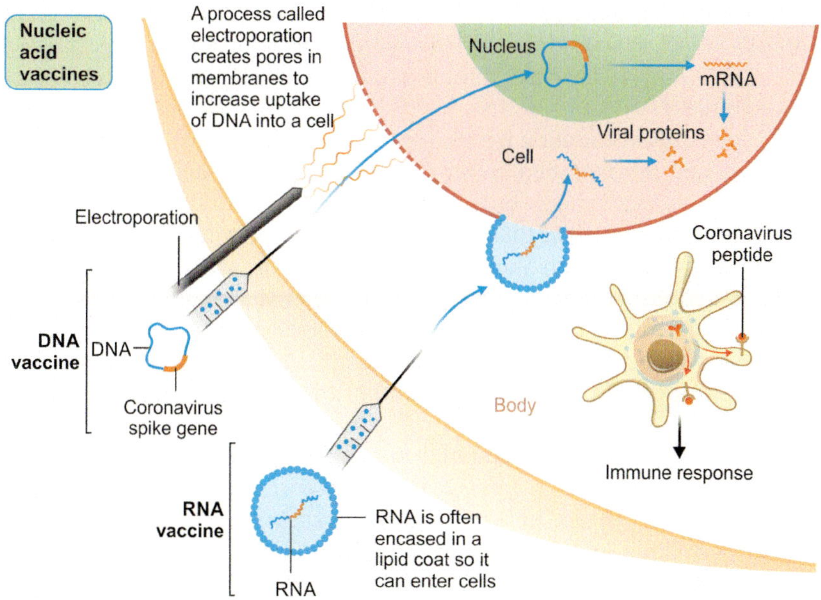

FIGURE 2: Mechanism of action of DNA vaccine versus RNA vaccine.[14]
(DNA: deoxyribonucleic acid; mRNA: messenger ribonucleic acid; RNA: ribonucleic acid)
Source: With permission from Callaway E (2020).[14]

time, and that the benefits of vaccination far outweigh the risks for most populations. It is recommended that recipients and caregivers receive the EUA Fact Sheet prior to vaccination. Patients should be informed about the potential systemic and local reactions associated with the Pfizer-BioNTech COVID-19 vaccine by their healthcare providers.[21]

As more information was gathered from ongoing trials, these recommendations continued to be updated. Recommendations were later extended to include guidance for pregnant women, patients who had contracted COVID-19 infection, and, as additional vaccines became available, guidance would be required for those who had received different pharmaceutical vaccines, particularly those with different mechanisms of action **(Fig. 2)**.

THE INITIAL SCARCITY OF VACCINES

Although we celebrated this historic milestone, we also acknowledged the challenges that lie ahead. The COVID-19 vaccine was in short supply in the US, but it was expected to increase in the weeks and months to come. In order to make vaccination against COVID-19 easy for everyone, large enough quantities of vaccine were to be made available as soon as possible.[22]

In an attempt to protect their populations, many countries expressed interest in financing and/or purchasing the COVID-19 vaccine as soon as it was available. By July 2020, 75 countries had already expressed an interest in joining COVAX, a facility intended to ensure rapid, equitable, and reasonable access to COVID-19 vaccines throughout the world, but the facility's efforts proved futile.[25]

Despite only accounting for 16% of the world's population, high-income countries had reserved 65% of all COVID-19 vaccines, according to Duke Global Health Innovation Center. In part, this is due to the fact that many wealthy countries, such as the United States and the United Kingdom, made bilateral agreements with vaccine manufacturers in early 2020. They have invested billions of dollars in developing novel vaccines and supporting their mass production prior to approval. These high-income countries are, in return, entitled to receive the first batches of vaccine doses once they have been approved by regulatory authorities and are available on the market.[26]

In addition to vaccine nationalism, the situation was also the result of vaccine nationalism. As a result of advanced marketing commitments, Canada and the UK had secured so much vaccine stock that their entire populations could have been vaccinated five times and three times over, respectively. It has been reported that nations such as Israel paid 50% more than the market price to guarantee early access to Pfizer/BioNTech vaccines and vaccinated 80% of their senior citizens before many other countries even began. A shipment of 250,000 doses of AstraZeneca vaccines to Australia was blocked by Italy in March 2021.[26]

About 4 months after the first vaccines were approved, >700 million vaccine doses had been administered worldwide by April 2021, with wealthier nations receiving >87%, and low-income countries receiving just 0.2%. Thus, one in four people in high-income countries received a vaccine, whereas one in >500 people in low-income countries did.[27]

In order to cover as many people as possible during this period of vaccine shortage, many strategies were proposed. As an example, consider the single dose proposal, which was supported by numerous Phase 3 trials demonstrating significant protection after the first dose. One dose of the Pfizer/BioNTech vaccine demonstrated 88.9% efficacy and one dose of the Moderna vaccine showed 80.2% efficacy.[26]

For countries such as the UK, giving more people some degree of protection was preferable to giving a limited number of people full protection. Another strategy was to delay the second dose. Additionally, they extended the interval between the two doses of all vaccines to 12 weeks instead of the original 4 weeks. This was an issue of controversy at the time, and many were concerned that immunity would diminish during this lengthy period between doses.[26]

Lastly, the mix and match strategy involved mixing different types of vaccines, such as the Pfizer/BioNTech vaccine followed by the Oxford-AstraZeneca vaccine, with one dose of each. It is not uncommon for routine vaccinations against the same pathogen to occur in this manner.

Unfortunately, there were no noninferiority trials supporting the idea at the time of this proposal, and it was not attractive to the population being vaccinated at the time.[26]

SIDE EFFECTS OF THE VACCINES: A DEEP VIEW ON MAJOR SIDE EFFECTS

There have been several documented adverse reactions to mRNA-based vaccines since they became available, these include myocarditis and pericarditis in the 15 months since they were first approved. Within 30 days of vaccination, signs of myocarditis and pericarditis were first detected in Israel, with the majority of cases occurring after the second dose. Numerous other countries have reported myocarditis and pericarditis after receiving mRNA COVID-19 vaccines. Both Pfizer-BioNTech (Comirnaty) and Moderna (Spikevax) have included these events in their product information.[28]

This safety signal was identified early in the vaccination program, indicating that young males were more likely to develop myocarditis or pericarditis after receiving the second dose of either of the mRNA-based COVID-19 vaccines. There is a very low incidence of myocarditis and pericarditis following the administration of the COVID-19 mRNA vaccine, with a frequency of 1–10 events per 100,000, and most cases make a full recovery after vaccination. Worldwide, vaccination programs differ in the type of vaccine and the manner in which they are administered. In general, vaccinations were prioritized for those most likely to experience severe complications from COVID-19, followed by healthy adults and children. All of these groups have approved and used mRNA vaccines in conjunction with adenovirus vector vaccines and inactivated virus vaccines.[28]

Comirnaty was estimated to have been administered to 26.2 million individuals in the UK as of March 2022. In a million vaccination recipients who received a minimum of one dose of Comirnaty, there were approximately 48.09 cases of myocarditis and pericarditis. As of the same date, approximately 1.6 million first doses and 1.5 million second doses of Spikevax had also been administered. Among those who received at least one dose of Spikevax in the UK, 203 cases of myocarditis and pericarditis were reported. US Vaccine Adverse Event Reporting System (VAERS) reported 2,986 events following Comirnaty and 1,640 events following Spikevax. Comirnaty had been fully vaccinated 124.12 million vaccines in the United States. These vaccines reported 14.70 cases of myocarditis per million fully vaccinated individuals and 9.36 cases of pericarditis, respectively, resulting in 12.03 cases of myocarditis and pericarditis per million fully vaccinated individuals. With 75.57 million people fully vaccinated with Spikevax, 12.35 cases of myocarditis have been reported per million fully vaccinated Spikevax recipients, and 9.36 cases of pericarditis have been reported per million fully vaccinated Spikevax recipients. This results in a reporting rate of 10.86 per million Spikevax vaccines for both myocarditis and pericarditis.[28]

Among the 1,824 myocarditis events reported by Comirnaty, 956 (52.41%) occurred following the second dose, whereas 383 (21.0%) occurred following a single dose. After two doses of Spikevax, 384 (41.16%) events of myocarditis were reported and 305 (43.14%) incidents of pericarditis were reported. Approximately 10% of myocarditis and pericarditis cases had been reported following a third dose for both vaccines as of March 2022. According to other studies, 64.72% of myocarditis and pericarditis events occurred after the second vaccine dose (range 25.00–91.78%).[28]

A higher incidence of myocarditis and pericarditis was seen in young males following COVID-19 mRNA vaccination. The majority of pericarditis cases reported in the USA and the majority of pericarditis cases reported in the European Union occurred in males, respectively. In all three regions evaluated, males reported more frequently than females. In the United States, 47.3% of myocarditis cases occurred among vaccines between the ages of 18 and 39 years, while in the European Union, 79.2% of reports were from people between the ages of 18 and 64 years.[28]

It has been reported that cases of myocarditis and pericarditis have resulted in fatalities. The UK reported four fatalities (0.25%), the USA reported 62 (1.3%), and the European Union/European Economic Area (EEA) reported 56 (0.6%). In total, 85.83% of fatal cases involved individuals aged 18 years or older; five fatal cases (4.17%) involved individuals aged under 18 years, and 10% did not specify the age; all of the cases involved myocarditis.[28]

OTHER POSSIBLE TREATMENTS

While the majority of the effort have been devoted to developing new vaccines there were also those who were looking at other possible preventive and treatment options. It was believed that a number of medications could be used to treat COVID-19, including azithromycin, hydroxychloroquine, and ivermectin. In spite of the lack of measurable evidence or studies, a large number of physicians supported their use based on clinical experience. But obtaining scientific evidence supporting the use of these medications would take some time.[29]

Several studies have indicated that the spike protein of SARS-CoV-2 attaches to glycoconjugates on red blood cells, thereby contributing to its infectivity and morbidity. Recently, a study was published about the use of ivermectin in the treatment of COVID-19. According to the study, ivermectin could be effective in preventing the progression of the disease to a more severe stage.[29]

The purpose of this study was to determine whether ivermectin could inhibit the binding of spike proteins to blood cells. Based on the results of the study, Ivermectin inhibited hemagglutination when added to red blood cells prior to spike protein and reversed it when added after. In light of the findings of this study, it appears that ivermectin may be a potential therapeutic option that might aid in elucidating the adverse effects associated with the COVID-19 mRNA vaccine.[29]

OVERCOMING CHALLENGES IN FIGHTING RESPIRATORY VIRUSES

The fight against respiratory viruses, which claim millions of lives each year worldwide, can only be won with effective vaccines and prevention strategies. It has been estimated that influenza is the deadliest vaccine-preventable viral respiratory disease, and current vaccines prove to be less than optimal in their effectiveness. In fact, their efficacy varies from year to year, with only 40–60% of vaccines successfully preventing infection. In addition to influenza A, SARS-CoV-2, endemic coronaviruses, respiratory syncytial virus (RSV), and other common cold viruses, other respiratory mucosa viruses present significant public health concerns due to their rapid replication and transmission. Since these viruses normally do not elicit complete or durable immunity, vaccines are ineffective in controlling them.[30]

A lack of natural protective immunity and viruses' ability to remain outside the reach of human innate and adaptive immunity make it challenging to develop durably protective vaccines against nonsystemic mucosal respiratory viruses that have a high mortality rate. In order to prevent deadly outbreaks and pandemics resulting from these viruses, researchers must think outside the box and rethink past assumptions and approaches.[30]

WAXING IMMUNITY

The RNA vaccines have proven to be effective in preventing SARS-CoV-2 infections, and high levels of neutralizing antibodies are crucial for vaccine-induced immunity. Recent findings regarding the immune response to mRNA COVID-19 vaccines, specifically Comirnaty from BioNTech/Pfizer and Spikevax from Moderna continue to reveal new information. A recent study found, e.g., that after the initial two doses, the immunoglobulin G (IgG) response mainly consisted of proinflammatory IgG1 and IgG3 subclasses. However, several months after the second vaccination, SARS-CoV-2-specific antibodies were found to be increasingly composed of noninflammatory IgG4, which were further boosted by a third mRNA vaccination and/or SARS-CoV-2 variant breakthrough infections. Flow cytometry revealed substantial frequencies of IgG4-switched B cells within the spike-binding memory B cell population. This class switch to IgG4 was associated with a reduced capacity of the spike-specific antibodies to mediate antibody-dependent cellular phagocytosis and complement deposition. These findings may have implications for the choice and timing of vaccination regimens using mRNA vaccines, including future booster immunizations against SARS-CoV-2.[31]

Another recent research indicates that bivalent vaccines are approximately 30% effective at protecting against SARS-CoV-2 infection, particularly if the predominant strains are Omicron BA.4/BA.5.[32]

Overall, these studies suggest that a more nuanced approach is required for assessing vaccination's impact, including the potential impact of multiple doses of the vaccine on future COVID-19 risk. Despite being highly effective in preventing COVID-19, the introduction of the Omicron variant has reduced natural immunity as well as vaccine-induced immunity from the original vaccine. Although vaccine boosting provides some protection against Omicron, it is not as effective as the original vaccine in terms of protecting against Omicron. As a result, there is a need to explore the effectiveness of newer vaccines such as bivalent COVID-19 mRNA vaccines, which contain antigens from the original vaccine and the BA.4/BA.5 lineages of Omicron. This also highlights the importance of further research into the effectiveness of multiple vaccine doses given over time.[32]

A RECENT VIEW OF THE VACCINES: FINAL THOUGHTS

The COVID-19 vaccine requires continual injections every 6 months with no end in sight. Even the most compliant patients are asking when this will end. The CDC reported that 79% of Omicron cases were fully vaccinated, which suggests the end of vaccine efficacy. A recent systematic review and meta-analysis showed that COVID-19 vaccines had <60% efficacy at 1, 3, 6, and 9 months, and <20% for later times. These results are disappointing for vaccine developers and program sponsors, which emphasizes the need for more efficacy studies.[33]

It is possible for epidemiologists to simulate events and to gain a better understanding of what might occur under various scenarios by using models, and vaccination against COVID-19 is not an exception to this rule.[34] A model used to estimate the impact of COVID-19 vaccinations has been shown to assist in the prevention of 14–20 million deaths by 2021, according to the epidemiological susceptible–exposed–infectious–recovered (SEIR) model.[34] However, after careful analysis, it was discovered that vaccination efficacy had been removed from the equation. Furthermore, these conclusions were based on partially simulated data applied to counterfactual scenarios.[34]

The data has been examined by several epidemiologists, and their conclusions regarding the effectiveness of the vaccines have differed.[34] According to prospective, randomized, double-blind, placebo-controlled trials, COVID-19 vaccines have not been effective in stopping infection, preventing transmission of the SARS-CoV-2 virus among fully vaccinated individuals, or reducing hospitalizations.[34]

It is pertinent to take into account the fact that the vast majority of the population has already been exposed to the infection at least once or multiple times, so there is a natural immunity effect, along with improvements in early therapeutics and in-hospital care.[34] In conclusion, it is clear that there is still much data to be analyzed before we can come to an informed conclusion as to whether the vaccine is beneficial or not. Critical realism should also be taken into consideration when making such a judgement.[34]

TIMELINE

Timeline of COVID-19 events is depicted in **Figure 3**.

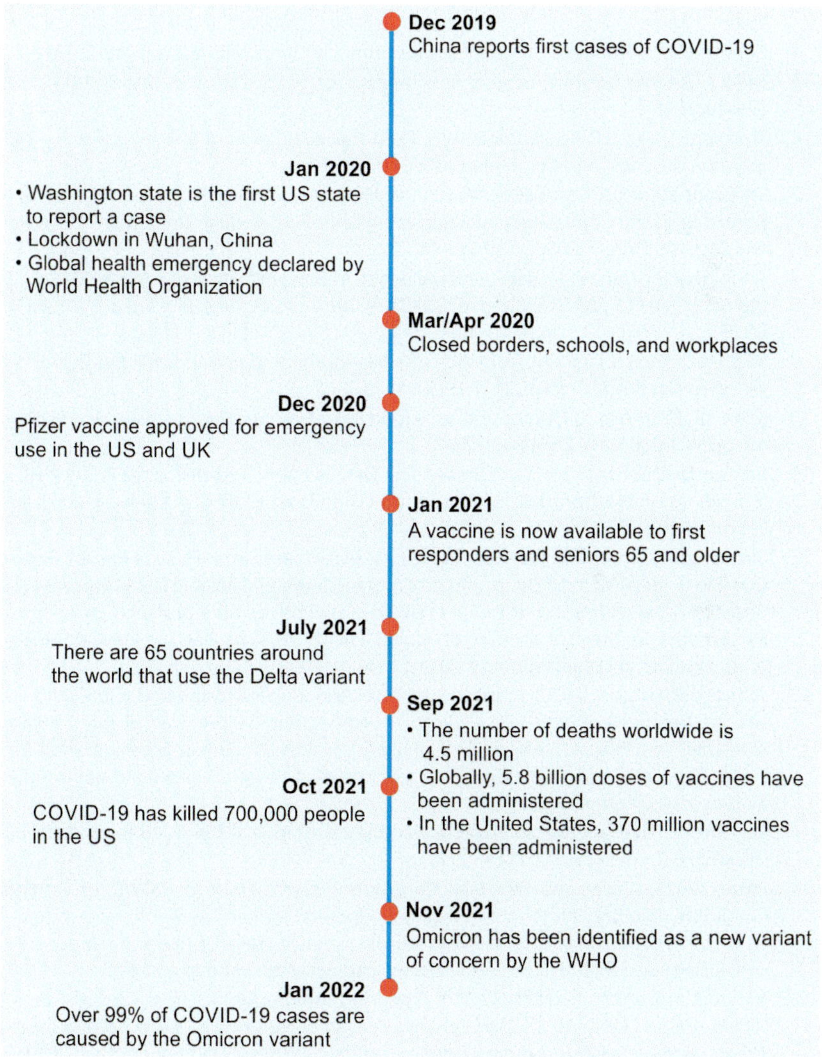

FIGURE 3: Timeline of coronavirus disease 2019 (COVID-19) events.[35]

REFERENCES

1. National Institutes of Health. (2020). NIH clinical trial of investigational vaccine for COVID-19 begins. [online] Available from https://www.nih.gov/news-events/news-releases/nih-clinical-trial-investigational-vaccine-covid-19-begins. [Last accessed February, 2024].
2. Centers for Disease Control and Prevention. (2021). ACIP Evidence to Recommendations for Use of Pfizer-BioNTech COVID-19 Vaccine. [online] Available from https://www.cdc.gov/vaccines/acip/recs/grade/covid-19-pfizer-biontech-etr.html. [Last accessed February, 2024].
3. Centers for Disease Control and Prevention. (2020). COVID Data Tracker. [online] Available from https://covid.cdc.gov/covid-data-tracker. [Last accessed February, 2024].
4. Cavanagh D. Coronavirus avian infectious bronchitis virus. Vet Res. 2007;38(2):281-97.
5. Saif LJ. Animal coronavirus vaccines: lessons for SARS. Dev Biol (Basel). 2004;119: 129-40.
6. Thurber ET, Bass EP, Beckenhauer WH. Field trial evaluation of a reo-coronavirus calf diarrhea vaccine. Can J Comp Med. 1977;41(2):131-6.
7. De Groot-Mijnes JDF, van Dun JM, van der Most RG, de Groot RJ. Natural History of a Recurrent Feline Coronavirus Infection and the Role of Cellular Immunity in Survival and Disease. J Virol. 2005;79(2):1036-44.
8. Abdelghany T, Ganash M, Bakri MM, Qanash H, Al-Rajhi AM, Elhussieny NI. SARS-CoV-2, the other face to SARS-CoV and MERS-CoV: Future predictions. Biomed J. 2021;44(1): 86-93.
9. Su S, Du L, Jiang S. Learning from the past: development of safe and effective COVID-19 vaccines. Nat Rev Microbiol. 2021;19(3):211-9.
10. Kahn JS, McIntosh K. History and recent advances in coronavirus discovery. Pediatr Infect Dis J. 2005;24(11 Suppl):S223-7.
11. Centers for Disease Control and Prevention. Details-Public Health Image Library (PHIL). [online] Available from https://phil.cdc.gov/Details.aspx?pid=23313. [Last accessed February, 2024].
12. Pfizer. (2020). Pfizer and BioNTech Dose First Participants in the U.S. as Part of Global COVID-19 mRNA Vaccine Development Program. [online] Available from https://www.pfizer.com/news/press-release/press-release-detail/pfizer_and_biontech_dose_first_participants_in_the_u_s_as_part_of_global_covid_19_mrna_vaccine_development_program. [Last accessed February, 2024].
13. Johnson & Johnson. (2020). Johnson & Johnson Announces Acceleration of its COVID-19 Vaccine Candidate; Phase 1/2a Clinical Trial to Begin in Second Half of July. [online] Available from https://www.jnj.com/johnson-johnson-announces-acceleration-of-its-covid-19-vaccine-candidate-phase-1-2a-clinical-trial-to-begin-in-second-half-of-july. [Last accessed February, 2024].
14. Callaway E. The race for coronavirus vaccines: a graphical guide. Nature. 2020;580 (7805):576-7.
15. Pfizer. (2022). Pfizer and BioNTech Conclude Phase 3 Study of COVID-19 Vaccine Candidate, Meeting All Primary Efficacy Endpoints. [online] Available from https://www.pfizer.com/news/press-release/press-release-detail/pfizer-and-biontech-conclude-phase-3-study-covid-19-vaccine. [Last accessed February, 2024].
16. National Institutes of Health. (2020). Promising Interim Results from Clinical Trial of NIH-Moderna COVID-19 Vaccine. [online] Available from https://www.nih.gov/news-events/news-releases/promising-interim-results-clinical-trial-nih-moderna-covid-19-vaccine. [Last accessed February, 2024].

17. ModernaTX, Inc. (2020). Clinical Study Protocol: A Phase 3, Randomized, Stratified, Observer-Blind, Placebo-Controlled Study to Evaluate the Efficacy, Safety, and Immunogenicity of MRNA-1273 SARS-CoV-2 Vaccine in Adults Aged 18 Years and Older. [online] Available from http://web.archive.org/web/20201018173405/https://www.modernatx.com/sites/default/files/mRNA-1273-P301-Protocol.pdf. [Last accessed February, 2024].
18. Doshi P. Will covid-19 vaccines save lives? Current trials aren't designed to tell us. BMJ. 2020;371:m4037.
19. Topol E. (2020). Paul Offit's biggest concern about COVID vaccines. [online] Available from https://www.medscape.com/viewarticle/936937. [Last accessed February, 2024].
20. U.S. Food and Drug Administration. (2020). FDA Takes Key Action in Fight Against COVID-19 By Issuing Emergency Use Authorization for First COVID-19 Vaccine. [online] Available from https://www.fda.gov/news-events/press-announcements/fda-takes-key-action-fight-against-covid-19-issuing-emergency-use-authorization-first-covid-19. [Last accessed February, 2024].
21. Woodworth KR, Moulia D, Collins JP, Hadler SC, Jones JM, Reddy SC, et al. The Advisory Committee on Immunization Practices' Interim Recommendation for Use of Pfizer-BioNTech COVID-19 Vaccine in Children Aged 5–11 Years—United States, November 2021. MMWR Morb Mortal Wkly Rep. 2021;70:1579-83.
22. Centers for Disease Control and Prevention. (2020). Media Statement from CDC Director Robert R. Redfield on Vaccine Milestone. [online] Available from https://www.cdc.gov/media/releases/2020/s1223-vaccine-milestone.html. [Last accessed February, 2024].
23. U.S. Food and Drug Administration. (2020). FDA Takes Additional Action in Fight Against COVID-19 By Issuing Emergency Use Authorization for Second COVID-19 Vaccine. [online] Available from https://www.fda.gov/news-events/press-announcements/fda-takes-additional-action-fight-against-covid-19-issuing-emergency-use-authorization-second-covid. [Last accessed February, 2024].
24. HHS. (2024). COVID-19 Vaccines. [online] Available from https://www.hhs.gov/coronavirus/covid-19-vaccines/index.html. [Last accessed February, 2024].
25. WHO. (2020). More than 150 countries engaged in COVID-19 vaccine global access facility. [online] Available from https://www.who.int/news/item/15-07-2020-more-than-150-countries-engaged-in-covid-19-vaccine-global-access-facility. [Last accessed February, 2024].
26. Choi EM. COVID-19 vaccines for low- and middle-income countries. Trans R Soc Trop Med Hyg. 2021;115(5):447-56.
27. United Nations. (2021). Low-income countries have received just 0.2 per cent of all COVID-19 shots given. [online] Available from https://news.un.org/en/story/2021/04/1089392. [Last accessed February, 2024].
28. Lane S, Yeomans A, Shakir S. Reports of myocarditis and pericarditis following mRNA COVID-19 vaccination: a systematic review of spontaneously reported data from the UK, Europe and the USA and of the scientific literature. BMJ Open. 2022;12(5): e059223.
29. Boschi C, Scheim DE, Bancod A, Militello M, Bideau ML, Colson P, et al. SARS-CoV-2 Spike Protein Induces Hemagglutination: Implications for COVID-19 Morbidities and Therapeutics and for Vaccine Adverse Effects. Int J Mol Sci. 2022;23(24):15480.
30. Morens DM, Taubenberger JK, Fauci AS. Rethinking next-generation vaccines for coronaviruses, influenzaviruses, and other respiratory viruses. Cell Host Microbe. 2023;31(1):146-57.
31. Irrgang P, Gerling J, Kocher K, Lapuente D, Steininger P, Habenicht K, et al. Class switch toward noninflammatory, spike-specific IgG4 antibodies after repeated SARS-CoV-2 mRNA vaccination. Sci Immunol. 2022;8(79):eade2798.

32. Shrestha NK, Burke PC, Nowacki AS, Simon JF, Hagen A, Gordon SM. Effectiveness of the Coronavirus Disease 2019 (COVID-19) Bivalent Vaccine. Open Forum Infect Dis. 2023;10(6):ofad209.
33. McCullough PA. (2023). COVID-19 Vaccines Fail in the Omicron Era. [online] Available from https://petermcculloughmd.substack.com/p/covid-19-vaccines-fail-in-the-omicron?publication_id=1119676&isFreemail=false. [Last accessed February, 2024].
34. McCullough PA. (2023). Modeling Study Makes False Conclusions on COVID-19 Vaccination. [online] Available from https://petermcculloughmd.substack.com/p/modeling-study-makes-false-conclusions?publication_id=1119676&isFreemail=true. [Last accessed February, 2024].
35. Macmillan Learning. (2022). Information about COVID-19. [online] Available from https://covid19.macmillanlearning.com/. [Last accessed February, 2024].

CHAPTER 17

Controversies Concerning the Immunology of the COVID-19 Adaptive Immunity Vaccines

Marian P Laderoute

PREFACE

There were many controversies concerning the immunology of the use of adaptive immunology coronavirus disease 2019 (COVID-19) vaccines to contain an RNA virus pandemic that focused on the development of antibodies to the spike protein. The spike protein is the molecule which mediates the binding of the virus to cells and antibodies to this determinant can often prevent virus entry referred to as neutralization. While in principle, one would ideally like to block the infection of cells which would correlate with resistance to acquisition of COVID-19 of the host and thus would play a role in herd immunity, this is not how it works for pandemic RNA viruses.

If you immunize the host to spike protein and cause the generation of spike-specific IgG1/3 particularly in the upper respiratory tract (URT), this does a number of things. First it causes selection of variants which are then transmitted to others. RNA viruses mutate at high rates and actually exist in the host not as one variant with the same identical RNA sequence but a swarm of mutated related sequences, called quasispecies. When the dominant quasispecies is blocked from replication by the antibodies, the nonblocked quasispecies emerges and then becomes dominant, which is then transmitted from the URT to third parties. This is referred to as "selection of new variants".

Unfortunately, this mismatching of the developed spike-specific (IgG1/3) antibodies with the newly selected variant causes antibody-dependent enhancement (ADE) of infection of the quasispecies into macrophages. This is because macrophages have receptors for these antibodies (that normally are used for phagocytosis), while macrophages do not express the angiotensin-converting enzyme 2 (ACE2) receptor. Now the quasispecies becomes *targeted to the protector macrophages* (and not the ACE2 positive cells in the body) and causes their conversion to disease-causing (pathogenic) macrophages (**Fig. 1**) in which the SARS-CoV-2 virus replicates.

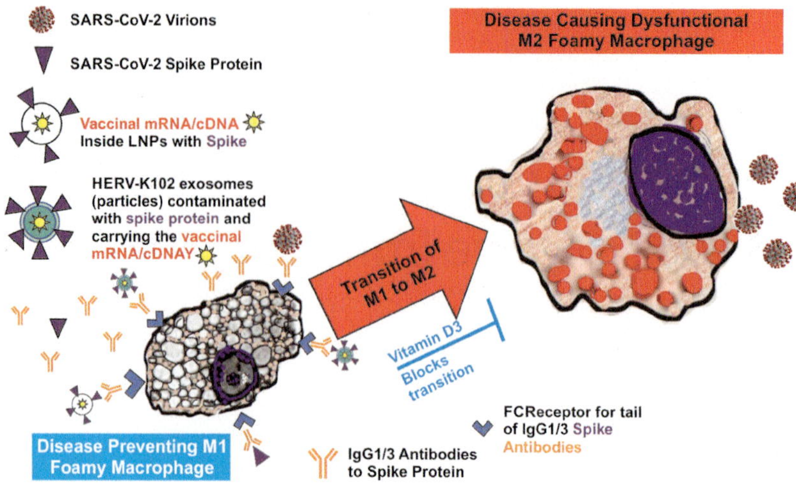

FIGURE 1: Antibody-dependent enhancement (ADE) of spike protein or spike-laden exosomes/particles/LNPs/SARS-CoV-2 virions into the protector M1 foamy macrophages (FM), causing their transition to disease-causing pathogenic and dysfunctional FM (immunosenescence of macrophages, ISM).
(LNPs: lipid nanoparticles)

It is theoretically possible too if the spike gene therapy mRNA/cDNA from the mRNA COVID-19 vaccines becomes integrated in the macrophage that spike protein could also be generated to high levels (with adverse effects on the host due to the toxicity of the spike protein, most importantly, causing macrophage dysfunction).

Note that the cell on the right is resistant to apoptosis induction and persists in the host for a long time. Severe acute respiratory syndrome coronavirus 2 (SARS-CoV-2) continuously replicates, produces, and releases SARS-CoV-2 virions from the M2 compromised cells. Alternatively, spike protein or other spike-laden particles/exosomes/lipid nanoparticles (LNPs) *are targeted to the protector FM* via the spike-specific IgG1/3 antibodies. Fortunately, optimal vitamin D3 levels block this transition explaining how vitamin D3 protects against COVID-19 severity, serious side effects of the mRNA gene therapy vaccines, and/or the more deadly vaccinal shedding. Vaccinal shedding may be the most dangerous as (1) it may carry the IgG1/IgG3 from the URT of the recently vaccinated donor (shedding may last up to 3–4 months), and (2) there is very high possibility of integrated vaccinal spike mRNA/cDNA due to hitching a ride with the HERV-K102 particles that contain and utilize functional reverse transcriptase and integrase for their own replication.

Lipid nanoparticles are used to transport the vaccinal spike mRNA/cDNA around the body.

As discussed at length and covered in this chapter, the foamy macrophages hold the *magical power* of deciding recovery or death from COVID-19. Even susceptibility to COVID-19 is determined at the level of the macrophage; those with dysfunctional foamy macrophages (referred to as immunosenescence of macrophages, ISM) are at much higher risk of developing severe COVID-19. This is because ISM causes age-associated chronic diseases (from cardiovascular diseases to cancer, autoimmunity, allergy, neurodegenerative disorders, metabolic syndrome, and so on). The COVID-19 disease caused by SARS-CoV-2 is undeniably also via the induction of ISM **(see Fig. 1)**.

It is for this reason, namely ADE, that safe and effective vaccines against emerging or pandemic RNA viruses have never been possible. In other words, they not only select for more transmissible variants, but the vaccinated are at much higher risk of developing severe illness and death in subsequent months or years when they encounter the vaccine selected descendants.

Fortunately, this evolution of dangerous descendants was interrupted by the emergence of the omicron variant in December 2021 and January 2020 globally. Omicron had putatively been selected through the common house mouse and apparently retained little or no affinity for human Basigin (BSG/CD147), but preferring mouse BSG. Before omicron, the severe cases of COVID-19 in the lower respiratory tract (LRT) involved a novel mechanism of ADE where the spike:ACE2 interaction was replaced by spike:BSG (probably via the emergence of the IgG4 isotype of the spike-specific antibodies which blocked SARS-CoV-2 binding to ACE2 on cells). The switch to the spike:BSG interaction was extremely dangerous as BSG is expressed by the macrophages and on several of the innate T and B cell types involved in the critical trained innate immunity needed for COVID-19 recovery. In other words, the switch targeted SARS-CoV-2 directly to the critical HERV-K102 host defense system.

Accordingly, it was said that omicron did not generate pneumonia in the LRT, and thus was less pathogenic although it was much more transmissible due to classical ADE in the URT. Classical ADE in the URT involved SARS-CoV-2 gaining entry to the foamy macrophages via spike-specific IgG1/3 binding to FCGR2A. These foamy macrophages are the sebocytes in sebaceous glands and represent specialized foamy macrophages constitutively producing and releasing HERV-K102 particles to the exterior of the body to coat the mucosal tissues. In the URT, there apparently is no conversion of the ADE promoting spike IgG1/3 to IgG4 despite repeated COVID-19 mRNA vaccination. This is why the multiply vaxed were at higher risk of infection proportional to the number of doses for the workers at the Cleveland Clinic, as it proportionally increased the amount of IgG1/3 to spike protein in the upper respiratory tract (URT).

Had the vaccination against SARS-CoV-2 stopped with two doses and/or upon the onset of omicron, there would have been far less death and injury. As it was, the use of adaptive immunity vaccines to the Wuhan original variant prolonged the COVID-19 pandemic beyond its natural course of extinction predicted to have been by May 2021. However, the use of omicron variants in the bivalent vaccines may have restarted the whole evolutionary process now with selection against the circulating mouse strain of SARS-CoV-2. Some have predicted this might have sudden dire consequences for the human race if, in fact, a mutation restores the affinity of the currently circulating SARS-CoV-2 variants for the human BSG. Let us hope not but this is an early warning that to avoid a catastrophic calamity, we must immediately ban all the so-called "gene therapy vaccines".

The main take-home message of this chapter is that *all the evidence* prior to the unexpected and questionable emergency use authorization (EUA) of the COVID-19 mRNA vaccines not only demonstrated but proved beyond a shadow of a doubt, that the development of the spike-specific IgG1/3 antibodies was associated with progression to *more severe disease*, and did *not ever result in the* "protection against COVID-19". This begs the question why the authorities proceeded with the EUAs for the mRNA COVID-19 vaccines, why these adaptive immunology vaccines were deemed "safe and effective", and why would these inherently dangerous vaccines would not only be highly recommended by public health authorities, but mandated!

KEY POINTS

Egregious aspects of the immunology of the COVID-19 mRNA adaptive immunity vaccines:

- *Gene therapy vaccine is an oxymoron.*
- *Adaptive immunity vaccine against pandemic viruses is also an oxymoron. It is impossible for spike IgG1/3 to protect against SARS-CoV-2 or provide herd immunity.*
- Gene therapy vaccination could kill the unvaccinated by shedding from the vaccinated albeit at reduced frequency when compared with the vaccinated (estimated that the mRNA COVID-19 *vaccinated* succumbed to shedding at about *116-fold higher rates* over the *unvaccinated* for England).
- *Stealth gene therapy shedding may have killed far more people than SARS-CoV-2* (at least 14-fold if not more as shedding likely also contributed to COVID-19 deaths).
- *Hiding the truth about risks of death and injury with the gene therapy products was unethical, immoral, and likely criminal.*
- *Using a gene therapy product fraudulently advertised as a safe and effective vaccine was likely criminal.*
- Failing to require proper studies on the risks of shedding of mRNA COVID-19 vaccines prior to awarding the EUAs was probably criminal. *The risk of shedding of gene therapy products was well known prior to the EUA of the mRNA gene therapy shots.*
- Failing to address the all-cause mortality test to establish the gold standard for the risk/benefit profile for the COVID-19 vaccines was likely criminal on behalf of the manufacturers and by the regulatory authorities. (This test should have been performed at 6 months, 12 months, 18 months, and 24 months prior to awarding the EUA.)

- *Saying the adaptive immunity/gene therapy vaccines were safe and effective was a bold-faced lie and was probably criminal as it led many people to their deaths and/or induced life-altering vaccine injuries.*
- Mandating of vaccines, particularly the COVID-19 gene therapy bioweapons of mass (stealth) destruction was akin to genocide.
- The indicator used for vaccine effectiveness (levels of spike IgG) had more to do with death and injury than the prevention of a transmissible disease. *The authorities knew this but granted EUAs anyway.*
- An adaptive immunology vaccine cannot protect against emerging pathogens or pandemics. *It is physically/immunologically impossible and the regulators and public health officials well knew and understood this, as did Dr Anthony Fauci.*
- The risk of shedding deaths was enhanced in the donor by the presence of spike-specific IgG1/3 in the URT (from the shedding donor) which was induced by the mRNA gene therapy vaccines and not present (to any great extent) in the unvaccinated.
- The risk of shedding deaths was also enhanced in the recipients of the shed gene therapy products when spike-specific IgG1/3 was systemically present such as in the blood. People who were infected first then received two or more doses of the COVID-19 mRNA vaccines were unlikely to convert to the tolerogenic IgG4, placing them at higher risks of shedding-induced death. The younger the age, the more likely they would have been infected first as the vaccines were distributed in descending order of age.
- The young adults who were at negligible risks of COVID-19 should not have received any COVID-19 vaccines. However, due to shedding there were large increases in excess deaths in the under 50 age groups particularly in the third and fourth quarters of 2021. Many of these deaths were known to involve myocarditis and sudden death (in their sleep or upon exertion). Shedding is likely a major contributor to myocarditis and sudden death exacerbated by having been infected first before the two doses of the mRNA vaccines. An example of a potential shedding incident causing ventricular tachycardia with sweating and high blood pressure during sleep in a 69-year-old female who was infected with SARS-CoV-2 prior to receipt of the two doses of the Pfizer-BioNTech in March 2024 is available online at *https://hervk102.substack.com/p/can-shedding-be-clinically-distinguished.*
- Testing for serum levels of vitamin D3, and topping up where needed, was an easy, safe, affordable, and attainable way to immunologically reduce the risks of severe COVID-19 and would have quenched or eliminated the need for risky vaccine interventions. This would have also reduced the risky congregation at large indoor venues which some noted were associated with SARS-CoV-2 infection especially at the time of the first injection.
- Similarly, ivermectin, hydroxychloroquine, and other repurposed drugs were not only cost effective but exemplary in their ability to promote

recovery as well as the prevention of COVID-19. These immune protector agents share a common immune enhancing and antiviral property of preventing and/or reversing *ISM* caused by a number of pathogenic agents including SARS-CoV-2.

- It was unlawful of the FDA to suggest ivermectin should not be used off-label to prevent SARS-CoV-2 infection or more severe COVID-19 disease.
- At the heart of COVID-19 disease and indeed most age and/or stress-associated diseases including infections involves the activity of alpha-fetoprotein (AFP) in the macrophages, which is commonly induced by pathogens and exacerbated by stress. AFP antagonists such as ivermectin, zinc, DHEA, or 7-keto-DHEA, genistein, and other isoflavonoids also target the estrogen receptor, and more recently, maraviroc is sure fire means for the prevention and recovery of COVID-19 and any future pandemics.
- There were attempts to validate innate immunity vaccines in clinical trials that started prior to the launch of the COVID-19 mRNA vaccines. But Big Pharma was able to convince Ethics Boards across the nation that no one should be denied the unlawful administration of an experimental intervention known or suspected of causing bodily harm especially where mandated. So, all these legitimate clinical trials were in fact ruined by interception by mRNA COVID-19 vaccines. Some of the reports of such trials concluded that the innate vaccines were ineffective against COVID-19 when in fact the trials were stopped early due to the unjustifiable interference by Big Pharma.
- The most abhorrent and reprehensible was the labeling of personal accounts of vaccine injury and death as disinformation or conspiratory theories, and thus, this abrogated the ability to warn others about the risks on social media. As well these people who needed immediate support allegedly caused by the governments' mandates were denied rapid compensation. Some in dire straits were instead offered medically assisted dying.
- Not only did the FDA and other regulators abandon the responsibility to report in real time on vaccine deaths and serious injuries, but in Canada just for these bioweapons only, the reporting structure was changed. The new system required reporting only to the municipal level which then was sent up to the provincial and federal levels which contradicted the point of rapid responses to faulty products on the market. Moreover, a Canadian citizen could no longer report a death or serious injury, while licensed physicians were afraid to lose their license if they reported COVID-19 gene therapy-associated deaths. Ergo virtually none were reported.
- The continued censorship on the reporting and discussion of the death and destruction caused by the COVID-19 vaccines especially the gene therapy shots is frankly undemocratic and unconstitutional. This will cause poor choices for future pandemics on how to immunologically handle the "next one".

- Saying that hybrid immunity was the best of both worlds was certainly not the case for people who were infected prior to receipt of the gene therapy shots. These people were at higher risk of SARS-CoV-2 and the shed gene therapy products transmitted via exosomes.
- Saying that the protection from the vaccines only lasted 6 months or less refers to the protection induced by innate immunity and little to do with waning of the spike IgG1/3 antibodies.
- Many researchers did not realize that using the pseudovirus assay in neutralization experiments which involves the culture of the pseudovirus in human cells instead of the green monkey Vero cell line actually detected innate neutralizing antibodies that reacted with HERV-K102 envelope present both on the particles and on the surface of such human but not nonhuman cell lines. The same is true for uncultured SARS-CoV-2 virus directly isolated from humans. Showing neutralizing antibody activity with these methods instead of the classical culture of the intact virus in green monkey cells and tested on green monkey cells as the indicator cell line misled some to conclude broader protection against SARS-CoV-2 variants. Some sloppy researchers actually reported spike neutralizing antibodies when by ELISA no antibodies to spike protein could be detected. Less commonly human cell lines were used as indicator cell lines which could led to false positive or false negative results due to the presence of the HERV-K102 particles in the plasma/serum, which is believed to cause lysis in susceptible human cell lines but not Vero cells at 24 hours.

INTRODUCTION

Single Cell RNA Sequencing has Revealed the Importance of Innate Immunity, Especially Macrophages

Single cell RNA (scRNA) sequencing has substantially revolutionized the ability to gauge cell fate and developmental programs such as for immune cells in sickness and in health.[1,2] Such investigations have revealed the importance of innate immune mechanisms in recovery from or protection against many common diseases.

For example, an initial investigation involving 39 cancer types and about 18,000 tumors unexpectantly determined in 2015 that the gamma-delta 2 (GD2) T cells and/or other innate T cells were frequently correlated with protection against many although not all cancers.[3] This discrimination was largely based on the expression of KLRB1 (CD161) on these innate T cells. KLRB1 is a lectin-like receptor that binds galactose-a-(1,3) galactose which is a carbohydrate marker of nonhuman cells and where humans have IgM against this moiety.[4] On the other hand, FOXM1 considered a marker of poor prognosis tended to identify neutrophil populations within many cancers.

More recently, using scRNA sequencing, M1-like proinflammatory macrophages have been implicated in remission from acute myeloid leukemia,[5] and as correlates of protection in patients with lung cancers.[6]

In addition, via scRNA sequencing, monocytes/macrophages have been identified as essential to a reduced risk of *Simian immunodeficiency virus/Simian-human immunodeficiency virus* (SIV/SHIV) acquisition in nonhuman primate (NHP) animal studies and were implicated in the partial vaccine efficacy against human immunodeficiency virus HIV-1 infection demonstrated in the RV144 trial.[7] At a more detailed level, the induction of hypoxia with inflammasome activation in CD14 monocytes has been associated with a decreased risk of SIV_{mac251} acquisition in NHP models.[8] It should be appreciated that hypoxia and inflammasome activation results in foam cell formation in M1-like proinflammatory macrophages.[9] Accordingly, it appears, proinflammatory foamy macrophages provide protection against HIV-1 acquisition, a conclusion reached earlier on entirely different evidence.[10,11]

Macrophages although long considered the central orchestrator of both innate and adaptive immunity, are primarily associated with innate immunity, the antigen nonspecific arm of the immune system involving interferon responses and intrinsic pathogen detection systems termed pattern recognition receptors (PRRs). Dendritic cells that are the antigen presenters for adaptive immune responses are derived from a separate set of bone marrow progenitors, called the common lymphoid progenitors (CLPs). Instead, macrophages (and monocytes) are derived from the common myeloid progenitors (CMPs) which then generate the granulocyte-macrophage progenitors (GMPs) and the megakaryocyte-erythroid progenitors (MEPs).[12] Accordingly, discussions of monocytes in the blood or macrophages in the tissues refer and pertain to innate immunity.

The Clue of Antibody Dependent Enhancement of Infection into Macrophages

Historically, a major line of evidence emphasizing the importance of macrophages in the control of infectious diseases and outcomes has been the concept of ADE of infection into monocyte/macrophages. Disease escalation involving antibodies that mediate the enhanced infection of macrophages through Fc receptors was first documented for dengue in 1967. Since that time ADE has been observed for various viral infections[13] such as measles, SARS-CoV, Middle East respiratory syndrome coronavirus (MERS-CoV), HIV-1, West Nile virus, Japanese encephalitis virus, Ross River virus, Ebola virus, respiratory syncytial virus, feline infectious peritonitis virus, porcine reproductive and respiratory syndrome virus, and now SARS-CoV-2.[14] Most notably, it has been suggested that COVID-19 disease progression from moderate to severe commonly relates to ADE-mediated infection of SARS-CoV-2 into monocytes/macrophages[14] (which will be examined and validated in more detail below). This view is, however, not supported by everyone, as some profess that ADE has not been observed clinically during COVID-19 infection.[15]

Despite the controversy in opinion, incontrovertible evidence had emerged that even before the COVID-19 vaccines were authorized for emergency use that demonstrated IgG antibodies to spike protein were not protective but instead were associated with progression to more severe COVID-19 disease including death during natural infection.[16-30] Despite this unanimous finding, three papers claimed exceptions to the consensus finding based on assumptions about neutralizing activity.[31-33] However, these could be discounted based on technical grounds. All three excursions were based on neutralizing antibody data generated from pseudotyped virus produced in human 293T cells rather than live SARS-CoV-2 virus grown and tested in the non-human, green monkey cell line and Vero cells. As virus pseudotyped in human cells likely carries human innate immunity target antigens, the authors did not address and exclude the possibility that the neutralization they observed was due to innate neutralizing antibodies rather than those reactive with spike protein.

As also noted by Ricke,[14] the main problem which led to more severe disease during natural infection was that the onset of IgG to spike protein preceded the clearance of SARS-CoV-2 by the innate immune system.[34-38] This earlier onset leading to more severe disease was also documented previously for spike IgG antibody to SARS-CoV-1.[39,40] In contrast when SARS-CoV-2 was neutralized or cleared from the URT before the onset of spike-specific IgG in the blood, this invariably resulted in mild COVID-19 disease.[41]

The problem of ADE following vaccination particularly for RNA viruses is believed in part to reflect the rapidity at which new variants are generated in the host following the introduction of antibodies to spike protein that can and do readily select for new variants. For example, in immunosuppressed high-risk individuals, it took 10 days on average for a neutralizing monoclonal antibody (MAb), bamlanivimab to spike protein to generate escape mutants and establish a rebound viremia.[42] Fortunately, in many instances but not all patients studied, convalescent plasma was able to provide recovery presumably related to innate neutralizing antibodies and other innate humoral immune mechanisms found in plasma.

Perhaps more importantly, a growing body of evidence implies for natural infection unless the case of COVID-19 was severe/critical, there were few IgG1 or IgG3 antibodies to spike RBD in the nasal secretions and none in the saliva.[43,44] However, with the second dose of COVID-19 vaccines (mRNA or virus vectored), these IgG1/3 antibodies to spike protein capable of mediating ADE were commonly detected at high levels in the URT.[43,44] Thus, the global mass vaccination with COVID-19 vaccines not only greatly increased the likelihood of the emergence of variants, but led to increased transmission and infection rates, all of which would and did prolong the pandemic beyond May 2021.[45]

Given the importance of the selection of SARS-CoV-2 variants and increased infection rates as salient proof of ADE, which in turn validates that the macrophage provides the most important correlate of protection against COVID-19, data supporting each of these statements will be briefly discussed.

Evidence from Canada for Selection of SARS-CoV-2 Variants Correlating with Vaccination Milestones

For both the Pfizer and Moderna mRNA COVID-19 vaccines, it was about 14 days after the second dose of vaccines, when the IgG antibodies to spike protein became significantly detectable in most individuals.[46,47] Also, it was known that the first dose which provoked trained innate immunity-induced heterologous protection against all-cause mortality. Negative excess all-cause mortality was clearly demonstrated in countries especially those that postponed the second dose (Canada[48] and the UK) at the time that the first dose was administered.[49] For the USA, a study of seven integrated healthcare organizations in the USA demonstrated that heterologous protection against non-COVID-19 mortality was induced upon the first dose and which was not appreciably altered upon receiving the second dose, at least for the first 7.5 months of the vaccination campaign.[50]

In Canada, the selection of variants (initial emergence or when the variant became dominant) was observed[51] either (1) when the percentage of the eligible population who received two doses over those who had only received one dose exceeded 0.5 **(Table 1)** or (2) when the negative excess all-cause mortality (heterologous protection against all-cause mortality comparing 2021 to the average for 2015–2019) reversed direction and started to trend positive **(Fig. 2)**. In either case, these parameters are alternative ways of looking at the relative impact of the induction of ADE-promoting, spike-specific IgG1/3 by the second dose relative to the heterologous protection by trained innate immunity of the first dose. Both sets of parameters examine and reflect ADE. As detailed elsewhere,[51] and reproduced here by the author, when the second dose to first dose ratio exceeded 0.5, this was associated with the initial emergence of the alpha variant and was also associated with the dominance of the delta variant **(Table 1)**. Conversely, when the negative excess all-cause mortality reversed direction (i.e., the heterologous protection of trained innate immunity against mortality became less, **Fig. 2**) this correlated with the alpha variant becoming dominant and with the initial emergence of the delta variant.

Accordingly, these tight correlations indicate a high likelihood that the COVID-19 vaccines through ADE mechanisms were causally related to selection of the alpha and delta variants. In further substantiation of this notion, the global selection of immune escape variants did not appreciably occur until the COVID-19 vaccines were introduced.[49] For clarification, the initial emergence of the alpha variant which occurred by December 2020 in the UK could have reflected that over 600,000 UK residents had taken part

TABLE 1: The two over one dose ratios for COVID-19 vaccination in Canada: December 22, 2020 to August 1, 2021 (from Our World in Data[49]).

Date	% at least one dose	% two doses	% one dose	Two/One ratio	Events	Notes
22-Dec	0.071	None	0.071	**N/A**		
29-Dec	*0.19*	None	*0.19*	**N/A**		
03-Jan	0.3	None	0.30	**N/A**		EACM decreases
10-Jan	0.84	0.1	0.74	**0.135**		
17-Jan	1.5	0.6	0.9	**0.667**		**EACM temporarily flattened**
24-Jan	2.03	0.15	1.88	**0.080**		
31-Jan	2.3	0.3	2	**0.150**		
07-Feb	2.4	0.47	*1.93*	**0.244**		
08-Feb	2.4	0.5	1.9	**0.263**		
10-Feb	2.5	0.6	1.9	**0.316**		**Enters Neg EACM**
14-Feb	2.59	0.81	1.78	**0.455**		
21-Feb	2.9	1.1	1.8	**0.611**		
22-Feb	3	1.2	1.8	**0.667**	Alpha emerges	
25-Feb	3.2	1.3	1.9	**0.684**		
26-Feb	3.4	1.4	2	**0.700**		
27-Feb	3.5	1.4	2.1	**0.667**	NACI intervention around Feb 27	
28-Feb	3.63	1.41	2.22	**0.635**		
07-Mar	4.85	1.52	3.33	**0.456**		Uptick in Neg EACM
08-Mar	5.1	1.6	3.5	**0.457**		
11-Mar	5.67	1.59	4.08	**0.390**		
14-Mar	6.5	1.6	4.9	**0.327**		
15-Mar	6.8	1.6	5.2	**0.308**		
21-Mar	8.83	1.7	7.13	**0.238**		Lowest Neg EACM (Nadir)
22-Mar	9.2	1.7	7.5	**0.227**	Alpha dominates	
28-Mar	11.81	1.81	10	**0.181**		Uptick in Neg EACM
04-Apr	15.07	1.92	13.15	**0.146**		
11-Apr	19.04	2.19	16.85	**0.130**		Uptick in Neg EACM
18-Apr	24	2.5	21.5	**0.116**		
19-Apr	25	2.5	22.5	**0.111**		

Continued

Continued

Date	% at least one dose	% two doses	% one dose	Two/One ratio	Events	Notes
25-Apr	29.18	2.75	26.43	**0.104**		
26-Apr	30	2.8	27.2	**0.103**		
28-Apr	31	2.9	28.1	**0.103**		Exit Neg EACM
02-May	33.58	3.05	30.53	**0.100**	Delta emerges	
03-May	34	3.1	30.9	**0.100**		
09-May	39	3.4	35.6	**0.096**		
16-May	45	3.8	41.2	**0.092**		
17-May	46	3.9	42.1	**0.093**	Max alpha at 59%	
23-May	51	4.05	46.95	**0.086**		
30-May	56.69	5.45	51.24	**0.106**		
02-Jun	58.8	6.11	52.69	**0.116**		
11-Jun	63.87	10.82	53.05	**0.204**		
14-Jun	64.86	13.11	51.75	**0.253**		
20-Jun	66.29	18.85	47.44	**0.397**		
26-Jun	67.38	26.47	40.91	**0.647**		
04-Jul	68.31	35.02	33.29	**1.052**		50% of the eligible receive 2nd dose
12-Jul	69.27	44.33	24.94	**1.777**	Delta dominant	
19-Jul	69.99	50.61	19.38	**2.611**		50% fully vaccinated
25-Jul	71	55	16	**3.438**		
01-Aug	71	59	12	**4.917**		

Note:

- Max alpha at 59% means the maximal portion of the sequenced variants was recorded at 59%.
- All of the data provided[49] is freely available for both academic and commercial use under Creative Commons Attribution 4.0 (CC-BY 4.0) license terms.

[EACM: excess all-cause mortality; NACI: National Advisory Committee on Immunization (Canada); Neg: negative; N/A: not applicable]

in vaccine clinical trials. Presumably, the use of neutralizing MAbs to spike protein and/or use of convalescent plasma may have also contributed to the earlier emergence of the alpha variant in the UK. Conversely, Canada did not participate in mRNA vaccine clinical trials. This enabled an assessment of both the emergence of the alpha and delta variants associated with mass immunization.

There is additional published data supporting the above conclusions that the COVID-19 vaccines were likely causally related to the selection of variants. SARS-CoV-2 variants sequenced from the two-dose vaccinated when compared with the unvaccinated had significantly higher percentages

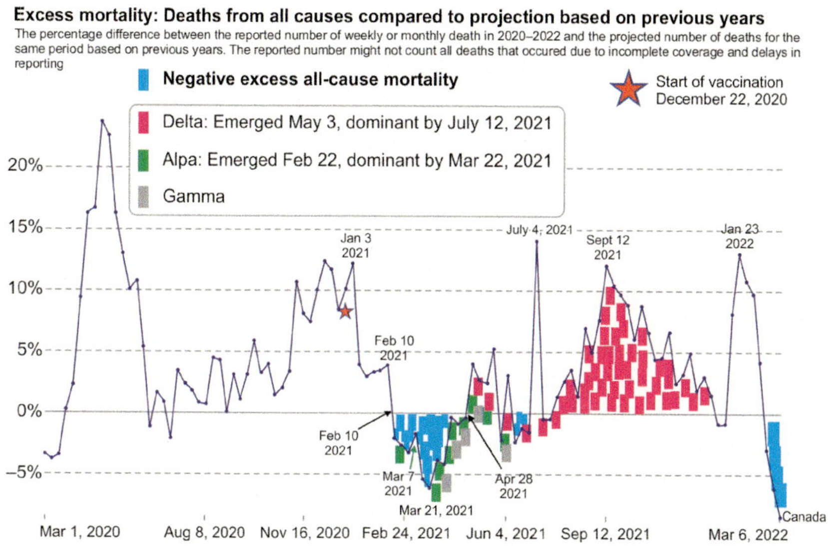

FIGURE 2: Negative excess all-cause mortality in spring 2021 (February 10–April 28) in Canada associated with postponement of second COVID-19 vaccine dose by up to 120 days.[48] Negative excess mortality relative to the average mortality per week for 2015–2019 is highlighted in turquoise as provided by Our World in Data.[49] Bright green highlights pertain to emergence and dominance of the alpha variant (emerged February 22, 2021 and became dominant by March 22, 2021 but never exceeded 57% of the total variants); hot pink highlights pertain to emergence (May 3, 2021) and dominance of the delta variant (July 12, 2021) and reached 99% of the total variants by Aug 30, 2021; and the gamma variant appearance is shown in gray and never reached higher than 26%. Mass vaccination started in Canada on December 22, 2020. There were no variants of concern selected prior to December 22, 2020, implicating mass vaccination as the cause. Note that the peak in excess all-cause mortality recorded on July 4 pertained to 619 heat wave related deaths from June 25 to July 1, 2021, in British Columbia[52] and thus are immaterial to the discussion.

Note: All of the data provided[49] is freely available for both academic and commercial use under Creative Commons Attribution 4.0 (CC-BY 4.0) license terms.

Source: Human Mortality Database (2022) and World Mortality Dataset (2022).

of immune escape variants as well as variants associated with higher infectivity.[53] Furthermore, in a separate report, boosted innate immunity (the first 6 days after the second dose) showed 100% vaccine effectiveness (VE) from April 2021 to August 2021 while during the same period the VE for adaptive immunity (7 days or longer after the second dose) declined from 78 to 48% as determined in a large integrated health system in the USA[54] (see their Supplemental Table 5c, in reference 54). The latter findings are consistent with the notion that the neutralizing antibodies of innate immunity can provide sterilizing or lasting herd immunity against SARS-CoV-2, whereas adaptive immunity neutralizing antibodies cannot. In other words, as expected due to ADE, adaptive immunity vaccines particularly producing IgG1 and IgG3 antibodies to spike protein are not very useful and may be harmful to control a pandemic.

Vaccination Increased SARS-CoV-2 Symptomatic Infection Rates in the UK Putatively by ADE

In the UK, most COVID-19 vaccines administered were the Pfizer-BioNTech mRNA COVID-19 vaccines. UK data consistent with the increased risk of symptomatic infection in the two dose COVID-19 vaccinated over the unvaccinated (unadjusted rates per 100,000) were first revealed in the 40+ age group.[55] This correlated with the onset of the dominance of the delta variant starting with the September 9, 2021, Week 36 report (reporting for the previous 4-week interval) released by Public Health England. It should be noted that the UK authorities did not release informative data concerning these risks prior to September 9, 2021.[55]

Over time these weekly vaccine surveillance reports[55] indicated that as the vaccines were rolled out to younger and younger age groups the increased risk of infection in the fully vaccinated (per 100,000) over unvaccinated affected younger and younger age groups, showing a cause-and-effect trend. For example, by week 41, reported on October 14, 2021, the fully vaccinated 30+ were additionally at increased risk. By week 50 reported on December 16, 2021, the 18+ age groups were at increased risks. This is consistent with ADE in the URT enhancing symptomatic infections in the vaccinated over the unvaccinated.

Vaccination which increases the risks of symptomatic infection particularly in the younger age groups who are generally at very low or insignificant risk (when compared to those over 65) clearly is the opposite goal of the intended public health measure of mass vaccination. This dilemma was predictable based on the known characteristics of ADE and the multitude of reports that universally showed the IgG antibodies to spike protein correlated with COVID-19 disease progression[13-30] especially when they emerged prior to the clearance of SARS-CoV-2[35-40,42] by innate immunity.[41]

However due to extreme transmissibility of the omicron SARS-COV-2 variants witnessed in January 2022 and after where the results of home testing were not reported to government authorities, the UKHSA reports on infection risk of the vaccinated over the unvaccinated ceased after the end of March 2022. By the last report on March 24, 2022,[56] the risk of symptomatic infection in the three dose vaccinated over the unvaccinated (unadjusted rates per 100,000) had reached 4.0-fold in the 30–39 age group which indicated the increased risks of infection related to vaccination were not trivial **(Table 2)**. As a rule of thumb in medical science, anything over 1.20-fold could be clinically significant.

In the USA, Shrestha et al. demonstrated that increasing doses of the COVID-19 shots were associated with an increasing risk of COVID-19 symptomatic infection in healthcare workers at the Cleveland Clinic,[57] in agreement with and as an extension of the UK government findings. Although it has been reported that there is an isotype switch following the third COVID-19 vaccine dose where the IgG1/3 antibodies in the blood to

TABLE 2: The United Kingdom Health Security Agency's COVID-19 vaccine surveillance report for week 12 reported on March 24, 2022, showed in all age groups over the age of 18 that the vaccinated were at increased risk of symptomatic infection.[56]

Unadjusted rates of COVID-19 infection, hospitalization and death in vaccinated and unvaccinated populations. Please note that the following table should be read in conjunction with pages 38 to 41 of this report, and the footnotes provided on page 45.

	Cases reported by specimen date between week 8 2022 (w/e 27 February 2022) and week 11 2022 (w/e 20 March 2022)		Cases presenting to emergency care (within 28 days of a positive test) resulting in overnight inpatient admission, by specimen date between week 8 2022 (w/e 27 February 2022) and week 11 2022 (w/e 20 March 2022)		Death within 28 days of positive COVID-19 test by date of death between week 8 2022 (w/e 27 February 2022) and week 11 2022 (w/e 20 March 2022)		Death within 60 days of positive COVID-19 test by date of death between week 8 2022 (w/e 27 February 2022) and week 11 2022 (w/e 20 March 2022)	
	(see information on population bases and unadjusted rates in footnotes 1 and 2 below this table)							
	Unadjusted rates among persons vaccinated with at least three doses (per 100,000)	Unadjusted rates among persons not vaccinated (per 100,000)[1,2]	Unadjusted rates among persons vaccinated with at least three doses (per 100,000)	Unadjusted rates among persons not vaccinated (per 100,000)[2]	Unadjusted rates among persons vaccinated with at least three doses (per 100,000)	Unadjusted rates among persons not vaccinated (per 100,000)[2]	Unadjusted rates among persons vaccinated with at least three doses (per 100,000)	Unadjusted rates among persons not vaccinated (per 100,000)[2]
Under 18	1,165.6	1,406.3	2.1	8.3	0.0	0.0	0.0	0.0
18–29	2,542.8	781.5	4.7	6.8	0.1	0.1	0.2	0.2
30–39	3,483.8	882.0	5.8	6.8	0.1	0.3	0.3	0.4
40–49	3,151.6	777.1	5.5	7.5	0.1	0.3	0.6	0.7
50–59	2,551.5	627.8	7.1	13.2	0.5	1.8	1.4	3.1
60–69	2,151.3	460.0	12.5	20.3	1.6	4.6	4.1	8.2
70–79	1,643.0	438.9	31.3	58.0	6.6	17.7	14.7	31.1
80 or over	1,569.8	637.9	100.0	112.5	42.3	85.6	90.0	134.3

Continued

Continued

[1]Comparing case rates among vaccinated and unvaccinated populations should not be used to estimate vaccine effectiveness against COVID-19 infection. Vaccine effectiveness has been formally estimated from a number of different sources and is summarized on pages 4 to 14 in this report.

The rates are calculated per 100,000 in people who have received either three doses of a COVID-19 vaccine or in people who have not received a COVID-19 vaccine. These figures are updated each week as the number of unvaccinated individuals and individuals vaccinated with three doses in the population changes.

The case rates in the vaccinated and unvaccinated populations are unadjusted crude rates that do not take into account underlying statistical biases in the data and there are likely to be systematic differences between these two population groups. For example:

- Testing behavior is likely to be different between people with different vaccination status, resulting in differences in the chances of being identified as a case.
- Many of those who were at the head of the queue for vaccination are those at higher risk from COVID-19 due to their age, their occupation, their family circumstances or because of underlying health issues.
- people who are fully vaccinated and people who are unvaccinated may behave differently, particularly with regard to social interactions and therefore may have differing levels of exposure to COVID-19.
- People who have never been vaccinated are more likely to have caught COVID-19 in the weeks or months before the period of the cases covered in the report. This gives them some natural immunity to the virus which may have contributed to a lower case rate in the past few weeks.

[2]Case rates are calculated using NIMS, a database of named individuals from which the numerator and the denominator come from the same source and there is a record of each individuals vaccination status. Further information on the use of NIMS as the source of denominator data is presented on page 40 of this report.

Unadjusted case rates among persons not vaccinated have been formatted in grey to further emphasize the caution to be employed when interpreting this data.

Source: CC-By 4.0 from https://www.nationalarchives.gov.uk/doc/open-government-licence/version/3/andreferencing bulletin.

the spike protein are converted to largely IgG4[58] which does not contribute to ADE, clearly this does not occur in the URT where risk of infection/transmission continues to escalate at three or more doses **(Table 2)**. Note by March 2022 most of the UK ever vaccinated had already received the third dose by December 2021.[49]

Indeed, as captured by 'Our World in Data'[49] the population of Canada and the United States as a whole, exhibited an increase in the reproductive rate (transmission reproductive rate) associated with the second and more so, the third dose associated also with the selection of variants **(Fig. 3)**. These findings corroborate the notion that the problem of ADE with the adaptive immunity spike vaccines leading to the selection of variants and higher infectivity was in fact, experienced globally.

From First Principles Adaptive Immunity is Not Able to Control Emerging Pathogens or Pandemics

Adaptive immunity antibodies particularly to spike protein would serve to prolong the pandemic by introducing new waves and making the newer selected variants more transmissible and more infectious as just reviewed. In addition, there are other fundamental reasons as to why adaptive immunity mechanisms are not well suited to handling pandemics or emerging pathogens. The adaptive response to a pathogen never seen before requires at least 14–21 days before levels of IgG antibody peak in most individuals.[41] Many pathogens can kill the host before the adaptive system ramps up. For

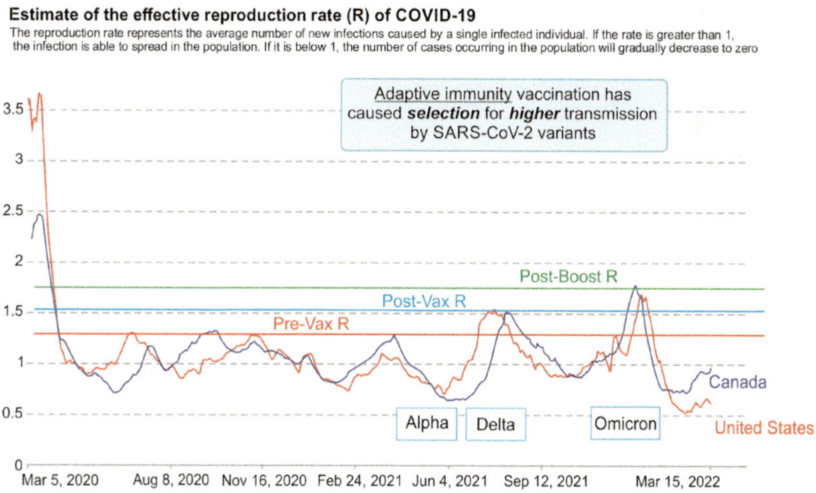

FIGURE 3: The effective reproduction rate "R" of severe acute respiratory syndrome coronavirus 2 (SARS-CoV-2) clearly indicates increased risk of transmission with two and more so, three doses of the adaptive COVID-19 vaccine for Canada and the United States.

Note: All of the data provided by Our World in Data[49] is freely available for both academic and commercial use under Creative Commons Attribution 4.0 (CC-BY 4.0) license terms.

SARS-CoV-2, the time to death was commonly pegged at 10 days.[59] Thus, from first principles, it is clear innate immunity which is the first line of defense, would and does play a pivotal role in COVID-19 disease outcomes, but adaptive immunity cannot and in fact could jeopardize the innate immunity critical to recovery via ADE.

Accordingly, adaptive immunity vaccines. such as the COVID-19 vaccines employing spike protein, were intrinsically unable to control SARS-CoV-2 infection at the individual and population level. This is because of the problem of ADE, which would increase transmissibility and lengthen the duration of the pandemic.

The ADE of SARS-CoV-2 in the URT, involved classical FCGR2A expression in macrophages which were labeled as the interferon responsive macrophages.[60] None of the five types of macrophages in the URT nasopharyngeal swab samples expressed angiotensin-converting enzyme 2 (ACE2) nor transmembrane protease serine 2 (TMPRSS2) indicating entry of SARS-CoV-2 into macrophages likely related to ADE. Many groups have indicated that macrophages in the lungs of severe COVID-19 patients but not those with mild or moderate disease are infected with SARS-CoV-2 where again ACE2 and/or TMPRSS2 are not expressed.[61-66] This corroborates the notion of SARS-CoV-2 entry into macrophages by ADE causing disease progression. In a very comprehensive study Ren et al.[61] uncovered in the LRT, a novel type of ADE involving a switch from the ACE2: spike interaction to BSG: spike. This focused the infections on the macrophages and other immune cells and away from lung epithelial cells. In the URT, macrophages which were judged to be sebocytes (specialized LB^- FMs) lost expression of BSG upon their activation and as mentioned appeared to instead use the classical FCGR2A for ADE-mediated entry of SARS-CoV-2.[60] Thus, there are two types of ADE associated with SARS-CoV-2 infection, classical in the URT and a novel switch type in the LRT involving BSG.

Aims of the Review

Given the importance of ADE as an impediment to the development of safe and effective vaccines against emerging and pandemic viruses including SARS-CoV-2, it is important to understand what is so special about the M1-like, proinflammatory foamy macrophages and to elucidate how they generate a *potent* virus-anti-virus (heterologous) response. HERV-K102 replication produces particles in M1-like macrophages and generates a foamy appearance when the particles bud into vacuoles **(Fig. 4)**.[10,11,67] We were first to suggest HERV-K102 is a replication competent live virus both *in vitro* and *in vivo*[10,67] and provided evidence that its replication may protect against HIV-1 acquisition, i.e., generates sterilizing immunity.[10,67] Other virologists have also unwittingly isolated HERV-K HML-2 *DNA* containing particles at the same low levels and frequencies from HIV-1 infected patients[68] in direct support of our findings as discussed elsewhere.[11] The goals of the present paper are to ask what host innate immunity mechanisms are abrogated by

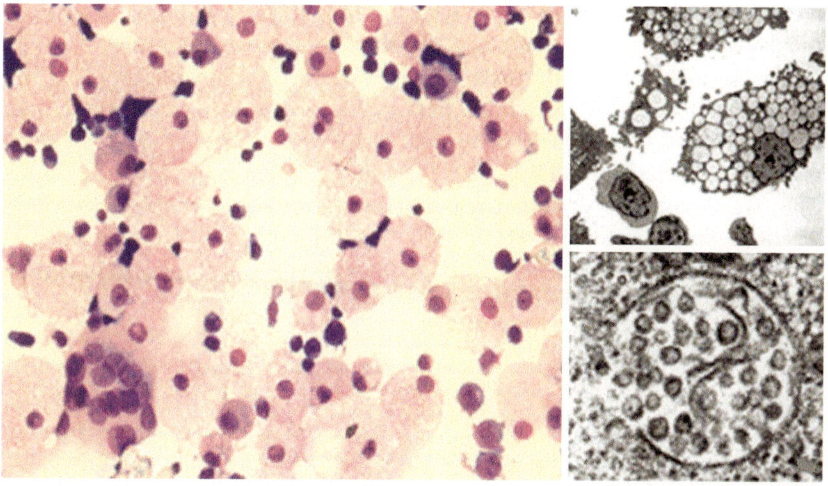

FIGURE 4: HERV-K102 particle production in cord blood mononuclear cells (CB) cultured in IMDM media.[10,11,67] Left image: H&E staining of a CB sample (cytospin slide) showing the dominant presence of highly vacuolated foamy macrophages amongst normal small lymphocytes (400×). Note the presence of a rare multinucleated giant macrophage. Right image top: Electron microscopy of vacuolating CB cells day 11 at 1,500×. Right image bottom: At 100,000× *immature* particles (the centers are not condensed) can be seen in the vacuoles which averaged about 100 nm. Envelope spikes are also noted. No cell surface budding was observed by EM. Instead, release of the particles occurred on day 6–7 by lysis. Note that when CB was cultured in traditional RPMI this aborted foam cell formation. Also, the addition of IL-2 and PHA aborted foam cell formation in IMDM cultures implying adaptive immunity may downmodulate HERV-K102 particle production. Blue arrow in right bottom image points to the preassembly of envelope with gag as aggregates in the trans-golgi network which then bud into the vacuoles.[69] This assembly which absolutely requires envelope protein is characteristic of foamy retroviruses but not orthoretroviruses.

(HERV-K102: human endogenous retrovirus-K102; H&E: hematoxylin and eosin; IMDM: Iscove's Modified Dulbecco's Medium; RPMI: Roswell Park Memorial Institute)

Source: Reproduced from "Laderoute MP. Clues to finding correlates of risk/protection for HIV-1 vaccines". F1000Research. 2018;6:868.[11]

ADE infection into macrophages and why does this cause and determine progression to more severe disease. Answers to these questions are relevant to all-cause mortality and thus human survival and so, are needed for preparation for future pandemics.

HERV-K102 PROTECTION SYSTEM OF PRO-INFLAMMATORY M1-LIKE FOAMY MACROPHAGES

HERV-K102 is a Type 1 HERV-K HML-2 Group Member

Human endogenous retrovirus-K102 , also named ERVK-7, is a member of the HERV-K (HML-2) group consisting of about 91 full length HERVs in the human genome.[70] HML-2 represents the most biologically active and most recently acquired of the 10 HERV-K groups in humans.[71] The letter K refers to the use of lysine-transfer RNA used to prime reverse transcription.

In the HML-2 group, there are two types of HML-2, those with (type 2) and without (type 1) a 292 nucleotide base pair region between the polymerase gene (*pol)* and envelope (*env*) genes.[71] The significance of this difference is yet to be determined. This sequence encodes Rec protein which results from an alternatively spliced transcript and is analogous to the Rev protein in HIV-1 and the Rex protein in HTLV used for encapsidation of proviral genomes in their particles.[71] HERV-K102 is a type 1 and lacks this region. The absence of Rec such as in HERV-K102 has led to the false notion that it is unlikely to be replication competent and thus has been largely ignored by virologists. However, the unconventional and nonpathogenic (foamy) spumaretroviruses also lack this domain yet remain fully replication competent.[72] Remarkably HERV-K102 has been shown to be replication competent in *in vitro*[10] and *in vivo*.[11,67] As might be anticipated, HERV-K102 fortunately exhibits all the hallmarks of the nonpathogenic category of retroviruses namely the spumaretroviruses.[10,67] Moreover, its replication has been associated with protection against HIV-1 acquisition in an HIV-1 exposed seronegative (HESN) cohort **(Fig. 5)**[10] cementing the notion that HERV-K102 replication is not pathogenic but protective.

HERV-K102 as the Elusive Foamy Retrovirus of Humans

Spumaretroviruses, commonly referred to as foamy viruses, are complex retroviruses belonging to the subfamily Spumaretrovirinae in the family Retroviridae. Foamy viruses are unconventional non-pathogenic retroviruses belonging to the oldest of virus phylogenies estimated at 400 million years old.[72,73] Simian foamy retroviruses have been coevolving with their primate hosts for over 60 million years[74] implying they provide major benefits to the host. While foamy viruses have been described in many species examined, until the documentation that replication competent HERV-K102 had all the hallmarks of foamy viruses,[10] the foamy virus of humans had remained elusive. In other words, our research group was the first to identify that humans indeed have a protector foamy virus, namely HERV-K102 encoded on chromosome 1, at 1q22.

It should be clarified that in the literature there has been reference to a human foamy virus (HFV) which was isolated from a human nasopharyngeal cell line. However, this virus originated in chimpanzees and when this was discovered it was therefore renamed prototype foamy virus (PFV) as by this time it had been well characterized.[72,73]

As mentioned, HERV-K102 has all the salient features of foamy viruses as exemplified by comparison with PFV (see extensive list in Supplemental Materials in reference 10). First and foremost, when the virus replicates in macrophages **(Fig. 4)** particles accumulate in vacuoles giving the cells a foamy cell appearance which is the primary tell-tale sign of foamy viruses.[72]

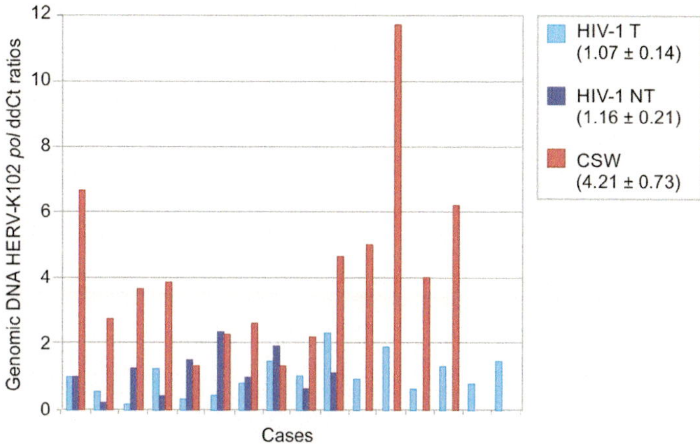

FIGURE 5: Evidence that HERV-K102 replicative activity is associated with sterilizing immunity (resistance to HIV-1 acquisition) in a HIV-1 exposed seronegative (HESN) cohort.[10] DNA was isolated from plasma. The ddCt real-time PCR method employed the 18S RNA gene to control for genomic equivalents and used uracil N-glycosylase (UNG) in the PCR buffer to digest the cDNA genomes of HERV-K102 particles which left only genomic DNA in the DNA extracted from plasma. The mean ddCt qPCR ratio (for HERV-K102 *pol*) of 30 normal healthy controls was 0.88 ± 0.37. In contrast, on average for the female commercial sex workers (CSW) HESN cohort it was 4.21 ± 0.73, with a $t < 0.0005$. This represents a substantial fivefold increase in genomic integration over normal healthy controls. The ratio for the total HIV-1 patients or as stratified based on the use of antiretroviral therapy (T) or not (NT), was not statistically different from the normal healthy controls.

(HERV-K102: human endogenous retrovirus-K102; PCR; polymerase chain reaction)

Source: Reproduced from Laderoute MP, Larocque LJ, Giulivi A, Diaz-Mitoma F. Further evidence that HERV-K102 is a replication competent foamy virus that may antagonize HIV-1 replication. Open AIDS J. 2015;9:112-22.

Another telltale sign of foamy viruses is that their genomes begin with "tgtg" which relates to how the genomes integrate into genomic DNA. Another distinguishing feature of foamy viruses is that the genomes are cDNA,[75] which has been clearly demonstrated for HERV-K102.[67] Rather than reverse transcribing upon entry into cells as is known for orthoretroviruses (the pathogenic retroviruses), instead foamy viruses reverse transcribe upon exit from cells[72,73,75] and so have a reverse life cycle to the orthoretroviruses. This could provide foamy viruses with a replication advantage over the orthoretroviruses which would be important for protecting the host. In addition, PFV is capable of multiple integrations in myeloid cells up to 20-fold[76] and multiple integrations into genomic DNA have also been demonstrated for HERV-K102 *in vivo* **(Fig. 5)**[10] and *in vitro* (unpublished observations).

Somewhat unexpectantly, and despite their nonpathogenic nature, foamy viruses such as PFV can undergo cytopathic infections in some fibroblast cell lines but not others.[72,73] This was also demonstrated for HERV-K102 particles **(Fig. 6)**. In fact, it turns out PFV is oncolytic meaning it causes cell lysis when

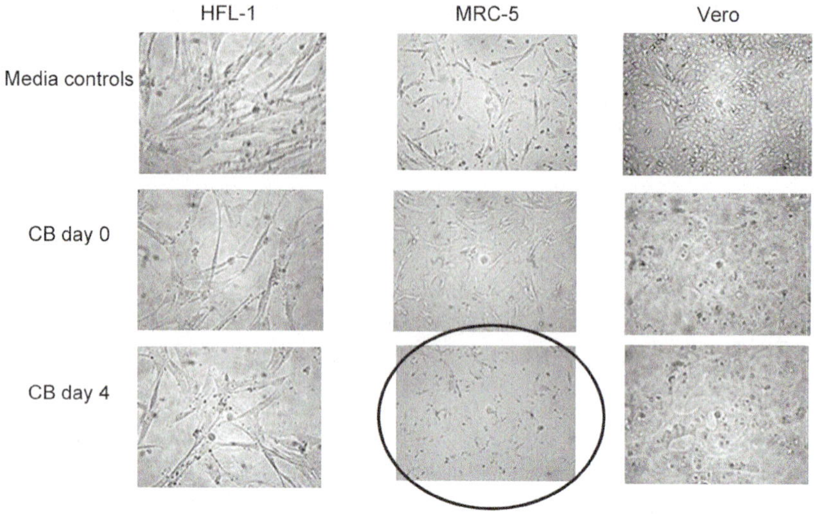

FIGURE 6: Human endogenous retrovirus-K102 (HERV-K102) particles liberated from cultured cord blood mononuclear cells (CB) by freeze-thaw lysis (but not from supernatants) may rapidly induce cell lysis at 24 hours but not at 16 hours in susceptible cells. HFL-1 = human fetal lung fibroblasts; MRC-5 = human fetal lung fibroblast; Vero = green monkey kidney epithelial cells. Representative of four full sets of data conducted in duplicate. Estimated multiplicity of infection (MOI) of 2. Supernatants from the cultured CB did not induce lysis as no HERV-K102 particles bud through the cell surface of the foamy macrophages by electron microscopy and because significant cell death did not occur until day 7. Freeze-thaw treated uncultured CB (day 0) which does not exhibit HERV-K102 particles does not lyse the MRC-5 cells, but day 4 cultured CB does. This demonstrates that the particles mediate lysis and is not a nonspecific factor of the culture media.

Source: From: Laderoute MP. (2022) What you need to know about the HERV-K102 innate immunity protector system of macrophages against RNA pandemic viruses. hervk102.substack.com. [online] Available from https://hervk102.substack.com/p/what-you-need-to-know-about-the-herv [Last accessed April, 2022].[79]

it replicates in tumor cells[77] while it merely integrates in normal cells. PFV infection also induces cell death in HIV-1 and HTLV-infected cells[78] implying foamy retroviruses may help provide immune surveillance against cancers as well as virally infected cells. Along these lines, it has been suggested that foamy viruses seem to have a peculiar relationship with or companionship with lentiviruses particularly in primates.[72,73] Thus, as suspected, foamy retroviruses do perform an important role defending the host, which may help explain its coevolution with the host.[74] However, it remains to be directly demonstrated if in fact HERV-K102 particles are oncolytic or induce lysis in virus infected cells.

The cell attachment receptor for PFV has been identified as heparan sulfate[80] which is the same for HERV-K HML-2[81] and which is widely expressed on cells. This explains the broad spectrum of permissive cells for foamy viruses and is consistent with their potentially protective nature broadly against viral infections and tumors.

Sebocytes of Sebaceous Glands Lining the Mucosa were Discovered to Produce HERV-K102 Particles

Another fascinating aspect of foamy viruses is that when they transmit to a new host, they replicate solely in the nonproliferating sebocytes of sebaceous glands and thus are deposited to the exterior mucosa causing no harm to the host.[73] An examination of hematoxylin and eosin-stained sections of sebaceous glands **(Fig. 7)**[82] reveals sebocytes have the exact same morphology as the M1-like foamy macrophages producing the HERV-K102 particles **(Fig. 4)**. A search of the expressed genes of sebocytes as available through GEO Profiles[83] revealed both *in vitro*[84] and *in vivo*[85] sebocytes are positive for the major antigens of M1-like foamy macrophages[86-88] including CD14, CD16, CD68, CD163, WDR74, and TNFSF10; for myeloid-specific enhancers

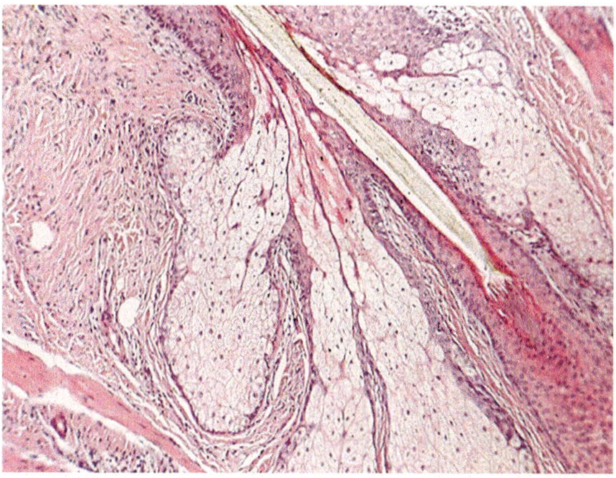

FIGURE 7: A human sebaceous gland[82] demonstrating sebocytes have the distinctive morphology of LB-FMs. Sebocytes are programmed to cell death on day 6/7[92] which generates sebum. This cell lysis involves a novel cytoplasmic-induced apoptosis around day 6–7 involving DNASE2 and LAMP1.100 These cells have the identical distinct morphology of the LB-FMs of Figure 4 and differentially express the same DEGs including ERVK-7 (HERV-K102), BSG, VDR, CD14, CD16, CD68, TP53, both in vivo and *in vitro*.[84,85] Thus, sebocytes constitutively express and release HERV-K102 particles providing a first line of innate immunity defense at the mucosa. This directly corroborates the significance of the HERV-K102 front-line response to emerging and/or pandemic pathogens.

(BSG: basigin; DEG: differentially expressed gene; ERVK: endogenous retrovirus-K; HERV-K102: human endogenous retrovirus-K102; LB-FM: lipid body negative foamy macrophage; VDR: Vitamin D receptor)

Source: From Wikimedia Commons. Insertion of sebaceous glands into hair shaft x10.jpg. [online] Available from https://commons.wikimedia.org/wiki/File:Insertion_of_sebaceous_glands_into_hair_shaft_x10.jpg [Last accessed April, 2024].[82]

SPI1 and CEBPB[88] which are also trained innate immunity enhancers;[89,90] for genes involved in foam cell formation [nuclear receptor subfamily 1 group H member 3 (NR1H3), low-density lipoprotein receptor (LDLR), SQLE, epidermal growth factor receptor (EGFR), hypoxia inducible factor 1 subunit alpha (HIF-1α), BSG, sterol regulatory element binding transcription factor ½ (SREBF1/2), peroxisome proliferator activated receptor gamma (PPARγ), and CD36)] which are also implicated in the induction of trained innate immunity;[90-96] for genes involved in the expression of HERV-K102 full length proviral genomes [interferon response factors 1 (IRF1), nuclear factor kappa B1 (NF-κB1), VDR, interferon gamma receptor 1/2 (IFNGR1/2), and nuclear receptor subfamily 3 group C member 1 (NR3C1) ± macrophage migration inhibitory factor (MIF)],[97-99] and genes associated with a novel day 6–7 apoptosis mechanism triggered in the cytoplasm (DNASE2, LAMP1, LCN2, and MX1).[92,100] Not only do macrophages that are M1 polarized express high levels of HERV-K102 proviral transcripts[99] but ERVK-7 (HERV-K102) was constitutively expressed in sebocytes[84] Thus, sebocytes are in fact programmed and phenotypically the same as M1-like foamy macrophages, and they respond the same way as macrophages do both *in vitro*[101] and *in vivo*,[60] except they constitutively express and release HERV-K102 particles. There is no doubt that sebocytes are specialized M1-like foamy macrophages that line the mucosa. This discovery makes it very plausible that the HERV-K102 protector system is in fact the first line of defense against infectious agents anticipating them in the mucosa and so, is critical to infectious disease outcomes.

The Origins of HERV-K102 also Provides a Major Clue to its Purpose

Accumulating phylogenetic evidence is consistent with a potential role of HERV-K HML-2 in limiting invasion of the human genome by orthoretroviruses.[102] Ancestral HML-2 elements emerged about 10.3 million years ago (Mya).[102] There has been a striking decline of insertions of ERVs in the last 10 million years (My) in the genomes of all sequenced hominids (great apes and gibbons), but not in old world monkeys (baboons and macaques), particularly regarding HERV-H.[102] HERV-H makes up 88% of all the ERV integrations into the human genome in the last 30 My and became extinct over the past 10 My. HERV-H is a gamma retrovirus, which integrated around 45–60 Mya and has about 962 copies in the human genome.[103] HERV-K, with 10 groups in the clade, only one of which is HML-2, on the other hand, entered the genome of ancestral catarrhines about 32–44 Mya, after the split from New World monkeys and before the split of hominids from the Old-World monkeys.[104] The sister lineages of HERV-K in most other catarrhines appear to have become extinct. Most remarkably, the HERV-K HML-2 group in humans is the only HERV-K that has continued to replicate since the origin of the catarrhines.[102] HERV-K102 is a member of the bioactive HERV-K HML-2 group and as mentioned appears to be the only known replication competent member both *in vitro* and *in vivo*.[10,67] Accordingly, since phylogenetic evidence supports an association of HERV-K HML-2 activity with protection against integration of orthoretroviruses, this substantiates the notion that modern day HERV-K102 particles, along with expression of proteins/transcripts from other HML-2 elements, might help prevent HIV-1 acquisition and provide sterilizing immunity **(Fig. 5)**.

On the Curious Origins of HERV-K102 in Humans

Somewhat ironically, humans apparently acquired the HERV-K102 defense mechanism from the same source of the modern HIV-1 pandemic strain; namely, chimpanzees,[105] possibly between 500,000 and up to 2 Mya.[70,106] The Homo-Pan split has been estimated at 6.6 Mya[104] or earlier at 7–8 Mya.[106]

As mentioned, the HERV-K HML-2 elements originated in primates about 10.3 Mya and the CERV-K102 sequence (DQ112149), which is 97% identical to HERV-K102, was estimated to have integrated into chimpanzees at a nonorthologous position about 10 (±3.3) Mya.[105]

Lentiviruses like HIV-1 may have been active in primates since the divergence of chimpanzees and humans.[107,108] Moreover, it has been suggested the ancestor to HIV-1 may have arisen in chimpanzees about 4 Mya.[109] Since it has been reported that subsets of chimpanzees with chronic HIV-1 infection showed progression analogous to humans, including greater expression of CD38 in CD8+ HLA-DR+ T cells.[110] this raises the notion that an HERV-K102 ancestor, as a potential antidote for HIV-1 infection may have been selected through evolution in chimpanzees before it was acquired by humans. The genus *Homo* arose about 2 Mya.[111] Accordingly, it is possible over about a 2-million-year window or longer, the HERV-K102 ancestor may have adapted to an HIV-1 like ancestor lentivirus(es) in chimpanzees prior to its acquisition by humans. Indeed, there is genetic evidence from a 5 amino acid deletion fixed in a human orthologue of tetherin that humans may have been afflicted by a lentivirus presence long before HIV-1, perhaps about 800,000 years ago, which may have caused changes in innate immune genes in humans.[112] Thus, the phylogenetic evidence raises the notion that HERV-K102 as a replication competent HERV-K HML-2 foamy retrovirus, may have evolved specific mechanisms to limit HIV/lentivirus replication and genome invasion in chimpanzees before being acquired in humans. Indeed, a high level of segmental duplication related to telomere like repeats, particularly at 1q21–1q22 in the human genome (i.e., HERV-K102 is located at 1q22) have been shown to be a causative factor in primate genome evolution.[113] This finding may further substantiate the role of HERV-K102 as being critical to hominin and *Homo sapiens'* survival and thus evolution.

Neanderthals and Denisovans appear to have lost HERV-K102 at the orthologous chromosome position at 1q22 **(Fig. 8)** and both went extinct. As mentioned, the *Homo* species which includes Neanderthals and Denisovans, arose about 2 million years ago.[111] The divergence of Neanderthal from anatomically modern humans (AHM) had been estimated at 550–760 thousand years before present (TYBP) but the mitochondrial DNA assessment suggests divergence only occurred around 400 TYBP.[114] Also, from sequencing of the Y chromosome, Denisovans split about 700 TYBP from AMH, and Neanderthal from AMH around 370 TYBP[115] implying first the divergence of Denisovans and then Neanderthals. That the Neanderthal genome contains a few more nucleotides surrounding the deleted HERV-K102 at 1q22 than the Denisovans (**Fig. 8**) may or may not be consistent with Denisovans separating earlier from AMH while Neanderthal split later.

It should be noted that the earliest modern human remains in Europe so far discovered was about 45,000 years ago.[116] Thus, at the time of HERV-K102 acquisition the common ancestor would have resided in Africa, and this makes it plausible that HERV-K102 may have been acquired from chimpanzees known to live in Africa but not Europe. The finding by Compton *et al.*[112] referenced above implicates an exposure to chimpanzee lentiviruses around the same time, consistent with co-mingling of humans and chimpanzees at that time that HERV-K102 crossed over and into humans. Whether lentivirus played a role in the loss of HERV-K102 in the extinct hominins and/or in their extinction remains to be determined.

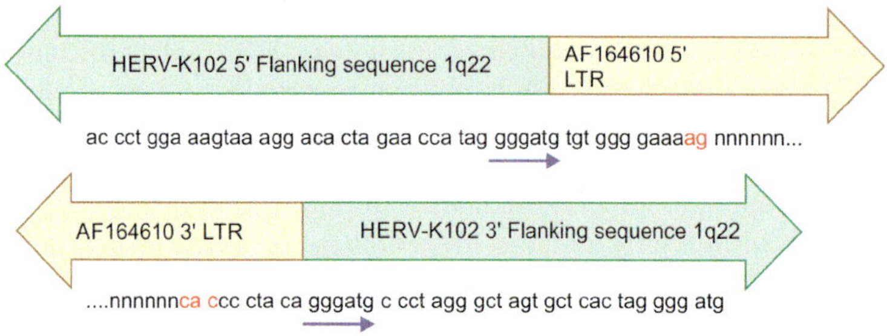

FIGURE 8: Evidence for past integration and excision of HERV-K102 at orthologous positions (1q22) in the Neanderthal and Denisovan genomes. Direct repeats (gggatg) flank the orthologous HERV-K102 sequence in the human and extinct hominin genomes. The nucleotides marked in red were missing from the Denisovan orthologous position but present in the Neanderthal genome. Most of the HERV-K102 provirus was missing in both extinct hominins with only a few nucleotides corresponding to the ends of the LTRs remaining intact. "n" stands for missing nucleotides. Inquiry was made of the Altai Neanderthal or Denisovan genome at http://bioinf.eva.mpg.de/fetchseq/ on chromosome 1 strand at 155,596,423 to 155,605,644. AF164610 GenBank LTR flanking sequences used: 5′ LTR sequence = AF095801 and 3′ LTR sequence = AF095802.

(HERV-K102: human endogenous retrovirus-K102; LTR: long terminal repeat)

Source: From Laderoute MP. (2022). What you need to know about the HERV-K102 innate immunity protector system of macrophages against RNA pandemic viruses. hervk102.substack.com. [online] Available from https://hervk102.substack.com/p/what-you-need-to-know-about-the-herv [Last accessed April, 2024].[79]

Nevertheless, RNA virus epidemics likely played some role in the demise of the extinct hominins as adaptively introgressed Neanderthal genes in humans frequently feature innate immunity genes against RNA viruses[117] or immune pathways against pathogens.[118] As well, innate immune reactions with pathogens affected human evolution between 0.6 and 2 Mya.[111] Consistent with a notion of a superior innate defense system of humans versus other interacting hominins was the finding of successful admixture between humans and Neanderthals but only when the female was human. This was deduced by showing mitochondrial DNA carried from the egg (i.e., female) in humans contained no introgressed Neanderthal genes.[119] However, it should be appreciated that there may have been other reasons for this one-way admixture aside from innate immunity. Nevertheless, it is tempting to speculate that at least in part, the HERV-K102 protection system *may have contributed* to the survival of *Homo sapiens* over Neanderthals given the known selection pressure from RNA viral epidemics at the time of admixture.

In summary, the phylogenetic history suggests HERV-K102 may have first coevolved in chimpanzees to protect against lentiviruses prior to being acquired by the *Homo species*. The remarkable observation that HERV-K102 replication was associated with sterilizing immunity to HIV-1 in the HESN sex trade workers (HESN) which manifested as protection against HIV-1 acquisition **(Fig. 5)**[10] becomes much more plausible and thus, credible.

Evidence for a Role of HERV-K HML-2 Activation in Innate Immunity

The HERV-K HML-2 group was discovered by hybridizing the cloned region of the reverse transcriptase of the Syrian hamster intracisternal A particles against a human cDNA genomic library.[120] Not long after, Lower et al. described the detection of antibodies to HERV-K HML-2 envelope (Env) in 45% of patients with testicular cancers, 26% of patients with lymphomas, 70% of HIV-1 patients, and 38% of pregnant women but in only 3% of normal healthy blood donors.[121] Since the antibodies that were found in 60% of patients with germ cell tumors disappeared upon resection,[122] these early observations were first to imply HERV-K HML-2 activity likely contributed to innate immune surveillance against tumors and pathogens. As a potential follow-up to antibodies to HERV-K HML-2 Env associated with pregnancy, HERV-K particles were subsequently identified as isolated from human placenta.[123] By 2015, Grow et al, discovered HML-2 was reactivated in human preimplantation embryos and pluripotent cells (including particles) to protect against exogenous viral infections.[124] For example, they also demonstrated that the Rec protein of type 2 HML-2 group members was found to induce IFITM1 which guides exogenous viruses into the lysosome for their destruction.[124]

As a side note, these findings of the activation of HERV-K HML-2 elements during early days of conception further substantiate the possibility that the HERV-K102 particles likely played a role generating successful progeny when females of the mating admixture between Neanderthals and AMH were of human origin.[119]

Presumptive evidence for HERV-K102-like particle production like **Figure 4**, had been published prior to our discovery. Morgan and Bodsky in 2004 described these immature HERV-K particles which budded into vacuoles in megakaryocytes in patients with essential thrombocytopenia.[125] An unknown virus appeared to be budding from the cell surface of the megakaryocytes suggesting a viral infection may have led to the induction of HERV-K immature particles putatively in the CMP that macrophages and megakaryocytes share.[12] Presumably, the release of the particles from the megakaryocytes would have also been through cell apoptosis, and this lysis and loss of megakaryocytes presumably would have resulted in thrombocytopenia.

The electron microscopy images of the megakaryocytes[125] also revealed the cytoplasmic "leopard spots" that congregated around the vacuoles as was shown for HERV-K102 replication in the foamy macrophages (**Fig. 4**, blue arrow in the right bottom image). These aggregates represent the telltale signature of the preassembly of Env with the Gag protein outside of vacuoles which is characteristic of nonpathogenic spumaviruses.[69] The pathogenic orthoretroviruses do not require the presence of Env for particle production explaining their proclivity for pseudotyping and their lack of the formation of 'leopard spots'. On the other hand, foamy retroviruses cannot be pseudotyped.[69,72,73]

Our group was first to identify and demonstrate that HERV-K102 particles were commonly and, in many instances, highly induced by viruses *in vivo*. The levels frequently reached 10^{12} particles per mL of plasma although not in HIV-1 infected patients.[10,11,67] It was only more recently that others have confirmed that HERV-K102 full length transcripts are strongly induced upon M1-like polarization of macrophages but not when M2-like polarizing protocols were used.[99] In HIV-1 patients there seemed to be direct antagonism with HERV-K102 replication where on average there may have been only 8,200–8,300 DNA containing particles per ml of plasma and about 70% of HIV-1 patients scoring positive.[11,67,68]

Further data implying a role of HERV-K activation in innate immunity host defenses was the finding of Morozov et al.[126] that the transmembrane region of HERV-K HML-2 Env suppressed adaptive immunity reactivity such as the Concanavalin-A T cell proliferative response. Along similar lines we found that PHA and IL-2 added to the IMDM media inhibited foam cell formation in the cultured cord blood mononuclear cells of **Figure 4** (unpublished data). Thus, innate immunity downregulates adaptive mechanisms and the converse is also true as would be expected.

Moreover, the HERV-K HML-2 envelope transmembrane region peptides strongly induced proteins related to M1-pro-inflammatory macrophages as assessed in peripheral blood mononuclear cells (PBMCs).[126] These cytokines and chemokines included IL-1α/β, IL-6, IL-8, CCL2-5, PLAUR, G-CSF, TNFRSF1B, and MMP1. Interestingly, the latter is a zinc dependent protease involved in the breakdown of the extracellular matrix, but which interestingly, also binds and *inactivates* the Tat protein of HIV-1. In addition, by microarray analysis of expressed genes, Morozov et al, demonstrated mRNA of various genes associated with M1-polarization were upregulated while those for M2-polarization[87] were downregulated.[126] An exception was that CXCL10, a chemokine of M1-polarized macrophages was found to be downregulated in the M1 macrophages. Interestingly in the list of down-regulated genes, HS3ST2 a heparan sulfate (glucosamine) 3-O-sulfotransferase 2 was also downregulated potentially implying a reduced entry of HERV-K102 particles in cells that might express HERV-K Env and/or HERV-K102 particles.

The 'Virus-Antivirus Properties' Associated with HERV-K HML-2 Activity

The full gamut of how the expression of HERV-K HML-2 RNA and proteins along with HERV-K102 particles may contribute to innate immunity and protect the host in an antigen nonspecific manner has not yet been realized. We have only seen the tip of the iceberg of the novel 'virus-antivirus responses' driven by expression of HERV-K HML-2 proteins/transcripts.

The ones that have been identified in addition to those already mentioned include (1) the protease of HML-2 may cut exogenous viruses in the wrong places, reducing their infectivity;[127] (2) HERV-K18 but not HERV-K102 Env may pseudotype the lentivirus HIV-1 reducing its ability to target and reduce certain cell populations such as CD4 T cells;[128] (3) HERV-K HML-2 Gag interferes with HIV-1 Gag again reducing infectivity,[129,130] and of primary clinical significance, while many pathogenic viruses including SARS-CoV-2 may block or delay the initial interferon response of the host;[131,132] and (4) HERV-K102 particles could upon infection of cells and release of their genomes and particle contents into the cytoplasm trigger innate PRRs including the RIG-1/MDA5/MAVS system, and/or the cGAS-STING response[133-135] to regain the protective interferon and other anti-viral responses through alternative pathways. This feature of how HERV-K HML-2 endogenous elements may trigger innate PRRs to amplify interferon and other antiviral responses has been called "viral mimicry".[136]

Additionally, there is some evidence to suggest that HERV-K long terminal repeat (LTR) elements may serve as enhancers for nearby immune response genes.[136] Moreover, it is not likely a coincidence that HERV-K LTR enhancers that bind the transcription factors (TFs) STAT1 and IRF1 response elements which are induced by interferon gamma (IFN-γ) are located in the vicinity of interferon (type I) stimulated genes (ISGs).[99] Thus, HERV-K elements may serve to convert the IFN-γ response to the type I innate immunity interferon response[99,136] which may be useful when an adaptive immunity response such as virus-specific antibodies might jeopardize the survival of the host by ADE.

The fact that HERV-K102 is replication competent and can quickly replicate itself reaching 2.55×10^{11} particles per mL of plasma from zero in about 84 hours,[11] indicates there can be a massive early induction and release of HERV-K102 to ensure the interferon and other innate antiviral responses prevail. In this regard, there is already evidence that HERV-K102 genomic sequences amplify the cGAS-STING response in COVID-19 patients resulting in mild disease.[137]

By examining scRNA sequencing data involving the activation of human macrophages with the TE count and Telescope software packages Russ et al.[99] were able to determine that with M1 polarization in response to LPS (TLR4) and IFN-γ proinflammatory signaling, HERV-K102 activation comprised the majority of HML-2 transcripts in direct substantiation of our work.[10,11,67] Moreover, the TFs STAT 1 and IRF1 critical for HERV-K102 induction by IFN-γ bound to a region called "LTR12F" which resides just upstream of the 5' LTR of HERV-K102. Genes subsequently induced by HERV-K102 expression in M1 macrophages included via cGAS: IRF1, IRF8, SOCS3, and ICAM1; via ISREs: MX1, ISG15, IFIT1-3, USP18, OAS1-3, OASL, and ISG20; and via cGAS and ISRE: STAT1/2, IRF9, IFITM1, BST2, TAP1, SOCS1, IFI35, HLA-G, ZC3HAV1, AIM2, and TRIM69.[99] Many of these genes are ISGs and confirms the finding of HERV-K102 in amplifying the critical type I interferon response *in vivo*.[136] Furthermore, in a humanized mouse model of mild COVID-19 disease, it was reported that macrophages somehow were able to amplify the interferon response critical to recovery.[138]

Russ et al.[99] also reported that VDR response elements and the glucocorticoid receptor response elements along with response elements for NF-κB1 and IRF-1 are contained within the 5' LTR of HERV-K102. Others have previously reported the response elements for these and other inflammatory TFs in the 5' LTR of HERV-K102.[97,98]

The Concept of Innate T and B Cell Responses Against HERV-K102 Envelope

The team of Feng Wang-Johanning and GL Johanning started their legacy of investigating the expression of HERV-K102 transcripts and proteins in common cancers with reports starting in 2001[139] in breast cancers and lasting up until 2017. In their seminal report which used northern blots, full length sequences referred to as proviral transcripts and spliced *env* transcripts were detected in the cancer samples and cell lines. Sequencing of these transcripts revealed type 1 HERV-K102 was strongly induced. Two years later using RT-PCR they published that both type 1 and type 2 HERV-K HML-2 *Env* transcripts were detected in breast cancers and were induced in breast cancer cell lines when treated with estrogen and progesterone.[140] That the 5' LTR contains response elements for these hormones was known at the time of initial sequencing of HERV-K HML-2.[120]

In 2008, this team published a comprehensive examination of the host immune response to the expression of HERV-K102 Env. About 88% of breast cancer tumors had detectable HERV-K102 Env by immunohistology which was not detected in normal breast tissue.[141] As well about 79% of the breast cancer patients and 5% of the normal healthy controls displayed IgG antibody to HERV-K102 Env. Furthermore, they investigated T cell responses to HERV-K102 Env surface unit antigens and found T cells proliferated and produced IFN-γ. During *in vitro* stimulation of PBMCs from breast cancer patients, an M1-like macrophage and a T helper 1 cytokine response were generated. T cell cytotoxic lymphocytes (CTLs) that lysed targets expressing HERV-K protein were found in breast cancer patients but not normal healthy controls.[141] This was the first time that the immunogenicity of HERV-K102 antigens had been investigated for T cell responses.

A most remarkable finding was subsequently reported by Wang-Johanning et al. in 2012.[142] In this report, they showed *in vitro*, a single-chain variable fragment (sc-Fv) MAb (that lacked the FC domain) which reacted with HERV-K102 Env surface unit was able to directly trigger apoptosis in the breast cancer cells without the need for complement or accessory cells such as those involved in antibody-mediated cytotoxicity. They confirmed that in breast cancer cells, HERV-K102 Env was directly wired to the host cell apoptosis machinery involving CIDEA, TP53, and caspase 3 and caspase 7 pathways.[142]

On the heels of the Wang-Johanning et al. success, interest in addressing T cell and B cell responses turned to HIV-1 patients. A T-cell clone from an HIV-1 elite suppressor (an HIV-1 infected person able to control HIV-1 replication *in vivo* and maintain near zero levels of HIV-1 in serum without pharmaceutical intervention) recognized a peptide in HML-2 Env that was 100% identical in sequence to HERV-K102. This T-cell clone was able to clear human cells infected with various monkey and human orthoretroviruses[143] showing innate T cells provide heterologous (antigen nonspecific) protection against cells infected with various viruses. However, this group was not able to identify a linear peptide sequence of HERV-K102 Env surface unit where antibodies from sera from HIV-1 patients were strongly or more commonly reactive over healthy controls.[144] They did discover antibodies to the transmembrane region of HERV-K102 Env albeit of unknown significance.

In our hands, we were able to determine that HIV-1 patients had significantly higher levels of antibodies to HERV-K102 surface unit peptides ML-4 and ML-5 than those with other viral infections and a higher percentage of positive reactivity (80% and 70% of the HIV-1 patients were positive for their reactivity, respectively).[67] This was similar to that reported in breast cancers.[141] While only 1/51 healthy normal controls (2%) were judged to be positive by peptide ELISA, these were very weak and only marginally positive reactions.

We had developed a very sensitive real-time quantitative polymerase chain reaction (PCR) HERV-K102 *pol* ddCt method performed on DNA isolated from plasma that contained an internal probe in *pol* to validate a true *pol* amplified fragment signal.[67] Moreover, unlike traditional PCRs because we measured the relative increase in plasma of a HERV-K102 *pol* signal over genomic equivalents detected with an 18S RNA probe this enabled a built-in validation that the isolation of DNA and PCR methods were working. With this method which was compared with a mean ddCt ratio of 0.88 ± 0.37 for 30 normal healthy controls, it was determined that 28/37 (75.7%) of HIV-1 patients were positive for HERV-K102 particles. However, 96% of the HIV-1 patients had a positive PCR and/or a positive serological test meaning HERV-K102 activation by these criteria was almost universal.[67]

The Concept of SELECT Epitopes Reactive to Innate Antibodies to HERV-K102 Env

The ML-4 and ML-5 peptides had been preselected for their immunogenicity, selectivity for HERV-K102 sequences and their likelihood of being cryptic on the HERV-K102 particles.[67] We were concerned that antibodies to the cell surface HERV-K102 protein (P61567 Env) expressed on the surface of tumor cells or virally infected cells which represent the product of a splice variant,[139,140] should not react with HERV-K102 particles. Otherwise, these protector antibodies would be self-defeating.

The particle associated type 1 Env encoded in the proviral transcript (P63135 Pol-Env) contains KRASTE which is absent in the type 2 Env. The ML4 sequence (KRASTEMVTPVTWMDN)[67] included the additional KRASTE leader sequence common to type 1 but not type 2 envelopes. It was possible that the addition of KRASTE could alter the conformation of the ML4 Env peptide on particles for example rendering the MVTPVTWMDN cryptic. The ML5 peptide (LETRDCKPFYTIDLNSS)[67] has a cysteine amino acid in the middle of the peptide sequence meaning depending on the conformation, the antibody-binding site might be obscured by a di-sulfide bridge. It also contains an N-glycosylation site (i.e., the NxS/T motif) which could also help render the ML5 sequence cryptic such as on particles. According to AlphaFold software[145,146] the conformation of P61567 is quite distinct from P63135 **(Figs. 9A and B)**.

As a side note, the fact that HERV-K102 uniquely has both the spliced Env protein sequence and a Pol-Env protein sequence associated with particles, provides further evidence substantiating that only HERV-K102 forms particles and could be replication competent.

We were not able to detect reactions of our affinity purified rabbit ML4 or ML5 antiserum with the foamy macrophages in **Figure 4** by flow cytometry

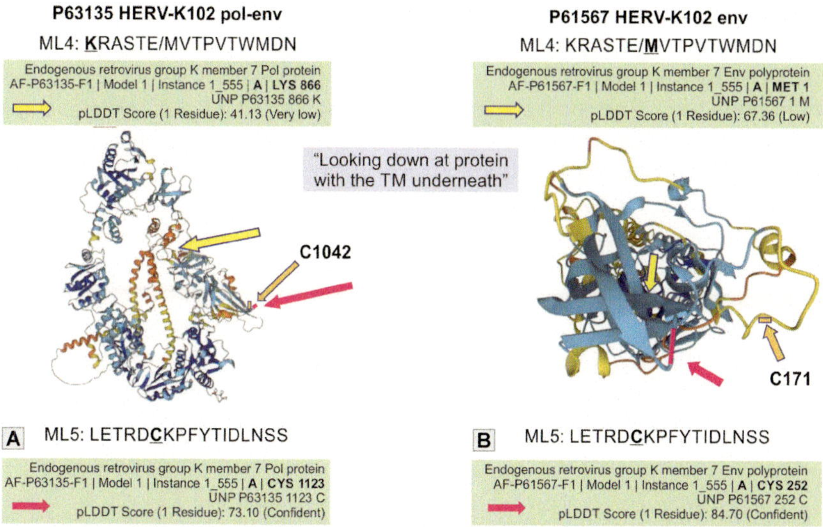

FIGURES 9A AND B: 3D visualization of human endogenous retrovirus-K102 (HERV-K102) Env by AlphaFold potentially reveals distinct conformations between the particle associated Env (P63135, left panel) and those putatively expressed at the cell surface of virally infected or tumor cells (P61567, right panel). The envelope protein (Env) of HERV-K102 becomes enzymatically cleaved into a transmembrane and a surface unit (TM and SU, respectively) domain at least when associated with particles. The conformation of the HERV-K102 Env protein after this cleavage maturation of particles has not been considered in the AlphaFold software[145,146] but could make the differences more pronounced. Nevertheless, here the view is that SU domain sits on top of the TM domain (still connected) as if one was looking down at the protein from the top of the plasma membrane. The P63135 (*pol-env*) Env produced from the expression of the proviral genomic sequence (of particles) begins with an additional KRASTE sequence which is not present in the P61567 sequence (spliced envelope). Yellow arrows indicate the location of the ML4 peptide epitope. Pink arrows indicate the location of the C amino acid in the ML5 peptide epitope. The orange arrows indicate the location of a C amino acid that may be closest to the C amino acid in the ML5 peptide that might be available for a disulfide bridge which may change the conformation of HERV-K102 Env. Note on the left side for the putative particle associated Env (P63135) the C amino acid of the ML5 peptide is very proximal to C1042 potentially consistent with a disulfide bridge. In contrast at the right, for the putative cell surface Env (P61567), the C amino acid of the ML5 peptide appears to be far away from the closest C amino acid at C171 consistent with the lack of a disulfide bridge. Thus, it is possible that the ML4 and ML5 epitopes on the cell surface Env are accessible but not on the particles, although this needs to be conclusively shown. Here it is proposed that the ML4 (the 5′ start of the Env protein) and ML5 epitopes are cryptic on the particles (left) but accessible on the cell surface of the virally infected or tumor cell (right). This conjecture is being made is because an antibody to HERV-K102 Env that can directly trigger apoptosis in virally infected or cancer cells[142] would not provide much good for the host if the same antibody cleared the protector HERV-K102 particles.

Note: All of the data provided is freely available for both academic and commercial use under Creative Commons Attribution 4.0 (CC-BY 4.0) licence terms.[145,146]

Source: From: AlphaFold Protein Structure Database. Background. [online] Available from https://alphafold.ebi.ac.uk/ [Last accessed April, 2024].

even when the cells were permeabilized (unpublished data). However, these antisera-labeled proteins by western blotting and stained intracellular particles by immunohistology on paraffin embedded samples of the foamy macrophages.[10] Thus, positive reactions involving HERV-K102 particles were only obtained when the particle proteins had been denatured. This suggested that the ML4 and ML5 epitopes were likely cryptic on the HERV-K102 particles as had been anticipated.

As shown in **Figure 10**, viruses that bud from the cell surface of *human* cells, the so-called enveloped viruses like HIV-1 and SARS-CoV-2 (that cloak themselves in the plasma membranes of cells), pick up HERV-K102 Env in the process meaning their virions carry HERV-K102 Env. Thus, antibodies to HERV-K102 Env are most probably neutralizing antibodies that can clear and inactivate exogenous virions as well as lyse virally infected cells. One of the earliest investigations of the SARS-CoV-2 pandemic had established in

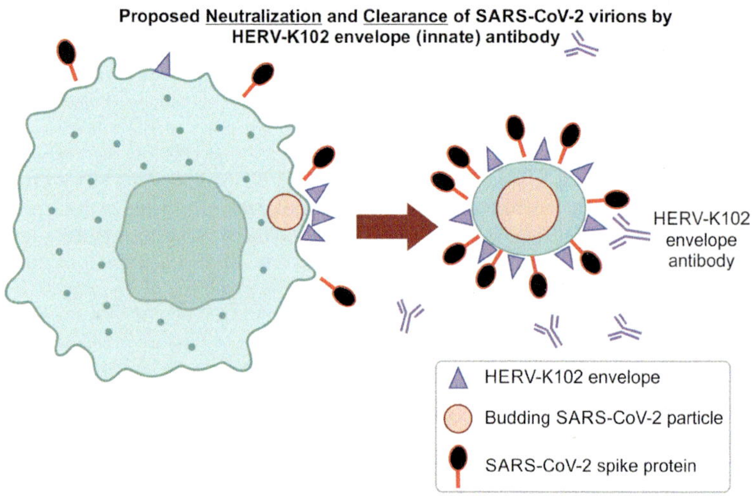

FIGURE 10: Antibodies to HERV-K102 envelope may neutralize and clear SARS-CoV-2 virions that bud from the surface of human cells but not from other species. Virus infected cells or tumor cells express HERV-K102 envelope protein on their cell surface which serves to induce clearance or apoptosis by envelope specific T cells and/or antibodies.[141,143] Antibodies to HERV-K102 Env have been demonstrated in HIV-1 patients and those with other viral infections.[67] In patients with mild COVID disease, both IgA and IgG antibodies reactive with HERV-K102/HERV-K18 envelope are universally detected in saliva.[147] Viruses like SARS-CoV-2 and HIV-1 that bud through the cell surface (the so-called *enveloped* RNA viruses) likely contain HERV-K102 envelope (or 95–97% identical HML-2 Env) in their virions which they acquire during the budding process. Thus, in mild COVID-19, the innate antibodies to HML-2 Env can neutralize and clear the virions in the URT before the onset of IgG to spike protein as was reported by Wolfel et al.[41] See text for discussion of ML4 and ML5 cryptic epitopes on the HERV-K102 particles but which were revealed by denaturation.

Note: New image created by author using cell and antibody icons from Biorender.com.

(HERV-K102: human endogenous retrovirus-K102; LTR: long terminal repeat)

mild disease that innate immunity neutralized and cleared SARS-CoV-2 from the URT prior to the onset of the spike-specific antibodies.[41] Therefore, the innate immunity SARS-CoV-2 neutralizing antibodies likely involve at least in part, antibodies to HERV-K102 Env.

Accordingly, it is tempting to speculate that monoclonal (sc-Fv) antibodies reactive with epitopes found on the P61567 HERV-K102 cell surface Env but not the particle associated P63135 pol-env, such as the ML4 and ML5 peptide sequences, could be used as novel treatments for viral infections especially against emerging and pandemic enveloped viruses. Although many of the MAbs against spike protein may have selected for new variants causing progression of disease and/or lost activity with the onset of immune escape variants,[42] there is little risk of this here as it is not the virus which encodes HERV-K102 Env and thus, there would be no viral selection. Moreover, these antibodies may also be useful for cancer patients especially those more recently diagnosed with "turbo cancer". Turbo cancers is a colloquial term used to describe cancers arising in individuals who have been injected with the mRNA gene therapy vaccines and where progression is rapid and/or onset is in a much younger population.[148]

The concept that the SARS-CoV-2 virions produced in human cells may carry HERV-K102 Env is quite intriguing. Arru et al.[149] described peptides corresponding to HERV-K102 Env surface unit peptide sequences that were able to induce TNF-α in T cells (the 19–37 peptide) that is, without the requirement for MHC. Also, the 19–37 and the 109–126 peptides of HERV-K102-induced IL-6, IFN-γ, CCL2, and CCL3 in B cells. This suggests innate T cells may be activated by HERV-K102 Env protein along with presumably innate B cells. Innate T cells include NKT cells, the mucosal associated invariant T (MAIT) cells, and the GD T cells.[150]

Recall that Morozov et al.[126] showed that the transmembrane region of HERV-K HML-2 Env strongly induced M1-activation cytokines and chemokines but not those for M2 when tested on PBMCs. When taken together these results imply that wherever the 'enveloped' exogenous virus goes, because it carries HERV-K102 Env, it will activate the HERV-K102 protector system (M1-like proinflammatory foamy macrophages and the innate T and B cells) providing yet another viral antivirus mechanism. This virus-anti-virus mechanism reveals nature to be quite ingenious with redundancy for innate immune activation relating to viral invasion.

While HERV-K HML-2 Env when expressed on tumor cells or virally infected cells appears to be an autoantigen that marks the cell for destruction, interestingly in neurons, the oppositive may be the case.

Bhat et al., suggested that HERV-K HML-2 Env increased neuronal cellular viability and prevented neurotoxicity mediated by HIV-1 Vpr.[151] In contrast in amyotrophic lateral sclerosis (ALS), Garcia-Montojo et al. reported that HML-2 Env protein expression in neurons was neurotoxic, but that antibodies to Env protected against neurodegeneration. Furthermore, these antibody levels correlated with survival times of patients with ALS.[152]

Interestingly, TDP-43 (gene card *TARDBP*) accumulation, which is associated with neuropathology in ALS, also induced HERV-K102 Env expression.[153] Clearly more work is needed to resolve these discrepancies as HERV-K102 Env and/or the IgG are protective in breast and other cancers.[154]

Epigenetic Control of HERV-K102 Expression and Trained Immunity

Systemic lupus erythematosus (SLE) is an autoimmune disease involving autoreactive T and B cells, immune complex disease, a systematic activation of type I interferon, and neutrophil activation with the formation of neutrophil extracellular traps (NETs). The strong induction of HERV-K102 Env RNA in whole blood (with minor contributions by HERV-K18, HERV-K106, and HERV-K115) was found in female SLE patients but not male[155] HML-2 RNA expression correlated with a lack of epigenetic silencing and where the antibody (largely IgG2) to HERV-K102 correlated with higher interferon I ISG expression.[155] HERV-K HML-2 regulation is through epigenetic control whereby DNA methylation and repressive histone methylation suppress ERV expression. The repressive marks are maintained by the Kruppel-associated box domain-zinc finger protein (KRAB-ZFP)-TRIM28 complex and human silencing complex (HUSH). Accordingly, HERV-K102 expression correlated inversely with TRIM28 expression.[155]

The epigenetic control of HERV-K102 expression is a segue into a discussion on trained (innate) immunity.

The term trained immunity was first coined by Professor Mihai Netea and colleagues in 2011 to describe the enhancement of a secondary innate immunity response after a primary infection or vaccination.[156] Unlike adaptive immunity, TI lacks specificity for any pathogen-specific antigens and thus, invariably involves heterologous protection or cross-protection against unrelated pathogens. TI was initially invoked to explain how vaccination with the live Bacillus Calmette–Guérin (BCG) vaccine (attenuated *Mycobacterium bovis*) in West Africa decreased childhood mortality from several different pathogens including tuberculosis. The protection furnished by the BCG vaccine was mediated by macrophages. Since in humans, macrophages cannot replicate (unlike mice), this has led to the concept of central TI in the hematopoietic stem and progenitor cells (HSPCs).[157-159] Accordingly, TI involves peripheral (monocytes-macrophages) and central (myeloid HSPCs) compartments. Most notably, the memory aspect of TI involves a metabolic switch to glycolysis and epigenetic changes. These involve changes in the histone methylation and acetylation in chromatin providing access to macrophage lineage and inflammatory genes.[159]

Trained immunity refers to a short-term enhancement (usually 3–12 months) of the release of cytokines (TNF-α, IL-1b, and IL-6) from M1-like macrophages upon rechallenge but which is also associated with enhanced heterologous antimicrobial and antitumor activity *in vivo*. How

TI in proinflammatory macrophages relates to enhanced pathogen and tumor control *in vivo* remains to be fully elucidated, however. As well, recent evidence indicates TI in macrophages occurs with or without the induction of inflammatory cytokines.[160,161] presenting somewhat of a conundrum for the functional definition of TI.

Commonly used inducers of TI include microbial products such as beta-glucan and muramyl dipeptide, but also ox-LDL, uric acid, the BCG vaccine, other live vaccines, and/or exposures to viruses.[159] The differences in epigenetic marks by the different TI inducers are reviewed elsewhere.[162] The myeloid-specific enhancers SPI1 and CEBPB[88] are in fact T-specific enhancers.[89,90]

The metabolic and epigenetic changes associated with TI are mediated via the Akt/mTOR/HIF-1α pathway[89,163] but where insulin resistance promotes an anti-inflammatory M2-like phenotype.[164,165] Glycolysis drives the PI3K/Akt/mTOR/HIF-1α pathway. In M1 macrophages, activation leads to the accumulation of succinate in the Krebs cycle which leads to the stabilization of the TF HIF-1α which induces the transcription of glycolysis genes.[163] In contrast, M2 macrophages primarily use oxidative phosphorylation.

Trained immunity associates with the induction of glycolysis which is similar to the Warburg effect described for tumors. At the risk of being an oversimplification, a reason why glycolysis is needed for tumorigenesis (the Warburg effect) is so the mitochondria can produce the substrate acetyl-CoA/citrate (from glycolysis) needed for cholesterol production through the mevalonate pathway.[166] Replenishing of the cell surface membrane and other membranes in the cell via higher cholesterol production would be needed in order to support tumor proliferation. Indeed, mevalonate initiates DNA synthesis and cell proliferation.[166] In human monocyte derived macrophages, which incidentally do not proliferate, excess cholesterol would be needed and utilized instead for foam cell formation pertaining to the replication of the protector foamy virus HERV-K102. Hence, glycolysis is linked to TI to support the generation of foam (HERV-K102 particles and vacuoles) during macrophage training.

TI involves foam cell formation in M1 macrophages.[93] Most notably the mevalonate (cholesterol) pathway is needed for TI in the monocyte/macrophage lineage as statins which inhibit HMG-CoA reductase (HMGCR) block TI induction.[94] Trained macrophages uptake lipids such as oxLDL through OLR1 to form foam cells and produce high levels of TNF-α, IL-6, IL-8, and IL-18 upon secondary challenge[167] associated with glycolysis.[96,168] Interestingly, SARS-COV-2 infection disrupts the mevalonate pathway[169] showing that it directly targets foam cell formation and thus, TI and thus, HERV-K102 particle production.

Hypoxia inducible factor 1 alpha plays a key role in initiating and promoting the formation of foam cells in macrophages.[170] NF-κB1 which induces the inflammatory response in macrophages is required for the transcription of HIF-1α.[171] A critical role of HIF-1α in foam cell formation in macrophages was demonstrated by the inhibition of foam cell formation by small interfering RNAs against HIF-1α.[172] Thus, it is very clear that TI critically involves the induction of foam in M1-like proinflammatory macrophages related to NF-κB1 and HIF-1α expression.

The PI3K/Akt/mTOR pathway plays a role in autophagy, apoptosis, metabolism, and cell growth but is commonly hyperactivated in tumors where it contributes to malignant potential.[173] It is also hyperactivated upon SARS-CoV-2 infection such as in the hepatocellular cell line Huh-7 associated with ERBB2 hyperactivity and alpha-fetoprotein (AFP) mRNA and protein expression (Professor Ujjwal Neogi, personal communication).[174] In macrophages, this pathway is used by the EGFR to generate foam cell formation.[175,176] For example, gene deletion of EGFR in macrophages in murine models limits the production of IL-6 and TNF-α, reduces lipid uptake by reducing the expression of the scavenger receptor CD36, and inhibits the development of atherosclerosis which involves foamy macrophages.[177] Similarly for human macrophages, the EGFR is activated by TLR4 and disruption of TLR4 or EGFR reduced inflammation and foam cell formation.[175-177] Triggering TLR4 activates HIF-1α, IRF1, VDR, S100A9, and NR3C1 (the glucocorticoid receptor) while downregulating PPARG and IFNGR1.[178] EGFR antagonists were also shown to block oxLDL induction of inflammation and foam cell formation with down-regulation of IL-6 and TNF-α.[177]

It should be noted that while the PI3K/Akt/mTOR pathway induces foam cell formation associated with BSG/CD147 expression in macrophages such as induced by oxLDL, interfering with NFkb1 does not block foam cell formation.[91] This means the inflammatory component such as by NFkb1 is not an absolute requirement for TI as has been recently noted by others.[160,161] Perhaps foam cell formation involving HERV-K102 particle production in foamy macrophages would better define and capture the essence of TI.

Recent evidence shows that upon lipopolysaccharide (LPS) and IFN-γ triggering of the M1 phenotype, AFP transfection into MO macrophages coinduces CD163 and IL-10 which are considered markers of M2.[179] However, CD163, IL-10, and the MI/M2 phenotype characterize the foamy macrophages illustrated in **Figure 4** which exhibit high levels of vacuoles and particles.[86] This may further substantiate the role of AFP in the training of macrophages associated with foam cell formation.

As mentioned, drivers of myeloid differentiation are the TFs SPI1 and CEBPB[88] which also drive TI.[89,90] SPI1 is considered a pioneering TF (also called lineage determining TFs) that opens up the chromatin in this case for macrophage differentiation which enables inflammation TFs to bind to response elements in the appropriate genes.[180] Macrophage inflammation involves networks of signal transducer and activator of transcription (STAT) factors, interferon response factors (IRFs) and NF-κB TFs.[180] Monocytes exposed to LPS and IFN-γ undergo classical M1-like (proinflammatory) macrophage activation with upregulation of SPI1, IRF1, IRF5, IRF8, STAT1,

STAT2, and NF-κB1. The alternative activation with IL-4 and IL-13 generates M2-like (anti-inflammatory) cells featuring SPI1, IRF4, STAT6, KDM6B, PPARγ, PPARδ, and CEBPB.[180] However, PPARγ plays an important role in the differentiation of monocyte to foamy macrophages[181] and CEBPB is a TI enhancer. Accordingly, the macrophages conferring TI express M1- and M2-like markers including CEBPB and PPARG which are associated with foam cell formation. As just mentioned, AFP expression may also contribute to M2 marker expression in the inflammatory M1-like macrophages.

It is noteworthy that IRF1 and NF-κB1 bind to two interferon stimulated response elements (ISREs) in the promoter of HERV-K102 which is found in the 5'LTR.[97,98] TNF-α is a potent activator of canonical NF-κB1 TF activity while IFN-γ and TNF-α synergize to activate IRF1. Indeed, newer evidence confirms that M1 polarization of macrophages in humans explicitly in response to IFN-γ signaling is promoted via HERV-K102 expression.[99] More recently the key role of IFN-γ in TI induction *in vivo* in response to BCG vaccination was affirmed by scRNA sequencing.[167]

In summary, TI critically involves EGFR/TLR4-induced foam cell formation in M1-like proinflammatory macrophages. LPS which triggers TLR4 along with IFN-γ induces M1-like proinflammatory foamy macrophages which is strongly associated with HERV-K102 proviral induction.[99] The evidence is incontrovertible that it is HERV-K102 replication in macrophages which generates trained (innate) immunity.

Figure 11 provides an illustration of the main cellular players involved in the HERV-K102 protector system and their targets. Thus, it is probable that TI heterologous protection extends to the innate T and B cells that recognize HERV-K102 Env. Indeed, Ren et al. indicated that T and B cells were also infected by SARS-CoV-2 associated with COVID-19 severity and that BSG, TFRC (transferrin receptor) and ISGs correlated with SARS-CoV-2 viral RNA in the different cell types.[61] BSG is an alternative or secondary receptor for SARS-CoV-2 entry into cells[182] and antibodies to BSG (CD147) block SARS-CoV-2 infection *in vitro*[182,183] and *in vivo* in BSG humanized mice.[183] The notion that SARS-CoV-2 specifically interacts with BSG was corroborated when the amino acids involved in mutual binding were mapped.[184] Curiously, in the PBMCs, CEBPB and SPI1 (TI enhancers thought to be specific to M1-like foamy macrophages) were also expressed in virus positive T cells and B cells.[61] This might imply that the innate T and B cells which express BSG may share some of the TI programming of foamy macrophages.

In summary, HERV-K HML-2 activation and HERV-K102 particle production in foamy macrophages constitute a "virus-anti-virus response" analogous to fighting fire with fire. Not only does the "virus mimicry" aspect help to amplify the interferon response through PRRs but innate T cells and antibodies that recognize HERV-K102 Env expressed on the surface of virus-infected cells are generated which kill virus infected cells. Indeed, in a twisted turn of events, it seems HERV-K102 Env expressed on the SARS-CoV-2 virions may alternatively stimulate M1-macrophages as well as innate

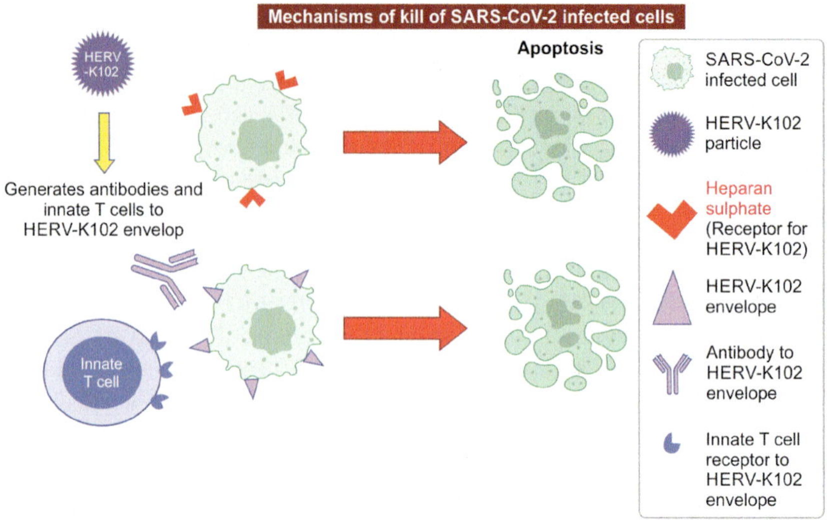

FIGURE 11: HERV-K102 particles may utilize heparan sulfate[81] to enter SARS-CoV-2 infected cells while innate antibodies and T cells recognize HERV-K102/HML-2 envelope (Env) and may directly trigger apoptosis. HERV-K102 particles enter cells through its receptor heparan sulfate which is widely expressed on most cell types[81] and is like other nonpathogenic foamy viruses. Entry of HERV-K102 particles into normal cells results in activation of the interferon system[136] and integration (arming)[10] while in virus-infected cells or tumors entry is proposed to be associated with lysis (see Fig. 6 for cytopathic effects of HERV-K102 particles). Most likely the relevant HERV-K HML-2 Env antibodies are to HERV-K102-specific epitopes like ML4 and ML5 accessible on the cell surface Env (P61567) but which are proposed to be cryptic on the particles (P63135 pol-env).

(HERV-K102: human endogenous retrovirus-K102; SARS-CoV-2: severe acute respiratory syndrome coronavirus 2)

Source: New image created by author using cell and antibody icons from Biorender.com.

T-cell and B-cell activation. Most significantly, the innate antibodies to HERV-K102 Env are postulated to neutralize and clear SARS-CoV-2 in mild cases as reported by Wolfel et al.[41] This feature helps to explain how boosting of innate immunity in the first 6 days following the second dose (before the adaptive IgG antibodies to spike protein are made) can be associated with sterilizing immunity (100% VE)[54] which is probably related to a recall or memory release of the antibody to HERV-K102 Env.

When Things Go Wrong with the HERV-K102 Protector System: Immunosenescence

It is equally important to discuss what happens when the HERV-K102 system fails and under what circumstances.

Clinical research concerning the study of putative HERV-K102/foamy macrophage immune parameters based on plasma amino acid profiling algorithms performed at immune system management led to the publication of the new immunosenescence paradigm (of macrophages) in 2015.[185] The new paradigm was then separately validated for cardiovascular disease.[186]

In brief, the new immunosenescence paradigm (of macrophages) was simply defined as the failed lytic release of HERV-K102 particles from the foamy macrophages **(Fig. 12)** which was causally related to AFP activity. The 67 kD AFP receptor which mediates the effects of AFP in macrophages was identified and characterized by 1991[187] In addition, active AFP or the AFP agonist MAbs to the 67 kD AFPr blocked apoptosis in human macrophages.[187,188] Since dehydroepiandrosterone (DHEA) binds and inactivates AFP.[185] and it was established that cortisol induces AFP expression in humans,[189] meant that as DHEA levels declined with age (faster in males) the cortisol/DHEA ratio would increase placing the host at higher risk of immunosenescence of macrophages and thus, disease. Most notably, high cortisol and low DHEA are commonly associated with chronic disease initiation and progression. For example, after adjustment for age, the cortisol/DHEAS ratio correlated with all-cause, cancer and noncancer mortality as shown in a prospective study of 4255 Vietnam army veterans over 15 years and where higher cortisol/DHEA ratios were associated with increased risk of death.[190]

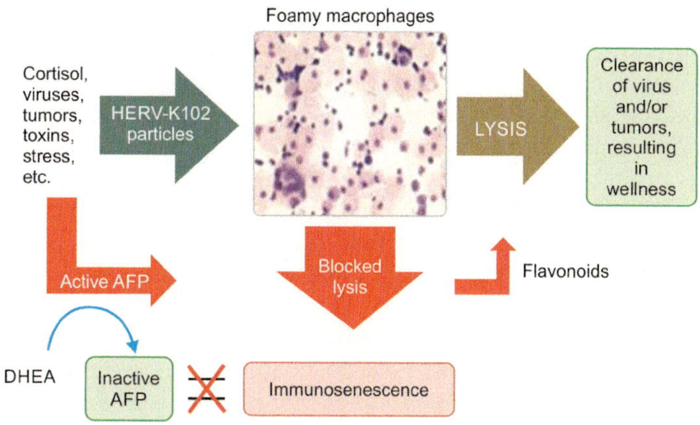

FIGURE 12: The new immunosenescence paradigm, 2015.[185] In the new immunosenescence paradigm, *active* alpha-fetoprotein (AFP) was proposed to mediate immunosenescence of macrophages, defined as the failed lytic release of human endogenous retrovirus-K102 (HERV-K102) particles from foamy macrophages.[185,186] AFP blocks apoptosis in macrophages.[187,188] The *activity* of AFP depends in part on the dehydroepiandrosterone (DHEA)/cortisol ratio which diminishes with age and/or stress. This is because cortisol induces AFP while DHEA binds and renders AFP inactive.[185] Thus, with age and/or stress there will be more active AFP in the system and a higher risk of immunosenescence. Flavonoids and zinc may reverse immunosenescence by binding and inhibiting AFP activity and thus, will appear to have antiviral properties. Recent evidence is also consistent with ivermectin reversing immunosenescence.[191]

Source: Reproduced with permission from Laderoute MP. A new paradigm about HERV-K102 particle production and blocked release to explain cortisol mediated immunosenescence and age-associated risk of chronic disease. Discov Med. 2015;20:379-91.

As shown in **Figure 12** cortisol is proposed to also induce HERV-K102 expression to generate the foamy macrophages as its LTR contains glucocorticoid response elements.[97-99] Oddly, it appears high dose dexamethasone may not induce HERV-K HML-2 such as tested in a breast cancer cell line.[192] However, whether methylprednisolone would induce these protector transcripts should be investigated since dexamethasone failed to reverse the SARS-CoV-2 interference of the IFN type 1 and IFN-γ innate responses while methylprednisolone did.[193,194] Moreover, methylprednisolone was associated with a much lower number needed to treat (nnt = 5) indicating higher proficiency. Alternatively, MIF which is known to counteract the anti-inflammatory effects of glucocorticosteroids, and which was inducible at low levels of dexamethasone but suppressed at higher levels,[195] potentially might additionally influence HERV-K102 proviral expression in macrophages secondary to corticosteroids. However, the differences between dexamethasone and methylprednisolone activation of HERV-K102 particle production requires further evaluation.

Critically, when AFP binds its receptor, it triggers a negative signal which abrogates any incoming signal whether it is for apoptosis, differentiation, proliferation, activation, adherence, etc.[187] AFP is well established to be intrinsically immunosuppressive, but this was corroborated with AFP agonistic MAbs to the 67 kD AFP receptor.[187] By the time the 67 kD AFP receptor becomes expressed, the macrophages are already expressing and releasing the proinflammatory cytokines, TNF-α, IL-1β, and IL-6. Thus, AFP prevents the ability to downregulate the expression of proinflammatory cytokines. Immunosenescence involves immunosuppression, a simultaneous proinflammatory state and apoptosis resistance, all mediated by AFP binding to its receptor.[187,188] Accordingly, the use of anti-inflammatories which are immunosuppressive, would only contribute to the problem of immunosenescence of macrophages and would not address the cause of disease, namely, AFP activity. Only AFP antagonists such as zinc, DHEA (or better, 7-keto-DHEA which cannot be converted to sex hormones), genistein, and more recently ivermectin,[191] are able to prevent and reverse immunosenescence. It is well appreciated that therapies can be curative if they target the cause of disease such as immunosenescence by AFP antagonists rather than just treating symptoms of disease such as inflammation with anti-inflammatories (which are immunosuppressive).

EFFECTS OF ADE ON THE LAUNCH OF THE CRITICAL HERV-K102 PROTECTOR SYSTEM IN M1-LIKE FOAMY MACROPHAGES

Figure 13 attempts to illustrate the harm of ADE-mediated entry of SARS-CoV-2 into the M1-like foamy macrophages that produce the HERV-K102 particles.[10,67,99] First, the entry of SARS-CoV-2 into the monocytes/macrophages causes them to convert to M2-like polarized macrophages with lipid

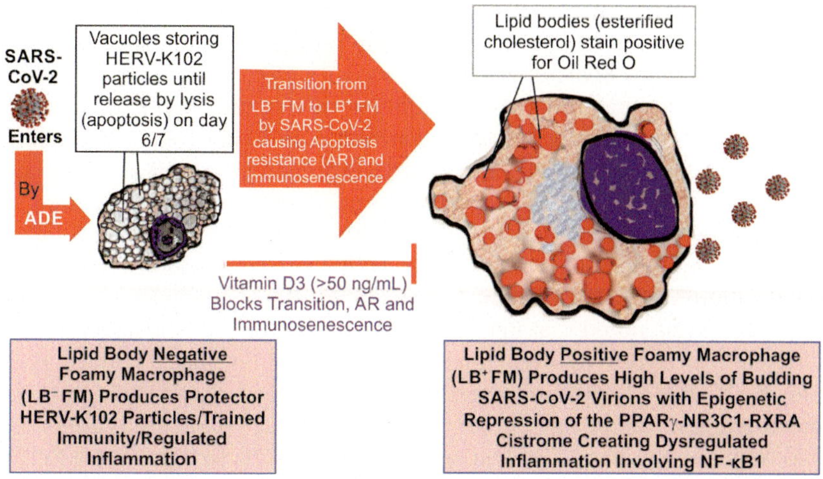

FIGURE 13: SARS-CoV-2 infection of the LB⁻ FMs by ADE causes the transition to LB⁺ FMs[196] blocked by the activated VDR.[171] SARS-CoV-2 converts the M1-like protector foamy macrophages (LB⁻ FMs) to M2-like LB⁺ FMs which upregulates PPARA,[61] and where the latter becomes a factory for SARS-CoV-2 replication.[196] When the levels of vitamin D3 are sufficient, the activated vitamin D receptor (VDR) can prevent the phosphorylation of MAPK8 blocking the transition from LB⁻ FMs to LB⁺ FMs.[165] Note it is possible that ivermectin may do the same as MAPK8 is on the ivermectin-protein string interaction network.[191] SARS-CoV-2 infection of the LB⁻ FMs by ADE blocks programmed cell death[197] abrogating the release of the HERV-K102 particles and at the same time inducing immunosenescence of the macrophages which exacerbates chronic illness. The conversion to LB⁺ FMs also does the same; but now SARS-CoV-2 particles are produced and released by cell surface budding and where NF-κB1 acts as the TF for the release of IL-1β, TNF-α, and CXCL8.[61] Note also that SARS-CoV-2 represses (epigenetically) the PPARγ-NR3C1-RXRA cistrome via SUMO1 which interacts with SARS-CoV-2 nucleoprotein and where SUMO1 is a partner of PPARγ.[199] This also contributes to uncontrolled inflammation. The main cause of the disruption resulting in immunosenescence and conversion to M2-like foamy macrophages (Fig. 12) is because SARS-CoV-2 induces AFP mRNA and protein expression.[174] (Dr Ujjwal Neogi, personal communication). Overall, this hijacking of the critical innate defense mechanism also creates an immunologically privileged site[196] possibly secondary to the fact that foamy macrophages may not express the spliced HERV-K102 envelope on their cell surface (unpublished flow cytometry data on the LB⁻ FMs).

(ADE: antibody-dependent enhancement; HERV-K102: human endogenous retrovirus-K102; NF-κB1: nuclear factor kappa subunit 1; PPAR: peroxisome proliferator activated receptor; SARS-CoV-2: severe acute respiratory syndrome coronavirus 2)

bodies[196] and would no longer express HERV-K102 transcripts.[99] Second, the S2 component of the spike protein interferes with p53 and BRCA which blocks apoptosis.[197] In this state of apoptosis resistance, SARS-CoV-2 is able to replicate and release virions by budding through the plasma membrane.[196] Apoptosis resistance means any HERV-K102 particles made are not being released by lysis, and so SARS-CoV-2 entry into M1-like macrophages directly and indirectly causes immunosenescence. Also p53 down modulates AFP[198] so the loss of p53 function would mean more AFP would be expressed again contributing to immunosenescence.

However, in the presence of adequate vitamin D3, the conversion of the M1-like LB⁻ FMs to the M2-like lipid body positive foamy macrophages[196] would not occur.[165] Second, as demonstrated in a *Mycobacterium tuberculosis* model involving macrophages, the addition of vitamin D3 upregulated the genes known to mediate M1-like polarization and HERV-K102 induction, including CD14, IL-8, IRG1, and CD163 expression, as well as foam cell formation.[200] While the mRNA for VDR was unaltered, the addition of Vitamin D3 nevertheless strongly induced VDR *protein*.[200] Thus, due to the presence of VDR response elements in the 5' LRT, HERV-K102 expression and M1-like polarization[99] are likely maintained by vitamin D3.

It should be noted that Ren et al.[61] established that of the 63 identified different cell types in bronchoalveolar lavage fluid (BALF) specimens, only the CD14+CD16+ monocytes and their progeny, the WDR74 positive macrophages (putatively producing HERV-K102 particles based on differentially expressed TFs) had highly activated VDR. In BALF, the WDR74 macrophages which were not induced in healthy uninfected controls were critical to recovery from mild-moderate COVID-19 but were lost with progression to severe disease consistent with ADE. The progenitors of the WDR74 macrophages the CD14+CD16+ (intermediate type) monocytes that are present in the BALF of healthy controls were similarly induced in progression to and recovery from moderate disease. Although they were depleted with progression to severe disease, they were highly activated in those who recovered. Autopsies of patients who died from COVID-19 revealed the inflammatory monocytes in lung samples expressed macrophage-associated markers such as CD68 and CD163[66] suggestive of emergency myelopoiesis. Thus, while the WDR74 macrophages per se did not promote recovery from severe COVID-19 their temporary expedited replacements (inflammatory monocytes) did. Interestingly, in the BALF, the GD2 T cells, which were present in healthy uninfected controls and expanded with progression and recovery from moderate disease, remained depleted during progression to severe disease and during recovery.[61]

In view of the above it is not surprising that optimal levels of vitamin D3 of at least 50 ng/mL of serum could prevent the onset of COVID-19 severity, as recently concluded from a systematic review and meta-analysis.[201] In addition to the prevention of COVID-19 mortality with >50 ng/mL vitamin D3 in plasma, SARS-CoV-2 infection could be prevented, and hypertension averted.[202] The latter implies vitamin D3 prevents or reverses immunosenescence raising the possibility that vitamin D3 might indirectly antagonize AFP activity. Moreover, the risk of death from myocardial infarction, cancer, type 2 diabetes, Alzheimer's disease, and more generally, all-cause mortality could be significantly decreased with vitamin D levels above 50 ng/mL.[202] These findings corroborate the notion that the HERV-K102 protective innate system that launches in M1-like foamy macrophages[99] which is strongly favored by optimal vitamin D3 levels plays a major role in human survival at the individual and population levels, including perhaps, phylogenetically **(Fig. 8)**.

INCONTROVERTIBLE EVIDENCE FOR ADE AS AN IMPEDIMENT TO THE SAFETY AND EFFECTIVENESS OF THE ADAPTIVE IMMUNITY COVID-19 VACCINES

In **Table 3**, the UK monthly mortality rate data released by the ONS on July 6, 2022,[203] has been recompiled into summaries of ratios of vaccinated mortality rates per 100,000 person-years over the same for the unvaccinated by month for all ages (14 plus), and categorized by all-cause, COVID-19 specific and non-COVID-19 mortality ratios covering January 1, 2021, to May 31, 2022. For this, the individual rates per 100,000 person years for each subcategory of vaccination and duration were separately added up to provide a total as the total for the ever vaccinated provided by the ONS appeared to be erroneous. Apparently, deaths before 2 weeks following an immunization dose may have been reclassified as unvaccinated as articulated by Fenton et al.[204] and which ONS confirmed on January 20, 2023.[205]

Upon examination of **Table 3**, first one notes that the only month in which the all-cause mortality showed vaccination benefit over risk was in February 2021 (ratio of ever vaccinated rates over unvaccinated of 0.61) but not in any other month from January 1, 2021, to May 31, 2022. Overall, the all-cause mortality test for risk versus benefit for the entire period was 6.37 with a p value of 0.0001 meaning that there were over six-fold higher all-cause deaths per 100,000 person years in the vaccinated over the unvaccinated which was highly significant. This also matched the results of the randomized clinical trials where none of the COVID-19 vaccines met the requirement for a statistically significant benefit over risk as demonstrated on all-cause mortality.[206] So overall the risks of COVID-19 vaccination did outweigh the benefits for the entire UK population measured over January 1, 2021–May 31, 2022 with the exception of February 2021.

In February 2021 but not at any other time in the mass vaccination campaign in the UK, the benefit of vaccination surprisingly outweighed the risks. However, upon closer examination the reason for the benefit over risk in February 2021 was because of those vaccinated by the end of February 2021, 95.6% had only received the first dose of vaccine but not yet the second (only 531,525 had received the second dose or about 4.4% of the 11,976,296 vaccinated mostly elders).[207] Recall that the first dose did not generate spike-specific IgG antibodies[46,47] but was known to generate heterologous protection against non-COVID-19 mortality.[50] In other words, it was likely the trained (innate) immunity that offered protection against COVID-19, non-COVID-19, and all-cause mortality in February 2021 in England.

As a separate issue, the reason why boosters were needed every 3–6 months was likely because TI is temporary usually lasting 3–12 months.[159]

TABLE 3: Office for National Statistics (ONS) UK mortality rates per 100,000 person-years: Rate ratios* of ever vaccinated (ever Vax) over unvaccinated (Unvax) January 1, 2021 to May 31, 2022.

		All-cause mortality			COVID-19 mortality			Non-COVID-19 mortality		
		Rate Unvax	Actual rate ever Vax	Ratio of Vax/ Unvax rates	RATE Unvax	Actual rate ever Vax	Ratio of Vax/ Unvax rates	Rate Unvax	Actual rate ever Vax	Ratio of Vax/ Unvax rates
2021	Jan	2,507.6	3,483.5	1.39	1,187	1,526	1.29	1,320	1,958	1.48
	Feb	5,261.5	3,205.4	0.61	2,174	456.8	0.21	3,087	2,689	0.87
	Mar	3,307.8	4,192.7	1.27	591.9	283.9	0.48	2,716	3,909	1.44
	April	2,298.4	5,039.7	2.19	145.8	184.0	1.26	2,153	4,855	2.25
	May	1,718.8	8,582.6	4.99	45.5	84.5	1.86	1,673	8,426	5.04
	June	1,589.7	10,060.0	6.33	55.6	87.7	1.58	1,534	9,916	6.46
	July	1,610.7	10,307.1	6.40	218.2	224.9	1.03	1,392	9,960	7.16
	Aug	1,711.6	10,340.7	6.04	404.2	402.9	1.00	1,307	9,266	7.09
	Sept	1,664.5	8,639.0	5.19	367.8	520.2	1.41	1,297	7,884	6.08
	Oct	1,623.7	12,456.3	7.67	322.3	568.6	1.76	1,302	11,845	9.10
	Nov	1,708	15,546.6	9.10	421.3	721.0	1.71	1,287	14,155	11.00
	Dec	1,878.5	16,974.3	9.04	520.5	1,121.9	2.16	1,358	15,501	11.41
2022	Jan	1,812	19,997.9	11.04	584.6	2,310.9	3.95	1,227	16,417	13.38
	Feb	1,384.5	12,474.4	9.01	258.7	1,128.4	4.36	1,126	11,346	10.08
	Mar	1,231.7	10,257.2	8.33	183.5	763.6	4.16	1,048	9,445	9.01
	April	1,204.6	12,423.2	10.31	204.7	800.8	3.91	1,000	11,622	11.62
	May	872.9	8,246.0	9.45	77.6	261.8	3.37	795	7,914	9.95

Note: Rates are per 100,000 person-years, and were re-compiled where all the rates for ever vaccinated were added up to provide totals (as the ever vaccinated total deaths reported by the ONS were erroneously undercalculated for unknown reasons).[203]

Source: CC-By 4.0 from Office for National Statistics (ONS). (2022). Deaths involving COVID-19 by vaccination status, England: deaths occurring between 1 January 2021 and 31 May 2022". [online] Available from https://www.nationalarchives.gov.uk/doc/open-government-licence/version/3/and referencing bulletin. [Last accessed April, 2024].

As well lingering spike protein from the mRNA vaccine may have abrogated TI potentially also via ADE or possibly by binding to TLRs. For example, a recombinant vaccine spike fragment (which lacks a trypsin cleavage site) was found in 50% of postvaccination plasma samples at 69 days and with a maximum of 187 days.[208] As well, spike protein (non-RBD) may trigger the TLR4/MyD88 activation pathway in macrophages leading to abnormal inflammation[209] potentially related to immunosenescence. In any case internalized spike protein through S2 interference with p53,[197] would have created immunosenescence **(Fig. 12)** abrogating trained innate immunity. Therefore, it is possible that critical protection against all-cause mortality by trained innate immunity may have been lost by persistent spike protein expression related to the use of mRNA gene therapy vaccines. Clearly this possibility needs to be investigated further.

Indeed, since in January 2021 the all-cause mortality test was 1.39, it could be reasonably argued that the COVID-19 vaccines should have been removed from the global market by the first week in February 2021 for which Dr Peter McCullough concurred based on the data in **Table 3**.[210] By a year later in February 2022, the all-cause mortality risk versus benefit ratio for the COVID-19 vaccines grew to a ratio of 11.04. This indicated with time the risk of mortality associated with the COVID-19 vaccines was becoming far worse rather than better. Thus, it is very clear from this comprehensive population data of England that the vaccines were not very good at saving lives from COVID-19, except for February 2021. The fact that the non-COVID-19 mortality rates in the vaccinated were exceptionally higher than the unvaccinated **(Table 3)** provides irrefutable proof that the Pfizer-BioNTech COVID-19 mRNA vaccine was toxic and deadly.[211] There were high proportions of sudden death following vaccination linked to myocarditis as determined through autopsies for the mRNA COVID-19 vaccines,[212,213] and abnormal clotting.[211] Other longer term issues of concern stemming from the COVID-19 mRNA vaccines are the associated 'turbo cancers'.[148]

It is doubtful that the spike-specific IgG antibodies could have helped anyone survive because a priori, they caused progression of disease.[16-30,34-38] The UK population mortality results in **Table 3** strongly corroborate and endorse this point that ADE was and remains a serious problem for disease associated with COVID-19 vaccines. This mortality data further corroborates the evidence cited earlier about immune escape variant selection and a higher risk of infection pertaining to ADE. Despite the notion that the third mRNA vaccine dose was associated with conversion of the spike-specific IgG1/3 which promoted ADE, to the spike-specific IgG4 which does not mediate ADE,[58] it is possible that (1) this conversion did not occur in the URT and (2) the lipid nanoparticles may have inadvertently targeted myeloid cells due to phagocytosis regardless.

FUTURE DIRECTIONS

The notion of developing innate immunity vaccines particularly for pandemic preparedness is not new given the general lack of success for adaptive immunity vaccines related to the problem of ADE. Based on BCG vaccines which enhance TI, others are trying to further optimize TI vaccines such as IMM-101 which involves heat killed *Mycobacterium obuense.* This vaccine induces M1 polarization of macrophages[214] and thus would induce HERV-K102 particle production;[99] and may promote the Vg9Vd2 T cells which help recover from SARS-CoV-2[214] as well as cancers. [3] Indeed, in addition to identifying M1-like foamy macrophages in recovery from COVID-19,[61] several papers have directly confirmed the role of HERV-K102 proviral expression or Env antibodies in recovery from COVID-19.[137,147,215,216] In addition, HERV-K HML-2 elements played a role in recovery from COVID-19 in children[217] and others have provided indirect evidence corroborating HERV-K102 activation in recovery.[218,219]

In terms of pandemic planning, the safest, most practical, and most effective means to prevent severe disease from pandemic viruses (and intracellular pathogens like *Mycobacterium tuberculosis*) is to top up the vitamin D3 levels by supplements and when possible, by suntanning. In addition, the benefits of 15-minute daily exposures to near-infrared rays for 7 days on COVID-19 recovery included a faster (1) reduction in the systolic and diastolic blood pressure, (2) reduction in neutrophils and leukocytosis, and (3) increased lymphocytes.[220] Note that the earlier normalization of hypertension by near-infrared light exposures indicates a faster reversal of the immunosenescence caused by SARS-CoV-2 which would greatly benefit the host and diminish all-cause mortality. In addition, the prevention and reversal of immunosenescence using AFP antagonists (zinc, genistein/isoflavones, 7-keto-DHEA, and ivermectin) especially in those with comorbidities may also help prevent moderate as well as more severe disease from developing.

Public health authorities should consider providing free annual vitamin D3 testing (and retesting when indicated). They need to provide encouragement to go outdoors, safely suntan and to closely monitor serum vitamin D3 levels. People can also reduce their risks of pandemic severity by employing various lifestyle improvements of maintaining an ideal weight, no or low sugar exposures, avoiding trans fats, being outdoors, exercising, reducing stress, and maintaining a normal blood pressure. In addition to Vitamin D3 and a multivitamin supplement, AFP antagonists such as zinc, genistein, 7 keto-DHEA (only legal in the USA) could be taken daily as a prophylactic. For those who may be at higher risk of poor outcomes, ivermectin which may also be an AFP antagonist[191] might be used for early treatment along with other measures of the early treatment protocols.[193,221] Note as mentioned, methylprednisolone is preferred over dexamethasone as dexamethasone failed to reverse the SARS-CoV-2 interference of the IFN-1 and IFN-γ

innate responses while methylprednisolone did.[193,194] Interestingly, it had been previously reported that high dose dexamethasone does not induce HERV-K102 transcripts *in vitro*[192] implying methylprednisolone might activate HERV-K102 proviral expression and replication. Clearly this also needs further investigation.

Finally, it is proposed that monoclonal sc-Fv antibodies that recognize the cell surface HERV-K102 Env (P61567 Env protein) but not the Env on HERV-K102 particles (P63135 Pol-Env protein), may provide novel therapeutics not only against pandemic viruses but also cancers. Unlike the MAbs to the spike protein, here there is little concern for loss of MAb effectiveness related to the emergence of viral variants **(Figs. 10 and 11)**.

SUMMARY AND CONCLUSION

Many novel findings of relevance to understanding the adverse effects of ADE on survival of humans to pandemic viruses are uncovered in this treatise.

First, overwhelming evidence strongly implies that HERV-K102 particle production in M1-like proinflammatory macrophages constitutes the core attributes of trained (innate) immunity related to epigenetic changes and glycolysis in macrophages. Accordingly, ADE-mediated infection of macrophages abrogates this potent protector mechanism and thus, it seems many human pathogens target HERV-K102. Second, for the first time, it is clarified that sebocytes in sebaceous glands that line the mucosa are specialized LB^- FMs that constitutively produce and release HERV-K102 particles by lysis. This validates that the HERV-K102 protector response is not only critical but always active at the front lines constituting critical host defense. Third, how trained (innate) immunity may generate a reduction in all-cause mortality (by reversing immunosenescence of macrophages which is causally related to chronic disease[185,186]) has been suggested. Fourth, a novel virus-anti-virus innate response has been uncovered and expanded upon which reveals how the body attempts to overcome pathogen mediated down-modulation of the protective interferon innate immunity response. This is by "virus mimicry"[136] amplified by high replication of HERV-K102 particles which enter normal cells and then integrate into the cell's genome additionally "arming the genome" with extracopies. Fifth, a more comprehensive explanation of how optimal blood levels of vitamin D3 can promote survival against pandemic viruses, as well as reduce all-cause mortality, is revealed, and involves the preservation of the HERV-K102 protection system of M1-like foamy macrophages. Six, novel evidence is provided implying the HERV-K102 protection system may be germane to overall human survival given the loss of HERV-K102 at the orthologous chromosomal positions in the extinct hominins. Finally, not only do HERV-K102 and/or M1-like macrophages appear to mediate recovery from mild-moderate COVID-19 disease, but it was previously reported that HERV-K102 high replication and integration was associated with resistance to HIV-1 acquisition[10] providing evidence of sterile immunity against pandemic viruses.

All in all, the evidence shows that pandemic *enveloped* RNA viruses like SARS-CoV-2 and/or HIV-1 target HERV-K102 particle production in foamy macrophages. In COVID-19 disease, severe pathogenesis appears to relate to ADE of infection into macrophages but where optimal levels of vitamin D3 prevents the transition to more severe disease.[222] This is accomplished by blocking the transition of the LB-FMs producing the protective HERV-K102 particles to LB+FMs[165] the latter that generate and secrete high levels of SARS-CoV-2 virions.[196] There is also much hope for the development innate immunity vaccines to preinduce the HERV-K102 protector system in the most vulnerable. However, for most adults, the reversal/prevention of immunosenescence in adults, especially elders, and maintaining vitamin D3 levels over 50 ng/mL would be main strategies to help prepare for the next pandemic.

There may be one additional strategy to prevent the next pandemic. In a direct comparison of viral evolution, SARS-CoV-2 was found to be adapted to humans upon its emergence whereas SARS-CoV-1 was not[223] suggesting a lab-leak versus zoonotic source (respectively) of these coronavirus pandemics. Allegedly, the Wuhan Institute of Virology could have serial passaged a SARS-CoV-2 progenitor virus through humanized mice using the new model published in October 2019 by Baric and colleagues.[224] These along with other arguments[225] strengthen the notion of a lab-leak source of SARS-CoV-2 including the notion presented here that SARS-CoV-2 targets a protection system only found in humans. This implies there was selection within the human immune system prior to release. Thus, a primary way to help deal with pandemics would be by banning gain-of-function virology research which in the USA, the House has recently approved.[226]

REFERENCES

1. Yuan GC, Cai L, Elowitz M, Enver T, Fan G, Guo G, et al. Challenges and emerging directions in single-cell analysis. Genome Biol. 2017;18(1):84.
2. Gao S, Yan L, Wang R, Li J, Yong J, Zhou X, et al. Tracing the temporal-spatial transcriptome landscapes of the human fetal digestive tract using single-cell RNA-sequencing. Nat Cell Biol. 2018;20(6):721-34.
3. Gentles AJ, Newman AM, Liu CL, Bratman SV, Feng W, Kim D, et al. The prognostic landscape of genes and infiltrating immune cells across human cancers. Nat Med. 2015;21(8):938-45.
4. Wikipidia. Galactose-alpha-1,3-galactose. [online] Available from https://en.wikipedia.org/wiki/Galactose-alpha-1,3-galactose [Last accessed April, 2024].
5. Mumme H, Thomas BE, Bhasin SS, Krishnan U, Dwivedi B, Perumalla P, et al. Single-cell analysis reveals altered tumor microenvironments of relapse- and remission-associated pediatric acute myeloid leukemia. Nat Commun. 2023;14(1):6209.
6. Zhang JT, Zhang J, Wang SR, Yan LX, Qin J, Yin K, et al. Spatial downregulation of CD74 signatures may drive invasive component development in part-solid lung adenocarcinoma. iScience. 2023;26(10):107699.

7. Shangguan S, Ehrenberg PK, Geretz A, Yum L, Kundu G, May K, et al. Monocyte-derived transcriptome signature indicates antibody-dependent cellular phagocytosis as a potential mechanism of vaccine-induced protection against HIV-1. Elife. 2021;10:e69577.
8. Vaccari M, Fourati S, Gordon SN, Brown DR, Bissa M, Schifanella L, et al. HIV vaccine candidate activation of hypoxia and the inflammasome in CD14+ monocytes is associated with a decreased risk of SIV_{mac251} acquisition. Nat Med. 201824(6):847-56.
9. Thomas C, Leleu D, Masson D. Cholesterol and HIF-1α: dangerous liaisons in atherosclerosis. Front Immunol. 2022;13:868958.
10. Laderoute MP, Larocque LJ, Giulivi A, Diaz-Mitoma F. Further evidence that human endogenous retrovirus K102 is a replication competent foamy virus that may antagonize HIV-1 replication. Open AIDS J. 2015;9:112-22.
11. Laderoute MP. Clues to finding correlates of risk/protection for HIV-1 vaccines [version 2; peer review: 2 approved with reservations]. F1000 Research. 2018;6:868.
12. Hussein HAM, Thabet AAA, Mohamed TIA, Elnosary ME, Sobhy A, El-Adly AM, et al. Phenotypical changes of hematopoietic stem and progenitor cells in COVID-19 patients: Correlation with disease status. Cent Eur J Immunol. 2023;48(2):97-110.
13. Sawant J, Patil A, Kurle S. A review: understanding molecular mechanisms of antibody-dependent enhancement in viral infections. Vaccines (Basel). 2023;11(7):1240.
14. Ricke DO. Two different antibody-dependent enhancement (ADE) risks for SARS-CoV-2 antibodies. Front Immunol. 2021;12:640093.
15. Gartlan C, Tipton T, Salguero FJ, Sattentau Q, Gorringe A, Carroll MW. Vaccine-associated enhanced disease and pathogenic human coronaviruses. Front Immunol. 2022;13:882972.
16. Zohar T, Alter G. Dissecting antibody-mediated protection against SARS-CoV-2. Nat Rev Immunol. 2020;20(7):392-4.
17. Chen W, Zhang J, Qin X, Wang W, Xu M, Wang LF, et al. SARS-CoV-2 neutralizing antibody levels are correlated with severity of COVID-19 pneumonia. Biomed Pharmacother. 2020;130:110629.
18. Chen X, Pan Z, Yue S, Yu F, Zhang J, Yang Y, et al. Disease severity dictates SARS-CoV-2-specific neutralizing antibody responses in COVID-19. Sig Transduct Target Ther. 2020;5:180.
19. Hashem AM, Algaissi A, Almahboub SA, Alfaleh MA, Abujamel TS, Alamri SS, et al. Early humoral response correlates with disease severity and outcomes in COVID-19 patients. Viruses. 2020;12(12):1390.
20. Zhao J, Yuan Q, Wang H, Liu W, Liao X, Su Y, et al. Antibody responses to SARS-CoV-2 in patients with novel coronavirus disease 2019. Clin Infect Dis. 2020;71(16):2027-34.
21. Shrock E, Fujimura E, Kula T, Timms RT, Lee IH, Leng Y, et al. Viral epitope profiling of COVID-19 patients reveals cross-reactivity and correlates of severity. Science. 2020;370(6520):eabd4250.
22. Choteau M, Scohy A, Messe S, Luyckx M, Dechamps M, Montiel V, et al. Development of SARS-CoV2 humoral response including neutralizing antibodies is not sufficient to protect patients against fatal infection. Sci Rep. 2022;12(1):2077.
23. Legros V, Denolly S, Vogrig M, Boson B, Siret E, Rigaill J, et al. A longitudinal study of SARS-CoV-2-infected patients reveals a high correlation between neutralizing antibodies and COVID-19 severity. Cell Mol Immunol. 2021;18(2):318-27.
24. Ren L, Fan G, Wu W, Guo L, Wang Y, Li X, et al. Antibody responses and clinical outcomes in adults hospitalized with severe coronavirus disease 2019 (COVID-19): a post hoc analysis of LOTUS China trial. Clin Infect Dis. 2021;72(10):e545-e551.
25. Wang K, Fan G, Wu W, Hu J, Gao QZ, Zhang GJ, et al. Longitudinal dynamics of the neutralizing antibody response to severe acute respiratory syndrome coronavirus 2 (SARS-CoV-2) infection. Clin Infect Dis. 2021;73(3):e531-e539.

26. Xu X, Nie S, Wang Y, Long Q, Zhu H, Zhang X, et al. Dynamics of neutralizing antibody responses to SARS-CoV-2 in patients with COVID-19: an observational study. Signal Transduct Target Ther. 2021;6(1):197.
27. Gao L, Zhou J, Yang S, Wang L, Chen X, Yang Y, et al. The dichotomous and incomplete adaptive immunity in COVID-19 patients with different disease severity. Sig Transduct Target Ther. 2021;6:113.
28. Huang AT, Garcia-Carreras B, Hitchings MDT, Yang B, Katzelnick LC, Rattigan SM, et al. A systematic review of antibody mediated immunity to coronaviruses: kinetics, correlates of protection, and association with severity. Nat Commun. 2020;11(1):4704.
29. Nair S, Chen X. Biology of severe acute respiratory syndrome coronavirus 2 (SARS-CoV-2) and the humoral immunoresponse: a systematic review of evidence to support global policy-level actions and research. Glob Health J. 2022;6(1):38-43.
30. Wu F, Liu M, Wang A, Lu L, Wang Q, Gu C, et al. Evaluating the association of clinical characteristics with neutralizing antibody levels in patients who have recovered from mild COVID-19 in Shanghai, China. JAMA Intern Med. 2020;180(10):1356-62.
31. Dispinseri S, Secchi M, Pirillo MF, Tolazzi M, Borghi M, Brigatti C, et al. Neutralizing antibody responses to SARS-CoV-2 in symptomatic COVID-19 is persistent and critical for survival. Nat Commun. 2021;12(1):2670.
32. Garcia-Beltran WF, Lam EC, Astudillo MG, Yang D, Miller TE, Feldman J, et al. COVID-19-neutralizing antibodies predict disease severity and survival. Cell. 2021;184(2):476-88.e11.
33. Gilbert PB, Montefiori DC, McDermott AB, Fong Y, Benkeser D, Deng W, et al. Immune correlates analysis of the mRNA-1273 COVID-19 vaccine efficacy clinical trial. Science. 2022;375(6576):43-50.
34. Zohar T, Loos C, Fischinger S, Atyeo C, Wang C, Slein MD, et al. Compromised humoral functional evolution tracks with SARS-CoV-2 mortality. Cell. 2020;183(6):1508-19.e12.
35. Tetro JA. Is COVID-19 receiving ADE from other coronaviruses? Microbes Infect. 2020;22(2):72-3.
36. Moorlag SJCFM, Taks E, Ten Doesschate T, van der Vaart TW, Janssen AB, Müller L, et al. Efficacy of Bacillus Calmette-Guérin vaccination against respiratory tract infections in the elderly during the Covid-19 pandemic. Clin Infect Dis. 2022;75(1):e938-e946
37. Bigay J, Le Grand R, Martinon F, Maisonnasse P. Vaccine-associated enhanced disease in humans and animal models: lessons and challenges for vaccine development. Front Microbiol. 2022;13:932408.
38. Munitz A, Edry-Botzer L, Itan M, Tur-Kaspa R, Dicker D, Marcoviciu D, et al. Rapid seroconversion and persistent functional IgG antibodies in severe COVID-19 patients correlates with an IL-12p70 and IL-33 signature. Sci Rep. 2021;11(1):3461.
39. Ho MS, Chen WJ, Chen HY, Lin SF, Wang WC, Di J. Neutralizing antibody response and SARS severity. Emerg Infect Dis. 2005;11:1730-7.
40. Liu L, Wei Q, Lin Q, Fang J, Wang H, Kwok H, et al. Anti-spike IgG causes severe acute lung injury by skewing macrophage responses during acute SARS-CoV infection. JCI Insight. 2019;4(4):e123158.
41. Wolfel R, Corman VM, Guggemos W, Seilmaier M, Zange S, Müller MA, et al. Virological assessment of hospitalized patients with COVID-2019. Nature. 2020;581(7809):465-9.
42. Jensen B, Luebke N, Feldt T, Keitel V, Brandenburger T, Kindgen-Milles D, et al. Emergence of the E484K mutation in SARS-COV-2-infected immunocompromised patients treated with bamlanivimab in Germany. Lancet Reg Health Eur. 2021;8:100164.
43. Guerrieri M, Francavilla B, Fiorelli D, Nuccetelli M, Passali FM, Coppeta L, et al. Nasal and salivary mucosal humoral immune response elicited by mRNA BNT162b2 COVID-19 vaccine compared to SARS-CoV-2 natural infection. Vaccines (Basel). 2021;9(12):1499.

44. Aksyuk AA, Bansal H, Wilkins D, Stanley AM, Sproule S, Maaske J, et al. AZD1222-induced nasal antibody responses are shaped by prior SARS-CoV-2 infection and correlate with virologic outcomes in breakthrough infection. Cell Rep Med. 2022;4:100882.
45. Kistler KE, Huddleston J, Bedford T. Rapid and parallel adaptive mutations in spike S1 drive clade success in SARS-CoV-2. Cell Host Microbe. 2022;30(4):545-55.e4.
46. Walsh EE, Frenck RW Jr, Falsey AR, et al. Safety and immunogenicity of two RNA-based Covid-19 vaccine candidates. N Engl J Med. 2020;383(25):2439-50.
47. Chu L, McPhee R, Huang W, et al. A preliminary report of a randomized controlled phase 2 trial of the safety and immunogenicity of mRNA-1273 SARS-CoV-2 vaccine. Vaccine. 2021;39(20):2791-9.
48. Miller A. (2021). Why Canada's decision to delay 2nd doses of COVID-19 vaccines may not work for everyone. [online] Available from https://www.cbc.ca/news/health/vaccine-dose-delay-canada-covid-19-research-1.5965996# [Last accessed April, 2024].
49. Our World in Data. Research and data to make progress against the world's largest problems. [online] Available from https://ourworldindata.org [Last accessed April, 2024].
50. Xu S, Huang R, Sy LS, Glenn SC, Ryan DS, Morrissette K, et al. COVID-19 vaccination and non–COVID-19 mortality risk—seven integrated health care organizations, United States, December 14, 2020–July 31, 2021. MMWR Morb Mortal Wkly Rep. 2021;70: 1520-4.
51. Laderoute MP. (2022). Did the Second Dose of mRNA COVID-19 Vaccines Select for the Alpha and Delta Variants Which Prolonged the Pandemic? [online] Available from https://hervk102.substack.com/p/did-the-second-dose-of-mrna-covid [Last accessed April, 2024].
52. Government of Canada. (2021). Surviving the heat: The impacts of the 2021 western heat dome in Canada. [online] Available from https://science.gc.ca/site/science/en/blogs/science-health/surviving-heat-impacts-2021-western-heat-dome-canada [Last accessed April, 2024].
53. Servellita V, Morris MK, Sotomayor-Gonzalez A, et al. Predominance of antibody-resistant SARS-CoV-2 variants in vaccine breakthrough cases from the San Francisco Bay Area, California. Nat Microbiol. 2022;7(2):277-88.
54. Tartof SY, Slezak JM, Fischer H, Hong V, Ackerson BK, Ranasinghe ON, et al. Effectiveness of mRNA BNT162b2 COVID-19 vaccine up to 6 months in a large integrated health system in the USA: a retrospective cohort study. Lancet. 2021;398(10309):1407-16.
55. UK. COVID-19 Weekly Surveillance Reports by Public Health England: COVID-19 Vaccine Surveillance Reports 2021 Weeks 19-38 at https://www.gov.uk/government/publications/covid-19-vaccine-surveillance-report and by UK Health Security Agency: COVID-19 Surveillance Reports for 2021 Week 39 to 2023 Week 23 at https://www.gov.uk/government/publications/covid-19-vaccine-weekly-surveillance-reports.
56. UK Health Security Agency. (2022). COVID-19 vaccine surveillance report Week 12. [online] available from https://assets.publishing.service.gov.uk/media/623c6ef0d3bf7f6ab9fe28bf/Vaccine-surveillance-report-week-12.pdf [Last accessed April, 2024].
57. Shrestha NK, Burke PC, Nowacki AS, Simon JF, Hagen A, Gordon SM. Effectiveness of the coronavirus disease 2019 bivalent vaccine. Open Forum Infect Dis. 2023;10(6):ofad209.
58. Irrgang P, Gerling J, Kocher K, Lapuente D, Steininger P, Habenicht K, et al. Class switch toward noninflammatory, spike-specific IgG4 antibodies after repeated SARS-CoV-2 mRNA vaccination. Sci Immunol. 2023;8(79):eade2798.
59. Our World in Data. (2024). Estimated cumulative excess deaths per 100,000 people during COVID-19, Jan 27, 2024. https://ourworldindata.org/explorers/coronavirus-data-explorer [Last accessed April, 2024].

60. Ziegler CGK, Miao VN, Owings AH, Navia AW, Tang Y, Bromley JD, et al. Impaired local intrinsic immunity to SARS-CoV-2 infection in severe COVID-19. Cell. 2021;184(18): 4713-33.e22.
61. Ren X, Wen W, Fan X, Hou W, Su B, Cai P, et al. COVID-19 immune features revealed by a large-scale single-cell transcriptome atlas. Cell. 2021;184(7):1895-913.e19.
62. Bost P, Giladi A, Liu Y, Bendjelal Y, Xu G, David E, et al. Host-viral infection maps reveal signatures of severe COVID-19 patients. Cell. 2020;181(7):1475-88.e12.
63. Chua RL, Lukassen S, Trump S, Hennig BP, Wendisch D, Pott F, et al. COVID-19 severity correlates with airway epithelium-immune cell interactions identified by single-cell analysis. Nat Biotechnol. 2020;38(8):970-9.
64. Wendisch D, Dietrich O, Mari T, von Stillfried S, Ibarra IL, Mittermaier M, et al. SARS-CoV-2 infection triggers profibrotic macrophage responses and lung fibrosis. Cell. 2021;184(26):6243-61.e27.
65. Grant RA, Morales-Nebreda L, Markov NS, Swaminathan S, Querrey M, Guzman ER, et al. Circuits between infected macrophages and T cells in SARS-CoV-2 pneumonia. Nature. 2021;590(7847):635-41.
66. Delorey TM, Ziegler CGK, Heimberg G, Normand R, Yang Y, Segerstolpe Å, et al. COVID-19 tissue atlases reveal SARS-CoV-2 pathology and cellular targets. Nature. 2021;595(7865):107-13.
67. Laderoute MP, Giulivi A, Larocque L, Bellfoy D, Hou Y, Wu HX, et al. The replicative activity of human endogenous retrovirus K102 (HERV-K102) with HIV viremia. AIDS. 2007;21(18):2417-24.
68. Bhardwaj N, Maldarelli F, Mellors J, Coffin JM. HIV-1 infection leads to increased transcription of human endogenous retrovirus HERV-K (HML-2) proviruses in vivo but not to increased virion production. J Virol. 2014;88(19):11108-20.
69. Yu SF, Eastman SW, Linial ML. Foamy virus capsid assembly occurs at a pericentriolar region through a cytoplasmic targeting/retention signal in Gag. Traffic. 2006;7(8): 966-77.
70. Subramanian RP, Wildschutte JH, Russo C, Coffin JM. Identification, characterization, and comparative genomic distribution of the HERV-K (HML-2) group of human endogenous retroviruses. Retrovirology. 2011;8:90.
71. van der Kuyl AC. HIV infection and HERV expression: a review. Retrovirology. 2012;9:6.
72. Linial ML. Foamy viruses are unconventional retroviruses. J Virol. 1999;73(3):1747-55.
73. Murray SM, Linial ML. Simian foamy virus co-infections. Viruses. 2019;11(10):902.
74. Switzer WM, Salemi M, Shanmugam V, Gao F, Cong ME, Kuiken C, et al. Ancient co-speciation of simian foamy viruses and primates. Nature. 2005;434:376-80.
75. Yu SF, Sullivan MD, Linial ML. Evidence that the human foamy virus genome is DNA. J Virol. 1999;73(2):1565-72.
76. Meiering CD, Comstock KE, Linial ML. Multiple integrations of human foamy virus in persistently infected human erythroleukemia cells. J Virol. 2000;74(4):1718-26.
77. Heinkelein M, Hoffmann U, Lücke M, Imrich H, Müller JG, Meixensberger J, et al. Experimental therapy of allogeneic solid tumors induced in athymic mice with suicide gene-transducing replication-competent foamy virus vectors. Cancer Gene Ther. 2005;12(12):947-53.
78. Mikovits JA, Hoffman PM, Rethwilm A, Ruscetti FW. In vitro infection of primary and retrovirus-infected human leukocytes by human foamy virus. J Virol. 1996;70(5): 2774-80.
79. Laderoute MP. (2022). What you need to know about the HERV-K102 innate immunity protector system of macrophages against RNA pandemic viruses. [online] Available from https://hervk102.substack.com/p/what-you-need-to-know-about-the-herv [Last accessed April, 2024].

80. Plochmann K, Horn A, Gschmack E, Armbruster N, Krieg J, Wiktorowicz T, et al. Heparan sulfate is an attachment factor for foamy virus entry. J Virol. 2012;86(18):10028-35.
81. Robinson-McCarthy LR, McCarthy KR, Raaben M, Piccinotti S, Nieuwenhuis J, Stubbs SH, et al. Reconstruction of the cell entry pathway of an extinct virus. PLoS Pathog. 2018;14(8):e1007123.
82. Wikimedia Commons. Insertion of sebaceous glands into hair shaft. [online] Available from https://commons.wikimedia.org/wiki/File:Insertion_of_sebaceous_glands_into_hair_shaft_x10.jpg [Last accessed April, 2024].
83. NCBI. GEO Profiles. [online] Available from https://www.ncbi.nlm.nih.gov/geoprofiles/ [Last accessed April, 2024].
84. Nelson AM, Zhao W, Gilliland KL, Zaenglein AL, Liu W, Thiboutot DM. Neutrophil gelatinase-associated lipocalin mediates 13-cis retinoic acid-induced apoptosis of human sebaceous gland cells. J Clin Invest. 2008;118(4):1468-78.
85. Nelson AM, Zhao W, Gilliland KL, Zaenglein AL, Liu W, Thiboutot DM. Isotretinoin temporally regulates distinct sets of genes in patient skin. J Invest Dermatol. 2009;129(4): 1038-42.
86. Stec M, Weglarczyk K, Baran J, Zuba E, Mytar B, Pryjma J, et al. Expansion and differentiation of CD14+CD16(-) and CD14+ +CD16+ human monocyte subsets from cord blood CD34+ hematopoietic progenitors. J Leukoc Biol. 2007;82(3):594-602.
87. Martinez FO, Gordon S, Locati M, Mantovani A. Transcriptional profiling of the human monocyte-to-macrophage differentiation and polarization: new molecules and patterns of gene expression. J Immunol. 2006;177(10):7303-11.
88. Maslova A, Ramirez RN, Ma K, Schmutz H, Wang C, Fox C, et al. Immunological genome project. Deep learning of immune cell differentiation. Proc Natl Acad Sci U S A. 2020; 117(41):25655-66.
89. Saeed S, Quintin J, Kerstens HH, Rao NA, Aghajanirefah A, Matarese F, et al. Epigenetic programming of monocyte-to-macrophage differentiation and trained innate immunity. Science. 2014;345(6204):1251086.
90. Arts RJW, Joosten LAB, Netea MG. The potential role of trained immunity in autoimmune and autoinflammatory disorders. Front Immunol. 2018;9:298.
91. Lv JJ, Wang H, Cui HY, Liu ZK, Zhang RY, Lu M, et al. Blockade of macrophage CD147 protects against foam cell formation in atherosclerosis. Front Cell Dev Biol. 2021;8:609090.
92. Zhang MF, Cai XL, Jing KP, Pi XX, Liao PY, Li SJ, et al. Differentiation model establishment and differentiation-related protein screening in primary cultured human sebocytes. Biomed Res Int. 2018;2018:7174561.
93. Bekkering S, Quintin J, Joosten LA, van der Meer JW, Netea MG, Riksen NP. Oxidized low-density lipoprotein induces long-term proinflammatory cytokine production and foam cell formation via epigenetic reprogramming of monocytes. Arterioscler Thromb Vasc Biol. 2014;34(8):1731-8.
94. Bekkering S, Arts RJW, Novakovic B, Kourtzelis I, van der Heijden CDCC, Li Y, et al. Metabolic induction of trained immunity through the mevalonate pathway. Cell. 2018;172(1-2):135-46.e9.
95. Wang J, Liu YM, Hu J, Chen C. Trained immunity in monocyte/macrophage: novel mechanism of phytochemicals in the treatment of atherosclerotic cardiovascular disease. Front Pharmacol. 2023;14:1109576.
96. Keating ST, Groh L, Thiem K, Bekkering S, Li Y, Matzaraki V, et al. Rewiring of glucose metabolism defines trained immunity induced by oxidized low-density lipoprotein. J Mol Med (Berl). 2020;98(6):819-31.
97. Manghera M, Ferguson-Parry J, Lin R, Douville RN. NF-κB and IRF1 induce endogenous retrovirus K expression via interferon-stimulated response elements in its 5′ long terminal repeat. J Virol. 2016;90(20):9338-49.

98. Manghera M, Douville RN. Endogenous retrovirus-K promoter: A landing strip for inflammatory transcription factors? Retrovirology. 2013;10:16.
99. Russ E, Mikhalkevich N, Iordanskiy S. Expression of human endogenous retrovirus group K (HERV-K) HML-2 correlates with immune activation of macrophages and type I interferon response. Microbiol Spectr. 2023;11(2):e0443822.
100. Fischer H, Fumicz J, Rossiter H, Napirei M, Buchberger M, Tschachler E, et al. Holocrine secretion of sebum is a unique DNase2-dependent mode of programmed cell death. J Invest Dermatol. 2017;137(3):587-94.
101. Törőcsik D, Kovács D, Póliska S, Szentkereszty-Kovács Z, Lovászi M, Hegyi K, et al. Genome wide analysis of TLR1/2- and TLR4-activated SZ95 sebocytes reveals a complex immune-competence and identifies serum amyloid A as a marker for activated sebaceous glands. PLoS One. 2018;13(6):e0198323.
102. Magiorkinis G, Blanco-Melo D, Belshaw R. The decline of human endogenous retroviruses: extinction and survival. Retrovirology. 2015;12:8.
103. Chuong EB, Elde NC, Feschotte C. Regulatory evolution of innate immunity through co-option of endogenous retroviruses. Science. 2016;351(6277):1083-7.
104. Kim YJ, Han K. Endogenous retrovirus-mediated genomic variations in chimpanzees. Mob Genet Elements. 2015;4(6):1-4.
105. Romano CM, Ramalho RF, Zanotto PM. Tempo and mode of ERV-K evolution in human and chimpanzee genomes. Arch Virol. 2006;151(11):2215-28.
106. Langergraber KE, Prüfer K, Rowney C, Boesch C, Crockford C, Fawcett K, et al. Generation times in wild chimpanzees and gorillas suggest earlier divergence times in great ape and human evolution. Proc Natl Acad Sci U S A. 2012;109(39):15716-21.
107. Katzourakis A, Pereira V, Tristem M. Effects of recombination rate on human endogenous retrovirus fixation and persistence. J Virol. 2007;81(19):10712-7.
108. Sawyer SL, Emerman M, Malik HS. Ancient adaptive evolution of the primate antiviral DNA-editing enzyme APOBEC3G. PLoS Biol. 2004;2(9):E275.
109. Gifford RJ. Viral evolution in deep time: lentiviruses and mammals. Trends Genet. 2012;28(2):89-100.
110. O'Neil SP, Novembre FJ, Hill AB, et al. Progressive infection in a subset of HIV-1-positive chimpanzees. J Infect Dis. 2000;182(4):1051-62.
111. Khan N, de Manuel M, Peyregne S, Do R, Prufer K, Marques-Bonet T, et al. Multiple genomic events altering hominin SIGLEC biology and innate immunity predated the common ancestor of humans and archaic hominins. Genome Biol Evol. 2020;12(7): 1040-50.
112. Compton AA, Malik HS, Emerman M. Host gene evolution traces the evolutionary history of ancient primate lentiviruses. Philos Trans R Soc Lond B Biol Sci. 2013;368(1626): 20120496.
113. Murphy WJ, Frönicke L, O'Brien SJ, Stanyon R. The origin of human chromosome 1 and its homologs in placental mammals. Genome Res. 2003;13(8):1880-8.
114. Posth C, Wißing C, Kitagawa K, Pagani L, van Holstein L, Racimo F, et al. Deeply divergent archaic mitochondrial genome provides lower time boundary for African gene flow into Neanderthals. Nat Commun. 2017;8:16046.
115. Petr HC, Wißing C, Kitagawa K, Essel E, Rougier H, Crevecoeur I, et al. The evolutionary history of Neanderthal and Denisovan Y chromosomes. Science. 2020;369(6511): 1653-6.
116. Hajdinjak M, Mafessoni F, Skov L, Vernot B, Hübner A, Fu Q, et al. Initial upper palaeolithic humans in Europe had recent Neanderthal ancestry. Nature. 2021;592(7853):253-7.
117. Enard D, Petrov DA. Evidence that RNA viruses drove adaptive introgression between neanderthals and modern humans. Cell. 2018;175(2):360-71.e13.
118. Gouy A, Excoffier L. Polygenic patterns of adaptive introgression in modern humans are mainly shaped by response to pathogens. Mol Biol Evol. 2020;37(5):1420-33.

119. Bücking R, Cox MP, Hudjashov G, Saag L, Sudoyo H, Stoneking M. Archaic mitochondrial DNA inserts in modern day nuclear genomes. BMC Genomics. 2019;20(1):1017.
120. Ono M. Molecular cloning and long terminal repeat sequences of human endogenous retrovirus genes related to types A and B retrovirus genes. J Virol. 1986;58(3):937-44.
121. Löwer R, Löwer J, Kurth R. The viruses in all of us: characteristics and biological significance of human endogenous retrovirus sequences. Proc Natl Acad Sci U S A. 1996;93(11):5177-84.
122. Bannert N, Kurth R. Retroelements and the human genome: new perspectives on an old relation. Proc Natl Acad Sci U S A. 2004;101 Suppl 2(Suppl 2):14572-9.
123. Simpson GR, Patience C, Löwer R, Tönjes RR, Moore HD, Weiss RA, et al. Endogenous D-type (HERV-K) related sequences are packaged into retroviral particles in the placenta and possess open reading frames for reverse transcriptase. Virology. 1996;222(2): 451-6.
124. Grow EJ, Flynn RA, Chavez SL, Bayless NL, Wossidlo M, Wesche DJ, et al. Intrinsic retroviral reactivation in human preimplantation embryos and pluripotent cells. Nature. 2015;522(7555):221-5.
125. Morgan D, Brodsky I. Human endogenous retrovirus (HERV-K) particles in megakaryocytes cultured from essential thrombocythemia peripheral blood stem cells. Exp Hematol. 2004;32(6):520-5.
126. Morozov VA, Dao Thi VL, Denner J. The transmembrane protein of the human endogenous retrovirus--K (HERV-K) modulates cytokine release and gene expression. PLoS One. 2013;8(8):e70399.
127. Padow M, Lai L, Fisher RJ, Zhou YC, Wu X, Kappes JC, et al. Analysis of human immunodeficiency virus type 1 containing HERV-K protease. AIDS Res Hum Retroviruses. 2000;16(18):1973-80.
128. Brinzevich D, Young GR, Sebra R, Ayllon J, Maio SM, Deikus G, et al. HIV-1 interacts with human endogenous retrovirus K (HML-2) envelopes derived from human primary lymphocytes. J Virol. 2014;88(11):6213-23.
129. Monde K, Contreras-Galindo R, Kaplan MH, Markovitz DM, Ono A. Human endogenous retrovirus K Gag coassembles with HIV-1 Gag and reduces the release efficiency and infectivity of HIV-1. J Virol. 2012;86(20):11194-208.
130. Monde K, Terasawa H, Nakano Y, Prohaska CC, Zhang L, Chelvanambi S,et al. Molecular mechanisms by which HERV-K Gag interferes with HIV-1 Gag assembly and particle infectivity. Retrovirology. 2017;14(1):27.
131. Minkoff JM, TenOever B. Innate immune evasion strategies of SARS-CoV-2. Nat Rev Microbiol. 2023:1-17.
132. Su HC, Jing H, Zhang Y, Casanova JL. Interfering with interferons: a critical mechanism for critical COVID-19 pneumonia. Annu Rev Immunol. 2023;41:561-85.
133. Kawai T, Akira S. Toll-like receptor and RIG-I-like receptor signaling. Ann N Y Acad Sci. 2008;1143:1-20.
134. Rehwinkel J, Gack MU. RIG-I-like receptors: their regulation and roles in RNA sensing. Nat Rev Immunol. 2020;20(9):537-51.
135. Decout A, Katz JD, Venkatraman S, Ablasser A. The cGAS-STING pathway as a therapeutic target in inflammatory diseases. Nat Rev Immunol. 2021;21(9):548-69.
136. Russ E, Iordanskiy S. Endogenous retroviruses as modulators of innate immunity. Pathogens. 2023;12(2):162.
137. Guo Y, Yang C, Liu Y, Li T, Li H, Han J, et al. High expression of HERV-K (HML-2) might stimulate interferon in COVID-19 patients. Viruses. 2022;14:996.
138. Kenney DJ, O'Connell AK, Turcinovic J, Montanaro P, Hekman RM, Tamura T, et al. Humanized mice reveal a macrophage-enriched gene signature defining human lung tissue protection during SARS-CoV-2 infection. Cell Rep. 2022;39(3):110714.

139. Wang-Johanning F, Frost AR, Johanning GL, Khazaeli MB, LoBuglio AF, Shaw DR, et al. Expression of human endogenous retrovirus K envelope transcripts in human breast cancer. Clin Cancer Res. 2001;7(6):1553-60.
140. Wang-Johanning F, Frost AR, Jian B, Epp L, Lu DW, Johanning GL. Quantitation of HERV-K env gene expression and splicing in human breast cancer. Oncogene. 2003;22(10): 1528-35.
141. Wang-Johanning F, Radvanyi L, Rycaj K, Plummer JB, Yan P, Sastry KJ, et al. Human endogenous retrovirus K triggers an antigen-specific immune response in breast cancer patients. Cancer Res. 2008;68(14):5869-77.
142. Wang-Johanning F, Rycaj K, Plummer JB, Li M, Yin B, Frerich K, et al. Immunotherapeutic potential of anti-human endogenous retrovirus-K envelope protein antibodies in targeting breast tumors. J Natl Cancer Inst. 2012;104(3):189-210.
143. Jones RB, Garrison KE, Mujib S, Mihajlovic V, Aidarus N, Hunter DV, et al. HERV-K-specific T cells eliminate diverse HIV-1/2 and SIV primary isolates. J Clin Invest. 2012;122(12): 4473-89.
144. Michaud HA, de Mulder M, SenGupta D, Deeks SG, Martin JN, Pilcher CD, et al. Trans-activation, post-transcriptional maturation, and induction of antibodies to HERV-K (HML-2) envelope transmembrane protein in HIV-1 infection. Retrovirology. 2014;11:10.
145. Jumper J, Evans R, Pritzel A, Green T, Figurnov M, Ronneberger O, et al. Highly accurate protein structure prediction with AlphaFold. Nature. 2021;596(7873):583-9.
146. Varadi M, Velankar S. The impact of AlphaFold Protein Structure Database on the fields of life sciences. Proteomics. 2022:e2200128.
147. Apostolou E, Rizwan M, Moustardas P, Sjögren P, Bertilson BC, Bragée B, et al. Saliva antibody-fingerprint of reactivated latent viruses after mild/asymptomatic COVID-19 is unique in patients with myalgic-encephalomyelitis/chronic fatigue syndrome. Front Immunol. 2022;13:949787.
148. Risch H. (2023). Rise in Aggressive "Turbo Cancers" And especially Among Younger People. [online] Available from https://www.theepochtimes.com/epochtv/dr-harvey-risch-rise-in-aggressive-turbo-cancers-and-especially-among-younger-people-atlnow-5489582?utm_source=prtnrhard&utm_campaign=vigilantf&src_src=prtnrhard&src_cmp=vigilantf [Last accessed April, 2024].
149. Arru G, Galleri G, Deiana GA, Zarbo IR, Sechi E, Bo M, et al. HERV-K modulates the immune response in ALS patients. Microorganisms. 2021;9(8):1784.
150. Lo Presti E, De Gaetano A, Pioggia G, Gangemi S. Comprehensive analysis of the ILCs and unconventional T cells in virus infection: profiling and dynamics associated with COVID-19 disease for a future monitoring system and therapeutic opportunities. Cells. 2022;11(3):542.
151. Bhat RK, Rudnick W, Antony JM, Maingat F, Ellestad KK, Wheatley BM, et al. Human endogenous retrovirus-K(II) envelope induction protects neurons during HIV/AIDS. PLoS One. 2014;9(7):e97984.
152. Garcia-Montojo M, Simula ER, Fathi S, McMahan C, Ghosal A, Berry JD, et al. Antibody response to HML-2 may be protective in amyotrophic lateral sclerosis. Ann Neurol. 2022;92(5):782-92.
153. Simula ER, Arru G, Zarbo IR, Solla P, Sechi LA. TDP-43 and HERV-K envelope-specific immunogenic epitopes are recognized in ALS patients. Viruses. 2021;13(11):2301.
154. Xue B, Sechi LA, Kelvin DJ. Human endogenous retrovirus K (HML-2) in health and disease. Front Microbiol. 2020;11:1690.
155. Tokuyama M, Gunn BM, Venkataraman A, Kong Y, Kang I, Rakib T, et al. Antibodies against human endogenous retrovirus K102 envelope activate neutrophils in systemic lupus erythematosus. J Exp Med. 2021;218(7):e20191766.
156. Netea MG, Quintin J, van der Meer JW. Trained immunity: a memory for innate host defense. Cell Host Microbe. 2011;9(5):355-61.

157. Mitroulis I, Ruppova K, Wang B, Chen LS, Grzybek M, Grinenko T, et al. Modulation of myelopoiesis progenitors is an integral component of trained immunity. Cell. 2018;172(1-2):147-61.e12.
158. Cirovic B, de Bree LCJ, Groh L, Blok BA, Chan J, van der Velden WJFM, et al. BCG vaccination in humans elicits trained immunity via the hematopoietic progenitor compartment. Cell Host Microbe. 2020;28(2):322-34.e5.
159. Al B, Suen TK, Placek K, Netea MG. Innate (learned) memory, J Allerg Clin Immunol. 2023.
160. Zhang B, Moorlag SJ, Dominguez-Andres J, Bulut Ö, Kilic G, Liu Z, et al. Single-cell RNA sequencing reveals induction of distinct trained-immunity programs in human monocytes. J Clin Invest. 2022;132(7):e147719.
161. Li W, Moorlag SJCFM, Koeken VACM, Röring RJ, de Bree LCJ, Mourits VP, et al. A single-cell view on host immune transcriptional response to in vivo BCG-induced trained immunity. Cell Rep. 2023;42(5):112487.
162. Drummer C 4th, Saaoud F, Shao Y, Sun Y, K, Lu Y, et al. Trained immunity and reactivity of macrophages and endothelial cells. Arterioscler Thromb Vasc Biol. 2021;41(3):1032-46.
163. Cheng SC, Quintin J, Cramer RA, Shepardson KM, Saeed S, Kumar V, et al. mTOR- and HIF-1α-mediated aerobic glycolysis as metabolic basis for trained immunity. Science. 2014;345(6204):1250684.
164. Ieronymaki E, Daskalaki MG, Lyroni K, Tsatsanis C. Insulin signaling and insulin resistance facilitate trained immunity in macrophages through metabolic and epigenetic changes. Front Immunol. 2019;10:1330.
165. Oh J, Weng S, Felton SK, Bhandare S, Riek A, Butler B, et al. 1,25(OH)2 vitamin D inhibits foam cell formation and suppresses macrophage cholesterol uptake in patients with type 2 diabetes mellitus. Circulation. 2009;120(8):687-98.
166. Coleman PS, Parlo RA. Warburg's ghost-cancer's self-sustaining phenotype: the aberrant carbon flux in cholesterol-enriched tumor mitochondria via deregulated cholesterogenesis. Front Cell Dev Biol. 2021;9:626316.
167. Arts RJW, Moorlag SJCFM, Novakovic B, Li Y, Wang SY, Oosting M, et al. BCG vaccination protects against experimental viral infection in humans through the induction of cytokines associated with trained immunity. Cell Host Microbe. 2018;23:89-100.e5.
168. Viola A, Munari F, Sánchez-Rodríguez R, Scolaro T, Castegna A. The metabolic signature of macrophage responses. Front Immunol. 2019;10:1462.
169. Gomez Marti JL, Wells A, Brufsky AM. Dysregulation of the mevalonate pathway during SARS-CoV-2 infection: An in silico study. J Med Virol. 2021;93(4):2396-405.
170. Gao L, Chen Q, Zhou X, Fan L. The role of hypoxia-inducible factor 1 in atherosclerosis. J Clin Pathol. 2012;65(10):872-6.
171. Rius J, Guma M, Schachtrup C, Akassoglou K, Zinkernagel AS, Nizet V, et al. NF- links innate immunity to the hypoxic response through transcriptional regulation of HIF-1alpha. Nature. 2008;453(7196):807-11.
172. Jiang G, Li T, Qiu Y, Rui Y, Chen W, Lou Y. RNA interference for HIF-1alpha inhibits foam cells formation in vitro. Eur J Pharmacol. 2007;562(3):183-90.
173. Fruman DA, Rommel C. PI3K and cancer: Lessons, challenges and opportunities. Nat Rev Drug Discov. 2014;13(2):140-56.
174. Appelberg S, Gupta S, Svensson Akusjärvi S, Ambikan AT, Mikaeloff F, Saccon E, et al. Dysregulation in Akt/mTOR/HIF-1 signaling identified by proteo-transcriptomics of SARS-CoV-2 infected cells. Emerg Microbes Infect. 2020;9(1):1748-60.
175. Orekhov AN, Oishi Y, Nikiforov NG, Zhelankin AV, Dubrovsky L, Sobenin IA, et al. Modified LDL particles activate inflammatory pathways in monocyte-derived macrophages: transcriptome analysis. Curr Pharm Des. 2018;24(26):3143-51.
176. Zeboudj L, Giraud A, Guyonnet L, Zhang Y, Laurans L, Esposito B, et al. Selective EGFR (epidermal growth factor receptor) deletion in myeloid cells limits atherosclerosis-brief report. Arterioscler Thromb Vasc Biol. 2018;38(1):114-9.

177. Wang L, Huang Z, Huang W, Chen X, Shan P, Zhong P, et al. Inhibition of epidermal growth factor receptor attenuates atherosclerosis via decreasing inflammation and oxidative stress. Sci Rep. 2017;8:45917.
178. Tallam A, Perumal TM, Antony PM, Jäger C, Fritz JV, Vallar L, et al. Gene regulatory network inference of immunoresponsive gene 1 (IRG1) identifies interferon regulatory factor 1 (IRF1) as its transcriptional regulator in mammalian macrophages. PLoS One. 2016;11(2):e0149050.
179. Zhang M, Liu K, Zhang Q, Xu J, Liu J, Lin H, et al. Alpha fetoprotein promotes polarization of macrophages towards M2-like phenotype and inhibits macrophages to phagocytize hepatoma cells. Front Immunol. 2023;14:1081572.
180. Platanitis E, Decker T. Regulatory networks involving STATs, IRFs, and NFκB in inflammation. Front Immunol. 2018;9:2542.
181. Tan L, Lu J, Liu L, Li L. Fatty acid binding protein 3 deficiency limits atherosclerosis development via macrophage foam cell formation inhibition. Exp Cell Res. 2021;407(1): 112768.
182. Wang K, Chen W, Zhang Z, Deng Y, Lian JQ, Du P, et al. CD147-spike protein is a novel route for SARS-CoV-2 infection to host cells. Signal Transduct Target Ther. 2020;5(1):283.
183. Geng J, Chen L, Yuan Y, Wang K, Wang Y, Qin C, et al. CD147 antibody specifically and effectively inhibits infection and cytokine storm of SARS-CoV-2 and its variants delta, alpha, beta, and gamma. Signal Transduct Target Ther. 2021;6(1):347.
184. Helal MA, Shouman S, Abdelwaly A, Elmehrath AO, Essawy M, Sayed SM, et al. Molecular basis of the potential interaction of SARS-CoV-2 spike protein to CD147 in COVID-19 associated-lymphopenia. J Biomol Struct Dyn. 2022;40(3):1109-19.
185. Laderoute MP. A new paradigm about HERV-K102 particle production and blocked release to explain cortisol mediated immunosenescence and age-associated risk of chronic disease. Discov Med. 2015;20(112):379-91.
186. Laderoute M. The paradigm of immunosenescence in atherosclerosis-cardiovascular disease (ASCVD). Discov Med. 2020;29(156):41-51.
187. Laderoute MP. The Characterization of a Novel, Widespread, PNA-Reactive Tumor Associated Antigen; The Alpha-fetoprotein Receptor/Binding Protein. Edmonton, Alberta, Canada: Ph.D. Thesis, University of Alberta; 1991.
188. Laderoute MP, Pilarski LM. The inhibition of apoptosis by alpha-fetoprotein (AFP) and the role of AFP receptors in anti-cellular senescence. Anticancer Res. 1994;14(6B): 2429-38.
189. Nakabayashi H, Koyama Y, Sakai M, Li HM, Wong NC, Nishi S. Glucocorticoid stimulates primate but inhibits rodent alpha-fetoprotein gene promoter. Biochem Biophys Res Commun. 2001;287(1):160-72.
190. Phillips AC, Carroll D, Gale CR, Lord JM, Arlt W, Batty GD. Cortisol, DHEA sulphate, their ratio, and all-cause and cause-specific mortality in the Vietnam Experience Study. Eur J Endocrin. 2010; 163(2):285-92.
191. Laderoute M. (2021). Ivermectin may prevent and reverse immunosenescence by antagonizing alpha-fetoprotein and downmodulating PI3K/Akt/mTOR hyper-activity. [online] Available from https://openheart.bmj.com/content/8/1/e001655.responses#ivermectin-may-prevent-and-reverse-immunosenescence-by-antagonizing-alpha-fetoprotein-and-downmodulating-pi3k-akt-mtor-hyperactivity [Last accessed April, 2024].
192. Ono M, Kawakami M, Ushikubo H. Stimulation of expression of the human endogenous retrovirus genome by female steroid hormones in human breast cancer cell line T47D. J Virol. 1987;61(6):2059-62.
193. Kory P, Meduri GU, Iglesias J, Varon J, Cadegiani FA, Marik PE. "MATH+" Multi-Modal Hospital Treatment Protocol for COVID-19 Infection: Clinical and Scientific Rationale. J Clin Med Res. 2022;14(2):53-79.

194. Draghici S, Nguyen TM, Sonna LA, Ziraldo C, Vanciu R, Fadel R, et al. COVID-19: disease pathways and gene expression changes predict methylprednisolone can improve outcome in severe cases. Bioinformatics. 2021;37(17):2691-8.
195. Leech M, Metz C, Hall P, Hutchinson P, Gianis K, Smith M, et al. Macrophage migration inhibitory factor in rheumatoid arthritis: evidence of proinflammatory function and regulation by glucocorticoids. Arthritis Rheum. 1999;42(8):1601-8.
196. Dias SSG, Soares VC, Ferreira AC, Sacramento CQ, Fintelman-Rodrigues N, Temerozo JR, et al. Lipid droplets fuel SARS-CoV-2 replication and production of inflammatory mediators. PLoS Pathog. 2020;16(12):e1009127.
197. Singh N, Bharara Singh A. S2 subunit of SARS-CoV-2 interacts with tumor suppressor protein p53 and BRCA: an in silico study. Transl Oncol. 2020;13(10):100814.
198. Lee KC, Crowe AJ, Barton MC. p53-mediated repression of alpha-fetoprotein gene expression by specific DNA binding. Mol Cell Biol. 1999;19(2):1279-88.
199. Desterke C, Turhan AG, Bennaceur-Griscelli A, Griscelli F. PPARγ cistrome repression during activation of lung monocyte-macrophages in severe COVID-19. iScience. 2020;23(10):101611.
200. Verway M, Bouttier M, Wang TT, Carrier M, Calderon M, An BS, et al. Vitamin D induces interleukin-1β expression: paracrine macrophage epithelial signaling controls M. tuberculosis infection. PLoS Pathog. 2013;9(6):e1003407.
201. Borsche L, Glauner B, von Mendel J. COVID-19 mortality risk correlates inversely with vitamin D3 status, and a mortality rate close to zero could theoretically be achieved at 50 ng/mL 25(OH)D3: results of a systematic review and meta-analysis. Nutrients. 2021;13(10):3596.
202. Grant WB, Al Anouti F, Boucher BJ, Dursun E, Gezen-Ak D, Jude EB, et al. A narrative review of the evidence for variations in serum 25-hydroxyvitamin D concentration thresholds for optimal health. Nutrients. 2022;14(3):639.
203. Office for National Statistics (UK). (2022). Deaths involving COVID-19 by vaccination status, England: Deaths occurring between 1 January 2021 and 31 May 2022. Age-standardised mortality rates and raw death numbers for deaths involving COVID-19 by vaccination status, broken down by age and /or sex group. [online] Available from https://www.ons.gov.uk/peoplepopulationandcommunity/birthsdeathsandmarriages/deaths/bulletins/deathsinvolvingcovid19byvaccinationstatusengland/deathsoccurringbetween1january2021and31may2022. [Last accessed April, 2024].
204. Fenton N, Neil M, Craig C, McLachlan S. (2022). What the ONS mortality COVID-19 surveillance data can tell us about vaccine safety and efficacy. [online] Available from https://d7694293-ffb8-4ed0-a014-.3581d49070e4.usrfiles.com/ugd/d76942_bd64e0ebb4754477afd3d9f00bb3dc0f.pdf [Last accessed April, 2024].
205. Fenton N, Campbell J. (2023). Is ONS data on mortality by vaccine status fit for purpose? [online] Available from https://www.youtube.com/watch?v=W-N-17_j_44 [Last accessed April, 2024].
206. Graña C, Ghosn L, Evrenoglou T, Jarde A, Minozzi S, Bergman H, et al. Efficacy and safety of COVID-19 vaccines. Cochrane Database Syst Rev. 2022;12(12):CD015477.
207. Table 10. Cumulative data up to week 9, 2021 for week ending March 7. [online] available from https://assets.publishing.service.gov.uk/government/uploads/system/uploads/attachment_data/file/968513/Weekly_Flu_and_COVID-19_report_w10.pdf [Last accessed April, 2024].
208. Brogna C, Cristoni S, Marino G, Montano L, Viduto V, Fabrowski M, et al. Detection of recombinant spike protein in the blood of individuals vaccinated against SARS-CoV-2: possible molecular mechanisms. Proteomics Clin Appl. 2023;17(6):e2300048.
209. Sahanic S, Hilbe R, Dünser C, Tymoszuk P, Löffler-Ragg J, Rieder D, et al. SARS-CoV-2 activates the TLR4/MyD88 pathway in human macrophages: a possible correlation with strong pro-inflammatory responses in severe COVID-19. Heliyon. 2023;9(11):e21893.

210. McCullough P. Sen. (2022). Ron Johnson Roundtable Discussion. COVID-19 Vaccines: What they are, how they work, and possible causes of injuries. [online] Available from https://twitter.com/SenRonJohnson/status/160050489272825037 [Last accessed April, 2024].
211. Seneff S, Nigh G, Kyriakopoulos AM, McCullough PA. Innate immune suppression by SARS-CoV-2 mRNA vaccinations: The role of G-quadruplexes, exosomes, and microRNAs. Food Chem Toxicol. 2022;164:113008.
212. Hulscher N, Hodkinson R, Makis W, McCullough P. Autopsy proven fatal COVID-19 vaccine-induced myocarditis. Preprints. 2023, 2023071198.
213. Schwab C, Domke LM, Hartmann L, Stenzinger A, Longerich T, Schirmacher P. Autopsy-based histopathological characterization of myocarditis after anti-SARS-CoV-2-vaccination. Clin Res Cardiol. 2023;112(3):431-40.
214. Kleen TO, Galdon AA, MacDonald AS, Dalgleish AG. Mitigating coronavirus induced dysfunctional immunity for at-risk populations in COVID-19: trained immunity, BCG and "new old friends". Front Immunol. 2020;11:2059.
215. Desingu PA, Nagarajan K. Unveiling HERV-K113-ENV as SARS-CoV-2 severity admissible biomarker by mining transcriptome data. J Med Virol. 2023;95(1):e28149.
216. Tovo PA, Garazzino S, Daprà V, Pruccoli G, Calvi C, Mignone F, et al. COVID-19 in children: expressions of type I/II/III interferons, TRIM28, SETDB1, and endogenous retroviruses in mild and severe cases. Int J Mol Sci. 2021;22(14):7481.
217. Temerozo JR, Fintelman-Rodrigues N, Dos Santos MC, Hottz ED, Sacramento CQ, de Paula Dias da Silva A, et al. Human endogenous retrovirus K in the respiratory tract is associated with COVID-19 physiopathology. Microbiome. 2022;10(1):65.
218. Utrero-Rico A, González-Cuadrado C, Chivite-Lacaba M, Cabrera-Marante O, Laguna-Goya R, Almendro-Vazquez P, et al. Alterations in circulating monocytes predict COVID-19 severity and include chromatin modifications still detectable six months after recovery. Biomedicines. 2021;9(9):1253.
219. Lieberman NAP, Peddu V, Xie H, Shrestha L, Huang ML, Mears MC, et al. In vivo antiviral host transcriptional response to SARS-CoV-2 by viral load, sex, and age. PLoS Biol. 2020;18(9):e3000849.
220. Pereira PC, de Lima CJ, Fernandes AB, Zângaro RA, Villaverde AB. Cardiopulmonary and hematological effects of infrared LED photobiomodulation in the treatment of SARS-COV2. J Photochem Photobiol B. 2023;238:112619.
221. McCullough PA, Alexander PE, Armstrong R, Arvinte C, Bain AF, Bartlett RP, et al. Multifaceted highly targeted sequential multidrug treatment of early ambulatory high-risk SARS-CoV-2 infection (COVID-19). Rev Cardiovasc Med. 2020;21(4):517-30.
222. Wimalawansa SJ. Infections and autoimmunity-the immune system and vitamin D: a systematic review. Nutrients. 2023;15(17):3842.
223. Zhan SH, Deverman BE, Chan YA. SARS-CoV-2 is well adapted for humans. What does this mean for re-emergence? BioRxiv. 2 2020 (preprint).
224. Wahl A, De C, Abad Fernandez M, Lenarcic EM, Xu Y, Cockrell AS, et al. Precision mouse models with expanded tropism for human pathogens. Nat Biotechnol. 2019;37(10): 1163-73.
225. Maxmen A, Mallaaty S. The COVID lab-leak hypothesis: what scientists do and don't know. Nature. 2021;594(7863):313-5.
226. Kaiser J. (2023). House approves ban on gain-of-function pathogen research. [online] Available from https://www.science.org/content/article/house-approves-ban-gain-function-pathogen-research [Last accessed April, 2024].

CHAPTER 18

The COVID-19 Vaccine

Suneela Garg, Shekhar Grover, Tanu Anand, Arvind Garg

IMMUNIZATION

Background

Immunization is unarguably one of the most important components of public health and disease prevention in our society today. Diseases that used to prevail with a significant impact on morbidity and mortality have now been pushed back due to development of vaccines. Immunization has made substantial contributions toward enhancing life expectancy and improved quality of life.[1]

The credit for developing vaccines goes to Edward Jenner, who in 1796 inoculated a 13-year-old boy with the virus responsible for cowpox, which resulted in enhanced immunity to smallpox. Subsequently, the first vaccine (smallpox) was created, ultimately leading to the eradication of smallpox in 1979. Over time, vaccine technology has improved, and enriched vaccines have been targeted to mitigate many diseases.[2]

For the World Health Organization (WHO), immunization has always been a priority, even including it as a fundamental component of health as per 2030 sustainable development goals (SDGs). The year 2012 saw the adoption of Global Vaccine Action Plan at the World Health Assembly (WHA), which focused on increasing access to and utilization of vaccines globally.

What is a Vaccine?

A vaccine is a pharmacologic compound having a complex chemical structure that improves a person's immunity to a particular disease. When a pathogenic bacterium or virus invades the human body, the body's defense mechanism (immune system) recognizes the bacterium/virus as a foreign material by antigens (antigens are usually protein structures of the invading organism). Vaccines actually possess a similar antigen in a weakened, killed, or inactivated version of the invading organism, or a protein from the surface of the microbe. This weakened exposure of the antigen to the immune system via vaccines allows it to recognize it as a foreign material and subsequently develop antibodies and memory T-lymphocytes against those antigens. This prepares the immune system for a more rapid and robust response if the body is exposed to the actual pathogenic organism in the future. If any vaccination is not provided, the first exposure to the pathogenic organism could be fatal before the body's defense mechanism can mount a sufficient immune response.[3]

Physiology of Vaccination

Vaccines work primarily by facilitating the development of B-lymphocytes and T-lymphocytes and their antigen recognition. Usually, the antigen response requires both B- and T-lymphocytes, termed T-cell dependent. Less commonly, antigens may stimulate immune response only through B-lymphocytes, termed T-cell independent. Initially, the foreign material introduced by vaccines is phagocytized and broken down by macrophages. This breakdown produces peptides as byproducts, which are displayed as antigens on the surface of macrophages using major histocompatibility complexes (MHC-I or MHC-II). This antigen presentation stimulates several inflammatory mediators, and an immune response is followed.

In T-cell-dependent immunity, helper T-cells recognize the antigen and stimulate the corresponding B-lymphocytes to proliferate and differentiate into antibody-forming plasma cells. These antibodies act as soldiers of the immune system and defend microbial attack by inactivating soluble protein toxins (antitoxins), damaging the bacterial membrane (lysins), and preventing the reproduction of pathogenic viruses (neutralizing antibodies) and bacterial adhesion to mucosal surfaces (antiadhesion). As a response to vaccines, the first antibodies produced are primarily immunoglobulin M (IgM), with a gradual switch to immunoglobin G (IgG) in the following weeks.[4]

Types of Immunity

There are two basic mechanisms for acquiring immunity: Active and passive.

Active Immunity

Active immunity is protection produced by a person's own immune system, which usually lasts for many years, often for a lifetime. One way to acquire active immunity is to survive infection (exposure) with the pathogenic organism, which will induce a lifelong immunity to that disease through memory B-cells.

Another way to produce active immunity is by vaccination. The process of generating an immune response has been explained above. However, several factors influence the immune response to vaccination. These include the presence of maternal antibodies, the nature and dose of antigen, the route of administration, and the presence of an adjuvant. In addition to this, host factors, such as age, nutrition, genetics, and coexisting disease, may also affect the immune response. The more similar a vaccine is to the disease-causing form of the organism, the better the immune response to the vaccine.[5]

Passive Immunity

Passive immunity is protection through antibody or antitoxin produced by one animal or human and transferred to another. Passive immunity provides immediate protection against infection, but that protection is usually temporary. The antibodies transferred, eventually, diminish over a few weeks or months, and the recipient will no longer be protected. A classic example of passive immunity is an infant receiving antibodies from the mother, primarily during the last 1–2 months of pregnancy. Passive immunity can also be acquired through blood/blood product transfusion as well as through concentrated inoculation of homologous-pooled human antibody, homologous human hyperimmune globulin, and heterologous hyperimmune serum.[6]

Classification of Vaccines

There are two basic types of vaccines:

1. Live, attenuated
2. Inactivated

   Their characteristics are different and determine how each type is used.

Live, Attenuated Vaccines

Live vaccines are derived from "wild" viruses or bacteria. These wild viruses or bacteria are weakened (attenuated) in a laboratory, usually by repeated culturing. The immune response is generated only when the live, attenuated microbe replicates in the vaccinated person, creating enough of the organism to stimulate the response. It usually results in disease that is much milder than the natural disease and is considered as an adverse reaction to the vaccine. However, administering a live, attenuated vaccine may cause a severe infection among individuals with weakened immune systems [e.g., human immunodeficiency virus (HIV) infected, leukemia].

Inactivated Vaccines

Inactivated vaccines are not live and cannot replicate, and hence can safely be administered in an immunodeficient person. However, inactivated antigens are less affected by circulating antibodies, so they are given when an antibody is present in the blood. The immunity achieved by inactivated vaccines is usually short lived as compared to live, attenuated vaccines, therefore requiring multiple doses over time in order to boost the diminishing antibody titers.[7]

CORONAVIRUS DISEASE 2019

COVID-19 Virus

Coronavirus disease 2019 (COVID-19) is a disease of the respiratory tract caused by the severe acute respiratory syndrome coronavirus 2 (SARS-CoV-2 virus), a ribonucleic acid (RNA) virus of the *Coronaviridae* family.[8] COVID-19 is primarily spread through respiratory droplets, aerosols, and direct person-to-person contact. Common symptoms include headache, fatigue, cough, and muscle aches. In severe cases, COVID-19 can lead to pneumonia, acute respiratory distress syndrome, multiple organ failure, and death. The long-term sequelae of COVID-19 infection involve varied symptoms, affecting most organ systems and impacting both physical and mental health.[9] As with other coronaviruses, SARS-CoV-2 encodes four major structural proteins, spike (S), membrane (M), envelope (E), and a helical nucleocapsid (N), of which S glycoprotein is identified as the main antigenic target.

COVID-19 Pandemic

Initial reports of severe respiratory infections of an unknown origin first arose in Wuhan, China, in late 2019, with infected lower respiratory tract samples subsequently detecting novel coronavirus. By March 2020, the WHO declared COVID-19 a global pandemic.[10] During the initial period of the disease, the efforts were concentrated on preventing and slowing down transmission. Global analysis of herd immunity warranted an urgent need for efficacious COVID-19-preventive measures. Major efforts were made to quickly develop means for its control, treatment, and prevention, including, most importantly, vaccines against COVID-19.[11]

India reported its first case on January 30, 2020, subsequently facing the pandemic in the country as well. The pandemic had an influence on practically every aspect of life, enforcing lockdowns, altering how people work, and overwhelming our existing healthcare system. Other than treating symptomatic patients, the prevention and control of the epidemic targeted monitoring asymptomatic infections, contact tracking, high-risk population screening, and disinfection of the epidemic source. However, an effective vaccination drive seemed to be the only way out.[12]

COVID-19 Vaccine Development in India (Fig. 1)

In early June 2020, the WHO facilitated engagement of vaccine manufacturer's network members giving rise to a dedicated facility called COVID-19 Vaccine Global Access Facility (COVAX). India became the largest producer of vaccines in the COVAX coalition. The Indian COVID-19 vaccine development mission known as the "COVID *Suraksha* Mission" was launched in November 2020, with a focus on accelerating end-to-end vaccine development starting from preclinical development to clinical trials

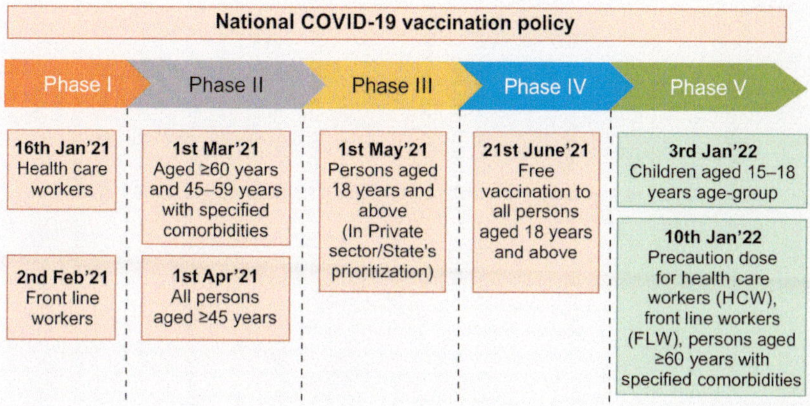

FIGURE 1: Timeline of national COVID-19 vaccination policy in India.
(FLW: frontline workers; HCW: healthcare workers)
Source: Ministry of Health and Family Welfare, Government of India.

to manufacturing and regulatory facilitation. The mission was envisaged for making available safe and efficacious COVID-19 vaccine which is affordable and accessible. The planning of the vaccination drive was initiated based on scientific evidence and global best practices **(Table 1)**.

A comprehensive strategy based on six key principles was evolved:
1. *Adoption of a universal program approach* to include those above 18 years of age and provision of "free of cost" vaccines at all government health centers
2. *"Aatmanirbharta"* or self-reliance based on which the government provided technology and funding support for the development of indigenous vaccines
3. *Prioritization of beneficiaries* or adoption of a "layered approach" based on global best practices and WHO guidelines
4. Development of a *digital interface* to facilitate the process of mass vaccination and to provide for registration, online certificate generation, and tracking of eligible beneficiaries
5. *"One earth, one health"* approach and proactive sharing of our experiences, expertise, and resources with the global community in this battle
6. *Consultative and collaborative approach* ensuring that all key stakeholders who had a role to play were engaged from day 1

In the latter half of 2020 in India, there were nearly 30 vaccine candidates in different stages of development [trials led by the Indian Council of Medical Research (ICMR) and the National AIDS Research Institute (NARI), Pune]. In addition to this, the Department of Biotechnology (DBT) and the Department of Science and Technology (DST) were supporting more than 20 vaccine candidates.[13] Such a variety of technology platforms

TABLE 1: Current status of COVID-19 vaccines in India.

Company and collaborating agency	Brand name	Vaccine design	Current status
Serum Institute of India (SII), Pune, India (in collaboration with University of Oxford, UK, and AstraZeneca)	Covishield	Nonreplicating chimpanzee adenovirus vaccine vector (ChAdOx1)	Available
Bharat Biotech Ltd, Hyderabad, India (in collaboration with the National Institute of Virology of ICMR, India)	Covaxin	Inactivated-virus vaccine	Available
Dr. Reddy's Laboratories, Hyderabad, India (vaccine developed by Gamaleya National Research Institute of Epidemiology and Microbiology, Moscow, Russia)	Sputnik V	Inactivated human adenovirus Ad5 and Ad26 with spike protein inserts	Available
Biological E. Limited (BioE) (vaccine developed by Texas Children's Hospital Center for Vaccine Development and Baylor College of Medicine in Houston, Texas and Dynavax Technologies based in Emeryville, California)	Corbevax	Protein subunit vaccine harvest from cultured yeast Pichia pastoris	DCGI approval for restricted use in emergency situations
Cadila Healthcare, Zydus Cadila, Ahmedabad, India [supported by the Department of Biotechnology (DBT), Government of India]	ZyCoV-D	Plasmid DNA vaccine	DCGI approval for restricted use in emergency situations
Bharat Biotech Limited in collaboration with DBT and Biotechnology Industry Research Assistance Council (BIRAC)	BBV154	Intranasal replication-deficient chimpanzee adenovirus vaccine	DCGI approval for restricted use in emergency situations
Indian Council of Medical Research in collaboration with Serum Institute of India	Covovax	Recombinant spike protein nanoparticle vaccine	DCGI approval for restricted use in emergency situations
Gennova Biopharmaceuticals Limited in collaboration with HDT Bio Corp and NIH, USA with DBT, India	HGC019	Novel mRNA-based vaccine	Phase 2/3 trials ongoing

(DCGI: Drug Controller General of India; DNA: deoxyribonucleic acid; ICMR: Indian Council of Medical Research; mRNA: messenger ribonucleic acid; NIH: National Institutes of Health)

TABLE 2: Clinical description of COVID-19 vaccines.

Brand name	Storage temperature	Number of doses	Administration route	Dose interval
Covishield	2–8°C	Two	Intramuscular	Day 0 + Day 28
Covaxin	2–8°C	Two	Intramuscular	Day 0 + Day 14
Sputnik V	−18°C	Two	Intramuscular	Day 0 + Day 21
Corbevax	2–8°C	Two	Intramuscular	Day 0 + Day 28
ZyCoV-D	2–8°C	Three	Intradermal	Day 0 + Day 28 + Day 56
BBV154	2–8°C	One	Intranasal	Day 0
Covovax	2–8°C	Two	Intramuscular	Day 0 + Day 21

were developed in order to build an effective COVID-19 vaccine including nucleic acid technologies [nucleoside-modified messenger RNA and Deoxyribonucleic acid (DNA)], nonreplicating viral vectors, peptides, recombinant proteins, live attenuated viruses, and inactivated viruses.[14] The top contenders were the Covishield, Covaxin, and Sputnik V **(Table 2)**.

COVISHIELD

In January 2021, India approved Oxford–AstraZeneca (Covishield) vaccine, the ChAdOx1 nCoV-19 (recombinant vector) replication-deficient adenoviral vector vaccine (Covishield™), manufactured by the Serum Institute of India. The vaccine comprised of 5×10^{10} virus particles replicated as a deficient chimpanzee adenovirus vector encoding the SARS-CoV-2 spike glycoprotein produced in the modified human embryonic kidney cells. The vaccination is injected in two doses of 0.5 mL into the deltoid muscle with a second dose followed at 4–12 weeks. Covishield can be securely maintained at temperatures ranging from 2 to 8°C and conveniently distributed in existing healthcare environments such as doctors' offices. Contraindications of Covishield include hypersensitive individuals, thrombosis, thrombocytopenia condition, and immune-compromised patients. Minor side effects such as pain at the site of injection, muscle ache, fatigue, dizziness, headache, fever, irregular heart rhythm, and diarrhea have been reported.[15]

The Ministry of Health and Family Welfare, Government of India, launched a massive, free vaccination program starting January 16, 2021, almost a year after the first reported case in the country, with more than 3,000 centers delivering Covishield or Covaxin across the nation.[16] However, the positivity rate was rising at the moment, leading to the catastrophic second wave of COVID-19 in March 2021 wherein the health system was overwhelmed by the scarcity of hospital beds, vaccines, oxygen supply, and other medical services across all Indian states. The available resources (oxygen, drugs, ventilators, etc.) got exhausted quickly and hospitals had no isolation wards left, thereby leading to a massive number of casualties.

Covishield was the first vaccine to receive emergency use authorization approval by the Drugs Controller General of India (DCGI) in early January 2021. A study (2020) showed that Covishield was 76% efficient after the first dose and 81.3% following the second dose.[17] Another study reported that the efficacy was 81% against B.1.1.7 (alpha variant) and 61% against B.1.617.2 (delta variant).[18]

COVAXIN

India's first indigenous SARS-CoV-2 inactivated vaccine, Covaxin (BBV152), was developed and manufactured by Bharat Biotech (a Hyderabad-based pioneering biotechnology company) in association with the National Institute of Virology (NIV), Pune. This homegrown vaccine has reported up to 93% efficacy against severe SARS-CoV-2 infection, 78% against symptomatic cases, and 65% against the newly emerged delta variant.[19] Covaxin was rolled out in the National COVID-19 Vaccination Program after receiving permission from the Central Drugs Standard Control Organization (CDSCO). This indigenous Indian vaccine gained authorization in some other nations such as Zimbabwe, Nepal, Philippines, Iran, Guyana, Venezuela, Guatemala, and Botswana.[20]

The inactivated virus in the vaccine is combined with Alhydroxiquim-II (Algel-IMDG), chemosorbed imidazoquinoline onto aluminum hydroxide gel, as an adjuvant to boost immune response and longer-lasting immunity. The two doses of Covaxin are separated by 4 weeks. The vaccine can be kept at temperatures ranging from 2 to 8°C. The vaccine had shown efficacy in neutralizing B.1.617 (delta variant) and zeta variant or P.2 (B.1.1.28) in investigations led by ICMR and NIV, Pune.[21]

SPUTNIK-V

Gam-COVID-Vac, also known as Sputnik V, is a COVID-19 vaccine developed by the Gamaleya National Center of Epidemiology and Microbiology of Moscow, Russia. It employs a harmless cold-type virus as a carrier to carry a small fragment of the coronavirus to the body. By exposing the body to a portion of the virus's genetic code in this way, it learns to recognize the antigen and develops a defense system. This vaccine can be stored at temperatures ranging from 2 to 8°C and conveniently transported as other vaccines.[11]

On April 12, 2021, DCGI granted emergency use approval to Sputnik-V in India. Dr Reddy's Laboratories, a Hyderabad-based pharmaceutical company, facilitated the import as well as large-scale manufacture of Sputnik-V in India. Sputnik V comprises two genetically modified E1 gene-deficient human adenoviruses: Ad26 and Ad5. These recombinant adenovirus types contain the SARS-CoV-2 S protein cDNA. Both of them are administered into the deltoid muscle. The Ad26-based vaccine is administered on day 1 and Ad5 on day 21 to boost immune responses.[22]

CORBEVAX

CORBEVAX™ SARS-CoV-2 (also named as Biological-E) vaccine is a protein subunit COVID-19 vaccine developed by Texas Children's Hospital Center for Vaccine Development and Baylor College of Medicine in Houston, Texas, and Dynavax Technologies based in Emeryville, California. It is licensed to the Indian biopharmaceutical firm Biological E. Limited (BioE) for development and production.

The vaccine is formulated from the virus's spike protein harvest from cultured yeast *Pichia pastoris* and is used in combination with adjuvants like aluminum hydroxide gel and CpG 1018.[15] The vaccine is intended for use in individuals above 12 years. The second dose of the vaccine is administered at least 4 weeks after the first dosage, and the related adverse effects in some individuals may include discomfort at the injection site, headache, high temperature, tiredness, nausea, and myalgia.

ZYCOV-D

ZyCoV-D, another domestic COVID-19 vaccine, by Zydus Cadila, Ahmedabad, is based on the new plasmid DNA vaccine technology. Plasmids are used as vectors to directly deliver the DNA encoding the target antigens into the body of the recipient. Sequence encoding for the pathogen's antigen is engineered into recombinant plasmid DNA. This vaccine is administered intradermally. Currently, the phase 2 human trials are going on for this vaccine.[11]

BBV154: INTRANASAL VACCINE

Bharat Biotech is conducting a multicentric study to evaluate the reactogenicity, safety, and immunogenicity of an intranasal adenoviral vector COVID-19 vaccine (BBV154) in healthy volunteers. BBV154 is an intranasal vaccine that stimulates a broad immune response—neutralizing IgG, mucosal IgA, and T-cell responses. Immune responses at the site of infection (in the nasal mucosa) are essential for blocking both infection and transmission of COVID-19. So far, phase 1 human trials are ongoing for this vaccine.[23]

COVOVAX

Indian Council of Medical Research and Serum Institute of India are jointly performing a phase 2/3, observer-blind, randomized controlled study to determine the safety and immunogenicity of COVOVAX [SARS-CoV-2 recombinant spike protein nanoparticle vaccine (SARS-CoV-2 rS) with Matrix-M1™ adjuvant] in Indian adults. This vaccine is currently undergoing phase 2/3 human clinical trials.[23]

mRNA-BASED VACCINE (HGCO19)

A randomized, phase 1/2, placebo-controlled, dose-ranging study is undergoing to evaluate the safety, tolerability, and immunogenicity of the candidate HGCO19 (COVID-19 vaccine) in healthy adult subjects. Gennova Biopharmaceuticals Limited is currently conducting the phase 1/2 trial.[23]

VACCINE ACCEPTANCE AND HESITANCY

With the development and availability of COVID-19 vaccines, there were some concerns regarding safety, efficacy, efficiency, negative aftereffects, and vaccine necessity among the Indian population.[24] The Strategic Advisory Group of Experts (SAGE), a working group of the WHO, has defined vaccine hesitancy as "the delay in acceptance or refusal of vaccines despite availability of vaccine service".

Vaccine hesitancy had been a major limiting factor in the initial times, contributing to a considerable challenge in attaining herd immunity. It is complicated and context specific, differing across time, place, and vaccine to vaccine. According to a systematic review conducted in February 2021, the global acceptability rate of COVID-19 vaccines ranged from 27.7 to 77.3%.[25] Consequently, the WHO has since listed vaccine hesitancy as one of the top 10 global health risks, even before the COVID-19 pandemic.

However, the Ministry of Health and Family Welfare, Government of India, helped improve vaccine acceptance through the development of trustworthy communication and information platforms to make general people aware of the benefits and availability of vaccines. Apart from this, the Government of India issued a portal named CoWIN for the function of registration, appointment scheduling, identity verification, vaccination, and certification of each vaccinated member. Understanding the vaccine hesitancy and the factors involved would be important for policymakers in planning competent strategies for the effective implementation of mass vaccination programs.

SUMMARY

With the introduction of COVID-19 vaccines, India has managed to control the epidemic; however, the loss cannot be quantified in any measure. India has been acknowledged as one of the chief contributors to the global COVID-19 vaccines. The country has an immense capacity for manufacturing and a robust mechanism for logistics, management, and distribution. However, organizing a national immunization program for preventing COVID-19 is challenging because of India's large population and overwhelmed health infrastructure. India and the world are at an important point in the history of the pandemic where the vaccines show a ray of hope for the end of COVID-19.

REFERENCES

1. DeStefano F, Bodenstab HM, Offit PA. Principal Controversies in Vaccine Safety in the United States. Clin Infect Dis. 2019;69(4):726-31.
2. Liebowitz D. Smallpox vaccination: An early start of modern medicine in America. J Community Hosp Intern Med Perspect. 2017;7(1):61-3.
3. Ginglen JG, Doyle MQ. Immunization. In: StatPearls [Internet]. Treasure Island (FL): StatPearls Publishing; 2023. [online] Available from https://www.ncbi.nlm.nih.gov/books/NBK459331/ [Last accessed February, 2024].
4. Baxter D. Active and passive immunity, vaccine types, excipients and licensing. Occup Med (Lond). 2007;57(8):552-6.
5. American Academy of Pediatrics. Active and passive immunization. In: Kimberlin DW, Brady MT, Jackson MA, Long SS (Eds). Red Book: 2018 Report of the Committee on Infectious Diseases, 31st edition. Itasca, IL: American Academy of Pediatrics; 2018. pp. 13-64.
6. Plotkin SA. Vaccines, vaccination, and vaccinology. J Infect Dis. 2003;187(9):1349-59.
7. Siegrist C. Vaccine immunology. In: Plotkin SA, Orenstein WA, Offit PA, Edwards KM (Eds). Plotkin's Vaccines, 7th edition. Elsevier; 2018. pp. 16-34.
8. Zhu N, Zhang D, Wang W, Li X, Yang B, Song J, et al. A novel coronavirus from patients with pneumonia in China, 2019. N Engl J Med. 2020;382(8):727-33.
9. Menni C, Valdes AM, Polidori L, Antonelli M, Penamakuri S, Nogal A, et al. Symptom prevalence, duration, and risk of hospital admission in individuals infected with SARS-CoV-2 during periods of omicron and delta variant dominance: A prospective observational study from the ZOE COVID Study. Lancet. 2022;399(10335):1618-24.
10. Cucinotta D, Vanelli M. WHO Declares COVID-19 a Pandemic. Acta Biomed. 2020;91(1):157-60.
11. Kumar VM, Pandi-Perumal SR, Trakht I, Panchatcharam Thyagarajan S. Strategy for COVID-19 vaccination in India: The country with the second highest population and number of cases. NPJ Vaccines. 2021;6(1):60.
12. Chauhan N, Manjunath BC, Yadav V, Kumar A, Sabbarwal B, Kumar JS. COVID-19 Vaccine Development in India during January 2021-December 2021: A Narrative Review. Saudi J Med. 2022;7(2):118-26.
13. Pathak D, Philo Magdalene A. COVID-19 Vaccine Development and Administration in India. In: Pachauri S, Pachauri A (Eds). Health Dimensions of COVID-19 in India and Beyond. Singapore: Springer; 2022. pp. 129-54.
14. Yan ZP, Yang M, Lai CL. COVID19 vaccines: A review of the safety and efficacy of current clinical trials. Pharmaceuticals (Basel). 2021;14(5):406.
15. Chavda VP, Vihol DR, Solanki HK, Apostolopoulos V. The Vaccine World of COVID-19: India's Contribution. Vaccines (Basel). 2022;10(11):1943.
16. Patel RB, Patel BB. An analysis of the COVID-19 situation in India in terms of testing, treatment, vaccine acceptance and national economic performance. Int J Public Health. 2022;67:1604975.
17. Voysey M, Costa Clemens SA, Madhi SA, Weckx LY, Folegatti PM, Aley PK, et al.; Oxford COVID Vaccine Trial Group. Single-dose administration and the influence of the timing of the booster dose on immunogenicity and efficacy of ChAdOx1 nCoV-19 (AZD1222) Vaccine: A pooled analysis of four randomised trials. Lancet. 2021;397(10277):881-91.

18. Sheikh A, McMenamin J, Taylor B, Robertson C; Public Health Scotland and the EAVE II Collaborators. SARS-CoV-2 Delta VOC in Scotland: Demographics, risk of hospital admission, and vaccine effectiveness. Lancet. 2021;397(10293):2461-2.
19. Ella R, Vadrevu KM, Jogdand H, Prasad S, Reddy S, Sarangi V, et al. Safety and Immunogenicity of an Inactivated SARS-CoV-2 Vaccine, BBV152: A double-blind, randomised, phase 1 trial. Lancet Infect Dis. 2021;21(5):637-46.
20. Sapkal GN, Yadav PD, Sahay RR, Deshpande G, Gupta N, Nyayanit DA, et al. Neutralization of delta variant with sera of Covishield vaccines and COVID-19-recovered vaccinated individuals. J Trav Med. 2021;28(7):taab119.
21. Sapkal G, Yadav PD, Ella R, Abraham P, Patil DY, Gupta N, et al. Neutralization of B.1.1.28 P2 Variant with sera of COVID-19 recovered cases and recipients of Covaxin an inactivated COVID-19 vaccine. J Trav Med. 2021;28(7):taab077.
22. Ali A, Kamaraju MM. A study on Covid-19 vaccination drive in India. BRICS J Educ Res. 2021;11(2):76-9.
23. COVID-19 Vaccine. Indian Council of Medical Research. [Internet]. Accessed at: https://vaccine.icmr.org.in/covid-19-vaccine
24. Xiao X, Wong RM. Vaccine hesitancy and perceived behavioral control: A meta-analysis. Vaccine. 2020;38(33):5131-8.
25. Patwary MM, Alam MA, Bardhan M, Disha AS, Haque MZ, Billah SM, et al. COVID-19 vaccine acceptance among low- and lower-middle-income countries: A rapid systematic review and meta-analysis. Vaccines (Basel). 2022;10(3):427.

3

SECTION

Special Issue of Interest

CHAPTER 19

The Art of Living

Kavitha Natarajan

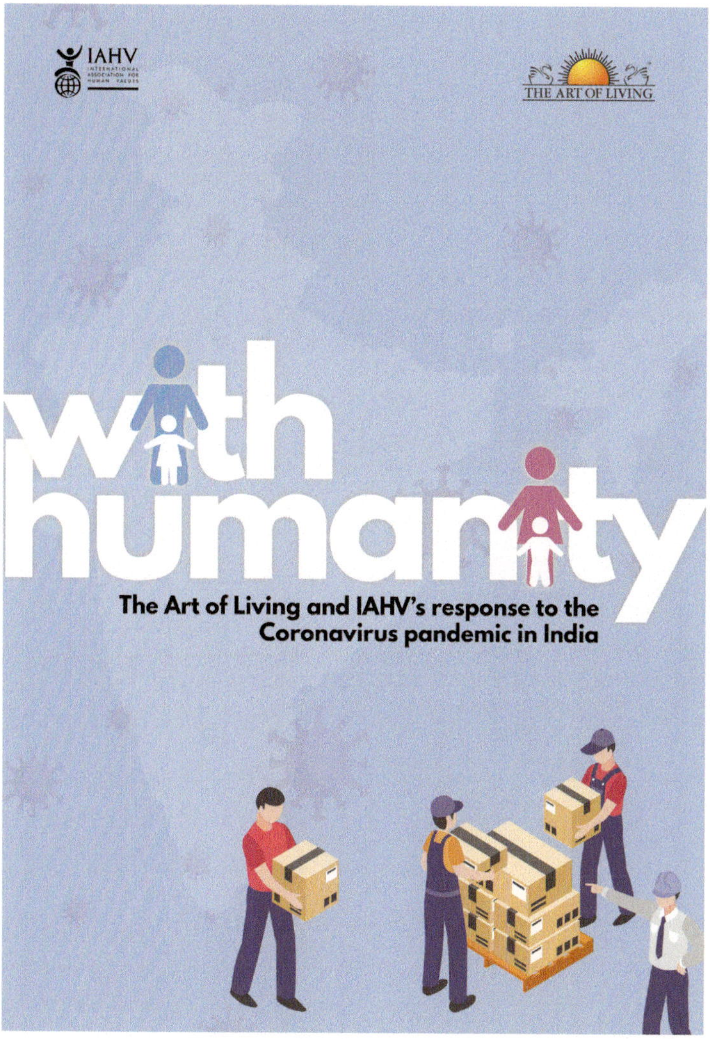

iStandwithHumanity

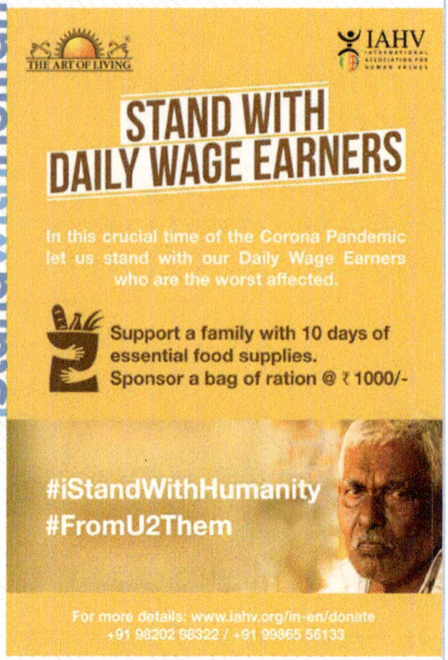
THE ART OF LIVING
IAHV
STAND WITH
DAILY WAGE EARNERS
In this crucial time of the Corona Pandemic let us stand with our Daily Wage Earners who are the worst affected.
Support a family with 10 days of essential food supplies.
Sponsor a bag of ration @ ₹ 1000/-
#iStandWithHumanity
#FromU2Them
For more details: www.iahv.org/in-en/donate
+91 98202 98322 / +91 99865 56133

7,51,22,069 meals

to over 25 lakh families

in India as of May 13th

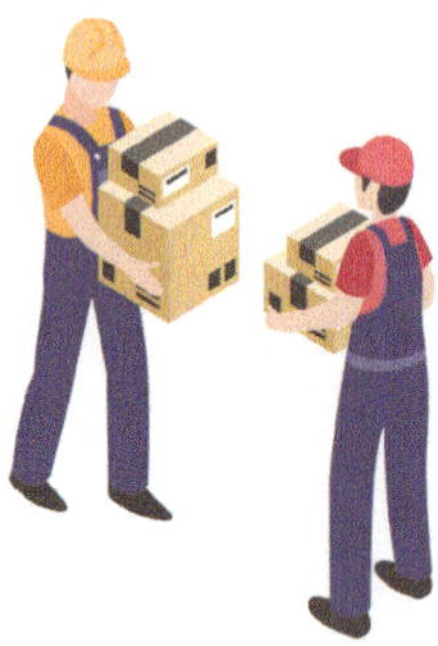

no one goes hungry

In the wake of the global pandemic COVID-19, daily wage workers have taken the hardest economic hit. India's immediate and unforeseen lockdown, while a necessary step in preventing the virus's spread, has caused desperate situations for this vast population of workers living hand to mouth across the country.

In order to ensure these people do not go hungry, the International Association for Human Values (IAHV) along with The Art of Living started a nation-wide initiative on 22nd March 2020 to provide food and essentials needed by this marginalized segment of the population.

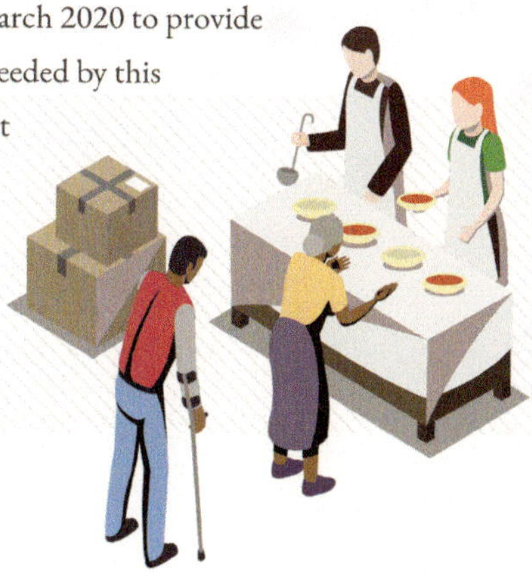

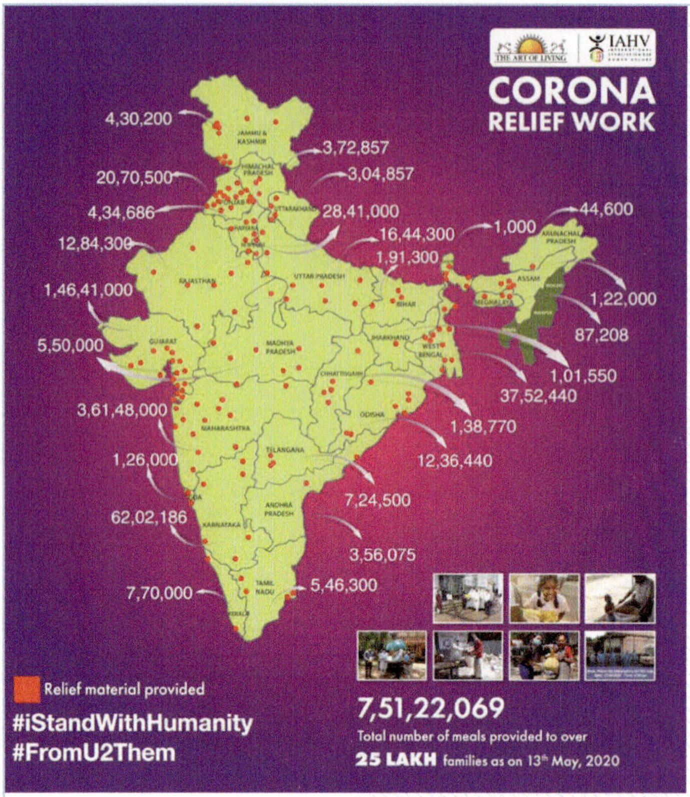

The Art of Living and IAHV teams immediately arranged for the distribution of ration kits, cooked food and PPEs. Each ration kit feeds a family of 4 for 10 days.

Safety of the volunteers and the community was maintained to the highest standards.

relief worth ₹40crore

Our volunteer teams, inspired by the message of *Gurudev* Sri Sri Ravi Shankar, responded swiftly to collect and distribute rations across the country in coordination with local authorities. The efforts of IAHV and The Art of Living have been critical in beginning the process of providing aid.

Gurudev Sri Sri Ravi Shankar prioritised the plight of the daily wage labourer since the beginning of the pandemic and ran an advocacy campaign called **#iStandWithHumanity**. This campaign had the support of national celebrities and reached an estimated audience of over 3 crores in 170 cities across India.

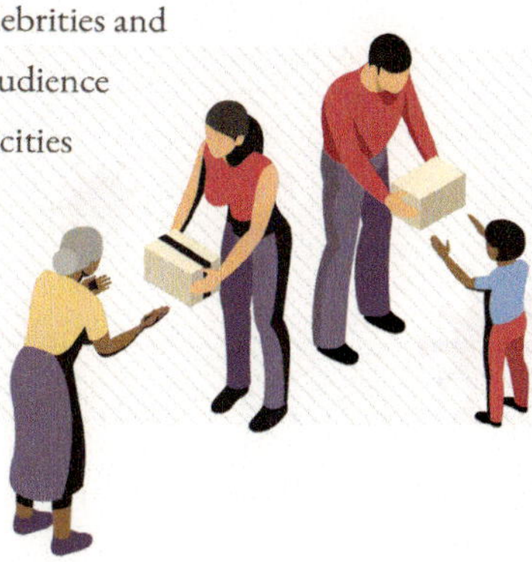

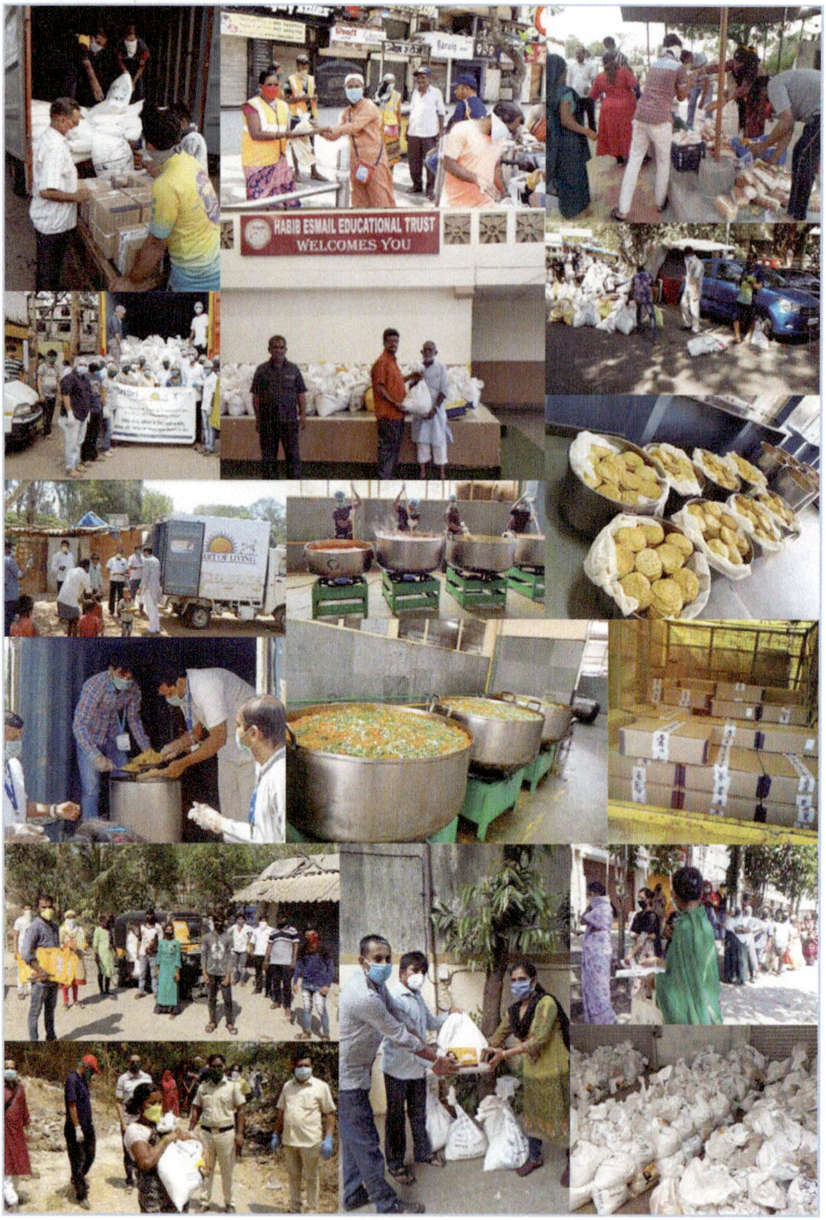
HABIB ESMAIL EDUCATIONAL TRUST
WELCOMES YOU

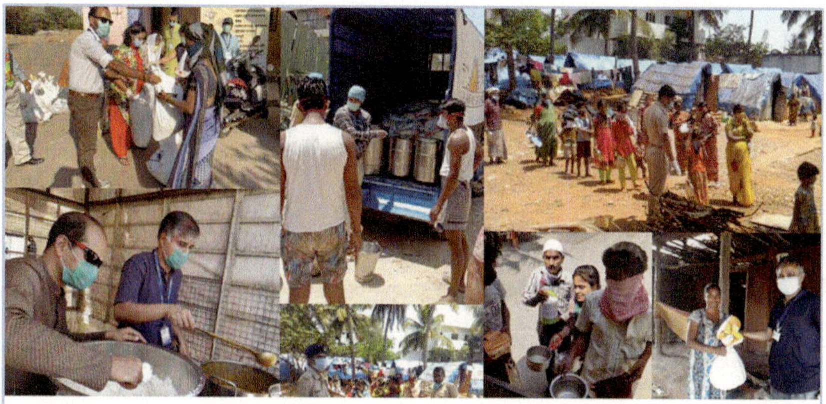

state wise response and relief (highlights)

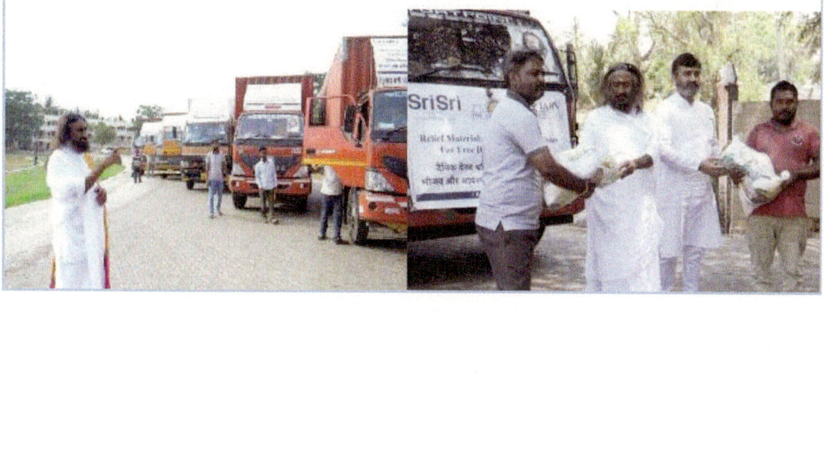

karnataka

34,000 cooked meals a day

provided by Art of Living Bangalore International Kitchen (ISO22000 certified) to migrant workers and nearby villages for the entire month

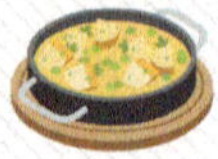

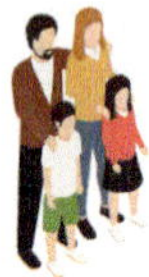

5,000 migrant families

from Bengaluru prevented from leaving the city with the provision of

12 tonnes of ration

over 10 days

5,500 containers of sanitizer

donated to District Administration

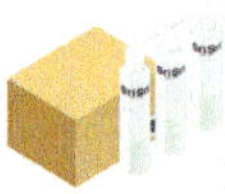

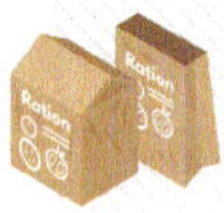

30,000 ration kits

distributed to the needy

325 ration kits

to the Kannada Film Artist Association

550PPE kits, 100 N95 masks & other medical aid

for COVID-19 preparedness provided to Bowring & Lady Curzon Hospital, Bengaluru

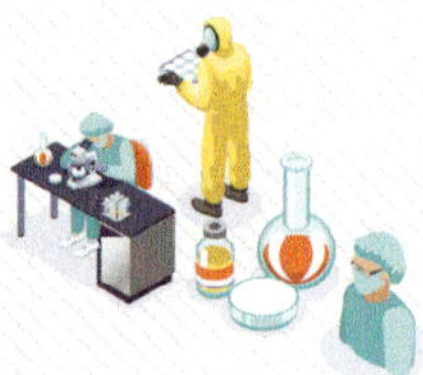

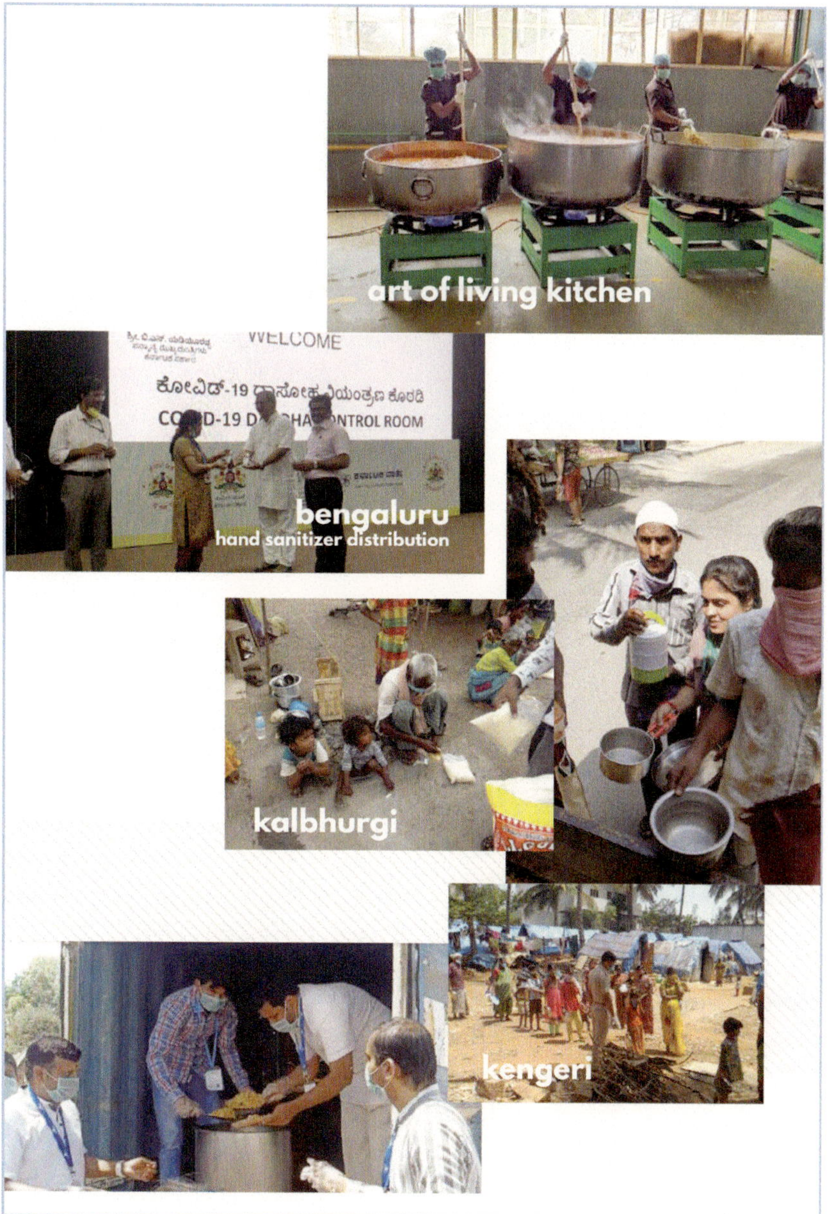
art of living kitchen
WELCOME
bengaluru
hand sanitizer distribution
kalbhurgi
kengeri

maharashtra

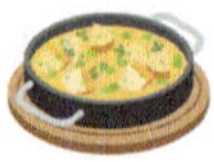

15,00,000 cooked meals
provided to migrant workers from Vasai, Virar, Nala Sopara, Govandi and Dharavi

2,000 ration kits within 30 mins
for migrant workers who flooded Mumbai's Bandra West railway station. Art of Living volunteers created public awareness, counselled and successfully persuaded them to stay back

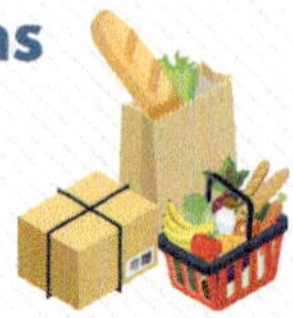

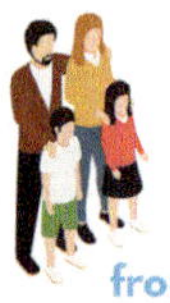

75,000 ration kits for 2,80,000 people
from labourer families (10 days of ration) to avoid a Delhi-like exodus due to starvation

2,000 ration kits (Nagpur)

12,500 ration kits (Pune)

1,000 ration kits
(in both Ahmednagar & Aurangabad)

100 ration kits (Shirpur)

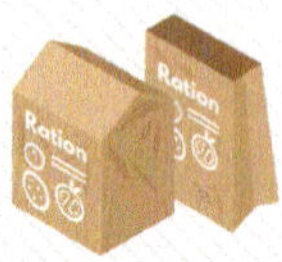

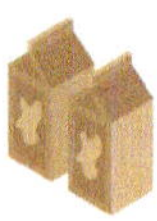

75,000 packets of biscuits
distributed in Mumbai

15,000 packets of biscuits
distributed in Nagpur

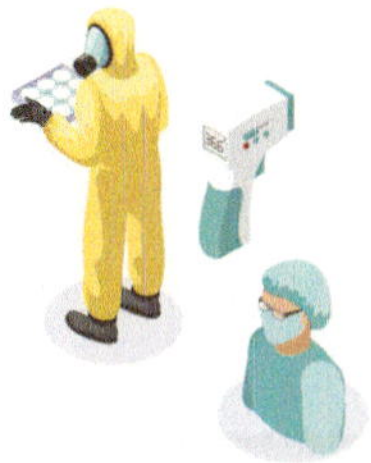

9,000 cloth masks

donated to Thane Municipal Corporation

300 infrared thermometers, 2000 N95 masks, 2000 PPE kits and 7 swab booths

donated to Pune Municipal Corporation

200 PPE kits, 5000 filter masks, 1950 N95 masks, 400 faceshields, 200 sanitizers and 10 infrared thermometers

provided to Sion Hospital through the Maharashtra Association for Residential Doctors

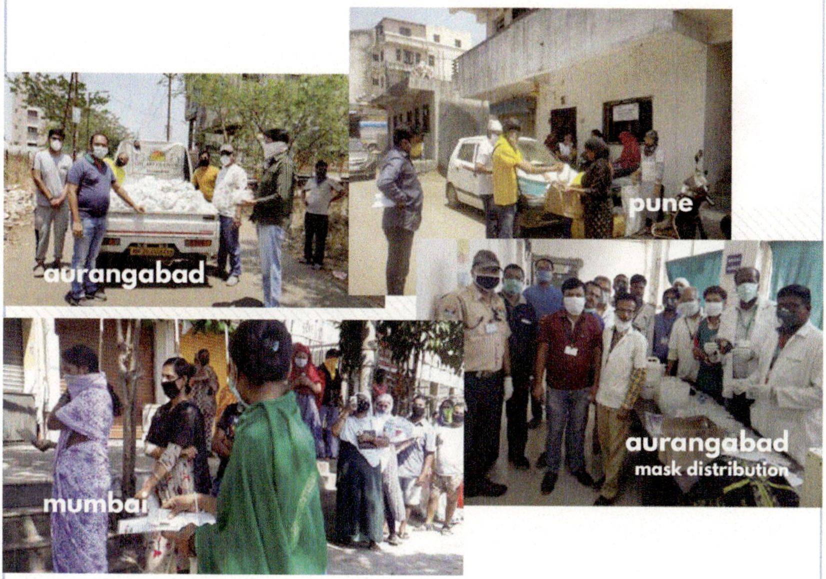

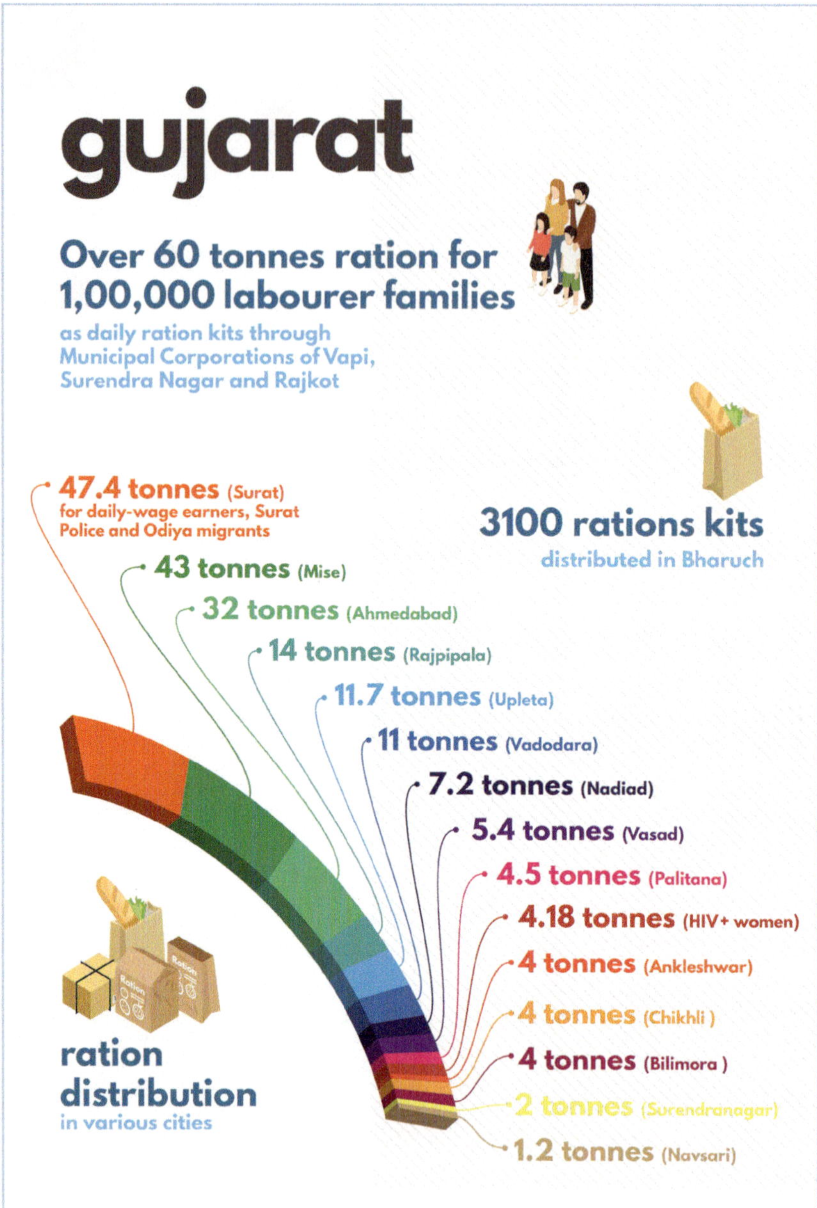
gujarat
Over 60 tonnes ration for 1,00,000 labourer families
as daily ration kits through Municipal Corporations of Vapi, Surendra Nagar and Rajkot
3100 rations kits
distributed in Bharuch
47.4 tonnes (Surat)
for daily-wage earners, Surat Police and Odiya migrants
43 tonnes (Mise)
32 tonnes (Ahmedabad)
14 tonnes (Rajpipala)
11.7 tonnes (Upleta)
11 tonnes (Vadodara)
7.2 tonnes (Nadiad)
5.4 tonnes (Vasad)
4.5 tonnes (Palitana)
4.18 tonnes (HIV+ women)
4 tonnes (Ankleshwar)
4 tonnes (Chikhli)
4 tonnes (Bilimora)
2 tonnes (Surendranagar)
1.2 tonnes (Navsari)
ration distribution
in various cities

Sanitization

Entire village of **Kalimakwana** in Rajpipala has been sanitized

2,000 PPE kits

and homeopathic medicines for **15,000 people** delivered to District Collector in Surat

3,100 masks

distributed in Dharampur

25,000 masks

distributed in Nadiad

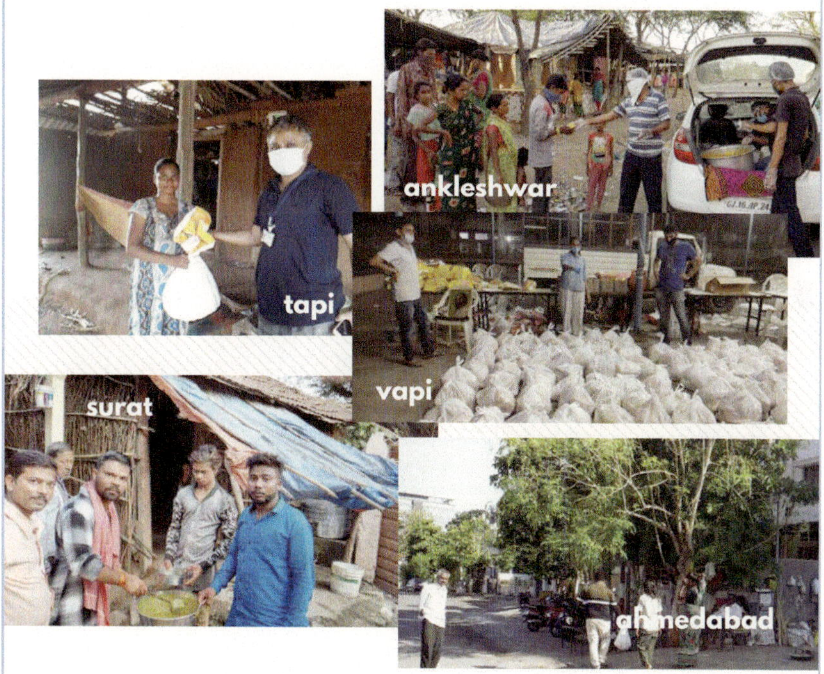

delhi

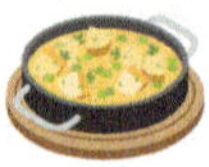

2,00,000 cooked food packets

distributed in slums of Anand Vihar and Pitampura. (Sangam Vihar, Sultanpuri, Sarita Vihar, Naharpur, Mehrauli, Mangol Puri, Alipore)

10,000 food packets

delivered to Delhi Police (Chawari Bazaar, Shastri Park, Yamuna Bank Metro, Nehru Place Metro, Special Branch, DCP office)

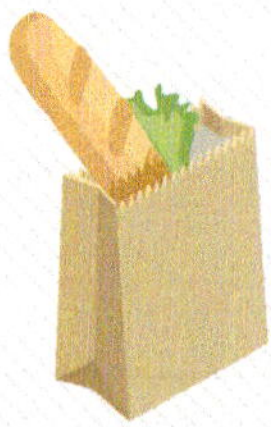

2,000 food packets

delivered to other social organizations including Idea of India & RSS

1,000 food packets

delivered to National Disaster Relief Force

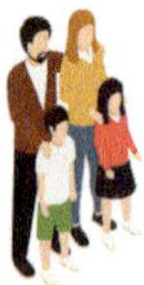

24,000 biscuit packets distributed in Delhi & 10,000 families

provided with **daily meals** in North, West and East Delhi, where thousands were stranded and in dire need of supplies. **Volunteer teams are helping police personnel** persuade people to stay put and not venture out of their area.

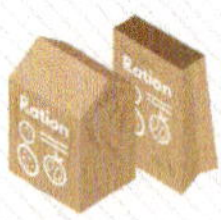

1,000 ration kits

handed to the deputy Mayor of Gurgaon for distribution

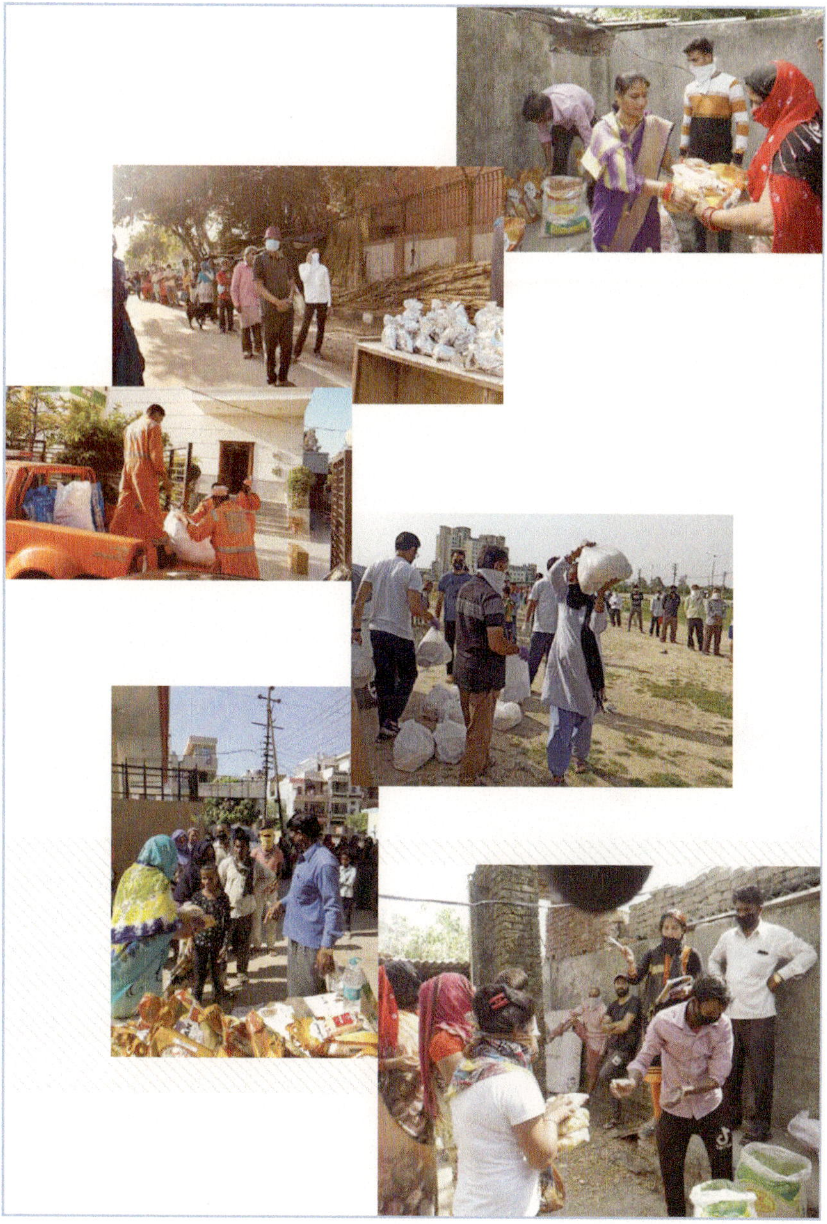

jammu

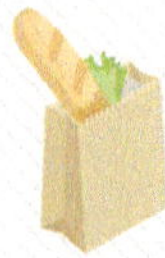

1,200 people

provided with food packets at Preet Nagar, Nanak Nagar, ChanniRama and ChanniHimat

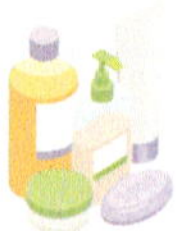

2,000 units of soap

have been distributed

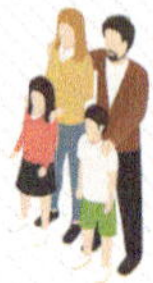

1,500 families

provided with daily rations

300 migrants

planning to leave were stopped and given ration by our volunteers

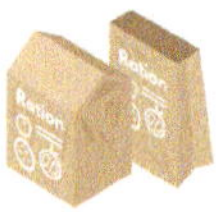

590 ration kits

for migrants distributed with the help of the Divisional Commissioner

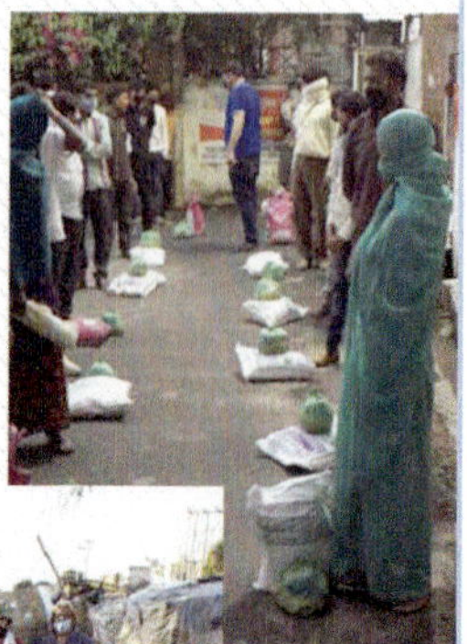

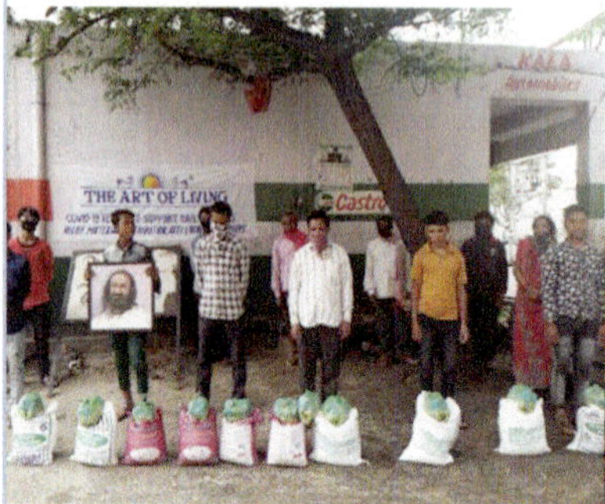

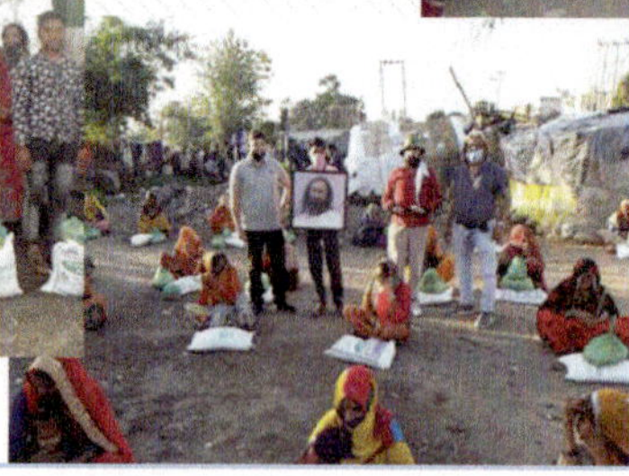

kashmir

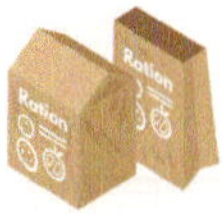

Over 200 children from 4 hostels

provided ration in Kargil

4.5 tonnes of ration

distributed among

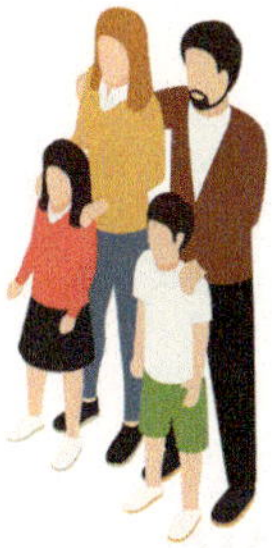

560 families in Chanpora,
110 families in Shergiri,
72 families in Pulwama,
67 families in Jawar Nagar,
62 families in Rambag,
31 families in Rajbag and Fatai Kadal **each**,
30 families in Karan Nagar,
21 families in Sorting, Lasjan and Vichar Nag **each**,
19 families in Bemina,
12 families in Nehru Park among Shikara Workers

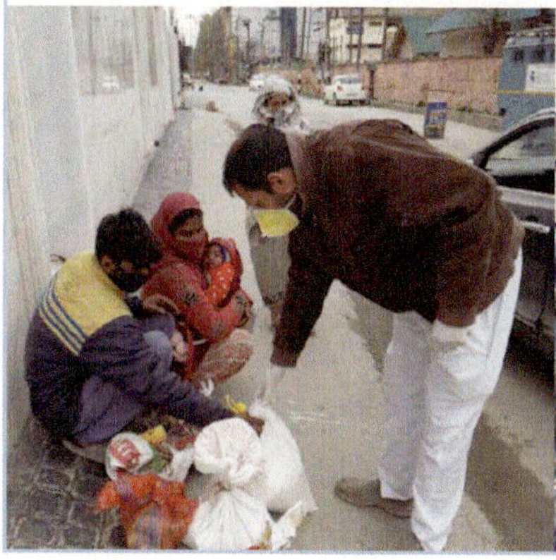

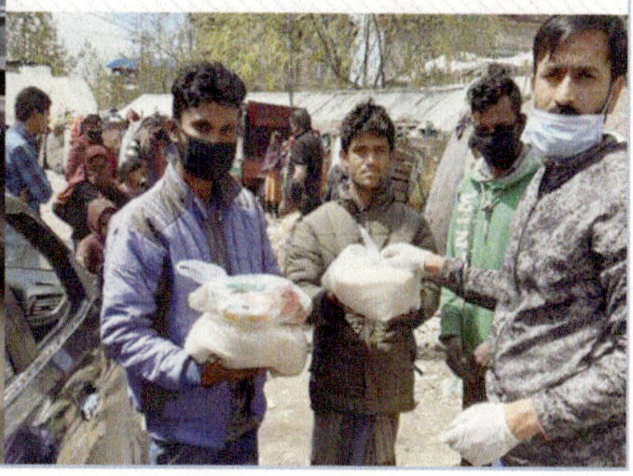

punjab

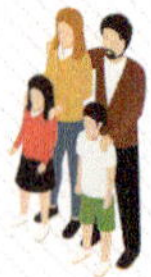

8,500 families

provided with ration for **10 days**

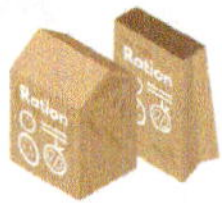

50 tonnes of food materials

have been provided to the local administrations in Bhatinda, Barnala, Faridkot, Muktasar, Nawanshahr, Rajpura, Chandigarh, Mandi Gobindgarh, Jagraon, Mohali, Nangal, Moga, Ferozpur, Ludhiana, Fazilka, Zira, Kapurthala

uttar pradesh

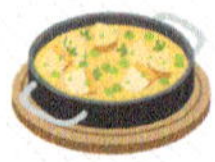

10,000 workers

given cooked food daily in Lucknow, Kanpur and Agra for **15 days**

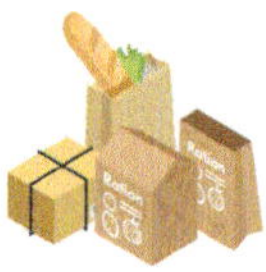

5,000 families

provided ration for **10 days**

haryana

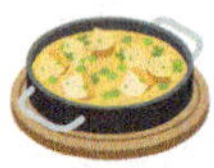

20,400 packets of cooked food

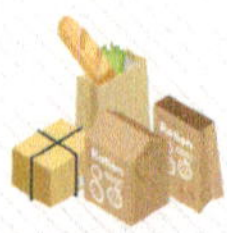

3000 ration kits & 19 tonnes of ration

himachal pradesh

10,000 families provided ration for **20 days**

15 tonnes ration distributed

15,000 packets of biscuits
distributed across the state

uttarakhand

1,15,000 ration kits
distributed across the state
(95,000 in Rishikesh, 20,000 in Dehradun)

50 tonnes ration & 30,000 meals
provided by the Art of Living ashram in Rishikesh

rajasthan

70 tonnes of food packets and cooked food
distributed through District Magistrate across **22 cities**

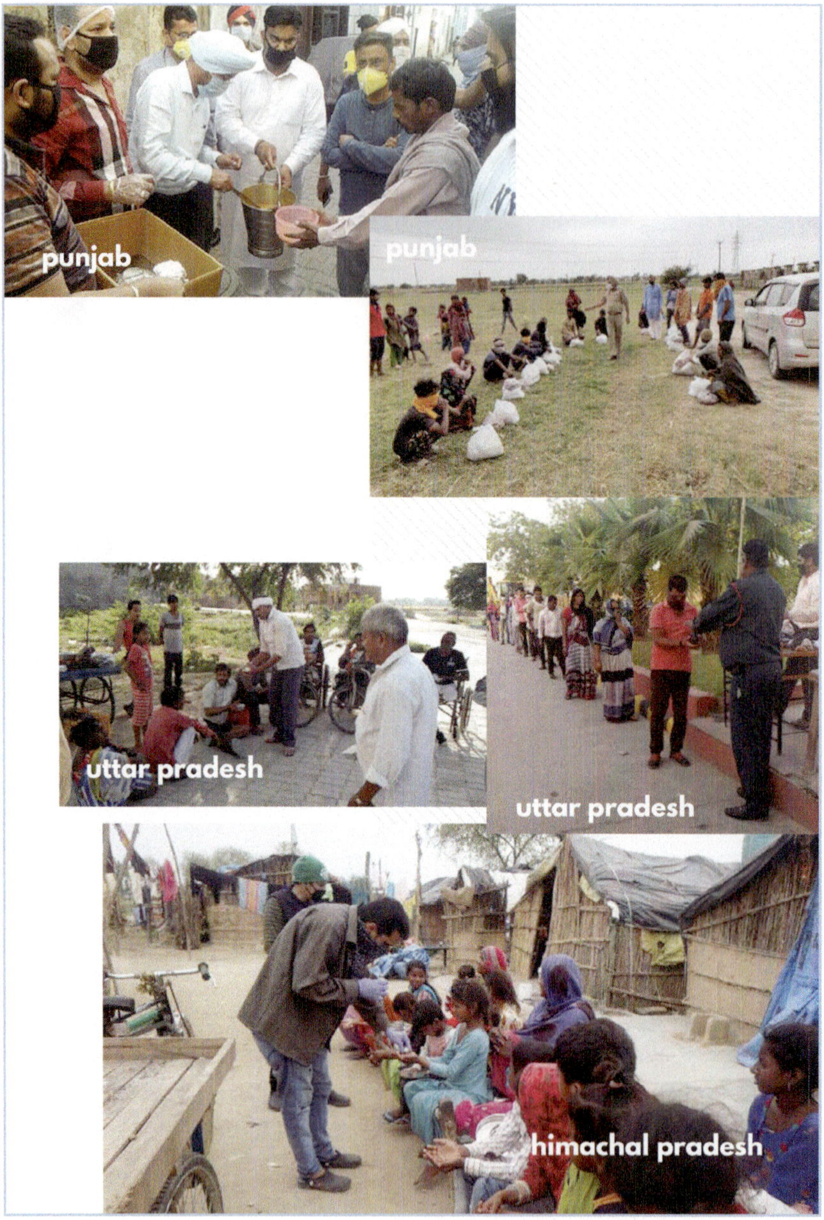
punjab
punjab
uttar pradesh
uttar pradesh
himachal pradesh

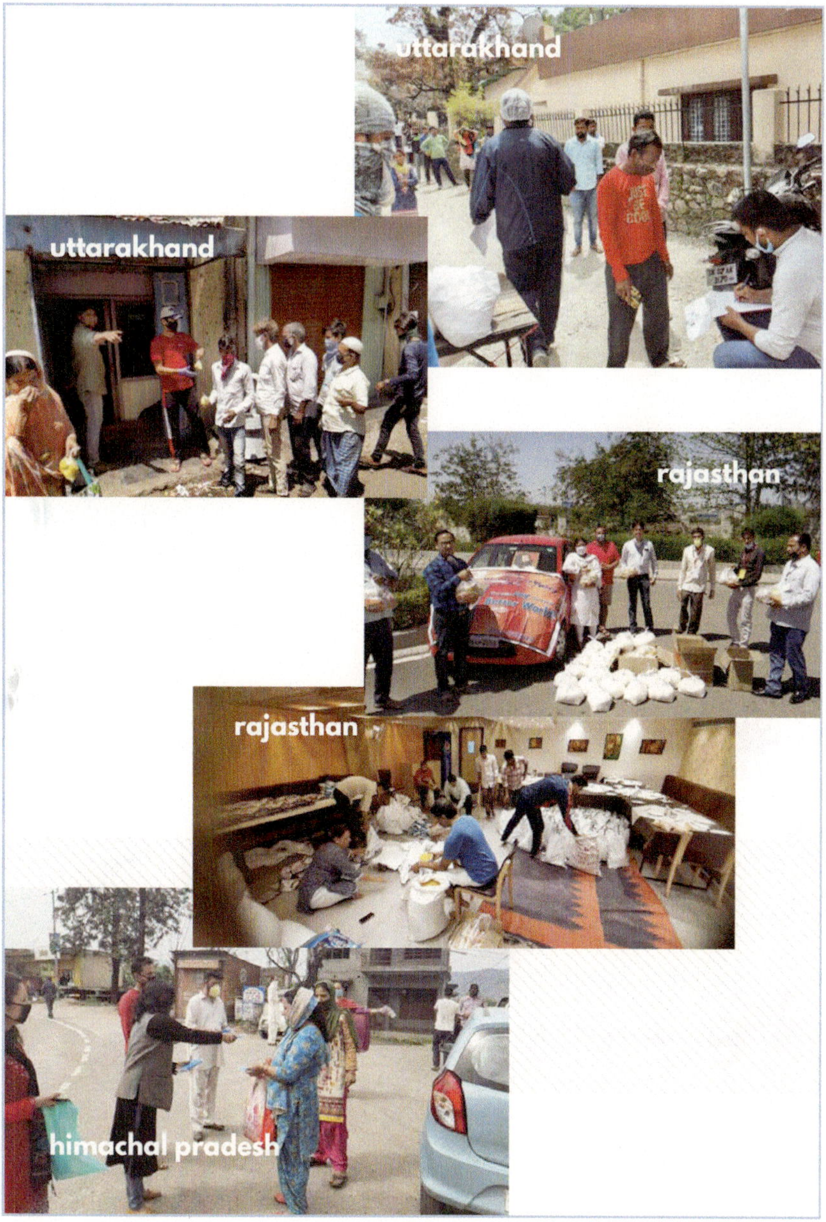
uttarakhand
uttarakhand
rajasthan
rajasthan
himachal pradesh

madhya pradesh

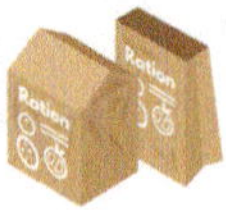

2,000 ration kits
provided across the state

65,000 meals
provided to families of daily wage labourers in Indore

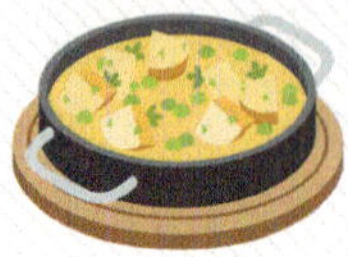

20,000 meals
provided in Gwalior, Seoni, Chhindwara

goa

600 ration kits
supplied to industry workers south Goa

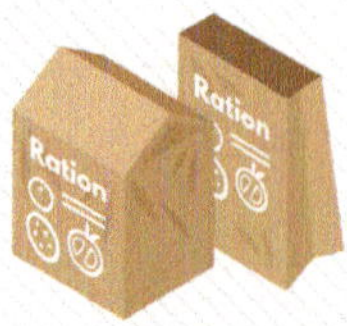

300 ration kits
provided at the Mapsa Police station, girls orphanage and MSG foundation for migrant workers

kerala

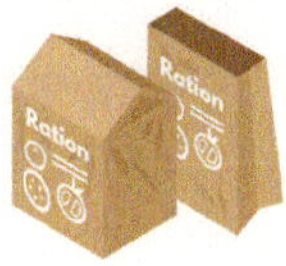

12 tonnes of food grains
distributed in Kasargod district to stop the labour exodus of over **3,000 families**

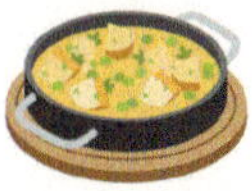

5,000 factory workers
provided cooked food for **15 days**

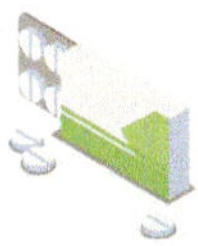

₹ 1 lakh worth medicines
provided to the Police Headquater in Trivandrum

meghalaya

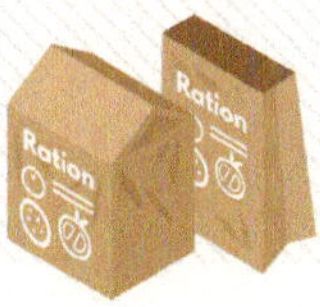

1.5 tonnes of ration
distributed to over **200 families** in Shillong

1 tonne of ration
distributed to **250 labourers** in Garo Hills

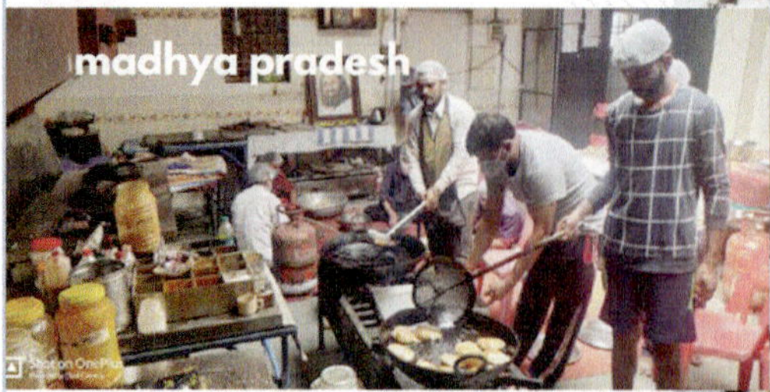
madhya pradesh

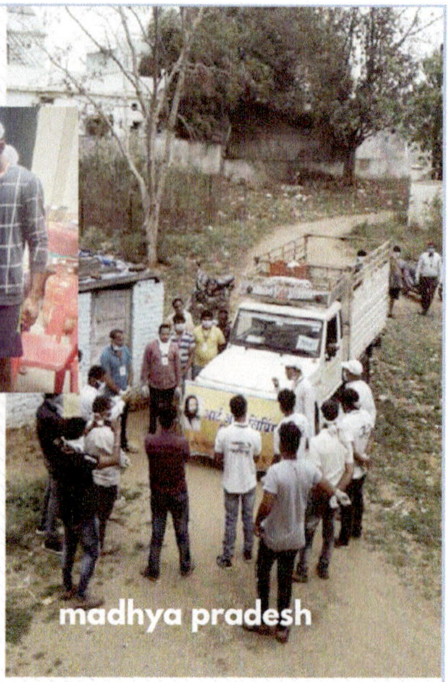
madhya pradesh

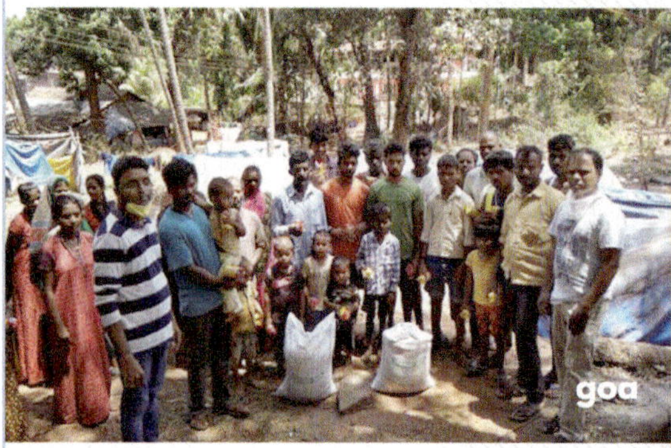
goa

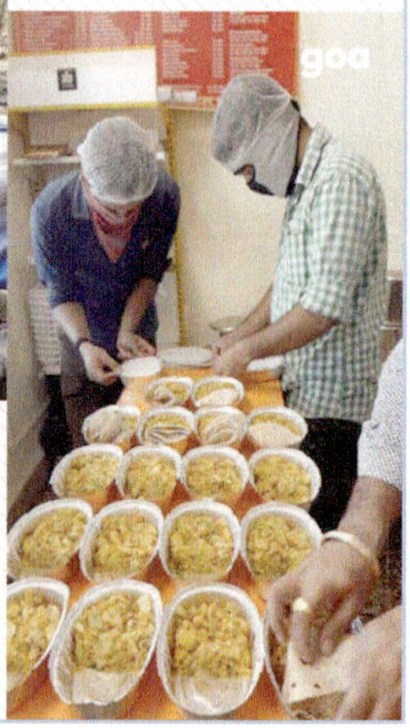
goa

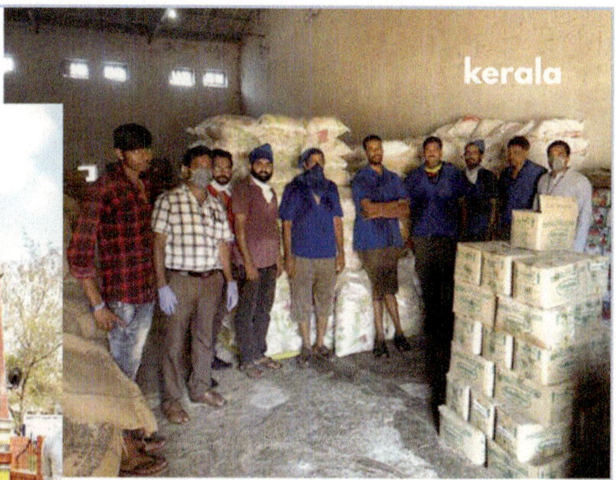
kerala

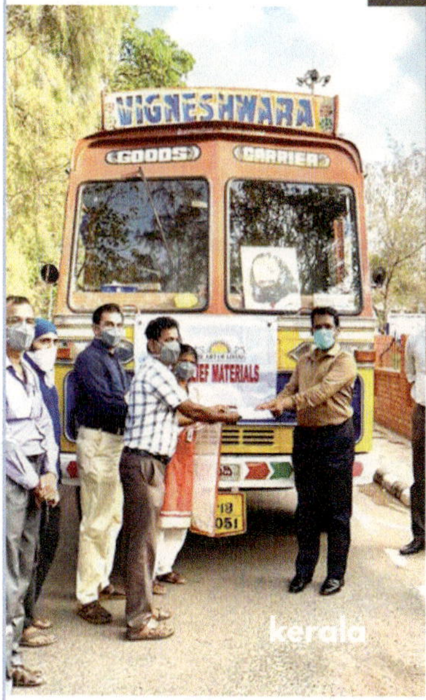
VIGNESHWARA
GOODS
CARRIER
kerala

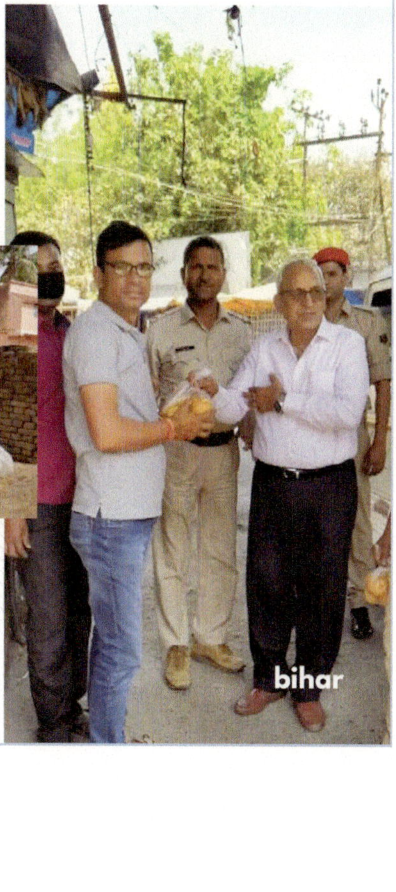
bihar

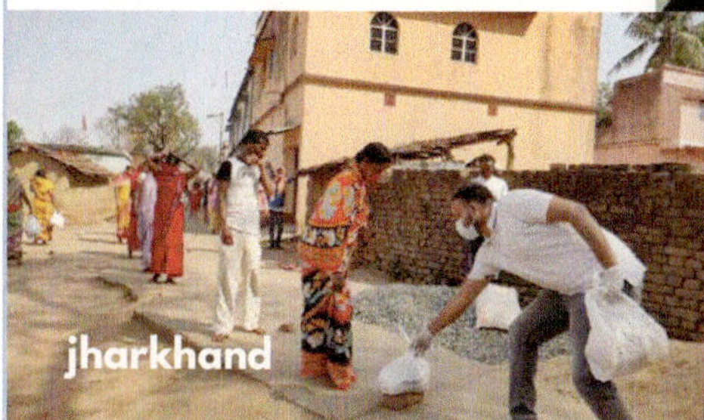
jharkhand

bihar

1,000 ration kits
distributed in Buxar

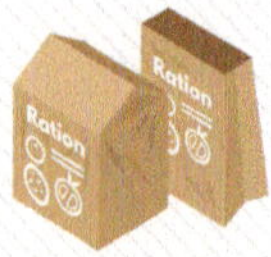

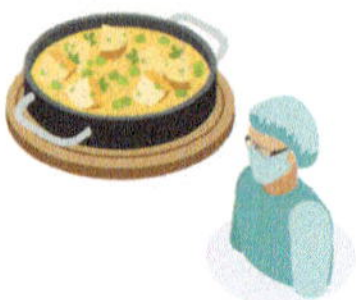

300 cooked food packets and 2,500 hand made masks
distributed in Muzaffarpur

75,000 cooked meals
distributed in one month in Patna

4,000 meals
distributed in Samastipur

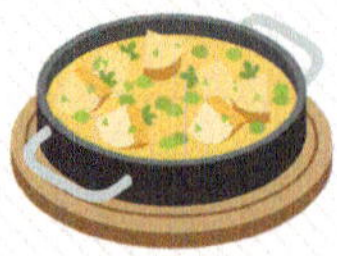

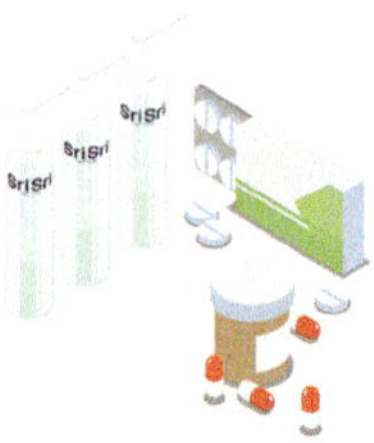

5,000 hand sanitizers & ₹ 8 lakh worth medicines
provided to district administration, health workers and police forces

odisha

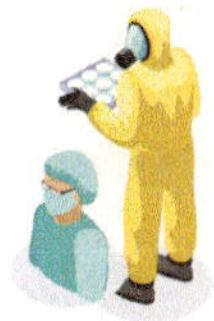

5,000 N95 masks & PPE kits
supplied to state government

500 masks supplied in Kalahandi

350 masks supplied to Bhubaneshwar Municipal Corp.

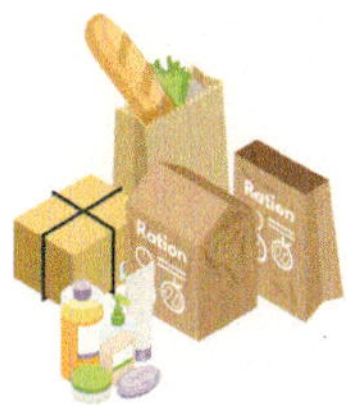

30,000 daily wage earners
provided with **40 tonnes rice, 30 tonnes Dal, 40,000 soaps, 1,50,000 packets of biscuits** sent from the Art of Living International Center, Bengaluru

2,000 ration kits supplied to Cuttack Municipal Corp.

500 ration kits supplied to Bhubaneshwar Municipal Corp.

434 ration kits distributed in Jeypore

248 ration kits distributed to families in Sambalpur

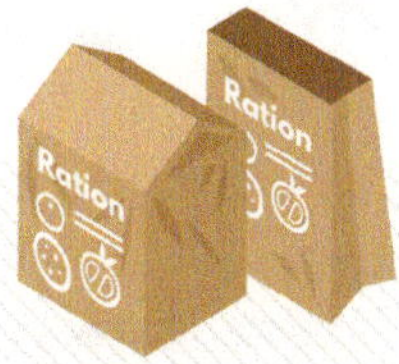

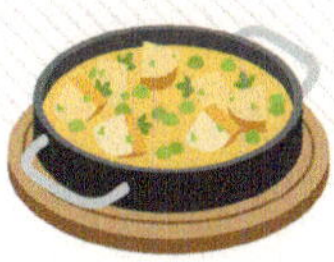

2,000 cooked meals
served daily in Bhubaneswar

100 families
being provided cooked meals in Puri

chhattisgarh

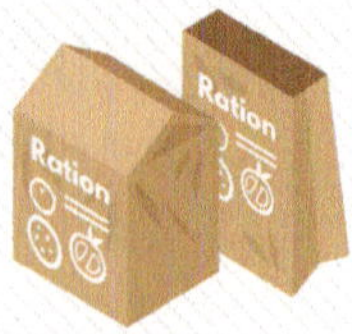

4 tonnes of ration
supplied to Raipur town authorities

Over 300 ration kits
distributed in nearby village and an orphanage

Ration for 10 days
to 500 families in Bhilai, Bilaspur, Dhamtari and Ambikapur

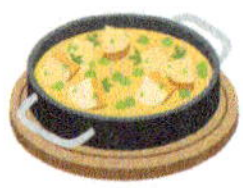

2,000 cooked meals
distributed to over **100 families** in Bilaspur

1500 gloves & 600 masks
distributed in the health care department

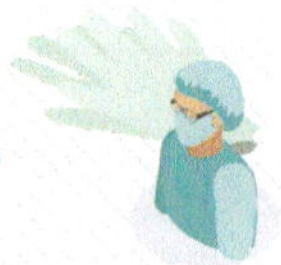

jharkhand

1,200 ration kits
distributed in Ranchi to tribal artisans

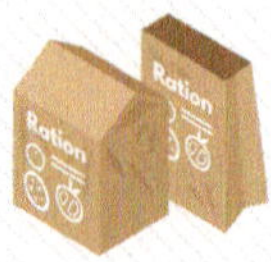

sikkim

25 labourers provided cooked food for 10 days

assam

700 ration kits
distributed in Guwahati, Maligao, Rangiya, Nalbari and Pandu village from the Art of Living ashram in Guwahati

7,000 packets of biscuits
distributed in Guwahati

arunachal pradesh

250 ration kits
distributed from the Art of Living Center in Itanagar

telangana

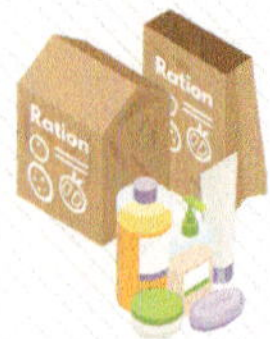

60 tonnes of ration and hygiene supplies

to **over 4,000 families**, mostly migrant labour in collaboration with GHMC Online & Police Department

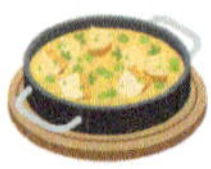

2,500 people

being given cooked food daily for **10 days**

andhra pradesh

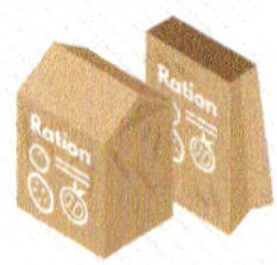

250 ration kits

distributed in Amaravati

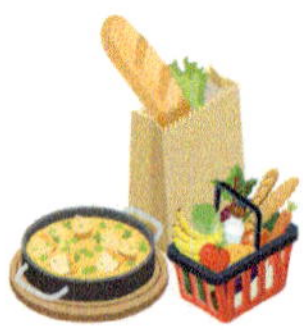

In Visakhapatnam

2,84,075 cooked meals, 22,800 liters of butter milk and 25,000 bananas have been served

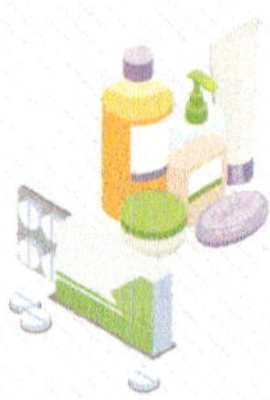

₹ 1 lakh worth medicines & 2000 hygiene kits

provided in Visakhapatnam

west bengal

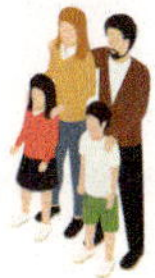

Ration & food supplied
to 500 families in Siliguri &
400 sex-worker families in Sonargachi

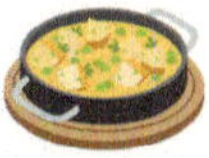

31,00,000 meals
given to 2,30,000 people all over West Bengal

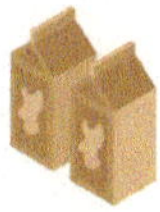

33,000 packets of biscuits
distributed across the state

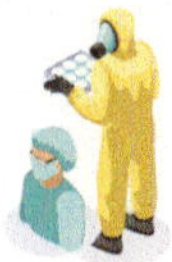

2,000 surgical masks & 50 PPE kits

tamil nadu

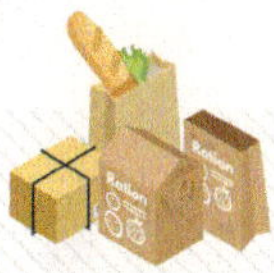

24 tonnes of provisions
for 2,175 families through Chennai Corporation

1,675 ration kits
supplied in Chennai and Coimbatore

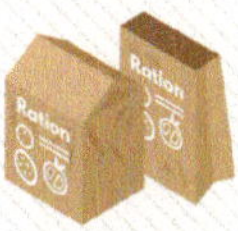

1.85 tonnes of rice
given to 370 sanitary workers in Udamalpet

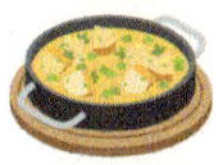

1,00,000 meals
provided to 3,000 daily wage workers
for 2 weeks in Coimbatore

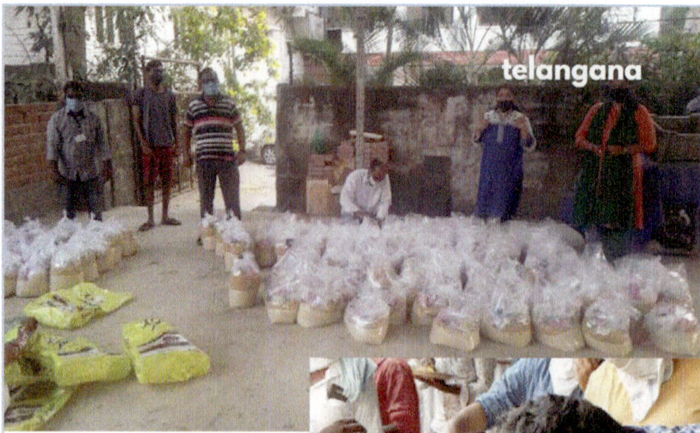
telangana

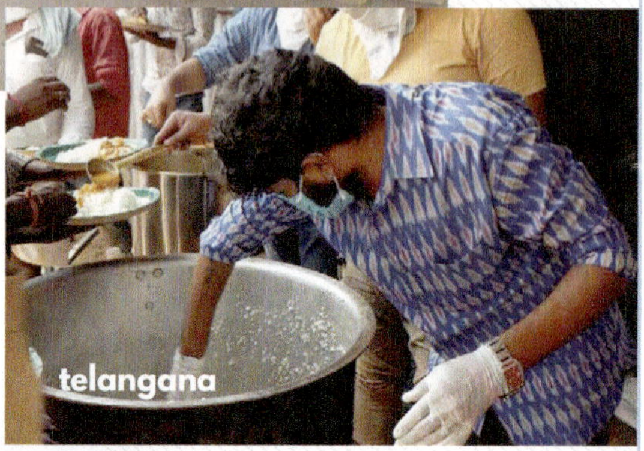
telangana

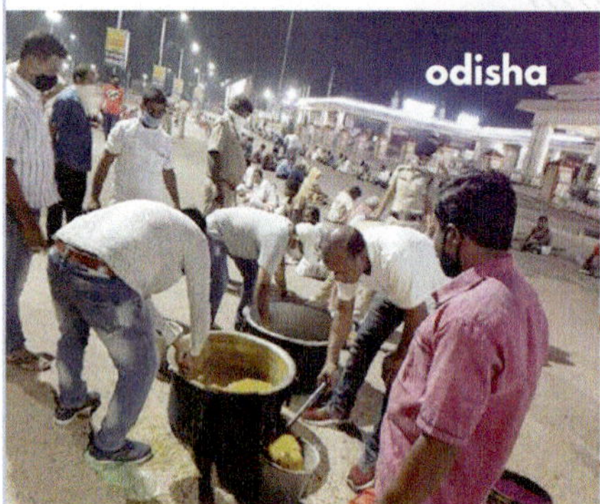
odisha

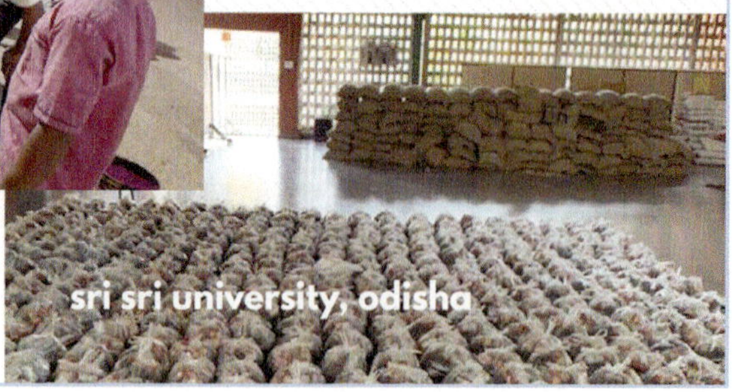
sri sri university, odisha

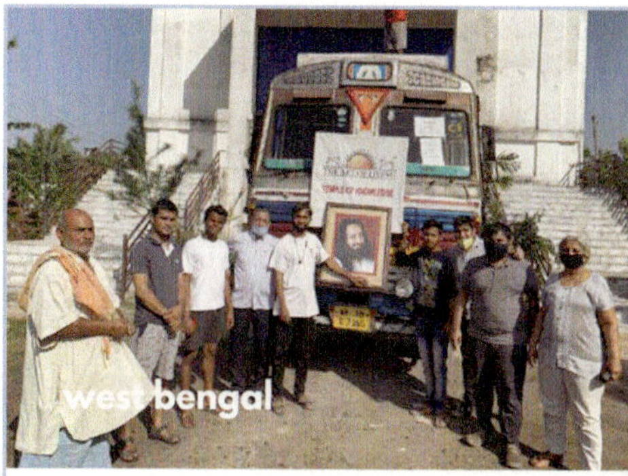
west bengal

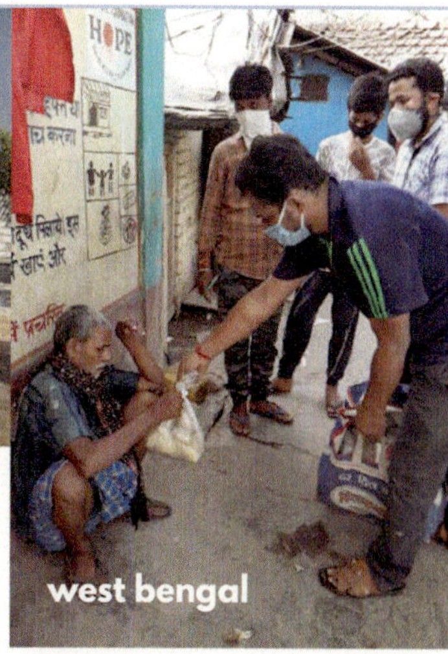
west bengal

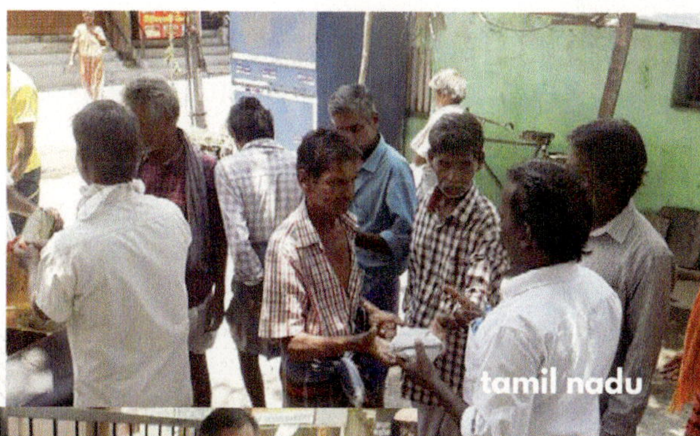
tamil nadu

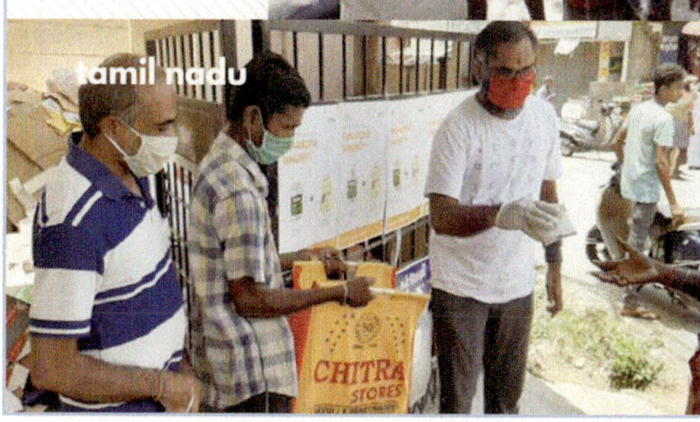
tamil nadu

Art of Living, IAHV volunteers help migrant labours, families with 500 tons of relief materials

- The organization is also setting up a hospital in Hyderabad while helping a Covid-19 hospital in Bengaluru.

International Business Times

Art of Living reaches out to sex workers in Sonagachi, distributes ration amid Covid-19 pandemic

- The Art of Living's Project Udaan volunteers have reached out to the community of sex workers situated in Sonagachi with essentials amid coronavirus pandemic.

आर्ट ऑफ लिविंग ने बढ़ाए मदद के हाथ, 100 परिवारों को पहुँचाई सहायता ..

Editor April 16, 2020

> *बिहार एपेक्स मेंबर दीपक कुमार पांडेय द्वारा आयोजित इस कार्यक्रम में दैनिक मजदूरी करने वाले परिवारों को चिन्हित करके राहत सामग्री का वितरण किया गया. साथ ही साथ संस्था के कार्यकर्ताओं द्वारा कोविड- 19 से बचाव के लिए सभी जरूरी बातें बताई गईं.*

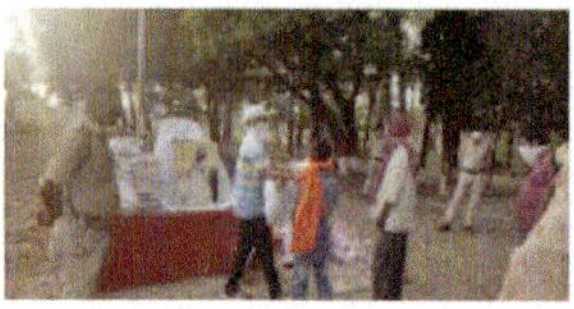

- वार्ड संख्या 9 के जरूरतमंदों को एक हफ्ते के लिए दी राहत सामग्री
- स्थानीय वार्ड पार्षद ने की प्रयास की सराहना

बक्सर टॉप न्यूज़, बक्सर: कोरोना संकटकाल की विषम परिस्थितियों में आर्ट ऑफ लिविंग परिवार ने स्थानीय हैप्पीनेस सेंटर के सामने वार्ड संख्या 9 में गृह रक्षा वाहिनी के फील्ड में लगभग 100 गरीब परिवारों के बीच हफ्ते भर का राशन वितरण किया. राशन किट में 5 किलो चावल, 5 किलो आटा, 500 ग्राम अरहर दाल, आधा लीटर सरसों तेल, मसाले, नमक और साबुन जैसे प्रतिदिन इस्तेमाल होने वाले सामान शामिल थे. बिहार एपेक्स मेंबर दीपक कुमार पांडेय द्वारा आयोजित इस कार्यक्रम में दैनिक मजदूरी करने वाले परिवारों को चिन्हित करके राहत सामग्री का वितरण किया गया. साथ ही साथ संस्था के कार्यकर्ताओं द्वारा कोविड- 19 से बचाव के लिए सभी जरूरी बातें बताई गईं.

THE ART OF LIVING

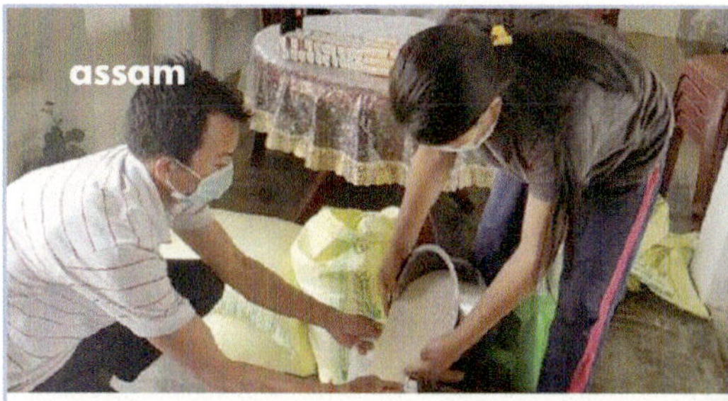
assam

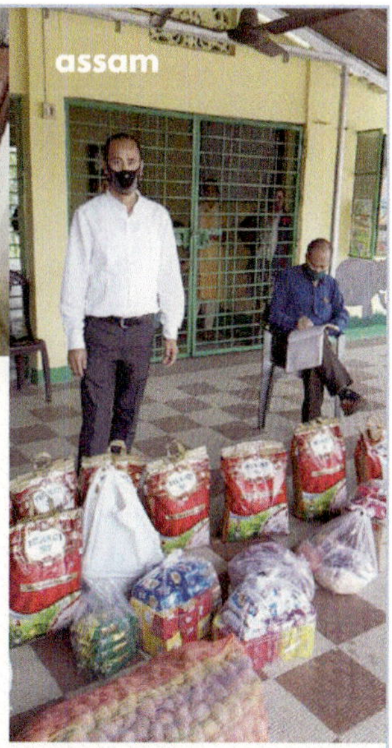
assam

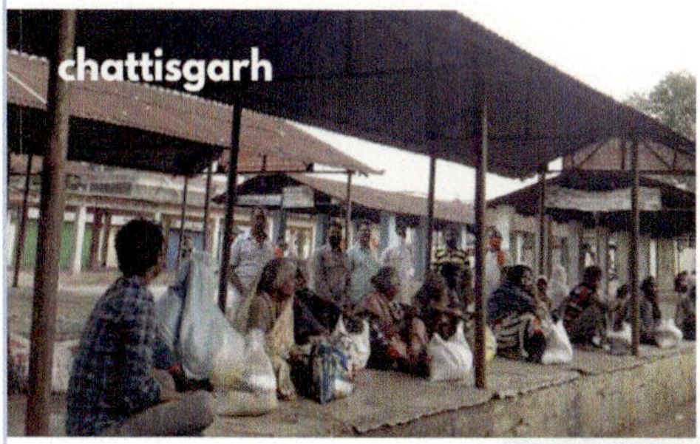
chattisgarh

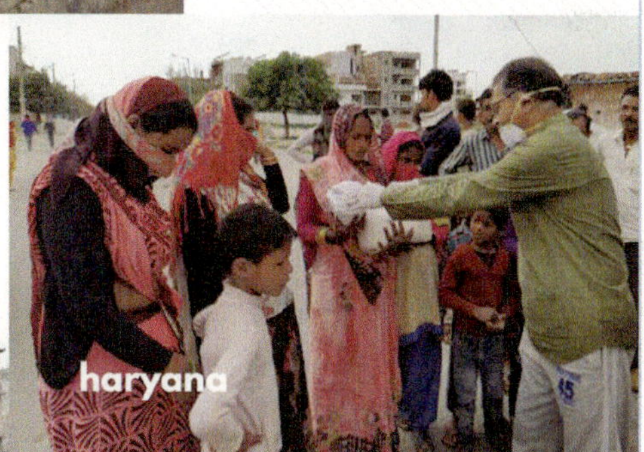
haryana

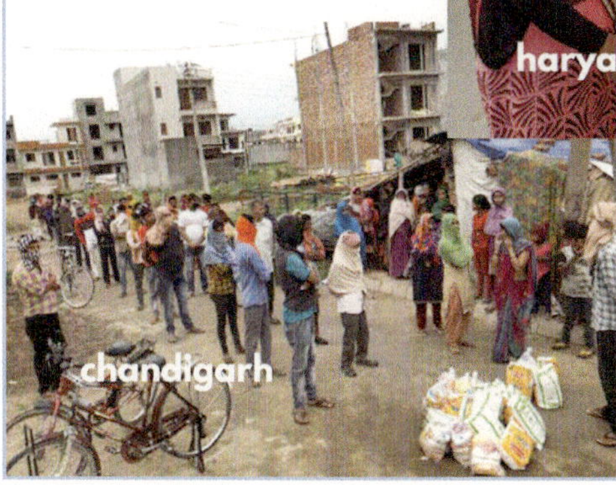
chandigarh

Supported by
(in alphabetical order)

ACG Associated
Adani Foundation
Advanced Vital Enzymes
Astapura
Atlas Copco
Avanee Foundation

Beeline Impex
BNY Mellon
BOSCH India

Capgemini
CloudMoyo
Colours of Life
CSI Software

Dharma Productions
Dynamic Prestress
Dynamic Projects

Ek Number Hospitality LLP
Emirates Shipping

Gateway Distripacks Ltd.
Global Insurance

Hikal Ltd.

Incred Fiancials
India Landtech Park

J K Industries
J M Financials
JDA software (Blue Yonder)

Karshev Diamonds
Kripa Stones & Granites

LIC Housing Finance
LIC of India
Luke Cuthino Holistic

MAA Foundation

Pfizer India
Phool Versha Foundation
Prabhat Dairy
Prasad Kock Technik

Sardarmal Charitable Trust
Screen Magic Mobile Media

The Hans Foundation

Vimochana Charitable Trust
Vishnu Aromatics

WIPRO Foundation

CHAPTER 20

Computed Tomography Thorax in COVID Management: A Rightfully Used or Misused Tool?

Prahlad Prabhudesai, Nafeesath, Swapnil Chopade, Abha Mahashur

INTRODUCTION

With over 900,000 infections and approximately 50,000 confirmed deaths in the first 3 months of 2020, the coronavirus disease of 2019 (COVID-19) has evolved into a staggering healthcare outbreak. The World Health Organization (WHO) declared the rapidly spreading COVID-19 a pandemic on March 11, 2020, and urged immediate international action in four key areas: To prepare and be ready; to detect, protect, and treat; to reduce transmission; and to innovate and learn.[1] During the pandemic, every patient with respiratory symptoms was suspected of having COVID-19, and it became imperative to effectively triage the patient and diagnose them so that timely management could be initiated to not only prevent potential complications but also curtail the ongoing rampant spread of the virus. The disease profile of COVID was found to be dynamic and evolve rapidly over time. Since there was no definitive treatment, the most effective control for COVID-19 relied upon early detection and isolation or quarantine of the infected patients. Early diagnosis was hindered, especially during the initial phase of the pandemic, due to challenges in the development and processing of reverse transcription-polymerase chain reaction (RTPCR), the standard diagnostic method to detect viral nucleotides.[2] Moreover, it was shown that RTPCR only had a sensitivity of 32–80%, which was negatively impacted by a number of factors such as quality and type of the specimen, handling of the specimen, and the stage of infection at the time of specimen collection.[1,3] In the first wave, the challenges were not only to procure the kit and get tested timely but also the false-negative rates of RTPCR, which were approximately 30–50%.[4] Thus, there were symptomatic patients being COVID RTPCR negative behaving like superspreaders and further increasing the load for healthcare facilities.

Due to the rapid rise in COVID-19 cases, doctors were struggling to cope with an overwhelming patient load and make a quick decision about which patients needed immediate hospitalization or critical care in order to prevent serious outcomes. For the medical fraternity, time was of the essence as early diagnosis was directly linked with controlling the spread, avoiding the progress to much severe forms, and reducing the patient load. In this dark tunnel of first wave, where COVID-19 was spreading like a storm, the only ray of light came from high-resolution computed tomography (HRCT) thorax where the early phase of disease also showed shadows irrespective of RTPCR status with such short turnaround time, and thus could help triaging the patients timely. By the second wave of COVID-19 in 2021, RTPCR was readily available all over, the awareness regarding the symptoms and confidence to deal with disease had emerged significantly. The timeline of infection was better understood by medical professionals. CT thorax helped us more to gauge the severity, progression and for prognostication than the diagnosis.

The significance of chest CT in the diagnosis, evaluation, and management of COVID-19 becomes crucial given the absence of a valid single diagnostic gold standard test for the disease. Off course, the rampant use of this diagnostic tool brought us to another aspect that was overuse or misuse of the same. Challenges of the first wave were limited working professionals with variable knowledge trying to support the shaken-up medical system. The word COVID had almost become a taboo in community. In places with poor or limited knowledge, inadvertent use of HRCT thorax was also noted. The threshold to do CT scan had come down drastically not only to pick up the disease the first time but also to monitor it time and again. To ascertain whether a CT thorax was rightfully indicated or misused on a larger scale, we need to go through the role of CT in different aspects of COVID management across the different waves of the pandemic.

ROLE OF RADIOLOGY IN COVID-19 PANDEMIC

Out of all the radiological tools available like chest X-ray (CXR), ultrasound, magnetic resonance imaging (MRI), and CT scan, HRCT emerged as the most useful adjunct for the early detection and prognostication of COVID-19 pneumonia in asymptomatic as well as symptomatic individuals.[5] The radiology always complemented to our knowledge to understand a possible infection, monitor the progression, rule out other diagnosis, and detect early complications. The first and the second waves had their own challenges and expectations from radiology inputs, where in the first wave, we wanted a supportive tool to detect a possible infection early, and in the second wave, with better knowledge and more microbiological support for detection, the focus in radiology shifted to severity and prognostication. Our understanding of the radiological features of COVID-19 is incomplete, and the emerging knowledge needs to be consolidated.[5]

CHEST X-RAY

Given that it is known to be accessible and economical, CXR has been used as the initial imaging modality to assess a patient with suspected respiratory ailments since ages. Attractive aspects like cost effectiveness, short turn-around times, easy availability even in interiors, and comparatively low radiation exposure have always made CXR the preferred investigative tool. Due to its portability, it is helpful for mechanically ventilated patients as well as immobile or bedridden patients in monitoring disease progression. However, the sensitivity of CXR ranges between 33 and 69%.[6] The most frequent CXR findings in COVID were bilateral, posterior, and peripheral shadows with a predominance in the lower lung fields. Reticular and reticulonodular patterns were the most frequently reported interstitial abnormalities, and hazy pulmonary opacities were the most frequently reported alveolar findings. According to a recent review of the literature on CXR findings in COVID, unilateral involvement was 22%, bilateral involvement was 80%, single infiltration was 48%, multiple infiltration was 52%, and interstitial infiltration was 7%. More widespread lung opacities and thicker interstitial marks were found to be signs of disease progression.[6] However, to combat the first wave's biggest concern which was prompt diagnosis, CXR with poor sensitivity could not play a significant role. Also, owing to low-density resolution, CXR could not pick early infection effectively and showed changes in moderate-to-severe disease primarily. The pattern of illness was mostly associated with soft alveolar opacities which were better delineated in CT scan than CXR. With the sharp rise of pandemic cases, a radiological tool was expected to detect infected patients so that they could be quarantined and further spread could be controlled. Interestingly, asymptomatic patients with normal CXR having silent hypoxemia and extensive parenchymal involvement in HRCT chest were not uncommon in COVID. However, CXR continued to serve its purpose in hospitalized patients where the progress had to be monitored time and again.

COMPUTED TOMOGRAPHY THORAX

Until the pandemic, as far as pulmonologists are concerned, a CT scan of the chest was never an investigation of choice before a CXR in the management of respiratory diseases. During the COVID-19 pandemic, CT scans were frequently used in patients for diagnosis and to judge the severity of the disease, even though they were not advised as a screening method for the illness. COVID-19 pneumonia with involvement of lung parenchyma showed diverse radiological features, which also depend on the clinical severity and the time elapsed since the onset of symptoms. Typical chest CT findings of COVID pneumonia included bilateral peripheral ground glass opacity (GGO), consolidation, reticulations, crazy paving patterns, etc., with bilateral involvement and a multifocal pattern in a peripheral, subpleural, and posterior distribution. GGOs were the most common pattern, followed by a mixed pattern of GGOs and consolidation.[6]

A small number of asymptomatic people did get benefited from the use of CT chest in detecting pneumonia and speeding up treatment.[1] Furthermore, the use of CT thorax helped in the evaluation of specific COVID-19 complications and sequelae such as pulmonary thromboembolism, lung abscess, acute respiratory distress syndrome (ARDS), myocarditis, and acute pulmonary edema which could be missed on CXR.[4]

In COVID-19 outbreak, the typical useful scenario with CT thorax was the diagnosis and the management of the disease in settings whenever the availability, turnaround times, and accuracy of RTPCR tests imposed limitations for the virologic diagnosis even though it was not a standard of practice.[7] In a retrospective study conducted by Long et al.[4] for the initial diagnosis of COVID pneumonia, the sensitivity of the CT thorax was 97.2%, while that of the initial RTPCR test was 83.3%.3 Hence, CT thorax was found extremely useful in high-risk patients, in those with severe disease, in areas where polymerase chain reaction testing was sparsely available, or in cases of strong clinical suspicion when the virological tests were reported negative.[9]

Computed Tomography Thorax Findings in Coronavirus Disease 2019

CT thorax in COVID aided not only in diagnosis but also in severity assessment or prognostication, assessment of post-COVID lung sequelae, and ruling out differential diagnosis.

Diagnosis

- *Anatomical distribution:* COVID-19 most commonly affected both lungs (82.2%), lower zones (54.5%), peripheral parts (87.1%), and multifocal areas (54.5%).[7]
- *Temporal progression:* Four stages of COVID-19 pneumonia were described by Pan et al. as depicted in **Table 1** and **Figure 1**. The development of GGOs was the primary characteristic of the early phase (0–4 days). There could be vascular expansion and the halo sign. The size and quantity of GGOs increased throughout the progressive phase (5–8 days), which was also marked by the appearance of a crazy paving pattern and the gradual conversion of GGOs into multifocal and consolidative patches. The more extensive lung involvement with dense consolidations, diffuse GGO, parenchymal bands, and crazy paving were characteristics of the peak stage (9–13 days). After the peak stage, there was the absorption stage where consolidations slowly disappeared and fibrotic bands, an indication of repaired lungs, appeared.[10]

TABLE 1: Clinicoradiological correlation of COVID with disease progression.

Stage	Early phase	Progressive phase	Peak phase	Resolving phase
Duration	0–4 days	5–8 days	9–13 days	>14 days
Symptoms	Mild constitutional symptoms, fever, and cough	Shortness of breath with or without hypoxia	ARDS, multi-system involvement, and cardiac failure	Resolving symptoms and recovery
HRCT findings	Scattered multiple GGO	Increase in GGO and crazy paving pattern	Extensive lung involvement with dense consolidations, diffuse GGO, parenchymal bands, and crazy paving	Fibrotic bands
	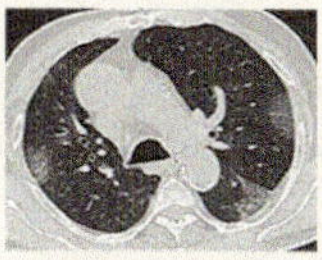	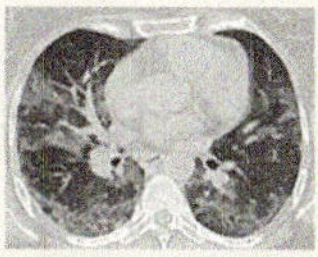	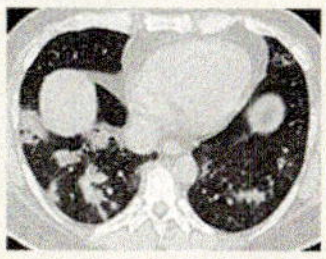	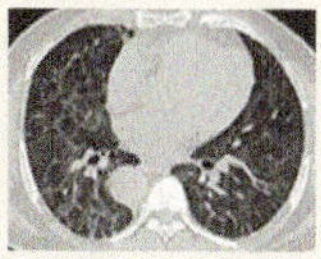

(ARDS: acute respiratory distress syndrome; GGO: ground glass opacity; HRCT: high-resolution computed tomography)

Common Imaging Patterns on Chest Computed Tomography Scan (Figs. 2 to 6)

Ground glass opacity: It was the most common as well as the earliest CT finding in patients infected with severe acute respiratory syndrome coronavirus-2 (SARS CoV-2). A hazy hyperattenuated area without obstruction of the underlying vasculature is known as ground glass opacity, and it is often brought on by interstitial thickening or partial filling of the airspaces.[11] Unilateral or bilateral GGO with peripheral and subpleural distribution are common signs of COVID-19 pneumonia. Up to 98% of patients appear to have GGO, making it the most frequent CT finding. Spider-web sign, which was first defined in this disease, showed a triangular or angular GGO under the pleura including thickened interlobular septa resembling a net **(Fig. 2)**.[12]

Consolidation: The complete filling of the alveolar airspaces results in consolidation, which is characterized by a hyperattenuated region with obscuration of the underlying arteries.[13] In individuals with COVID-19 pneumonia, multifocal, spotty, or segmental consolidations were seen in 2–64% of cases. Peripheral and subpleural lesions were more common compared with central peribronchovascular lesions.[7] Consolidation usually appears later than GGO and peaks in days 10–12 after the onset of the disease.[7]

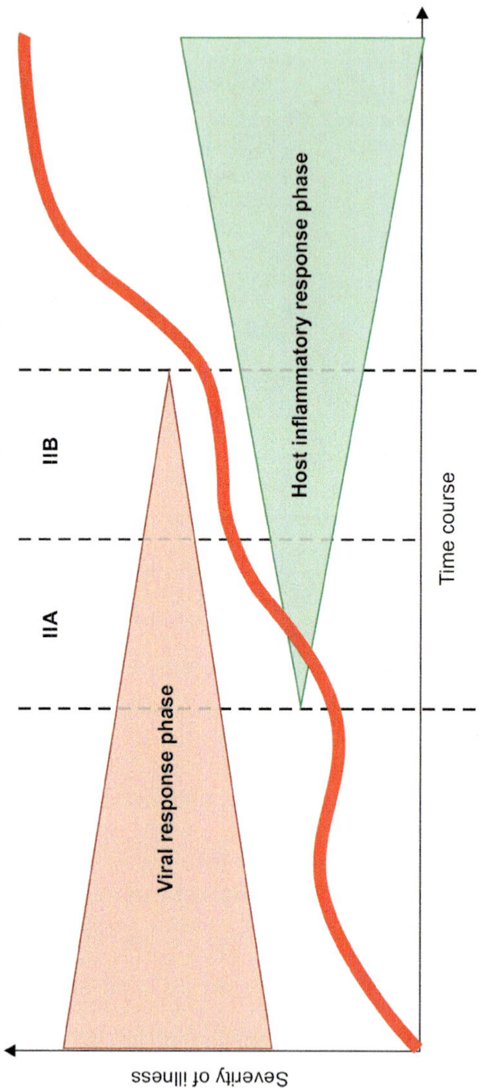

FIGURE 1: The three escalating phases of COVID-19 pneumonia progression.[11]

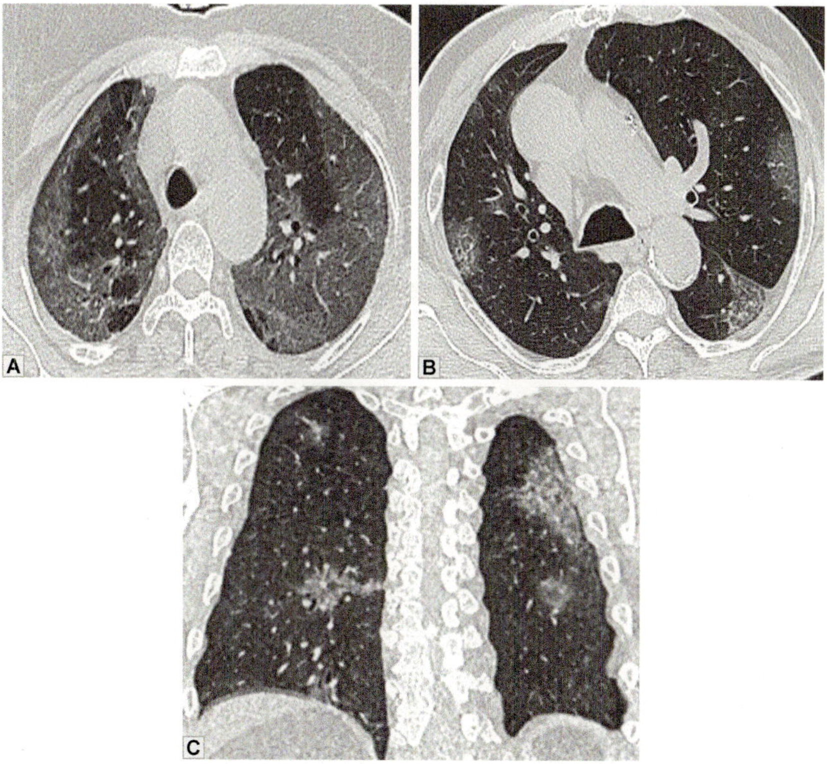

FIGURES 2A TO C: (A) Thin section axial CT image of a 45-year-old, asymptomatic male patient with history of contact with COVID-19 pneumonia patient. His RTPCR for COVID-19 from nasopharyngeal swab was negative. CT scan shows bilateral extensive GGO. (B and C) Thin section axial and coronal CT images of a 50-year-old male patient who presented with fever and dyspnea. CT scan taken on day 5 of symptoms show bilateral multifocal subpleural and peribronchial GGO.

(CT: computed tomography; GGO: ground glass opacity; RTPCR: reverse transcription-polymerase chain reaction)

Reticulations: Reticulation is defined as thickened interlobular septa and intralobular lines, which appear as linear opacities on CT.[13] Reticulation was found to be the third most common CT appearance and it usually appears late.

Crazy paving pattern: It is defined as thickened interlobular septa or intralobular lines superimposed on GGO, resembling paving stones. This sign may refer to the alveolar edema and acute interstitial inflammation presented also in severe acute respiratory syndrome (SARS).[12]

Other findings in COVID included airway changes like air bronchogram, air trapping, bronchiectasis, bronchial wall thickening. The assumed pathological mechanism was bronchial obstruction and bronchial wall inflammatory damage, both leading to the destruction of bronchial wall

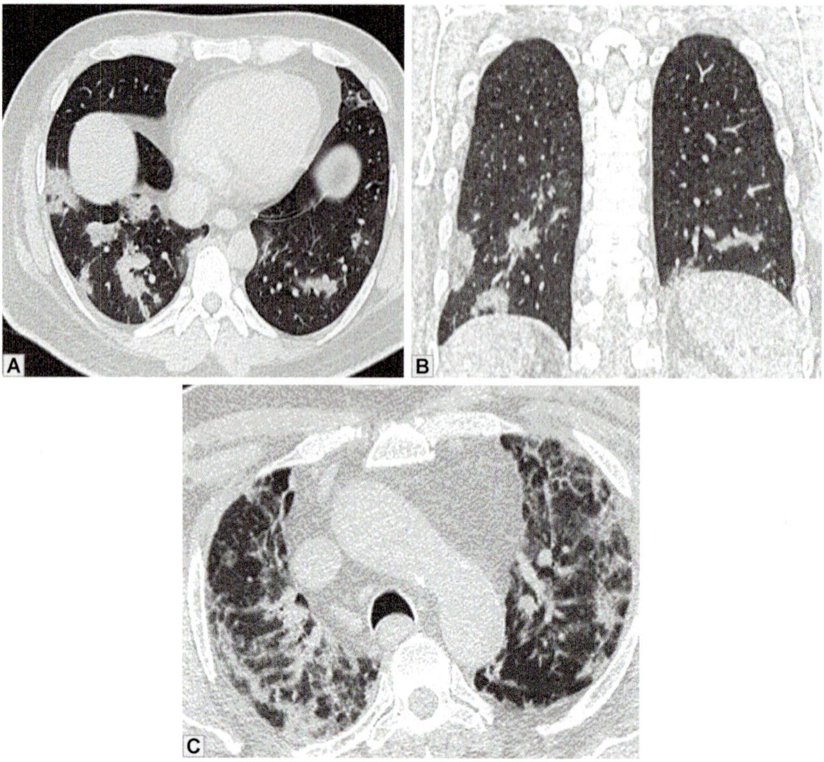

FIGURES 3A TO C: (A and B) A 56-year-old female, COVID RTPCR positive, presented with fever and worsening hypoxia. Axial and coronal CT images done on day 7 of symptoms show bilateral multifocal areas of consolidation with an air bronchogram in both lower lobes. (C) Axial CT image shows thickened pulmonary interstitial structures with a reticular pattern and fibrous stripes in upper lobes. The patient was a 60-year-old female who had COVID-19 pneumonia 3 weeks back. Symptoms have resolved since then except dyspnea.

(CT: computed tomography; RTPCR: reverse transcription-polymerase chain reaction)

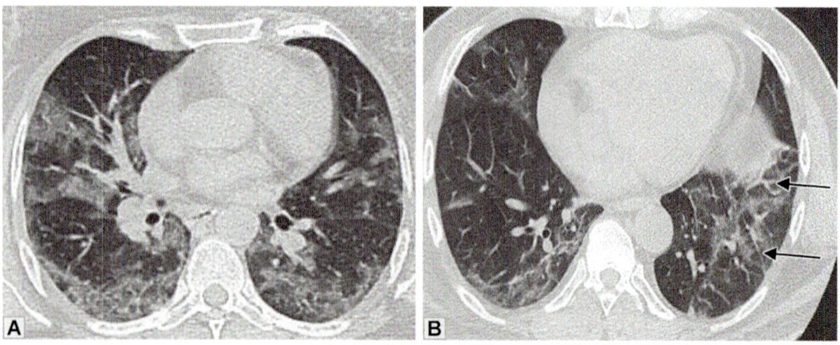

FIGURES 4A AND B: (A) Axial HRCT chest image shows crazy paving pattern. (B) Axial CT image shows vascular ectasia in involved lung parenchyma (black arrows).

(HRCT: high-resolution computed tomography)

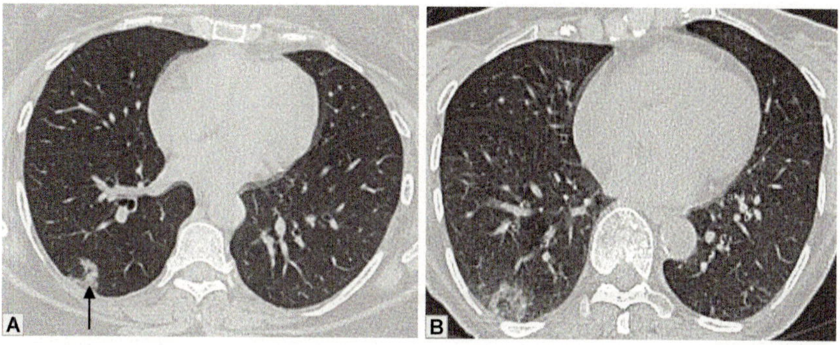

FIGURES 5A AND B: Axial HRCT images in two different patients showing focal area of GGO delimited by a peripheral ring with consolidation "reverse halo sign" (black arrow).
(GGO: ground glass opacity; HRCT: high-resolution computed tomography)

structures, to the development of fibrosis, and to consequent bronchiectasis. The most common pleural changes were pleural thickening (32%) and pleural effusion (5%).[13] A pulmonary nodule is defined as a rounded or irregular parenchymal opacity of<3 cm in diameter. Multifocal solid irregular nodules were found in 3–13% of COVID-19 patients.[13] Architectural distortion, vascular enlargement, perilobar pattern, nodules, vascular ectasia, lymphadenopathy, pericardial effusion, etc., were less common findings. A mass or nodule covered in GGOs is referred to as a "halo sign", while the presence of a specific ring-like area of consolidation with one superimposed rounded GGO is referred to as an "atoll sign" or a "reversed halo sign". These signs in COVID-19 pneumonia were believed to be linked to either a healing lesion with a lower-density core or an emerging lesion encircling an already-existing GGO.[14]

Prognostication (Severity Assessment)

The extent of lung involvement and the severity of the disease were estimated by several scoring systems. Yang et al. introduced the CT severity scoring (CT-SS) system based on the degree of lung involvement. In CT-SS proposed by Yang et al., the 18 segments of both lungs were divided into 20 regions. The lung opacities in all of the 20 regions were subjectively evaluated on chest CT images using a system attributing scores of 0, 1, and 2 if parenchymal opacification involved 0%, < 50%, or ≥50% of each region, respectively. The CT-SS was defined as the sum of the individual scores in the 20 lung segment regions, which may range from 0 to 40 points.[15] Pan et al. proposed a semiquantitative scoring system to estimate the pulmonary involvement as depicted in **Table 2**. The Dutch Radiological Society developed the COVID-19 reporting and data system (CO-RADS) **(Table 3)** for categorical assessment of suspicion of pulmonary involvement, wherein they included clinical and laboratory data in addition to the lung involvement in CT.[15,16]

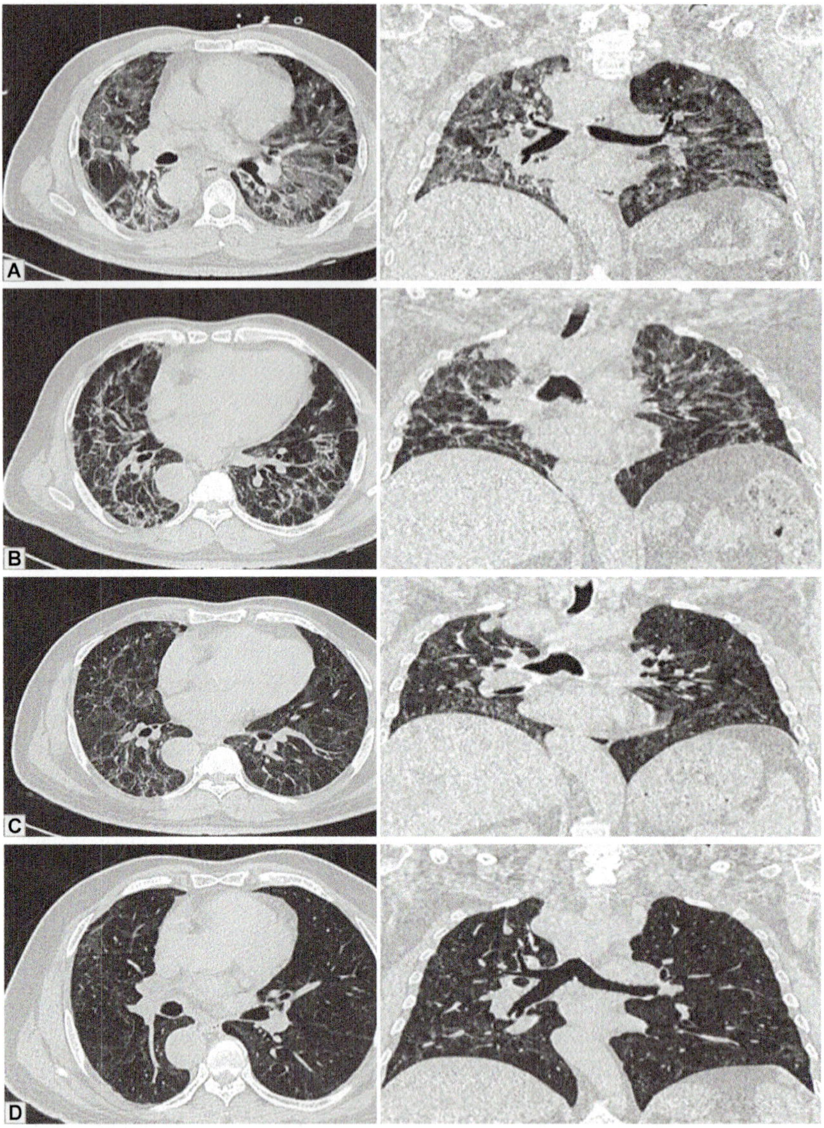

FIGURES 6A TO D: Sequential CT scan taken (A) 2 weeks, (B) 4 weeks, (C) 11 weeks, and (D) 56 weeks after COVID infection of a 49-years-old male patient. Axial and coronal CT images show reduction in ground glass opacities, atelectatic bands, associated crazy paving, and forming consolidation. There were only few subtle ground glass opacities and atelectatic bands at the end of 56 weeks.

Follow-up

The knowledge about the long-term lung radiographic changes in patients who recovered from COVID-19 pneumonia is still limited. Serial CTs in

TABLE 2: CT severity scoring (CT-SS) system.[10,17]

% of lobar involvement	CT score of each lobe
No lung involvement	0
<5	1
5–25	2
26–49	3
50–75	4
>75	5
Total CT score	25
CT severity grading	*Total CT score*
Mild	<8
Moderate	9–15
Severe	>15

(CT: computed tomography)

TABLE 3: COVID-19 Reporting and Data System (CO-RADS).[16]

CO-RADS score	Level of suspicion for pulmonary involvement	Summary
0	Not interpretable	Scan technically insufficient for assigning a score
1	Very low	Normal or noninfectious
2	Low	Typical for other infections but not COVID-19
3	Equivocal	Features compatible with COVID-19 but also other diseases
4	High	Suspicious for COVID-19
5	Very high	Typical for COVID-19
6	Proven	RTPCR positive for SARS CoV-2

(RTPCR: reverse transcription-polymerase chain reaction; SARS CoV-2: severe acute respiratory syndrome coronavirus-2)

the follow-up of patients were considered only in selected cases with post-COVID sequalae or suspected complications. It was not recommended routinely in clinically stable patients as the risk of repeated radiation exposure outweighed the benefit.[2] In a retrospective study of 51 hospitalized patients about 4 weeks after discharge, there was substantial improvement in CT findings in most patients, but 54% had persistent abnormalities, most commonly interlobular septal thickening and focal or multifocal GGO.[18]

Differential Diagnosis

The differential diagnosis of COVID-19 on chest CT presents one of the primary hurdles in COVID-19 imaging. A definitive distinction among various causes of pneumonia is still not possible based solely on CT, as similar findings can be seen in other conditions such as alveolar infectious etiologies (both viral and nonviral), interstitial and vascular pathologies, inspiration/motion artifacts, and trauma. Prior to making a diagnosis, it is also crucial to always take into account the patient's epidemiological history and their symptoms, in addition to the objective laboratory and imaging data.

When the pandemic first started, there was a lot of uncertainty and anticipation about the illness. As the disease spread like a wildfire during the first wave, health organizations faced enormous difficulties in the diagnosis and management. For the sake of curbing the rapidly spreading coronavirus, early detection with a CT scan played a pivotal role. But due to the absence of defined criteria at that time, chest CT scans were also misused at certain instances. The ferocious second wave brought in fear and anxiety among patients, leading to unregulated prescriptions for medications and a plethora of interventions that were not supported by evidence. Unfortunately, in many regions indiscriminate use and reliance on CT scan images rather than clinical and molecular methods for the diagnosis as well as prognostication of the disease was widely practiced. CT scan was used as a screening tool and as a point of care for the diagnosis of COVID, even though they were not recommended as per standard guidelines. Patients were subjected to CT scans in the early course of the disease, where the parenchymal involvement stays minimal, leading to false-negative results. Multiple chest CT scans were performed on many patients, which were not clinically warranted. CT exposed patients to harmful ionizing radiation, which is known to be carcinogenic. Although low-dose CT protocols were reliable for the diagnosis, they were not adopted in many institutions. Indiscriminate use of multiphase scans and contrast-enhanced scans multiplied the radiation dose delivered to the patients.[19]

Looking back at how the COVID pandemic evolved and progressed over the course of more than 3 years highlights the unwavering dedication of health professionals and researchers around the world to enhance our knowledge on COVID-19. As the virus mutated and evolved into several variants, the clinical spectrum also shifted. The omicron variant was associated with more upper respiratory tract symptoms and less lung involvement as compared to the delta variant. In the second wave, with better knowledge and more microbiological support for detection of the disease, various radiological societies and health organizations, including WHO and Indian Council of Medical Research (ICMR) advised strongly against the routine use of CT scans as it is not a COVID screening tool. However, in certain clinical scenarios, such as symptomatic patients with negative RTPCR but high clinical suspicion, COVID-19 patients exhibiting unexplained clinical deterioration, or when other concurrent lung pathology such as pulmonary thromboembolism, pulmonary edema needs to be excluded, a CT scan is crucial in overall management. In our vast experience of handling so many COVID-19 patients, in long run, most of the patients, even those with severe

COVID-19 pneumonia, showed encouraging physiological improvement on follow-up pulmonary function test. We realized that most of the pulmonary scars also cleared from the lung parenchyma. Thus, a follow-up CT chest should be thought of in those patients where pulmonary function test reveals persistent abnormality over a period of time.

It is vital for healthcare professionals to be knowledgeable about the proper utilization of CT chest in COVID-19 given the ongoing rise in COVID-19 patients across the world. The hazards of CT scan in terms of radiation exposure should be judiciously weighed upon prior to projecting a patient for the scan. At this juncture, the use of CT chest has become minimal as the involvement of lung has reduced considerably with the current strain of SARS CoV-2. Thus, we can confidently conclude that CT chest should be performed not with the thought of diagnosing the COVID-19 infection but to understand and intervene in a scenario of clinical deterioration in terms of hypoxia and respiratory distress over the course of illness. Performing a CT scan should rely upon clinical discretion, where it is expected to significantly contribute in the management of patient and not merely to enhance the knowledge of treating team. Also, follow-up of COVID-19 does not warrant a CT necessarily, but if the clinical scenario demands a better delineation of anatomic picture, a CT should be done in those selected few.

REFERENCES

1. Rubin GD, Ryerson CJ, Haramati LB, Sverzellati N, Kanne JP, Raoof S, et al. The Role of Chest Imaging in Patient Management during the COVID-19 Pandemic. Chest. 2020;158(1):106-16.
2. Pezzutti DL, Wadhwa V, Makary MS. COVID-19 imaging: Diagnostic approaches, challenges, and evolving advances. World J Radiol. 2021;13(6):171-91.
3. Wiersinga WJ, Rhodes A, Cheng AC, Peacock SJ, Prescott HC. Pathophysiology, transmission, diagnosis, and treatment of coronavirus disease 2019 (COVID-19): A review. JAMA. 2020;324(8):782-93.
4. Kohli A, Joshi A, Shah A, Jain RD, Gorlawar A, Dhapare A, et al. Does CT help in reducing RT-PCR false negative rate for COVID-19? Indian J Radiol Imaging. 2021;31(Suppl 1): S80-6.
5. Di Paolo M, Iacovelli A, Olmati F, Menichini I, Oliva A, Carnevalini M, et al. False-negative RT-PCR in SARS-CoV-2 disease: Experience from an Italian COVID-19 unit. ERJ Open Res. 2020;6(2):00324-2020.
6. Rousan LA, Elobeid E, Karrar M, Khader Y. Chest X-ray findings and temporal lung changes in patients with COVID-19 pneumonia. BMC Pulmonary Medicine. 2020;20(1): 245.
7. Güneyli S, Atçeken Z, Doğan H, Altınmakas E, Atasoy KÇ. Radiological approach to COVID-19 pneumonia with an emphasis on chest CT. Diagn Interv Radiol. 2020;26(4):323-32.
8. Long C, Xu H, Shen Q, Zhang X, Fan B, Wang C, et al. Diagnosis of the Coronavirus disease (COVID-19): rRT-PCR or CT? Eur J Radiol. 2020;126:108961.
9. Floridi C, Fogante M, Agostini A, Borgheresi A, Cellina M, Natella R, et al. Radiological diagnosis of coronavirus disease 2019 (COVID-19): A practical guide. Acta Biomed. 2020;91(Suppl 8):51-9.

10. Pan F, Ye T, Sun P, Gui S, Liang B, Li L, et al. Time Course of Lung Changes on Chest CT during Recovery from 2019 Novel Coronavirus (COVID-19) Pneumonia. Radiology. 2020;295:715-21.
11. Siddiqi HK, Mehra MR. COVID-19 illness in native and immunosuppressed states: A clinical–therapeutic staging proposal. J Heart Lung Transplant. 2020;39(5):405-7.
12. Wu J, Wu X, Zeng W, Guo D, Fang Z, Chen L, et al. Chest CT findings in patients with coronavirus disease 2019 and its relationship with clinical features. Invest Radiol. 2020;55(5):257-61.
13. Hansell DM, Bankier AA, MacMahon H, McLoud TC, Müller NL, Remy J. Fleischner Society: Glossary of terms for thoracic imaging. Radiology. 2008;246(3):697-722.
14. Sales AR, Casagrande E de M, Hochhegger B, Zanetti G, Marchiori E. The reversed halo sign and COVID-19: Possible histopathological mechanisms related to the appearance of this imaging finding. Arch Bronconeumol. 2021;57:73-5.
15. Yang R, Li X, Liu H, Zhen Y, Zhang X, Xiong Q, et al. Chest CT Severity Score: An imaging tool for assessing severe COVID-19. Radiol Cardiothorac Imaging. 2020;2(2):e200047.
16. Zayed NE, Bessar MA, Lutfy S. CO-RADS versus CT-SS scores in predicting severe COVID-19 patients: Retrospective comparative study. Egypt J Bronchol. 2021;15(1):13.
17. Sharma S, Aggarwal A, Sharma RK, Patras E, Singhal A. Correlation of chest CT severity score with clinical parameters in COVID-19 pulmonary disease in a tertiary care hospital in Delhi during the pandemic period. Egypt J Radiol Nucl Med. 2022;53(1):166.
18. Liu C, Ye L, Xia R, Zheng X, Yuan C, Wang Z, et al. Chest Computed Tomography and Clinical Follow-up of Discharged Patients with COVID-19 in Wenzhou City, Zhejiang, China. Ann Am Thorac Soc. 2020;17(10):1231-7.
19. Khashoo R, Vimalesvaran S, Tewari D, Khashu S, Khashu M. Indiscriminate use of CT chest imaging during the COVID-19 pandemic. Clin Radiol. 2022;77(4):316-7.

CHAPTER 21

Surgical Education and Training during the COVID-19 Pandemic

Aishan Patil, Konstantinos Giannopolos, Tanvir Hussain

SURGICAL EDUCATION AND TRAINING DURING THE COVID-19 PANDEMIC

The coronavirus disease 2019 (COVID-19) pandemic led to unprecedented changes in surgical training and healthcare in general. With the development of safety protocols and regulations by international organizations, elective theater operations were significantly reduced to protect patients against infection by the novel virus. Conferences, examinations, and hands-on training workshops were continually rescheduled or canceled, causing significant disruptions in teaching and learning. As such, surgical training in the COVID-19 era was not up to standard because surgery is a skill that must be learned through inhospital clerkships, hands-on experience, apprenticeship, and practice.[1] Although innovative strategies such as online learning and simulation platforms promoted continuing education, they could not adequately replace on-site learning. The few surgical learning opportunities and operative experiences that took place in the theater environment were mainly dominated by senior surgical professionals, leaving medical students, surgical residents, and fellows with limited exposure time.[2] The global surgical community has undergone significant changes and adapted to the rapidly changing healthcare environment to maintain surgical education and training amidst the COVID-19 pandemic.

COVID-19 DECLARED A PANDEMIC

March 11, 2020, will forever remain etched in the history of the world; this is the day when the World Health Organization (WHO) declared COVID-19 a global pandemic, resulting in various unprecedented changes, especially in healthcare.[3] One of the most affected specialties in healthcare was surgical training. In a matter of days, the specialty had drastically changed, and elective surgical procedures were suspended to increase hospital capacity for COVID-19 admissions and critical care.[4] Most teaching and learning events were also canceled as healthcare facilities redeployed healthcare trainees to other sections, including the intensive care unit (ICU).[5,6] Various surgical organizations issued timely guidelines on service prioritization, the use of various personal protective equipment, and safe practice.[7-9]

Surgical education and training bodies altered their processes of recruiting, appraising, licensing, and certifying trainees in response to the rapidly changing situation to maintain and sustain career progression.[10-12] Many healthcare training centers canceled postgraduate medical examinations to allow clinicians to perform clinical duties while reducing COVID-19 transmission among trainees.[13,14] In the United Kingdom, the General Medical Council (GMC) encouraged healthcare providers to work intelligently and flexibly, thus fostering innovation for optimal health outcomes.[15] Consequently, trainers and trainees created novel learning opportunities to promote adaptability to the new healthcare environment.[16] Since March 2020, the rising cases of COVID-19 necessitated more changes in surgical training.

UNIQUENESS OF MEDICAL AND SURGICAL TEACHING

Medical and surgical training is best conducted using the traditional in-person approach because the two fields involve hands-on experience and skills that may not be effectively gained through simulation and alternative approaches. During the COVID-19 pandemic, the traditional teaching approach was indefinitely disrupted due to safety requirements, such as social distancing. Thus, trainees could not congregate in healthcare training facilities. Instead, novel teaching methods, such as online or virtual teaching programs, were utilized, thanks to the increased availability of video conferencing and telecommunication software, such as Zoom and Google Meet.[17,18]

The development and modification of online video conferencing platforms made peer-to-peer teaching increasingly popular, thus allowing more learners to attend than would have been possible in person.[19,20] Online platforms developed and became increasingly interactive by incorporating polling, breakout rooms, and workshops. These attributes of online learning platforms simulated actual learning experiences and allowed greater participation by the audience. On the other hand, social media platforms, such as Twitter, were used to create awareness of available teaching and learning resources, host open discussions on various topics, and disseminate diverse learning materials. Additionally, instant messaging and social media platforms allowed trainers and trainees to create accessible and engaging educational videos.[21]

Virtual conferences allowed clinicians and trainees globally to attend teaching and learning sessions at minimal expense and enabled the exchange of medical and surgical research and knowledge.[22] Organizers of these virtual conferences ensured that the social aspects of conferences were accommodated through industry exhibitions and networking areas. These conferences have created a foundation for the hybrid conference model that incorporates virtual and face-to-face aspects, making the events more accessible and robust.[23] Novel online teaching platforms are accessible to more significant audiences worldwide at their convenience while enhancing attendees' safety against the pandemic.[24] Even with the reduction in COVID-19 cases worldwide, the training events and resources utilized at the pandemic's peak continue to be utilized.

With each successfully practiced and mastered skill, surgical trainees are equipped to carry out more complex procedures. Shah et al.[25] established that most trainees practicing with virtual reality surgical kits relay positive feedback regarding their experience. Learners can transfer the skills they learn from simulated sessions to actual operating theaters, thus improving their coordination, confidence, and participation. Thus, integrating simulation into surgical education and training improves students' hand–eye coordination, boosts their confidence, and supplements their experience through exposure.

CONTINUING SURGICAL TRAINING

Since surgery is mainly learned through apprenticeship, the current surgical workforce has a responsibility to train upcoming surgeons, notwithstanding the impact of COVID-19 on surgical training. Most surgical training centers attempted to remain operational by providing surgical training and services even though most elective surgical cases were canceled due to the initial COVID-19 spike.[11] Private healthcare institutions came in handy during the COVID-19 peak by relieving public hospitals from the overwhelming burden of elective and emergency operations. In some places, private hospitals were considered "light sites" or "COVID-free sites", thus placing them at a vantage point to provide surgical training to healthcare trainees.[26]

While elective theaters were suspended during the COVID-19 peak, life-saving emergency operations were maintained. However, many cases were managed conservatively (nonoperatively) where possible. For instance, some cases of acute appendicitis were managed by antibiotic therapy. While reducing the care burden at healthcare facilities, this approach significantly reduced surgical trainees' learning opportunities.[27] Nevertheless, surgical trainees and trainers were required to establish learning objectives in operating theaters and discuss them during and after the procedure. Every surgical procedure is a learning opportunity for the trainees, who must demonstrate progression by logging their activities in their portfolio throughout the training program. Structured frameworks and reflective models help the trainees to maximize available learning opportunities and develop as surgeons.[1]

As stated, digital simulation and virtual reality software foster clinical and procedural skills among trainees by utilizing simulation trainers.[28] A multidisciplinary team (MDT) approach to participation improves both nontechnical and clinical skills, thus mitigating the impact of changes in surgical training opportunities due to the COVID-19 pandemic.[29,30]

CLINICAL SUPERVISION

COVID-19 significantly hindered the supervision of trainees. Supervising competent trainees during actual operations enhances their surgical skills and ability to perform them independently. Nevertheless, course materials and other resources, such as the Non-Technical Skills for Surgeons (NOTSS), are freely available online, allowing surgical trainees at various levels to develop surgical skills further.[31,32] Teaching ward rounds led by senior consultants allows surgical trainees to learn to apply specialist knowledge to diverse clinical scenarios. Most importantly, postadmission and post-operative ward rounds provide ample learning opportunities that foster case-based discussions between trainers and trainees. Deployment of surgical trainees to other sections, such as the ICU, maximizes their learning by exposing them to new cases.[33] Such "less familiar" clinical specialties expose learners to new training opportunities that enhance their development as holistic healthcare providers.

EXAMINATIONS

Surgical examinations at both undergraduate and postgraduate levels of training were significantly affected by the pandemic, resulting in adjustments to their delivery. For example, the international examination by the Intercollegiate Membership of the Royal College of Surgeons (MRCS) was computerized to allow candidates to complete the assessment through online platforms.[34] This approach was a safety measure aimed at curbing the spread of COVID-19 due to the congregation of candidates in busy in-person exam halls. The computerization of examinations in surgery not only reduced the risk of transmission but also reduced the considerable accommodation and travel costs associated with physical MRCS exams.[35]

Surgical examination bodies continually discussed the best delivery methods for objective structured clinical examinations (OSCE) during the COVID-19 pandemic. This is because some aspects of surgical training and examination, including procedural skill testing, clinical assessment, and nonverbal communication (body language), are challenging to simulate via online platforms.[36] However, the GMC approved an examination methodology by the Fellowship of the Royal College of Surgeons (FRCS) involving trainee assessment without physically examining the patient, thus enabling career progression.[26]

Multiple surgical organizations, including the Association of Program Directors in Surgery, the Association for Academic Surgery, and the Society of Gastrointestinal and Endoscopic Surgeons, played a significant role in ensuring that surgical residency programs transited well during the unprecedented COVID-19 pandemic.[37] These organizations offered alternative approaches to teaching and learning, including free access to various surgical video libraries and shared resources by qualified and accredited surgical educators. Regionalizing educational teleconferences ensured that surgical trainees from various training institutions had access to quality education.

PROFESSIONAL DEVELOPMENT

The COVID-19 pandemic also necessitated more personal protective equipment while causing new team dynamics with implications on patient safety. With the raging pandemic and redeployment of surgical staff, some healthcare providers in theaters were unfamiliar with the theater environment, and others needed to gain the technical know-how of specialist operations. Therefore, an indirect impact of the pandemic on surgical training is that it significantly compromised patient safety, thus necessitating effective communication and situational awareness.[38]

The risk of medical and surgical errors in operating theaters was enhanced further by dehydration, hunger, fatigue, and burnout.[39] Identifying human factors associated with medical error and conducting appropriate training promote optimal health outcomes and reduce the risks of errors.[40] These challenges called for surgical departments at various healthcare training centers to reflect on team dynamics and allow trainees and other junior health professionals to raise concerns regarding patient safety without the fear of retribution.[41]

NEED FOR CHANGES IN SURGICAL TRAINING

According to Chick et al.,[42] the COVID-19 pandemic uniquely challenged surgical residency programs and rapidly changed the educational landscape in surgery. Additionally, the time course for surgical education and training programs remained significantly undefined. This is especially true, considering the restrictions recommended by healthcare-affiliated institutions, such as the Centers for Disease Control and Prevention (CDC). To establish the scope of the impact of the COVID-19 pandemic, many healthcare training facilities maintained surgical education while promoting the safety of educators, residents, and patients.[43]

Innovative solutions were established to maintain rigorous surgical education in the wake of limited in-person gatherings, limited inhospital rotations, and postponement or cancellation of elective theater operations.

Examples of innovative solutions in surgical education and training included online practice questions, procedural simulation, surgical videos, teleconferencing, and telemedicine clinics. These technology-utilizing solutions bridge the surgical educational gap for healthcare trainees, including surgical trainees, in this unprecedented situation. Again, it is worth emphasizing that these alternative approaches to surgical training cannot substitute hands-on learning that is best attained through direct patient care and operative experience.[42]

The profound changes in surgical training and service provision aimed at mitigating the associated risk of viral transmission while improving the quality of care and promoting patient safety. Even in the wake of the COVID-19 pandemic, characterized by reduced learning opportunities for surgical trainees, involving these trainees in decision-making and other processes fosters their leadership and management skills as they prepare to be surgeons.[44] Additionally, research opportunities related to the COVID-19 pandemic and their impact on service delivery in surgical centers allow greater participation by learners. While virtual learning had already been incorporated into healthcare training to create blended learning before the pandemic, the COVID-19 pandemic saw an exponential increase in the use of such platforms.

As the effects of the pandemic raged and the risk of transmission increased, many healthcare training institutions, including medical schools, withdrew their learners from inhospital learning experiences and clerkships.[45] This was due to safety guidelines by organizations, such as the Association of American Medical Colleges (AAMC). The AAMC requires medical students to undertake approximately 8 weeks of clerkship in surgery before graduating. As such, most medical institutions faced the challenge of training students in surgery without exposure to COVID-19. Medical schools mitigated the impact of halting inhospital clerkships using virtual learning platforms.[2] Some platforms, including Aquifer–Wise MD, were interactive and went beyond the delivery of didactic online learning materials to confer clinical skills alongside decision-making exercises, thus ensuring the continuous flow of information and career progression.

Most interactive online learning platforms provide walkthroughs of surgical procedures, reviews of surgical anatomy, intricate patient cases, and practice test questions. These resources allowed students to improve their clinical reasoning skills and ability to develop differential diagnoses.[2] Utilizing virtual learning in surgical clerkships yielded noninferior learning outcomes and improved students' satisfaction. Despite providing access to didactic learning resources, the virtual learning platform could not bridge some gaps in surgical education and training due to the lack of inhospital intraoperative experiences.[46] Whereas virtual learning in surgery does not necessarily replace students' hands-on experiences, it mitigates lost intraoperative time by providing continuing education and allowing students to practice with home-based surgical kits.[47,48]

REDUCED ELECTIVE THEATER CASES

The pandemic inadvertently caused significant declines in elective theater cases in surgical residency programs due to shortages of personal protective equipment and concerns about exposure to COVID-19. Most surgical training institutions adjusted their residency programs and infrastructure to address obstacles to surgical education and training and mitigate unnecessary disruption.[49] As mentioned earlier, the pandemic also caused emotional exhaustion and burnout among surgical residents, evidenced by limited self-care. Thus, more healthcare training centers advocated for mental health improvement among surgical trainees through mindfulness and self-care.[50]

Reduction in elective surgical cases limited residents' time to complete procedural quotas and familiarize themselves with other clinical specialties, thus generating more difficulty when residents contemplate specialty selections.[51] Thus, medical institutions should re-evaluate their delivery methods for educational experiences through other platforms, including simulation. Simulations allow residents to practice various surgical skills under supervision. Surgical residents' schedules were redesigned and adjusted to allow them more exposure to other specialties.[52] It suffices to say that the most significant burdens experienced in resident training involved decreased time in the operating theater and honing surgical techniques. Interactive online courses allow trainees to review surgical knowledge and technical skills, including ultrasound techniques and laparoscopic skills. Thus, the utilization of virtual learning resources when traditional teaching and learning were disrupted enabled students to prime their surgical skills in preparation for the resumption of inhospital clerkships and training.[53] It is essential to incorporate blended learning at various levels of surgical education and training to allow continuous exposure to technology.

With the cancellation of most elective surgical clinics, surgical consultations moved toward and became increasingly dependent on telehealth clinics via online video conferencing software. This approach helps surgical residents to be continually involved with clinical work, thus maintaining their educational experience. Telehealth clinics rely on functional software and stable internet connectivity.[54] Thus, remote consultation services for surgical patients are hindered by limited technological and internet capabilities. Additionally, these platforms lack the physical exam dimension, raise patient information security concerns, and fail to establish a rapport with patients as with in-person encounters.[55] Nevertheless, access to nonhospital-based simulations provides surgical residents with opportunities to hone their clinical and surgical skills through deliberate and goal-directed service.

Aziz et al.[56] evaluated the effect of the COVID-19 pandemic across the United States and found statistically significant changes in the volume of surgical cases before and during the pandemic. Before the pandemic, many

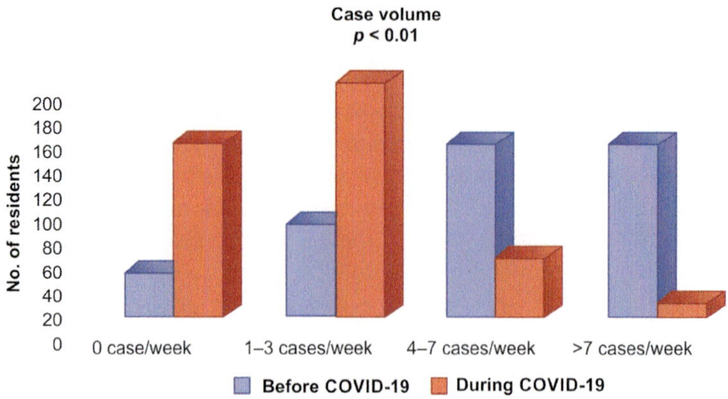

FIGURE 1: Change in resident operative experience.
Source: Adapted from Aziz et al. (2021).[56]

surgical residents attended surgical clinics. Conversely, approximately 80.67% of residents did not attend any surgical clinic during the peak COVID-19 period. There was a significant decline in the number of operative cases that residents performed per week, as shown in **Figure 1**.

CT OF COVID-19 ON RESIDENT WELL-BEING

The COVID-19 pandemic also had profound effects on the well-being of surgery residents, causing them to take more days off. Before the pandemic, most surgery residents took an average of 4 days off per month. Conversely, during the pandemic, more than 65% of surgery residents reported taking more than 4 days off every month. Additionally, more respondents reported increased burnout during the pandemic and raised concerns about potentially transmitting COVID-19 to friends and family. Other residents feared contracting the viral illness.[56]

Figure 2 shows the most significant stressors among surgical residents during the pandemic.

In the United Kingdom, changes to surgical training were due to the need to minimize healthcare personnel in theaters, causing most operative procedures to be senior-led and locking out medical students and surgical residents. Additionally, canceling elective theater procedures prevented the unnecessary exposure of "well" patients to COVID-19. There were also significant changes in surgical shift schedules and the redeployment of residents to other areas, such as the ICU.[25] In a study to identify critical concerns among junior trainees in general surgery regarding surgical training during the COVID-19 pandemic, Shah et al.[25] established that respondents unanimously decried the shortage of learning opportunities, especially in operating theaters. Nevertheless, the use of simulation boxes conferred a safe training method without compromising the safety of patients. Most

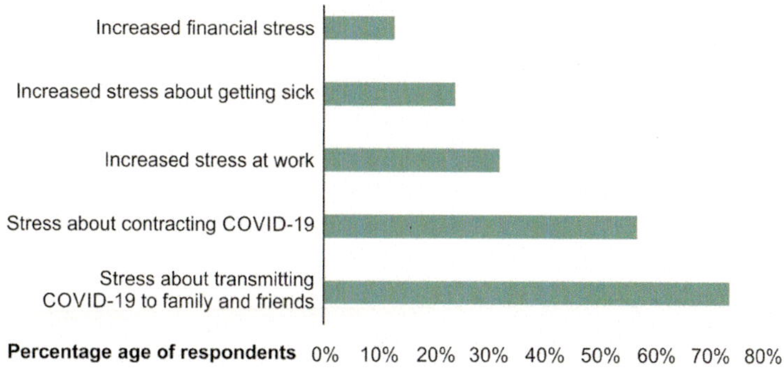

FIGURE 2: Significant stressors among surgical residents.
Source: Adapted from Aziz et al. (2021).[56]

training facilities that took up surgical training through simulation also provided students with individualized online databases for recording their progress.[35]

OVERALL IMPACT OF THE PANDEMIC ON SURGICAL TRAINING

Disrupted teaching and learning across surgical training centers raised serious concerns about the ability of surgical fellows and residents to achieve the expectations of the training program. Surgical trainees were also worried about adequate preparation and unnecessary delays in sitting board examinations.[57] Surgical training prepares trainees for independent practice (operative autonomy), but such readiness is only sometimes reflected in case numbers. Nevertheless, case numbers provide preliminary information regarding a surgical fellow's or resident's surgical exposure and experience. Thus, competency-based education models, including video-based (virtual) platforms, provided learning opportunities for addressing concerns about operative autonomy and technical competence.[58,59]

The surgical specialties most affected by the disruption in elective theater operations include general surgery, ophthalmology, neurosurgery, and orthopedic surgery. Both cadaver laboratories and simulation centers had limited accessibility during the COVID-19 pandemic but increased students' exposure to surgical skills.[60] Many hospitals continually struggled to provide the usual surgical training due to decreased surgical volume as they freed beds for a possible surge in COVID-19 infections with consequently increased admissions. Some patients with elective surgical conditions also avoided the procedures during this period without clearly understood reasons.[61]

The COVID-19 pandemic resulted in didactic innovations that implemented distant learning through virtual platforms, and anecdotal experiences strongly suggest that these platforms will still be valuable for teaching and learning in the post-COVID era. An adequate response to the pandemic's impact on surgical education and training fostered the development of evidence-based strategies to mitigate future disruptions. Disrupted surgical training during the COVID-19 era suggests that most institutions were not prepared to address the impact of the pandemic on surgical training.[62] Healthcare training institutions should be sufficiently prepared to handle such unprecedented crises and promote alternative avenues for summative evaluation, decision-making, remediation, and independent practice.[63] In similar future pandemics, surgical educators can design innovative strategies for continued training and technical competence to minimize disruptions.

CONCLUSION

Globally, surgical training has been significantly affected by the unprecedented COVID-19 pandemic. The hallmark of the pandemic's impact on surgical training entails reduced surgical activity (reduced elective theater cases) and disrupted learning opportunities (reduced inhospital clerkships, rescheduled examinations, and canceled workshops and conferences). The traditional learning method, involving inhospital clerkships and hands-on experience, was limited by safety measures aimed at mitigating viral transmission. The circumstances surrounding the COVID-19 pandemic necessitated expanded and improved curriculums sustained by technological innovations. The innovative utilization of videoconferencing and other virtual platforms promoted learning while safeguarding the safety of educators, learners, and patients. These online learning platforms were a timely response to the impact of the pandemic and provided alternative avenues of surgical training, evaluation, and certification. Although simulations and other platforms cannot sufficiently replace the traditional surgical training method, interactive resources enrich surgical trainees and promote their skills that significantly contribute to their career progression. The main concern about surgical training during COVID-19 is the standard of professional competence of trainees who undergo surgical training via simulations and virtual platforms.

REFERENCES

1. Ellis R, Scrimgeour DSG, Brennan PA. Surgical training during the COVID-19 pandemic: Preparing for future uncertainty. Br J Oral Maxillofac Surg. 2022;60(1):42-5.
2. Ehrlich H, McKenney M, Elkbuli A. We asked the experts: Virtual learning in surgical education during the COVID-19 pandemic—shaping the future of surgical education and training. World J Surg. 2020;44(7):2053-5.
3. White EM, Shaughnessy MP, Esposito AC, Slade MD, Korah M, Yoo PS. Surgical education in the time of COVID: Understanding the early response of surgical training programs to the novel coronavirus pandemic. J Surg Educ. 2021;78(2):412-21.

4. The Royal College of Surgeons. (2020). Statement on COVID-19 and its effect on surgical training. [online] Available from https://www.rcsed.ac.uk/news-public-affairs/news/2020/march/statement-on-covid-19-and-its-effect-on-surgical-training. [Last accessed February, 2024].
5. The Association of Surgeons in Training. (2020). ASiT Response Letter: Implications of COVID-19 in delivery of care and training. [online] Available from https://www.asit.org/news/asit-and-the-15-speciality-associations-joint-letter-to-surgical-trainees-on-covid-19-the-implications-for-surgical-tra/nwc11195 [Last accessed February, 2024].
6. Hourston GJM. The impact of despecialisation and redeployment on surgical training in the midst of the COVID-19 pandemic. Int J Surg. 2020;78:1-2.
7. Al-Jabir A, Kerwan A, Nicola M, Alsafi Z, Khan M, Sohrabi C, et al. Impact of the coronavirus (COVID-19) pandemic on surgical practice-Part 1. Int J Surg. 2020;79:168-79.
8. Al-Jabir A, Kerwan A, Nicola M, Alsafi Z, Khan M, Sohrabi C, et al. Impact of the Coronavirus (COVID-19) pandemic on surgical practice-Part 2 (surgical prioritisation). Int J Surg. 2020;79:233-48.
9. Royal College of Surgeons of England. (2020). COVID-19 Information Hub. [online] Available from https://www.rcseng.ac.uk/coronavirus/. [Last accessed February, 2024].
10. Health Education England. (2020). COVID-19 Statement for applicants recruitment update. [online] Available from https://www.hee.nhs.uk/sites/default/files/documents/COVID-19%20Statement%20for%20applicants%20recruitment%20update.pdf. [Last accessed February, 2024].
11. Health Education England. (2020). The need to reinstate training. [online] Available from www.hee.nhs.uk/sites/default/files/documents/AoMRC%20Four%20Nation%20The%20need%20to%20reinstate%20training%203%20June%202020_1.pdf [Last accessed February, 2024].
12. Joint Committee on Surgical Training. (2020). Surgery specific management of ARCPs during COVID-19. [online] Available from https://www.entuk.org/sites/default/files/Surgery%20specific%20management%20of%20ARCPs%20during%20COVID-19.pdf [Last accessed February, 2024].
13. Royal College of Surgeons of England, Royal College of Physicians and Surgeons of Glasgow, The Royal College of Surgeons of Edinburgh. (2020). Joint policy statement from the Royal Surgical Colleges. [online] Available from https://www.intercollegiatemrcsexams.org.uk/-/media/files/rcs/coronavirus/joint-policy-statement-on-covid19.pdf [Last accessed February, 2024].
14. James HK, Pattison GTR. Disruption to surgical training during Covid-19 in the United States, United Kingdom, Canada, and Australasia: A rapid review of impact and mitigation efforts. J Surg Educ. 2021;78(1):308-14.
15. Marx DC. General Medical Council. (2020). Doctors will stop at nothing to provide care in this crisis–our job is to support them video transcript. [online] Available from https://www.gmc-uk.org/news/news-archive/doctors-will-stop-at-nothing-to-provide-care-in-this-crisis-our-job-is-to-support-them [Last accessed February, 2024].
16. Hollander JE, Carr BG. Virtually perfect? Telemedicine for COVID-19. N Engl J Med. 2020;382(18):1679-81.
17. Fonseka T, Ellis R, Salem H, Brennan PA, Terry T. The effects of COVID-19 on training within urology: Lessons learned in virtual learning, human factors, non-technical skills and reflective practice. J Clin Urol. 2021;14(1):29-35.
18. Sharif S, Sherbino J, Centofanti J, Karachi T. Pandemics and innovation: How medical education programs can adapt extra clinical teaching to maintain social distancing. ATS Sch. 2020;1(4):344-7.
19. Jeong L, Smith Z, Longino A, Merel SE, McDonough K. Virtual peer teaching during the COVID-19 pandemic. Med Sci Educ. 2020;30(4):1361-2.

20. Roberts V, Malone K, Moore P, Russell-Webster T, Caulfield R. Peer teaching medical students during a pandemic. Med Educ Online. 2020;25(1):1772014.
21. Chan AKM, Nickson CP, Rudolph JW, Lee A, Joynt GM. Social media for rapid knowledge dissemination: Early experience from the COVID-19 pandemic. Anaesthesia. 2020;75(12):1579-82.
22. Vervoort D, Dearani JA, Starnes VA, Thourani VH, Nguyen TC. Brave new world: Virtual conferencing and surgical education in the Coronavirus Disease 2019 era. J Thorac Cardiovasc Surg. 2021;161(3):748-52.
23. Khan S, Mian A. Medical education: COVID-19 and surgery. Br J Surg. 2020;107(8):e269.
24. Clements JM, Burke J, Nally D, Rabie M, Kane E, Barlow E, et al. COVID-19 impact on Surgical Training and Recovery Planning (COVID-STAR)-A cross-sectional observational study. Int J Surg. 2021;88:105903.
25. Shah R, Carty I, Ugwu F. Surgical Training during the COVID-19 Pandemic. Pak J Med Sci. 2021;37(2):610-1.
26. Health Education England, NHS England, Independent Healthcare Provider Network. (2020). Joint Position Statement: Ensuring Education and Training in the Independent Sector. [online] Available from https://www.jcst.org/-/media/files/jcst/key-documents/position-statement-independent-sector-training-nhsei-hee-sept-20.pdf. [Last accessed February, 2024].
27. Javanmard-Emamghissi H, Boyd-Carson H, Hollyman M, Doleman B, Adiamah A, Lund JN, et al. The management of adult appendicitis during the COVID-19 pandemic: An interim analysis of a UK cohort study. Tech Coloproctol. 2021;25(4):401-11.
28. Ahmed S, Dann S. The virtual future of education and training. The Bulletin of the Royal College of Surgeons of England. 2015;97(10):431-2.
29. Hintz GC, Duncan KC, Mackay EM, Scott TM, Karimuddin AA. Surgical training in the midst of a pandemic: A distributed general surgery residency program's response to COVID-19. Can J Surg. 2020;63(4):E346-8.
30. McKechnie T, Levin M, Zhou K, Freedman B, Palter VN, Grantcharov TP. Virtual surgical training during COVID-19: Operating room simulation platforms accessible from home. Ann Surg. 2020;272(2):e153.
31. El-Ghandour NMF, Ezzat AAM, Zaazoue MA, Gonzalez-Lopez P, Jhawar BS, Soliman MA. Virtual learning during the COVID-19 pandemic: A turning point in neurosurgical education. Neurosurg Focus. 2020;49(6):E18.
32. Ellison EC, Spanknebel K, Stain SC, Shabahang MM, Matthews JB, Debas HT, et al. Impact of the COVID-19 pandemic on surgical training and learner well-being: Report of a survey of general surgery and other surgical specialty educators. J Am Surg. 2020;231(6):613-26.
33. Dickinson KJ, Gronseth SL. Application of universal design for learning (UDL) principles to surgical education during the COVID-19 pandemic. J Surg Educ. 2020;77(5):1008-12.
34. Hau HM, Weitz J, Bork U. Impact of the COVID-19 pandemic on student and resident teaching and training in surgical oncology. J Clin Med. 2020;9(11):3431.
35. Okland TS, Pepper JP, Valdez TA. How do we teach surgical residents in the COVID-19 era?. J Surg Educ. 2020;77(5):1005-7.
36. Popa C, Schlanger D, Zaharie F, Al Hajjar N. Impact of the COVID-19 pandemic on the training of general surgery residents. Eur Surg. 2022;54(6):295-300.
37. Co M, Chu KM. Distant surgical teaching during COVID-19-A pilot study on final year medical students. Surg Pract. 2020;24(3):105-9.
38. Ellis R, Hay-David AGC, Brennan PA. Operating during the COVID-19 pandemic: How to reduce medical error. Br J Oral Maxillofac Surg. 2020;58(5):577-80.
39. Parry D, Oeppen RS, Gass H, Brennan PA. Impact of hydration and nutrition on personal performance in the clinical workplace. Br J Oral Maxillofac Surg. 2017;55(10):995-8.

40. O'Connor T, Papanikolaou V, Keogh IJ. Safe surgery, the human factors approach. The Surgeon. 2010;8(2):93-5.
41. Brennan PA, Davidson M. Improving patient safety: We need to reduce hierarchy and empower junior doctors to speak up. BMJ. 2019;366:l4461.
42. Chick RC, Clifton GT, Peace KM, Propper BW, Hale DF, Alseidi AA, et al. Using technology to maintain the education of residents during the COVID-19 pandemic. J Surg Educ. 2020;77(4):729-32.
43. Daodu O, Panda N, Lopushinsky S, Varghese Jr TK, Brindle M. COVID-19–Considerations and implications for surgical learners. Ann Surg. 2020;272(1):e22-3.
44. Adesoye T, Davis CH, Del Calvo H, Shaikh AF, Chegireddy V, Chan EY, et al. Optimization of surgical resident safety and education during the COVID-19 pandemic–lessons learned. J Surg Educ. 2021;78(1):315-20.
45. Ali US, Sukhia RH, Ghandhi D. Effect of coronavirus pandemic on oral and maxillofacial surgical education and training: Developing standards for effective online training. Adv Oral Maxillofac Surg. 2022:100246.
46. Bali RK, Chaudhry K. Maxillofacial surgery and COVID-19, The Pandemic!! J Maxillofac Oral Surg. 2020;19(2):159-61.
47. Bernardi L, Germani P, Del Zotto G, Scotton G, de Manzini N. Impact of COVID-19 pandemic on general surgery training program: An Italian experience. Am J Surg. 2020;220(5):1361-3.
48. Brar B, Bayoumy M, Salama A, Henry A, Chigurupati R. A survey assessing the early effects of COVID-19 pandemic on oral and maxillofacial surgery training programs. Oral Surg Oral Med Oral Pathol Oral Radiol. 2021;131(1):27-42.
49. Bishop R, Woerner JE, Stavropoulos F. Effects of the COVID-19 pandemic on the professional career of women in Oral and maxillofacial surgery. Oral Maxillofac Surg Clin North Am. 2021;33(4):475-80.
50. Ellison EC, Nagler A, Stain SC, Matthews JB, Spanknebel K, Shabahang MM, et al. Impact of the COVID-19 pandemic on surgical trainee education and well-being spring 2020–winter 2020: A path forward. Am J Surg. 2022;223(2):395-403.
51. Barca I, Cordaro R, Kallaverja E, Ferragina F, Cristofaro MG. Management in oral and maxillofacial surgery during the COVID-19 pandemic: Our experience. Br J Oral Maxillofac Surg. 2020;58(6):687-91.
52. Co M, Chung PH, Chu KM. Online teaching of basic surgical skills to medical students during the COVID-19 pandemic: A case–control study. Surg Today. 2021;51(8):1404-9.
53. Chigurupati R, Panchal N, Henry AM, Batal H, Sethi A, D'innocenzo R, et al. Considerations for oral and maxillofacial surgeons in COVID-19 era: Can we sustain the solutions to keep our patients and healthcare personnel safe? J Oral Maxillofac Surg. 2020;78(8):1241-56.
54. Coe TM, Jogerst KM, Sell NM, Cassidy DJ, Eurboonyanun C, Gee D, et al. Practical techniques to adapt surgical resident education to the COVID-19 era. Ann Surg. 2020;272(2):e139.
55. Huntley RE, Ludwig DC, Dillon JK. Early effects of COVID-19 on oral and maxillofacial surgery residency training—Results from a national survey. J Oral Maxillofac Surg. 2020;78(8):1257-67.
56. Aziz H, James T, Remulla D, Sher L, Genyk Y, Sullivan ME, et al. Effect of COVID-19 on Surgical Training Across the United States: A National Survey of General Surgery Residents. J Surg Educ. 2021;78(2):431-9.
57. Tassé N, Auger-Dufour E. The Impact of COVID-19 on Surgical Education: A Monocentric Survey of Residents Training in Surgical Specialties. Research Square. 2021.
58. Reolon LZ, de Oliveira RB, H Junior OL. Oral and maxillofacial surgery in front of Covid-19. Open Dent J. 2020;14(1).

59. Verma A, Verma S, Garg P, Godara R. Online teaching during COVID-19: Perception of medical undergraduate students. Indian J Surg. 2020;82(3):299-300.
60. Nagaraj MB, Weis HB, Weis JJ, Cook GS, Bailey LW, Shoultz TH, et al. The impact of COVID-19 on surgical education. J Surg Res. 2021;267:366-73.
61. Patel NA, Ji YD, Odera SL. The role of oral and maxillofacial surgeons in COVID-19 response. J Oral Maxillofac Surg. 2020;78(7):1052.
62. Wise CE, Merrell SB, Sasnal M, Forrester JD, Hawn MT, Lau JN, et al. COVID-19 impact on surgical resident education and coping. J Surg Res. 2021;264:534-43.
63. International Virtual Medical Conference. (2020). Finding a way. Conference Program. [online] Available from https://drive.google.com/file/d/1h46eYFVCTy2a0c2e-rqTxvskd--yJsPV/view [Last accessed February, 2024].

4

SECTION

Therapies

CHAPTER 22

The Need to Revisit Hydroxychloroquine in Early Treatment Strategies of COVID-19

Adriana Luzariaga, Jose Iglesias

INTRODUCTION

As no effective medicines were available during the early phases of the coronavirus disease 2019 (COVID-19) pandemic in March 2020, when the virus spread quickly and the healthcare systems were under extreme stress, the central focus was providing supportive care.[1] This approach was a somewhat nihilistic view that could translate to *"stay home and come to the hospital when you cannot breathe"*. Physicians began exploring the repurposing of the Food and Drug Administration (FDA) approved medicines for the off-label therapy of COVID-19.[2-4] Due to their in vitro and animal model antiviral effects against severe acute respiratory syndrome coronavirus 1 (SARS-CoV-1) and Middle East Respiratory Syndrome (MERS) virus, the first drugs to show promise were chloroquine (CQ) and hydroxychloroquine (HCQ).[5-9] This chapter will focus on HCQ as this agent became the central focus of controversy and confusion. It is the opinion of the authors that several issues are essential in attempting to understand the confusion and lack of clarity in discerning the benefit or lack thereof of repurposed drugs in general and HCQ in specific in the management of COVID-19. First is the politicization of HCQ and studies such as the scandalous Surgisphere studies, unwarranted safety concerns by health officials, the internet, the blogosphere, and mainstream media censoring and sensationalism.[4,10-18] Secondly, the lack of clinical trialists and public health officials not correctly considering the possibility that pre-hospitalized and hospitalized patients with COVID-19 represent different clinical phenotypes and pathophysiologic stages of the disease.[14,16,17,19-22] We will mainly concern ourselves with the latter.

It is pertinent to note that in <1 month of HCQ receiving emergency use authorization and unpopular world leaders endorsing HCQ, the therapeutic potential of HCQ in the early outpatient therapy was shipwrecked on politics.[13,18,23,24] In the United States, the Health and Human Services (HHS) department requested an early use expanded IND (Investigational New Drug) evaluating outcomes employing the Oracle platform, potentially leading to widespread rollout for HCQ early outpatient use.[17,22,24,25] However, some scientists and high-level bureaucrats at the FDA, skeptical of early data and concerned about drug safety (an agent that has been used safely for over 65 years), resisted HHS requests. Janet Woodcock MD and Richard Bright urged for a EUA limiting HCQ use to hospitalized patients under a healthcare provider's supervision.[17,24,25] The FDA authorized the emergency therpeutic use (EUA) of CQ and HCQ in certain hospitalized adults and teens on March 29, 2020.[17,22,24,25] Under the EUA, these medications could be used by licensed healthcare providers on patients who have been confirmed to have COVID-19, weigh >110 pounds, and are unable to participate in a clinical trial.[21,22,24,25] This EUA limited early outpatient treatment outside of randomized clinical trials.[21,22,25]

Interestingly, an agent employed safely in many settings for over half a century was raising safety concerns.[22,26] The basis for this was based on studies that used extremely high doses of HCQ and CQ in hospitalized critically ill patients, and two retracted studies of highly questionable validity.[10,11,26,27] Mehra et al.'s paper in The Lancet, published on May 22, suggested that CQ/HCQ therapy was ineffective and increased the risk of harm due to cardiac toxicity in COVID-19 patients.[10,28,29] The WHO suspended clinical trials involving these medications as a result.[26] However, The Lancet later published an Expression of Concern due to "serious scientific questions" and unverifiability and errors in the paper.[11,30] Shortly after that, the authors requested the paper's retraction due to issues with the data provided by the company responsible for data collection and analysis, Surgisphere.[11] An article in the New England Journal of Medicine on the safety of CQ, which also used data from Surgisphere, faced similar issues and was subsequently retracted.[10] Despite these flawed studies and evidence to the contrary, the FDA narrative continued.

Most adverse events reported during the height of HCQ use occurred in severely ill hospitalized patients.[21] The FDA has advised against using HCQ or CQ to treat COVID-19 outside of a hospital or clinical trial due to the risk of cardiotoxicity.[17,21] The warning is based on a review of the safety of these medications when used to treat hospitalized COVID-19 patients, which revealed severe cardiac issues and other safety concerns such as hematologic and immune system disorders, renal injuries, and hepatocellular toxicity and failure.[17,20,22,31] The FDA has not evaluated the safety of these medications for treating high-risk outpatients with COVID-19, and therefore, the effects and potential side effects seen in hospitalized patients cannot be applied to outpatient treatment. It is uncertain whether the FDA has data on the potential side effects of HCQ in outpatients.[21] A small percentage of COVID-19 patients at high risk of serious illness may have reasons why they should not take HCQ alone or in combination with agents known to prolong QT interval. This percentage is likely to be <5%.[21,22,31] However, it is up to individual doctors to decide whether to prescribe HCQ to their patients based on the patient's overall health and any potential contraindications. This process is a normal part of evaluating the suitability of medications for individual patients and does not necessarily mean that HCQ should not be used in general. Of note that in the majority, if not all, of the early outpatient treatment trials involving thousands of patients, there were no significant life-threatening arrhythmias.[5,32-35] As emphasized, applying safety concerns due to adverse events in critically ill hospitalized patients to early outpatient HCQ use is erroneous and unwarranted, e.g., consider the Solidarity and Recovery Trials. The WHO SOLIDARITY trial was a randomized controlled trial (RCT) that evaluated the efficacy of HCQ as a treatment for COVID-19.[36] The study enrolled 954 individuals who were in very late stages of the illness with a significant percentage of patients receiving oxygen or ventilation support.[36] The results of the trial showed that HCQ did not significantly reduce mortality compared to standard care (SC).[36]

The dose used in the Solidarity trial was very high, with patients receiving 1,600 mg in the first day and 9,600 mg over 10 days. It is pertinent to note that due to HCQ half-life, this dose may result in drug toxicity.[36] The authors of the trial did not report the weight or obesity status of the individuals, so it is not possible to determine whether toxicity may have been increased in individuals of lower weight.[36]

The trial's Kaplan-Meier (KM) curves demonstrate an increase in HCQ mortality between days 5 and 7, corresponding to about 90% of the excess mortality seen on day 28. Almost all of the excess mortality was seen in patients who were receiving mechanical ventilation.[36] It is no surprise that the trial results suggest that HCQ may not be an effective therapy for COVID-19 and may be linked with increased mortality in specific patient groups.[36]

Similarly, the RECOVERY trial was an RCT that assessed the efficacy of HCQ as a treatment for COVID-19.[37] The trial enrolled very sick patients who were at least nine days after symptom onset. The trial demonstrated that HCQ did not significantly decrease mortality compared to SC.[37]

The HCQ dosage used in the trial was very high, with patients receiving a 9,200 mg over 10 days.[37] As in the Solidarity trial, the authors did not report the results based on patient weight, body mass index (BMI), or comorbidities, which may have provided additional insight into the potential for toxicity.[37] There was no weight based dose adjustment, so that toxicity may have been higher in patients with a lower weight.[37]

The KM curves for the trial show an increase in HCQ mortality between days 5 and 8, which corresponds to about 85% of the excess mortality seen on day 28.[37] The authors of the trial noted that they did not detect an excess in mortality in first 24–48 hours of therapy. However, they did not consider the long half-life of HCQ or the dosing regimen, which may have been a factor in the increased mortality.[37] Other studies, such as the one by Borba et al., have shown that increased mortality can occur after 2 days of treatment with high doses of HCQ.[38]

In order to fully appreciate the controversy of repurposed drugs in general and HCQ in particular, it is essential to emphasize that COVID-19 infection has several clinical stages resulting in a multitude of pathophysiologic aberrations ranging from a pre-symptomatic viral replication phase, a viremic phase when patients become symptomatic, followed in some to later stages of pulmonary involvement and in a smaller percentage to a late inflammatory pulmonary phase acute respiratory distress syndrome (ARDS), cytokine storm, and organ failure. Most patients accounting for progression to severe disease hospitalization, excess morbidity, and mortality are usually elderly and have underlying comorbidities. During the first two waves of the pandemic, individuals hospitalized already manifested severe illness and late presentation.[39-43] In this setting, it is improbable that administering any antiviral agent such as HCQ would be therapeutic. Due to the multiphasic pathophysiology of the disease, which involves virally mediated, prothrombotic, and inflammatory injury, there is unlikely one silver bullet for therapy; rather multimodal early therapeutic approach would be much more prudent.[34,39,41,42] Thus, any repurposed agent to treat COVID-19 should be used with other therapeutic agents such as zinc, antibiotics with immune-modulating properties such as azithromycin (AZ) or doxycycline, ivermectin, anticoagulant-antithrombotic agents, and vitamins.[34,39,41,42,44] Glucocorticoids such as methylprednisolone, dexamethasone, prednisone, or inhaled budesonide if high-risk patients progress to the pulmonary phase of the disease.[42] In addition, administering agents to hypoxemic critically ill patients would increase the potential for adverse effects, thus raising safety concerns. Recognizing these factors is essential in the analysis and totality of evidence involving the use of HCQ, medication dosing, the timing of drug administration, and the patient population studied. Thus, early COVID-19 and late diseases can be viewed as two diseases requiring a focus and deployment of different treatment strategies. We propose revisiting HCQ studies based on an early treatment paradigm in high-risk patients.

TOTALITY OF EVIDENCE

For the last several decades, physicians have emphasized what is now called evidence-based medicine (EBM), which relies heavily on RCT to be the basis of clinical decision-making. However, RCTs are not the best and end-all when making clinical decisions at the bedside of critically ill patients. RCTs are a common type of study design used in research to assess the effectiveness of a treatment or intervention. However, RCTs have limitations and are subject to potential flaws and biases, are subject to the limitations of statistical power, and may not always apply to real-world experience. In addition, RCTs can be designed to fail.[45-48]

Nonrandomized trials and large observational studies, another type of study design, can provide valuable evidence and sometimes show similar results to RCTs.[49] Anglemyer et al. performed a large meta-analysis on several thousands of individual studies and determined that the overall effect estimate, as measured by the pooled relative risk ratio (RRR), was similar for both studies.[49] Thus, the results of well-conducted observational studies, which do not use random assignment to assign participants to treatment groups, are similar to those of RCTs.

A more rewarding course of action should be based on the totality of evidence that takes into consideration the pathophysiology of the disease, the natural history of the disease, i.e., who is at risk for severe disease, the status of the patient, the molecular pharmacology of agents which may be of benefit, the real-world experience with treating the disease ranging from individual case series, large observational studies, and open-label trials, nonrandomized and randomized clinical trials. In the following section, we will briefly review the vital evidence which will make a case for revisiting HCQ in the early therapeutic management of the disease.

The antiviral effects of HCQ are multifactorial **(Fig. 1)**. The fusion of SARS-CoV-2 to the endosomal membrane, a necessary step for viral components to enter the cytosol, depends on an acidic endosomal pH.[50-52] HCQ is a weak base that has been found to raise endosomal pH, thus inhibiting endosomal pathways and enzymes necessary for viral entry into the cytosol.[50-53] In silico docking experiments by Baildya et al. have demonstrated that HCQ binds to the principal protease of SARS-CoV-2 and alters the structure of the protease, thus potentially inhibiting protease activity.[6] Fantini et al., employing Silico experiments, demonstrated that HCQ binds to cell surface sialic acid glycoproteins and gangliosides, inhibiting viral S protein attachment to the angiotensin-converting enzyme 2 (ACE2) receptor and restriction of pH-dependent S protein cleavage at the ACE2 receptor site.[54] HCQ is a known zinc ionophore and increases lysosomal zinc concentrations in lysosomes, thus potentiating the antiviral effects of zinc.[55]

Yao et al., employing SARS-CoV-2 infected Vero cells, demonstrated that HCQ was more potent than CQ. After evaluating five different dosing models, the potentially safest and most effective dose to treat SARS-CoV-2 infection was to start with 400 mg twice a day on the first day of treatment, proceeded by 200 mg twice daily for 4 more days.[8] In a small nonrandomized open-label trial in which the primary endpoint was virological clearance at day 6, Gautret et al. reported a statistically significant decrease in viral load on day 6 in patients who received 600 mg of HCQ daily compared to controls.[56] Lagier et al. in a retrospective analysis propensity-matched study involving over 3,735 COVID-19 patients comparing 3,119 patients who received early treatment with HCQ 600 mg daily for 5 days and AZ to patients who received other treatment.[57] Treatment with HCQ/AZ resulted in a statistically significant decrease in transfer to the intensive care unit (ICU), less hospitalization, and faster viral clearance. It is pertinent to note that 3,064 patients were essentially outpatients treated in a daycare hospital.[57]

In contrast, Rodrigues et al., in a double-blinded randomized trial, was conducted to test the efficacy of HCQ and AZ in treating early and mild cases

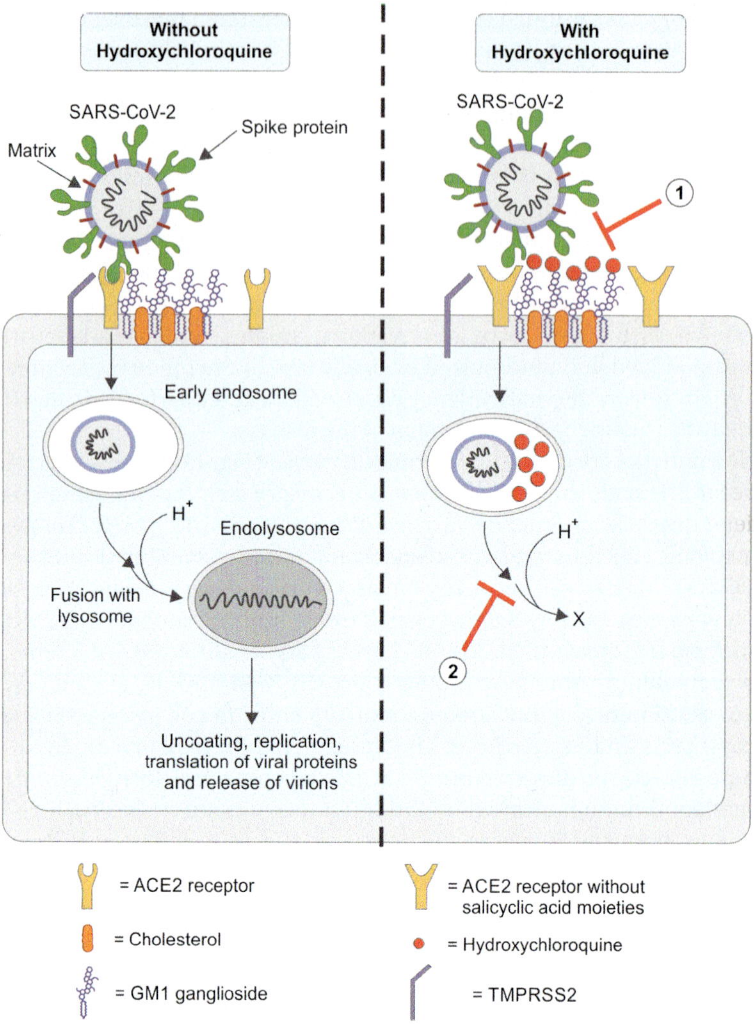

FIGURE 1: Multifactorial antiviral mechanisms of action of hydroxychloroquine in preventing coronavirus disease 2019 (COVID-19) infection. (1) Blocking entry of severe acute respiratory syndrome coronavirus 2 (SARS-CoV-2) by binding to GM1 gangliosides present on the cell membrane, preventing the interaction of viral spike protein with them. In addition, by inhibiting synthesis of sialic acid moieties on the angiotensin-converting enzyme 2 (ACE2) receptor, it reduces binding of the viral ligand to its target receptor. (2) Hydroxychloroquine is concentrated in the endosomes and lysosomes of the cell. Due to their basic nature, they lower the pH in the endosomes, thus preventing the maturation of early endosomes into endolysosomes and preventing the activity of cathepsin B and L.[52]

Source: Adapted with permission from Agarwal M, Ranjan P, Baitha U, Mittal A. Hydroxychloroquine as a Chemoprophylactic Agent for COVID-19: A Clinico-Pharmacological Review. Front Pharmacol. 2020;11:593099.

of disease.[58] The trial included 84 patients who were randomly assigned to receive either the treatment or a placebo.[58] The study's primary endpoint was viral clearance within nine days, and the secondary endpoints included viral load reduction, clinical evolution, hospitalization rates, and chest CT evolution.[58] The results showed no significant difference in viral clearance rates between the treatment and placebo.[58] It is of note that the average age of these individuals was 36 years old, thus representing a relatively low-risk group.[58] There was only one hospitalization in the HCQ AZ group.[58] Likewise, Avezum et al., in a reasonably large double-blind RCT outpatient trial (COPE trial) involving relatively young patients, median age 45 (35–56), which included 1,372 randomly assigned to receive either HCQ or a placebo.[5] Over 60% were randomized at >4 days from the onset of symptoms, with results demonstrating no difference in the risk of hospitalization between those treated with HCQ or placebo.[5] In the Avezum et al. study, the investigators also included a small meta-analysis of six published studies suggesting there was no significant benefit of HCQ in reducing hospitalization among patients, although not reaching statistical significance, higher efficacy was observed when therapy was initiated <4 days from onset, relative risk (RR) of 0.61.[5] Of note that this meta-analysis included three studies which were essentially late treatment trials one of which was terminated early.[5] Johnston et al. conducted an RCT that compared therapy with ascorbic acid + folic acid, HCQ + folic acid, and HCQ + AZ.[59] The study was terminated early, and enrollment occurred at a median time of 5.9 days after individuals became symptomatic.[59] The study demonstrated a trend in differences in hospitalization rates between the treatment groups, with a trend toward lower hospitalization rates in the HCQ and HCQ + AZ groups. The study demonstrated that HCQ was associated with a trend to faster viral clearance compared to the other treatment groups.[59] The published paper reported a median time to viral clearance of 7 days for the ascorbic acid + folic acid group.[59] The study included primarily low-risk patients (although the study title states high risk, with a median age of 37 and no deaths, and post-hoc analyses were performed to obscure the statistically significant rapid viral clearance of HCQ).[59] The investigators identified low and high-risk groups but did not give results on viral shedding or symptom resolution for these groups.[59] A RCT conducted by Omrani and colleagues compared the use of HCQ + AZ and HCQ alone to a control group in low-risk patients.[60] The investigators demonstrated any difference between the groups in terms of clinical outcomes.[60] The authors noted that the results might not apply to higher risk individuals, and the presence of detectable levels of the virus [as measured by polymerase chain reaction (PCR)] may not necessarily indicate active infection, and that alternative dosing regimens for HCQ may be more effective. Medication adherence was not assessed in the study.[60] The HCQ dosing in the study was 600 mg/day for 1 week, and it is probable that therapeutic levels of the drug were not achieved for several days.[60] No deaths or serious adverse events were reported in the study, and although the investigators observed a 12% lower hospitalization rate in the treatment groups, the result was not statistically significant.[60] It is possible that the study was underpowered to detect a difference. Lastly Schwartz et al. conducted a small RCT comparing the use of HCQ to a control group.[61] The study was terminated early and demonstrated no differences between the treatment groups.[61] The HCQ group had a median of 7 days from symptomatic disease onset, but it is not clear if this includes the delay in delivering the medication.[61] The study reported that four HCQ hospitalizations occurred, but only one of these hospitalizations was included in the per-protocol analysis.[61] It is not specified in the study whether patients received and took any HCQ before being hospitalized, which occurred one day after randomization.[61]

It is important to consider the power of a RCT when interpreting its results, mainly when the study is unable to reject the null hypothesis (a "negative trial"). In order to accurately determine the effectiveness of a treatment, RCTs should be powered to detect meaningful outcomes such as hospitalizations and mortality and should be conducted in high risk individuals.

Catteau et al. evaluating a large hospital registry that involved 4,542 patients receiving a total of 2,400 mg of HCQ over 5 days and SC and 3,533 patients receiving SC, demonstrated that treatment with HCQ was associated with a significant difference in both early treatments ≤ 5 days or late treatment ≥ 5 days after symptom onset.[62]

A Dutch multicenter observation study involving over 1,000 non-ICU patients treated with HCQ within 1 day of admission (mean dose of 2,020 mg during admission) resulted in a 53% decrease in transfer to ICU. However, the study did not demonstrate a significant decrease in mortality.[63]

Matthieu et al. evaluated the mortality rate of individuals treated as outpatients and received HCQ and AZ as part of their therapy.[34] The primary outcome was 6-week mortality, with the secondary outcome being the transfer rates to the ICU and hospitalization. The study included 10,429 patients, with a median age of 45 and 53.7% women.[34] Out of these, 16 patients died, giving a mortality rate of 0.15%, and the infection fatality rate, or the proportion of infected individuals who died, was 0.06% among the 8,315 patients who received HCQ + AZ treatment.[34] There were no deaths among the 8,414 patients under the age of 60.[34] The study demonstrated that older age and being male were linked to a higher risk of death, ICU transfer, and hospitalization.[34] HCQ + AZ treatment was linked to a lower risk of death, regardless of age, gender, or the episode of the epidemic.[34]

Skipper et al., in a multinational internet, mail-order double-blind RCT, evaluated the early treatment with HCQ in adults who were not hospitalized and had four days or less of symptomatic disease.[64] Participants in the treatment group received a dose of HCQ (800 mg once, followed by 600 mg in 6–8 hours, then 600 mg daily for 4 more days), while participants in the control group received a placebo of folic acid 400 μg per day.[64] This study involved many low-risk patients (median age 40 years, 65% of patients with no comorbidities) and was grossly underpowered to detect a difference in the primary outcome.[64] After interim analysis, the primary endpoint was changed from hospitalization, ICU admission, and mortality within 14 days of treatment to a change in overall symptom severity within 14 days.[64] The findings of the study imply that the treatment being evaluated may be associated with a lower risk of death or hospitalization due to COVID-19, a lower risk of hospitalization due to COVID-19, a decreased risk of death or hospitalization due to all causes, a lower risk of hospitalization due to all causes, and a lower risk of not recovering by day 14 compared to the control group.[64] The differences in risk between the treatment and control groups were not significant for any of these outcomes ($p > 0.05$).[64] This article sparked some degree of controversies that transcend this chapter, and we refer to the comments section of the published article and Pullen et al.[64,65] Suffice to say there are limitations to the current study, among them the low-risk population recruited and the self-resolution of disease in low-risk subjects. In the case of Skipper et al., self-resolution is a confounder which is the natural history of the disease in low-risk patients that dilutes the potential benefit of active treatment **(Figs. 2A and B)**.[64,66]

Similarly, Mitjà et al. suffers from the same issues, as this is a low-risk patient population with a median age of 42 years.[22,67] The study enrolled 136 patients who received HCQ 3,200 mg over 7 days (800 mg day 1, 400 mg days 2–7) and 157 control patients who did not receive any treatment, with a median time from the onset of symptomatic disease to enrollment was 3 days in both groups; however, the authors report a delay of up to 120 hours and results are not stratified according to time to treatment.[67] The primary endpoint was decreased nasal pharyngeal viral load by PCR, which may or

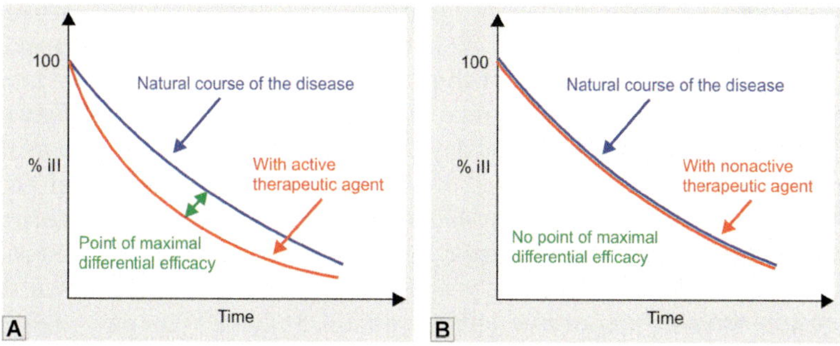

FIGURES 2A AND B: Self-resolution is a confounder which is the natural history of the disease in low risk patients and dilutes potential benefit of active treatment. (A) The effect of treatment in a high-risk patient without self-resolution; (B) Low-risk patient with self-resolution of disease.

Source: Adapted with permission from Skipper CP, Pastick KA, Engen NW, Bangdiwala AS, Abassi M, Lofgren SM, Williams DA, et al. Hydroxychloroquine in nonhospitalized adults with early COVID-19: A Randomized Trial. Ann Intern Med. 2020;173(8):623-31.

may not represent a viable virus.[67] The study found that the control group had a hospitalization rate of 7.0%, while the treatment group had a hospitalization rate of 5.9%.[67] The study is considered uninformative because the study involved mostly low-risk individuals, and the low risk is demonstrated by the relatively low hospitalization rates in both groups.[22] In another trial, Mitjà et al. conducted an open-label, cluster-randomized post-exposure prophylaxis (PEP) study comparing HCQ (800 mg on day 1, then 400 mg on days 2–7) to no treatment in asymptomatic COVID-19 patients' contacts.[68] The primary outcome was PCR-confirmed symptoms within 14 days, and the secondary outcome was SARS-CoV-2 infection with or without symptoms. Adverse events were also recorded for 28 days.[68] Individuals were randomly assigned to the HCQ or the control groups. Although one must consider the caveats of subgroup analysis, an exciting finding involving a subgroup of nursing home patients, which are high-risk individuals, revealed a more significant effect of the treatment on positive, symptomatic cases of the disease in nursing home residents compared to the overall population.[22,68] However, the sample size was too small for statistical significance. If the trend continued, the result would be significant with a larger number of patients.

In an early treatment trial, Cadegiani et al. compared the effectiveness of three treatments (HCQ, nitazoxanide, and ivermectin) to a historical control group of untreated patients from the same population were studied retrospectively for COVID-19 in terms of overall clinical outcomes.[69] The study found that these treatments were similarly effective when used within 7 days of symptom onset, and were superior to no treatment, even for outcomes that are not influenced by the placebo effect, especially when combined with AZ, ascorbic acid, vitamin D, and zinc.[69] The study included 585 individuals with an average treatment delay of 2.9 days, and there were no hospitalizations ($p = 0.001$), mechanical ventilation ($p = 0.001$, or deaths ($p = 0.21$) among the treated group.[69]

The Hapvida Brazil outpatient treatment study was conducted between May and June 2020 and involved 717 patients over 40 who had tested positive and were receiving treatment at the Hapvida HMO in Brazil.[70] The study examined the effectiveness of a range of medications, including HCQ (400 mg BID on day 1, then 400 mg daily on days 2–5), prednisone, AZ, and ivermectin, in the treatment of COVID-19.[70] The study found that the use of HCQ (400 mg BID on day 1 followed by 400 mg daily on days 2–5) and prednisone together was associated with a lower risk of hospitalization; while the use of HCQ alone or prednisone alone was also associated with a decreased risk of hospitalization, prednisone alone, and HCQ alone.[70] Therapy with AZ showed a small, though not statistically significant, additional benefit, while ivermectin did not show any additional benefit.[70] No cardiac arrhythmia events required medication termination in any of the patients, and no deaths were attributed to such arrhythmias.[70]

A study was conducted by Ip et al. among outpatients in New Jersey to examine the effect of HCQ on C outcomes, and the study included 1,274 patients, with 75% of patients being high risk with nonadmission emergency room (ER) visits who had confirmed SARS-CoV-2 infection by PCR testing. Of these patients, 97 received HCQ, and the remaining 1,177 were matched to the HCQ group based on age, demographic variables, and various comorbidity factors.[33] The study found that treatment with HCQ significantly reduced the risk of hospitalization by 46% compared to the matched control group.[33] The retrospective study used propensity score matching to control for potential confounders. Therapy with HCQ decreased the risk of hospitalization by 46% ($p = 0.038$).[33]

A nonrandomized observational study conducted in 24 nursing homes in Marseille found that among 226 infected nursing home residents (51.4% patients received HCQ) with AZ and were monitored as described in previous studies for at least 3 days, the study adjusted for factors such as gender, age, oxygen therapy, and the method of detection. There was an associated 63% reduced risk of mortality $p = 0.02$.[71] The study results suggest that HCQ and AZ may effectively reduce the mortality risk in this patient population.

Heras et al. evaluated HCQ in high-risk patients from a skilled nursing facility; this study analyzed 100 confirmed cases, with the majority of patients being elderly (median age 85 and female, and the case fatality rate was 20%).[72] Male gender, fever, pulmonary symptoms, dementia, a low Barthel Index (a measure of functional independence), and lymphocytopenia were associated with a higher risk of death. Receiving treatment with HCQ plus AZ was associated with a higher chance of survival.[72] After adjusting for other factors, male gender, a low Barthel Index, no pharmacological treatment, and lymphocytopenia were identified as independent risk factors for mortality.[72] Therapy with HCQ + AZ versus only other antibiotics improved survival OR = 0.044 (95% CI 0.006–0.35), $p = 0.004$, while treatment with HCQ + other antibiotics versus other antibiotics alone did not.[33]

An observational study conducted by Cangiano et al. investigated the association between COVID-19 mortality and vitamin D and HCQ treatment in a nursing home in Milan, Italy; among the 157 residents, 98 tested positive for COVID-19 and were included in the study.[73] The average age of the study patients was 90 years.[73] Of the 96 PCR-positive patients, supplementation with vitamin D was associated with 70% lower mortality RR 0.30, $p = 0.04$.[73] In addition, the administration of HCQ to this high-risk group was also associated with a sevenfold reduced mortality risk.[73] The administration of HCQ was limited to individuals with better electrocardiogram results and those receiving fewer medications which potentially cause electrocardiographic changes, such as antipsychotics and antidepressants.[73] However, it is unclear whether these medications explain entirely the considerable decrease in mortality risk seen with HCQ use.[73]

Sulaiman et al., whose study is still in preprint and not peer-reviewed, evaluated 7,892 patients with PCR-confirmed COVID-19 outpatients who attended fever outpatient clinics and had confirmed clinical outcomes at day 28.[74] The study group was divided into two groups: A HCQ group and a SC group.[74] At baseline, the HCQ group was more likely than the SC group to be male and not have hypertension or chronic lung disease compared to the SC group, and the HCQ group also had higher rates of symptoms (fever, headache, and cough) at presentation.[74] The study found that early HCQ-based therapy had less hospital admissions within 28 days [9.4% vs. 16.6%, relative risk reduction (RRR) 43%, $p < 0.001$].[74] The composite outcome of ICU admission and/or mortality at 28 days was also lower in the HCQ group compared to the SC group (1.2% vs. 2.6%, RRR 54%, $p = 0.001$).[74] Controlling for age, gender, and significant comorbidities, the probability of hospitalization was lower in the HCQ group.[74]

Mokhtari et al., conducted a multicenter, retrospective cohort study of adults with mild disease involving 28,759 patients, who diagnosed either RT-PCR (79%) or by clinical parameters and chest imaging (21%).[75] The therapy group ($n = 7{,}295$) received HCQ at a dose of 400 mg twice daily on day 1 and 200 mg twice daily for the following 4 days, and the control group received supportive care only.[75] The groups were similar in age and gender, but the treated group had a slightly higher incidence of coexisting conditions.[75] After adjusting for age, gender, BMI, hypertension, and comorbidities, treatment with HCQ was associated with a 38% reduction in the risk of being hospitalized and a 70% reduction in the risk of mortality.[75] These risk reductions were significant and similar in individuals diagnosed by PCR or by clinical factors and chest imaging.[75]

Early outpatient treatment of high-risk COVID-19 patients with HCQ with or without multimodal therapies such as corticosteroids, zinc, and other agents may improve hard clinical outcomes such as hospitalization and death. Based on an early outpatient treatment paradigm, HCQ use should be revisited. We review all the major early studies with hospitalizations and/or mortality as endpoints in **Figures 3 and 4** represent Forrest plots demonstrating early treatment outcomes.

Similar to outpatient treatment, the use of HCQ in pre-exposure prophylaxis (PrEP) and PEP has been fraught with uncertainty.[76] During the prevaccine period of the pandemic, HCQ was initially considered as a potential prophylactic agent for COVID-19. However, due to concerns regarding dosing regimens and after trials reported a nonstatistically significant lower risk associated of infection with HCQ prophylaxis, HCQ was generally considered by the medical community as ineffective for COVID-19 prophylaxis.[76] The extensive although early belief about HCQ's lack of efficacy impeded the enrollment of patients into ongoing trials of HCQ prophylaxis.[76] As Garcia-Albeniz et al. point out in their recent meta-analysis, key decisions were made based on insufficient evidence during the prevaccine period of the pandemic.[76] Garcia-Albeniz conducted a meta-analysis of 11 completed

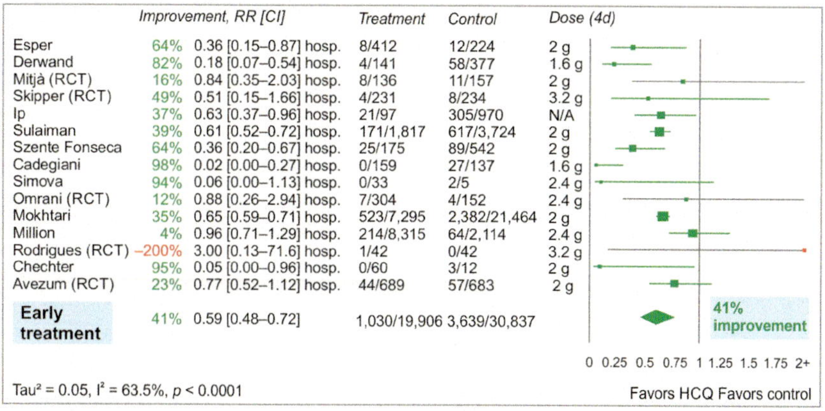

FIGURE 3: Meta-analysis of all 15 early treatment trials and hospitalization.[29,32,33,34,44,48,58,60,64,69,70,75,172,173]

(HCQ: hydroxychloroquine; RCT: randomized controlled trial; RR: relative risk)

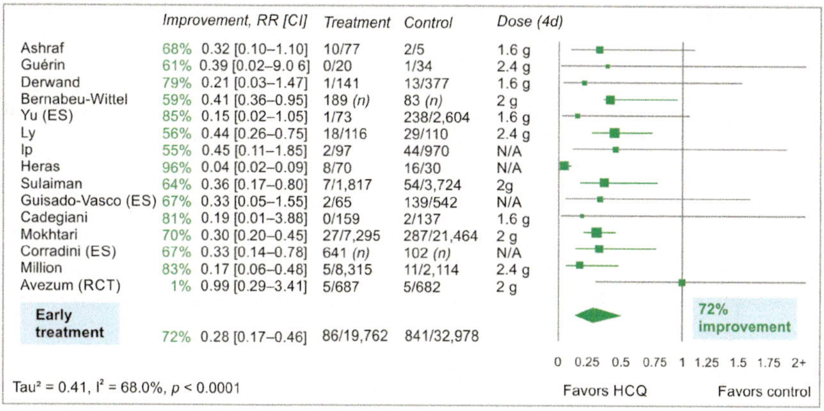

FIGURE 4: Meta-analysis of all early treatment trials and mortality.[5,44,33,71,72,75,173]

(HCQ: hydroxychloroquine; RCT: randomized controlled trial; RR: relative risk)

randomized trials studying the effectiveness of HCQ to prevent COVID-19 observing that a benefit of HCQ as prophylaxis for COVID-19 cannot be excluded based on the current evidence.[76] The pooled risk ratio estimate of the PrEP trials was 0.72 and for the PEP trials was 0.91.[76] All trials found a similar rate of serious adverse effects in the HCQ and no HCQ groups.[76] However, the "not statistically significant" interpretation of early prophylaxis trials as evidence of HCQ's lack of effectiveness disrupted the timely completion of remaining trials, which hindered the generation of precise estimates for pandemic management before the development of vaccines.[76] A summary of PrEP and PRP studies is summarized in **Table 1**.

TABLE 1: Hydroxychloroquine pre-exposure studies including subjects with autoimmune disorders and prophylaxis studies.	
[Abella], 9/30/2020, randomized controlled trial, USA, peer-reviewed[77]	Risk of case, 5.0% lower, RR 0.95, $p = 1.00$, treatment 4 of 64 (6.2%), control 4 of 61 (6.6%), NNT 325
[Agarwal], 9/14/2021, prospective, India, preprint[78]	Risk of hospitalization, 94.8% lower, RR 0.05, $p = 0.61$, treatment 0 of 29 (0.0%), control 17 of 455 (3.7%), NNT 27, relative risk is not 0 because of continuity correction due to zero events (with reciprocal of the contrasting arm)
	Relative severity, 26.9% better, RR 0.73, $p = 0.21$, treatment 29, control 455
	Risk of case, 4.6% higher, RR 1.05, $p = 0.81$, treatment 6 of 29 (20.7%), control 90 of 455 (19.8%)
[Ahmed], 11/23/2021, retrospective, Saudi Arabia, peer-reviewed[79]	Risk of case, 99.3% lower, OR 0.007, $p = 0.08$, treatment 0 of 50 (0.0%) cases, 13 of 50 (26.0%) controls, NNT 1.7, case control OR
[Alegiani], 4/15/2021, retrospective, case control, database analysis, Italy, peer-reviewed[80]	Risk of death, 8.0% higher, OR 1.08, $p = 0.64$, HCQ vs. other cDMARDs, RR approximated with OR
	Risk of hospitalization, 18.0% lower, OR 0.82, $p = 0.03$, HCQ vs. other cDMARDs, RR approximated with OR
	Risk of death, 19.0% higher, OR 1.19, $p = 0.32$, HCQ vs. MTX, RR approximated with OR
	Risk of hospitalization, 12.0% lower, OR 0.88, $p = 0.17$, HCQ vs. MTX, RR approximated with OR
[Alzahrani], 4/15/2021, retrospective, Saudi Arabia, peer-reviewed[81]	Risk of death, 58.7% lower, RR 0.41, $p = 1.00$, treatment 0 of 14 (0.0%), control 1 of 33 (3.0%), NNT 33, relative risk is not 0 because of continuity correction due to zero events (with reciprocal of the contrasting arm)
	Risk of mechanical ventilation, 81.0% lower, RR 0.19, $p = 0.54$, treatment 0 of 14 (0.0%), control 3 of 33 (9.1%), NNT 11, relative risk is not 0 because of continuity correction due to zero events (with reciprocal of the contrasting arm)
	Risk of severe case, 32.7% lower, RR 0.67, $p = 0.70$, treatment 2 of 14 (14.3%), control 7 of 33 (21.2%), NNT 14
[Arleo], 10/27/2020, retrospective, USA, preprint[82]	Risk of death, 50.0% lower, RR 0.50, $p = 0.67$, treatment 1 of 20 (5.0%), control 5 of 50 (10.0%), NNT 20, all patients
	Risk of death, 52.0% lower, RR 0.48, $p = 0.64$, treatment 1 of 10 (10.0%), control 5 of 24 (20.8%), NNT 9.2, inpatients

Continued

Continued

[Badyal], 6/7/2021, prospective, India, peer-reviewed[83]	Risk of case, 60.1% lower, RR 0.40, $p < 0.001$, treatment 247 of 617 (40.0%), control 611 of 1,473 (41.5%), adjusted per study, odds ratio converted to relative risk, ≥6 weeks, logistic regression
	Risk of case, 35.1% lower, RR 0.65, $p = 0.003$, treatment 88 of 185 (47.6%), control 611 of 1,473 (41.5%), adjusted per study, odds ratio converted to relative risk, 4–5 weeks, logistic regression
	Risk of case, 23.2% lower, RR 0.77, $p = 0.04$, treatment 80 of 181 (44.2%), control 611 of 1,473 (41.5%), adjusted per study, odds ratio converted to relative risk, 2–3 weeks, logistic regression
[Bae], 2/20/2021, retrospective, propensity score matching, South Korea, peer-reviewed[84]	Risk of case, 30.3% lower, RR 0.70, $p = 0.18$, treatment 16 of 743 (2.2%), control 91 of 2,698 (3.4%), NNT 82, odds ratio converted to relative risk, PSM
	Risk of case, 19.5% lower, RR 0.81, $p = 0.50$, treatment 16 of 743 (2.2%), control 91 of 2,698 (3.4%), odds ratio converted to relative risk, PSM, adjusted for region
	Risk of case, 30.3% lower, RR 0.70, $p = 0.30$, treatment 16 of 743 (2.2%), control 91 of 2,698 (3.4%), NNT 82, odds ratio converted to relative risk, PSM, adjusted for immunosuppressant use
	Risk of case, 40.2% lower, RR 0.60, $p = 0.09$, odds ratio converted to relative risk, PSM, HCQ ≥ 6 months
[Becetti], 8/5/2022, retrospective, Qatar, peer-reviewed, mean age 43[85]	Risk of case, 36.8% lower, RR 0.63, $p = 0.17$, treatment 26 of 314 (8.3%), control 49 of 386 (12.7%), NNT 23, adjusted per study, odds ratio converted to relative risk, multivariable
	Risk of case, 52.0% lower, RR 0.48, $p < 0.001$, treatment 16 of 46 (34.8%), control 29 of 40 (72.5%), NNT 2.7, patients with close contact to cases, close contact
[Behera], 11/3/2020, retrospective, India, peer-reviewed[86]	Risk of case, 27.9% lower, RR 0.72, $p = 0.29$, treatment 7 of 19 (36.8%), control 179 of 353 (50.7%), NNT 7.2, adjusted per study, odds ratio converted to relative risk, model 2 conditional logistic regression
	Risk of case, 26.3% lower, RR 0.74, $p = 0.25$, treatment 7 of 19 (36.8%), control 179 of 353 (50.7%), NNT 7.2, odds ratio converted to relative risk, matched pair analysis
[Belmont], 10/6/2021, prospective, USA, preprint, clinical trial NCT04354870 (history)[87]	Risk of symptomatic case, 78.6% lower, RR 0.21, $p = 0.21$, treatment 1 of 56 (1.8%), control 2 of 24 (8.3%), NNT 15
	Risk of case, 14.3% lower, RR 0.86, $p = 1.00$, treatment 4 of 56 (7.1%), control 2 of 24 (8.3%), NNT 84
[Bhatt], 8/4/2021, prospective, India[88]	Risk of case, 49.3% higher, RR 1.49, $p = 0.02$, treatment 167 of 731 (22.8%), control 30 of 196 (15.3%)

Continued

Continued

[Bhattacharya], 6/9/2020, retrospective, India[89]	Risk of case, 80.7% lower, RR 0.19, $p = 0.001$, treatment 4 of 54 (7.4%), control 20 of 52 (38.5%), NNT 3.2
[Cassione], 5/12/2020, retrospective, Italy, peer-reviewed, survey, median age 52.5, patients excluded in exclusion analyses: not fully adjusting for the different baseline risk of systemic autoimmune patients[90]	Risk of case, 49.6% higher, RR 1.50, $p = 0.59$, treatment 10 of 127 (7.9%), control 2 of 38 (5.3%)
[Chatterjee], 5/28/2020, retrospective, India, peer-reviewed, survey[91]	Risk of case, 66.8% lower, RR 0.33, $p < 0.001$, treatment 12 of 68 (17.6%), control 206 of 387 (53.2%), NNT 2.8, full course vs. unused
[Cordtz], 8/27/2021, retrospective, population-based cohort, Denmark, peer-reviewed, study period 1 March, 2020 to 2 February, 2021[92]	Risk of hospitalization, 40.0% lower, HR 0.60, $p = 0.39$, treatment 1,170, control 1,363, adjusted per study
[Cordtz (B)], 12/28/2020, retrospective, population-based cohort, Denmark, peer-reviewed[93]	Risk of hospitalization, 24.0% lower, HR 0.76, $p = 0.67$, treatment 3 of 2,722 (0.1%), control 38 of 26,718 (0.1%), NNT 3124, adjusted per study, time-dependent exposure model
	Risk of hospitalization, 55.0% lower, HR 0.45, $p = 0.28$, treatment 3 of 2,722 (0.1%), control 38 of 26,718 (0.1%), adjusted per study, time-fixed exposure model
[Datta], 11/6/2020, retrospective, India, peer-reviewed[94]	Risk of case, 22.1% lower, RR 0.78, $p = 0.47$, treatment 16 of 146 (11.0%), control 19 of 135 (14.1%), NNT 32
[lopez-de la Iglesia], 9/2/2020, retrospective, database analysis, Spain, preprint, patients excluded in exclusion analyses: not fully adjusting for the different baseline risk of systemic autoimmune patients[95]	Risk of hospitalization, 50.0% higher, RR 1.50, $p = 1.00$, treatment 3 of 687 (0.4%), control 2 of 688 (0.3%)
	Risk of case, 42.6% higher, RR 1.43, $p = 0.15$, treatment 42 of 648 (6.5%), control 30 of 660 (4.5%), suspected COVID-19
	Risk of case, 7.8% lower, RR 0.92, $p = 0.84$, treatment 12 of 678 (1.8%), control 13 of 677 (1.9%), NNT 665, confirmed COVID-19
[Desbois], 7/20/2020, retrospective, France, preprint, mean age 58.8[96]	Risk of case, 16.9% lower, RR 0.83, $p = 1.00$, treatment 3 of 27 (11.1%), control 23 of 172 (13.4%), NNT 44
[Dev], 3/24/2021, retrospective, India, peer-reviewed[97]	Risk of case, 26.0% lower, RR 0.74, $p = 0.003$, treatment 260, control 499, any number of HCQ doses vs. no HCQ prophylaxis
[Erden], 1/23/2022, retrospective, Turkey, peer-reviewed, 11 authors, excluded in exclusion analyses: unadjusted results with no group details[98]	Risk of death, 150.0% higher, RR 2.50, $p = 1.00$, treatment 1 of 6 (16.7%), control 0 of 3 (0.0%), continuity correction due to zero event (with reciprocal of the contrasting arm)
	Risk of hospitalization, 75.0% lower, RR 0.25, $p = 0.23$, treatment 1 of 6 (16.7%), control 2 of 3 (66.7%), NNT 2.0

Continued

Continued

[Ferriera], 6/29/2020, retrospective, population-based cohort, database analysis, Portugal, peer-reviewed[99]	Risk of case, 47.1% lower, RR 0.53, $p < 0.001$, adjusted per study, odds ratio converted to relative risk
[Ferri], 8/27/2020, retrospective, Italy, peer-reviewed, survey, 29 authors Submit Corrections or Updates[100]	Risk of COVID-19 case, 63.0% lower, RR 0.37, $p = 0.01$, treatment 9 of 994 (0.9%), control 16 of 647 (2.5%), NNT 64
[Fitzgerald], 2/5/2021, retrospective, USA, preprint, 34 patients excluded in exclusion analyses: not fully adjusting for the baseline risk differences within systemic autoimmune patients[101]	Risk of case, 8.5% lower, RR 0.91, $p = 0.54$, treatment 65 of 1,072 (6.1%), control 200 of 3,594 (5.6%), adjusted per study, odds ratio converted to relative risk
[Fung], 10/1/2021, retrospective, population-based cohort, USA, peer-reviewed, patients excluded in exclusion analyses: not fully adjusting for the different baseline risk of systemic autoimmune patients[102]	Risk of death, 13.0% lower, HR 0.87, $p = 0.15$, vs. past use (better match for systemic autoimmune diseases)
	Risk of hospitalization, 3.0% lower, HR 0.97, $p = 0.63$, vs. past use (better match for systemic autoimmune diseases)
	Risk of case, 9.0% lower, HR 0.91, $p = 0.02$, vs. past use (better match for systemic autoimmune diseases)
	Risk of death, 8.0% higher, HR 1.08, $p = 0.26$, vs. never used
	Risk of hospitalization, 6.0% higher, HR 1.06, $p = 0.13$, vs. never used
	Risk of case, 5.0% lower, HR 0.95, $p = 0.03$, vs. never used
[Gendebien], 6/25/2020, retrospective, Belgium, peer-reviewed, survey, patients, excluded in exclusion analyses: not fully adjusting for the baseline risk differences within systemic autoimmune patients[103]	Risk of case, 3.9% lower, RR 0.96, $p = 0.93$, treatment 12 of 152 (7.9%), control 6 of 73 (8.2%), NNT 308
[Gendelman], 5/5/2020, retrospective, database analysis, Israel, peer-reviewed, patients excluded in exclusion analyses: not fully adjusting for the different baseline risk of systemic autoimmune patients[104]	Risk of case, 8.1% lower, RR 0.92, $p = 0.88$, treatment 3 of 36 (8.3%), control 1,314 of 14,484 (9.1%), NNT 135

Continued

Continued

[Gentry], 9/21/2020, retrospective, database analysis, USA, peer-reviewed[105]	Risk of death, 91.3% lower, RR 0.09, $p = 0.10$, treatment 0 of 10,703 (0.0%), control 7 of 21,406 (0.0%), NNT 3,058, relative risk is not 0 because of continuity correction due to zero events (with reciprocal of the contrasting arm), COVID-19 mortality within all patients
	Risk of death, 90.7% lower, RR 0.09, $p = 0.19$, treatment 0 of 31 (0.0%), control 7 of 78 (9.0%), NNT 11, relative risk is not 0 because of continuity correction due to zero events (with reciprocal of the contrasting arm), mortality for infected patients
	Risk of case, 20.9% lower, RR 0.79, $p = 0.27$, treatment 31 of 10,703 (0.3%), control 78 of 21,406 (0.4%), NNT 1338, odds ratio converted to relative risk
[Gianfrancesco], 5/28/2020, retrospective, database analysis, multiple countries, peer-reviewed, patients excluded in exclusion analyses: not fully adjusting for the baseline risk differences within systemic autoimmune patients[106]	Risk of hospitalization, 3.3% lower, RR 0.97, $p = 0.82$, treatment 58 of 130 (44.6%), control 219 of 470 (46.6%), NNT 50, odds ratio converted to relative risk
[Goenka], 10/24/2020, retrospective, India, preprint[107]	Risk of IgG positive, 87.2% lower, RR 0.13, $p = 0.03$, treatment 1 of 77 (1.3%), control 115 of 885 (13.0%), NNT 8.6, adjusted per study, odds ratio converted to relative risk
[Grau-Pujol], 9/21/2020, randomized controlled trial, Spain, peer-reviewed[108]	Risk of case, 10.6% lower, RR 0.89, $p = 1.00$, treatment 1 of 142 (0.7%), control 1 of 127 (0.8%), NNT 1202
[Gönenli], 12/16/2020, retrospective, Turkey, peer-reviewed, survey, mean age 36.0, study period 14 May, 2020 to 13 June, 2020[109]	Risk of pneumonia, 29.7% lower, RR 0.70, $p = 0.77$, treatment 3 of 148 (2.0%), control 12 of 416 (2.9%), NNT 117
	Risk of case, 18.9% higher, RR 1.19, $p = 0.58$, treatment 8 of 148 (5.4%), control 20 of 416 (4.8%), odds ratio converted to relative risk
[Huang], 6/16/2020, retrospective, China, peer-reviewed, patients excluded in exclusion analyses: significant unadjusted confounding possible[110]	Risk of hospitalization, 80.0% lower, RR 0.20, $p < 0.001$, treatment 8, control 1,247
[Huh], 12/19/2020, retrospective, database analysis, South Korea, peer-reviewed, 8 authors, excluded in exclusion analyses: not fully adjusting for the different baseline risk of systemic autoimmune patients[111]	Risk of progression, 251.0% higher, RR 3.51, $p = 0.11$, treatment 5 of 8 (62.5%), control 873 of 2,797 (31.2%), adjusted per study, multivariate
	Risk of case, 6.0% lower, RR 0.94, $p = 0.82$, treatment 17 of 122 (13.9%), control 7,324 of 43,924 (16.7%), adjusted per study, multivariate

Continued

Continued

[Isnardi], 10/6/2022, retrospective, Argentina, peer-reviewed, mean age 51.4, 199 authors, study period 13 August, 2020 to 31 July, 2021, trial NCT04568421 (history)[112]	Risk of death, 33.9% lower, RR 0.66, $p = 0.23$, treatment 11 of 361 (3.0%), control 72 of 1,554 (4.6%), NNT 63, odds ratio converted to relative risk
	Risk of severe case, 48.0% lower, RR 0.52, $p = 0.02$, treatment 14 of 361 (3.9%), control 117 of 1,554 (7.5%), NNT 27, odds ratio converted to relative risk
	Risk of hospitalization, 17.0% lower, RR 0.83, $p = 0.09$, treatment 83 of 512 (16.2%), control 429 of 1,554 (27.6%), NNT 8.8, odds ratio converted to relative risk
[Juneja], 1/7/2022, retrospective, India, peer-reviewed, study period 2 April, 2020 to 3 September, 2020, patients excluded in exclusion analyses: excessive unadjusted differences between groups[113]	Risk of severe case, 141.8% higher, RR 2.42, $p = 0.59$, treatment 2 of 996 (0.2%), control 1 of 1,204 (0.1%)
	Risk of case, 6.4% higher, RR 1.06, $p = 0.67$, treatment 103 of 996 (10.3%), control 117 of 1,204 (9.7%)
[Jung], 12/11/2020, retrospective, South Korea, peer-reviewed[114]	Risk of death, 59.3% lower, RR 0.41, $p = 1.00$, treatment 0 of 649 (0.0%), control 1 of 1,417 (0.1%), NNT 1417, relative risk is not 0 because of continuity correction due to zero events (with reciprocal of the contrasting arm)
	Risk of case, 13.1% higher, RR 1.13, $p = 0.86$, treatment 15 of 649 (2.3%), control 31 of 1,417 (2.2%), adjusted per study
[Kadnur], 7/22/2020, prospective, India, peer-reviewed, mean age 31.2, study period 23 April, 2020 to 11 June, 2020[115]	Risk of case, 62.3% lower, RR 0.38, $p = 0.01$, treatment 10 of 258 (3.9%), control 15 of 100 (15.0%), NNT 9.0, odds ratio converted to relative risk, multivariate logistic regression
[Kamstrup], 6/1/2021, retrospective, population-based cohort, Denmark, peer-reviewed, patients excluded in exclusion analyses: not fully adjusting for the different baseline risk of systemic autoimmune patients[116]	Risk of hospitalization, 44.0% higher, OR 1.44, $p = 0.25$, treatment 5,488, control 54,846, RR approximated with OR.
	Risk of case, 10.0% lower, HR 0.90, $p = 0.23$, treatment 188 of 5,488 (3.4%), control 2,040 of 54,846 (3.7%), NNT 340, adjusted Cox proportional hazards regression
[Khoubnasabjafari], 1/13/2021, retrospective, Iran, peer-reviewed[117]	Risk of case, 16.7% lower, RR 0.83, $p = 0.59$, treatment 34 of 1,436 (2.4%), control 12 of 422 (2.8%), NNT 210
[Khurana], 7/24/2020, retrospective, India, preprint, survey[118]	Risk of case, 51.0% lower, RR 0.49, $p = 0.02$, treatment 6 of 22 (27.3%), control 88 of 159 (55.3%), NNT 3.6, odds ratio converted to relative risk

Continued

Continued

[Konig], 5/7/2020, retrospective, database analysis, multiple countries, peer-reviewed, patients excluded in exclusion analyses: not fully adjusting for the baseline risk differences within systemic autoimmune patients[119]	Risk of hospitalization, 3.0% lower, RR 0.97, $p = 0.88$, treatment 16 of 29 (55.2%), control 29 of 51 (56.9%), NNT 59
[Korkmaz], 6/1/2021, retrospective, Turkey, preprint[120]	Risk of death, 82.1% lower, RR 0.18, $p = 0.19$, treatment 0 of 385 (0.0%), control 2 of 299 (0.7%), NNT 150, relative risk is not 0 because of continuity correction due to zero events (with reciprocal of the contrasting arm)
	Risk of case, 93.7% lower, RR 0.06, $p < 0.001$, treatment 2 of 395 (0.5%), control 24 of 299 (8.0%), NNT 13
[Küçükakkaş], 7/20/2021, retrospective, Turkey, preprint, patients excluded in exclusion analyses: minimal details of groups provided[121]	Risk of ICU admission, 42.9% higher, RR 1.43, $p = 1.00$, treatment 1 of 7 (14.3%), control 1 of 10 (10.0%)
[Laplana], 9/9/2020, retrospective, Spain, peer-reviewed, survey, patients excluded in exclusion analyses: not fully adjusting for the different baseline risk of systemic autoimmune patients[122]	Risk of case, 56.0% higher, RR 1.56, $p = 0.24$, treatment 17 of 319 (5.3%), control 11 of 319 (3.4%)
[Llanos-Cuentas], 2/28/2023, randomized controlled trial, Peru, peer-reviewed, mean age 39.2, 10, study period July 2020 to November 2020, trial NCT04414241 (history)[123]	Risk of case, 69.0% higher, RR 1.69, $p = 0.46$, treatment 5 of 36 (13.9%), control 3 of 32 (9.4%), adjusted per study
[Loucera], 8/16/2022, retrospective, Spain, preprint, study period January 2020 to November 2020[124]	Risk of death, 69.3% lower, HR 0.31, $p < 0.001$, treatment 320, control 15,648, Cox proportional hazards, day 30
[MacFadden], 3/29/2022, retrospective, Canada, peer-reviewed, 9 authors, study period 15 January, 2020 to 31 December, 2020 Submit Corrections or Updates[125]	Risk of case, 12.0% lower, OR 0.88, $p = 0.01$, RR approximated with OR

Continued

Continued

[Macias], 5/16/2020, retrospective, database analysis, Spain, preprint, patients excluded in exclusion analyses: not fully adjusting for the baseline risk differences within systemic autoimmune patients[126]	Risk of hospitalization, 25.5% lower, RR 0.74, $p = 1.00$, treatment 1 of 290 (0.3%), control 2 of 432 (0.5%), NNT 846
	Risk of case, 49.0% higher, RR 1.49, $p = 0.53$, treatment 5 of 290 (1.7%), control 5 of 432 (1.2%)
[Mahto], 2/15/2021, retrospective, India, peer-reviewed, excluded in exclusion analyses: unadjusted results with no group details[127]	Risk of IgG positive, 26.9% lower, RR 0.73, $p = 0.38$, treatment 9 of 89 (10.1%), control 84 of 600 (14.0%), NNT 26, unadjusted, odds ratio converted to relative risk
[Mathai], 11/6/2020, retrospective, India, peer-reviewed[128]	Risk of case, 89.5% lower, RR 0.10, $p < 0.001$, treatment 10 of 491 (2.0%), control 22 of 113 (19.5%), NNT 5.7
	Risk of case, 88.5% lower, RR 0.12, $p < 0.001$, treatment 5 of 491 (1.0%), control 10 of 113 (8.8%), NNT 13, symptomatic
[Mathew], 2/28/2023, prospective, India, peer-reviewed, study period April 2020 to October 2021[129]	Risk of death, 20.0% lower, OR 0.80, $p = 0.80$, treatment 23, control 41, RR approximated with OR
	Risk of hospitalization, no change, OR 1.00, $p = 0.94$, treatment 23, control 41, RR approximated with OR
	Risk of severe case, 40.0% lower, OR 0.60, $p = 0.37$, treatment 23, control 41, RR approximated with OR
[Mitchell], 5/5/2020, retrospective, multiple countries, preprint, patients excluded in exclusion analyses: excessive unadjusted differences between groups[130]	Risk of death, 99.0% lower, RR 0.01, $p < 0.001$
[Naggie], 8/25/2021, double-blind randomized controlled trial, placebo-controlled, USA, peer-reviewed, mean age 43.6, study period April 2020 to November 2020, trial NCT04334148 (history) (HERO-HCQ)[131]	Risk of symptomatic case, 23.5% lower, RR 0.76, $p = 0.18$, treatment 41 of 683 (6.0%), control 53 of 676 (7.8%), NNT 54, odds ratio converted to relative risk, logistic regression
	Risk of symptomatic case, 29.3% lower, RR 0.71, $p = 0.18$, treatment 41 of 683 (6.0%), control 53 of 676 (7.8%), NNT 54, odds ratio converted to relative risk, Mantel–Haenszel
	Risk of symptomatic case, 50.5% lower, RR 0.49, $p = 0.34$, treatment 3 of 683 (0.4%), control 6 of 676 (0.9%), NNT 223, PCR confirmed

Continued

Continued

[Nasri], 1/27/2023, randomized controlled trial, Iran, peer-reviewed, mean age 29.7, 11 authors, study period 11 August, 2020 to 11 November, 2020, trial IRCT20200414047076N1[132]	Risk of symptomatic case, 92.2% lower, RR 0.08, $p = 0.03$, treatment 0 of 70 (0.0%), control 6 of 73 (8.2%), NNT 12, relative risk is not 0 because of continuity correction due to zero events (with reciprocal of the contrasting arm), severe cases
	Risk of symptomatic case, 85.1% lower, RR 0.15, $p = 0.003$, treatment 2 of 70 (2.9%), control 14 of 73 (19.2%), NNT 6.1, moderate or severe cases
	Risk of symptomatic case, 47.9% lower, RR 0.52, $p = 0.16$, treatment 7 of 70 (10.0%), control 14 of 73 (19.2%), NNT 11, all cases
[Obrişcă], 9/28/2022, prospective, Romania, peer-reviewed, mean age 39.0, 12 authors, study period 26 February, 2020 to 1 May, 2021[133]	Risk of case, 86.7% lower, RR 0.13, $p = 0.01$, treatment 10 of 81 (12.3%), control 5 of 14 (35.7%), NNT 4.3, adjusted per study, odds ratio converted to relative risk, multivariable
[Oku], 9/6/2022, retrospective, Japan, peer-reviewed, study period 3 June, 2020 to 30 June, 2021[134]	Risk of death, 92.2% lower, RR 0.08, $p = 1.00$, treatment 0 of 14 (0.0%), control 11 of 206 (5.3%), NNT 19, unadjusted, relative risk is not 0 because of continuity correction due to zero events (with reciprocal of the contrasting arm)
	Risk of hospitalization, 11.5% lower, RR 0.88, $p = 0.34$, treatment 9 of 14 (64.3%), control 177 of 206 (85.9%), NNT 4.6, adjusted per study, odds ratio converted to relative risk, multivariable
[Opdam], 2/23/2022, retrospective, Netherlands, peer-reviewed[135]	Risk of hospitalization, 45.0% lower, OR 0.55, $p = 0.18$, treatment 8 of 81 (9.9%) cases, 59 of 396 (14.9%) controls, NNT 17, case control OR
[Oztas], 3/21/2022, retrospective, Turkey, peer-reviewed, patients excluded in exclusion analyses: not adjusting for the different baseline risk of systemic autoimmune patients; excessive unadjusted differences between groups[136]	Risk of hospitalization, 215.1% higher, RR 3.15, $p = 0.36$, treatment 3 of 317 (0.9%), control 1 of 333 (0.3%)
	Risk of symptomatic case, 40.1% higher, RR 1.40, $p = 0.44$, treatment 16 of 317 (5.0%), control 12 of 333 (3.6%)
	Risk of case, 5.0% higher, RR 1.05, $p = 0.88$, treatment 22 of 317 (6.9%), control 22 of 333 (6.6%)
[Patel], 7/15/2022, retrospective, USA, preprint, mean age 60.0, patients excluded in exclusion analyses: unadjusted results with no group details[137]	Risk of case, 46.3% lower, RR 0.54, $p = 0.001$, treatment 28 of 18,358 (0.2%), control 223 of 78,509 (0.3%), cases vs. total person-months, unadjusted
[Patil], 8/24/2021, prospective, India, 20 authors[138]	Risk of death, 65.9% lower, RR 0.34, $p = 0.10$, treatment 5,266, control 3,946
	Risk of case, 9.1% lower, RR 0.91, $p = 0.43$, treatment 167 of 5,266 (3.2%), control 147 of 3,946 (3.7%), NNT 181, adjusted per study

Continued

Continued

[Pham], 3/2/2021, retrospective, USA, peer-reviewed[139]	Risk of death, 19.7% lower, RR 0.80, $p = 0.77$, treatment 2 of 14 (14.3%), control 5 of 28 (17.9%), NNT 28, odds ratio converted to relative risk, univariate
	Risk of ICU admission, 35.5% higher, RR 1.35, $p = 0.61$, treatment 4 of 14 (28.6%), control 6 of 28 (21.4%), odds ratio converted to relative risk, univariate
[Polo], 8/5/2022, double-blind randomized controlled trial, placebo-controlled, Spain, peer-reviewed, median age 38.0, trial NCT04334928 (history) (EPICOS)[140]	Risk of symptomatic case, 51.0% lower, RR 0.49, $p = 0.79$, treatment 3 of 224 (1.3%), control 5 of 211 (2.4%), NNT 97
	Risk of case, 27.0% lower, RR 0.73, $p = 0.31$, treatment 21 of 224 (9.4%), control 23 of 211 (10.9%)
[Raabe], 7/3/2022, prospective, USA, preprint, 7 authors, trial NCT04354870 (history)[87]	Risk of symptomatic case, 82.2% lower, RR 0.18, $p = 0.17$, treatment 1 of 59 (1.7%), control 2 of 21 (9.5%), NNT 13
	Risk of symptomatic case, 88.4% lower, RR 0.12, $p = 0.07$, treatment 0 of 59 (0.0%), control 2 of 21 (9.5%), NNT 10, relative risk is not 0 because of continuity correction due to zero events (with reciprocal of the contrasting arm), fever
	Risk of case, 28.8% lower, RR 0.71, $p = 0.65$, treatment 4 of 59 (6.8%), control 2 of 21 (9.5%), NNT 36, seroconversion
[Rajasingham], 9/21/2020, randomized controlled trial, USA, peer-reviewed, trial NCT04328467 (history) (COVID PREP)[141]	Risk of hospitalization, 50.1% lower, RR 0.50, $p = 1.00$, treatment 1 of 989 (0.1%), control 1 of 494 (0.2%), NNT 987
	Risk of case, 27.0% lower, HR 0.73, $p = 0.12$, treatment 58 of 989 (5.9%), control 39 of 494 (7.9%), NNT 49
[Rangel], 1/10/2021, retrospective, USA, peer-reviewed, patients excluded in exclusion analyses: not fully adjusting for the different baseline risk of systemic autoimmune patients[142]	Risk of death, 25.1% lower, RR 0.75, $p = 0.77$, treatment 4 of 50 (8.0%), control 11 of 103 (10.7%), NNT 37, from all patients
	Risk of hospitalization, 22.2% lower, RR 0.78, $p = 0.29$, treatment 17 of 50 (34.0%), control 45 of 103 (43.7%), NNT 10
	Hospitalization time, 41.2% lower, relative time 0.59, $p = 0.12$, treatment 21, control 54
[Rao], 12/4/2021, prospective, India, peer-reviewed, excluded in exclusion analyses: unadjusted results with minimal group details[143]	Risk of case, 11.0% lower, RR 0.89, $p = 0.68$, treatment 16 of 273 (5.9%), control 67 of 1,021 (6.6%), NNT 143

Continued

Continued

[Rentsch], 9/9/2020, retrospective, population-based cohort, database analysis, United Kingdom, peer-reviewed, patients excluded in exclusion analyses: not fully adjusting for the baseline risk differences within systemic autoimmune patients; medication adherence unknown and may significantly change results[144]	Risk of death, 3.0% higher, HR 1.03, $p = 0.83$, treatment 70 of 30,569 (0.2%), control 477 of 164,068 (0.3%), adjusted per study
[Revollo], 11/21/2020, retrospective, propensity score matching, Spain, peer-reviewed[145]	Risk of case, 23.0% lower, RR 0.77, $p = 0.52$, treatment 16 of 69 (23.2%), control 65 of 418 (15.6%), adjusted per study, PSM, risk of PCR+
	Risk of case, 43.0% higher, RR 1.43, $p = 0.42$, treatment 17 of 60 (28.3%), control 62 of 404 (15.3%), adjusted per study, PSM, risk of IgG+
[Rojas-Serrano], 5/16/2021, double-blind randomized controlled trial, Mexico. Trial NCT04318015 (history). Submit Corrections or Updates[146]	Risk of symptomatic case, 82.0% lower, RR 0.18, $p = 0.12$, treatment 1 of 62 (1.6%), control 6 of 65 (9.2%), NNT 13, adjusted per study
[Sahebari], 9/7/2022, retrospective, Iran, peer-reviewed[147]	Risk of case, 56.0% lower, RR 0.44, $p = 0.02$, treatment 10 of 108 (9.3%), control 56 of 368 (15.2%), odds ratio converted to relative risk
[Salvarani], 8/6/2020, retrospective, population-based cohort, Italy, peer-reviewed, patients excluded in exclusion analyses: not fully adjusting for the different baseline risk of systemic autoimmune patients[148]	Risk of case, 6.0% lower, OR 0.94, $p = 0.75$, RR approximated with OR
[Samajdar], 11/17/2021, retrospective, India, peer-reviewed, study period 1 September, 2020 to 31 December, 2020, dosage not specified, patients excluded in exclusion analyses: minimal details provided; unadjusted results with no group details; results may be significantly affected by survey bias[149]	Risk of case, 74.5% lower, RR 0.25, $p < 0.001$, treatment 12 of 129 (9.3%), control 29 of 81 (35.8%), NNT 3.8, odds ratio converted to relative risk, physician survey
	Risk of case, 48.6% lower, RR 0.51, $p = 0.03$, treatment 11 of 109 (10.1%), control 39 of 200 (19.5%), NNT 11, odds ratio converted to relative risk, combined ivermectin or HCQ in community

Continued

Continued

[Santos], 7/27/2020, prospective, Spain, peer-reviewed, median age 78.4, mean age 75.3, study period 1 March, 2020 to 1 June, 2020, patients excluded in exclusion analyses: unadjusted results with no group details[150]	Risk of death, 92.5% lower, RR 0.08, $p = 0.19$, treatment 0 of 7 (0.0%), control 10 of 31 (32.3%), NNT 3.1, relative risk is not 0 because of continuity correction due to zero events (with reciprocal of the contrasting arm)
[Satti], 4/22/2022, retrospective, Qatar, peer-reviewed, patients excluded in exclusion analyses: unadjusted results with no group details[151]	Risk of case, 61.5% lower, RR 0.39, $p = 0.04$, treatment 10 of 63 (15.9%), control 7 of 17 (41.2%), NNT 4.0
[Seet], 4/14/2021, Cluster randomized controlled trial, Singapore, peer-reviewed, dosage 400 mg day 1, 200 mg days 2–42, this trial compares with another treatment—results may have been better when compared to placebo, trial NCT04446104 (history)[152]	Risk of symptomatic case, 35.1% lower, RR 0.65, $p = 0.047$, treatment 29 of 432 (6.7%), control 64 of 619 (10.3%), NNT 28
	Risk of case, 32.0% lower, RR 0.68, $p = 0.009$, treatment 212 of 432 (49.1%), control 433 of 619 (70.0%), NNT 4.8, adjusted per study, odds ratio converted to relative risk, model 6
[Shahrin], 12/7/2022, retrospective, Bangladesh, peer-reviewed, median age 34.0, study period 31 March, 2020 to 12 July, 2020[153]	Risk of case, 87.8% higher, RR 1.88, $p = 0.09$, treatment 43 of 230 (18.7%), control 11 of 106 (10.4%), adjusted per study, odds ratio converted to relative risk, multivariable
	Risk of case, 8.0% lower, OR 0.92, $p = 0.89$, adjusted per study, excluding the first 14 days and including participants that worked for at least 16 days, multivariable, RR approximated with OR
[Shaw], 7/1/2021, retrospective, USA, peer-reviewed, study period 1 March, 2020 to 15 May, 2020[154]	Risk of case, 13.0% lower, OR 0.87, $p = 0.006$, treatment 45, control 99, adjusted per study, propensity score matching, multivariable, RR approximated with OR
[Shukla], 12/13/2022, retrospective, India, peer-reviewed, survey, study period July 2021 to October 2021, trial CTRI/2021/06/034255[155]	Risk of PASC, 5.0% lower, RR 0.95, $p = 0.78$, treatment 22 of 76 (28.9%), control 184 of 603 (30.5%), NNT 64, odds ratio converted to relative risk
[Singer], 8/5/2020, retrospective, database analysis, USA, peer-reviewed, patients excluded in exclusion analyses: not fully adjusting for the baseline risk differences within systemic autoimmune patients[156]	Risk of case, 9.0% higher, RR 1.09, $p = 0.62$, treatment 55 of 10,700 (0.5%), control 104 of 22,058 (0.5%)

Continued

Continued

[Barnabas], 12/7/2020, randomized controlled trial, USA, peer-reviewed, trial NCT04328961 (history)[166]	Risk of hospitalization, 3.7% higher, RR 1.04, $p = 1.00$, treatment 1 of 407 (0.2%), control 1 of 422 (0.2%). Included a modified intention to treat analysis (miTT) Primary end point PCR + day1–14, secondary endpoint PCR + symptomatic
	Risk of case, 27.0% higher, HR 1.27, $p = 0.33$, treatment 43 of 353 (12.2%), control 33 of 336 (9.8%), adjusted per study
	Risk of case, 23.0% higher, HR 1.23, $p = 0.41$, treatment 40 of 317 (12.6%), control 32 of 309 (10.4%), adjusted per study
	Risk of case, 10.0% higher, HR 1.10, $p = 0.66$, treatment 53 of 353 (15.0%), control 45 of 336 (13.4%), adjusted per study
	Risk of case, 1.0% lower, HR 0.99, $p = 0.97$, treatment 46 of 317 (14.5%), control 43 of 309 (13.9%), adjusted per study
	Risk of case, 19.0% lower, HR 0.81, $p = 0.23$, treatment 82 of 387 (21.2%), control 99 of 393 (25.2%), NNT 25, adjusted per study
[Boulware], 6/3/2020, randomized controlled trial, USA, peer-reviewed, this trial compares with another treatment—results may be better when compared to placebo[167]	Risk of case, 17.0% lower, RR 0.83, $p = 0.35$, treatment 49 of 414 (11.8%), control 58 of 407 (14.3%), NNT 41
	Risk of case, 25.1% lower, RR 0.75, $p = 0.22$, treatment 32 of 414 (7.7%), control 42 of 407 (10.3%), NNT 39, probable COVID-19 cases
[Dhibar], 1/7/2023, double-blind randomized controlled trial, placebo-controlled, India, peer-reviewed, mean age 35.0, 14 authors, study period 22 March, 2021 to 17 June, 2021, trial NCT04858633 (history)[168,169]	Risk of symptomatic case, 26.7% lower, RR 0.73, $p = 0.32$, treatment 17 of 574 (3.0%), control 24 of 594 (4.0%), NNT 93
	Risk of case, 21.2% lower, RR 0.79, $p = 0.21$, treatment 16 of 574 (2.8%), control 21 of 594 (3.5%), NNT 134, PCR+
	Risk of case, 8.0% lower, RR 0.92, $p = 0.21$, treatment 24 of 574 (4.2%), control 27 of 594 (4.5%), NNT 275
[Dhibar], 11/6/2020, prospective, India, peer-reviewed, trial NCT04408456 (history)[169]	Risk of symptomatic case, 43.9% lower, RR 0.56, $p = 0.21$, treatment 6 of 132 (4.5%), control 15 of 185 (8.1%), NNT 28, adjusted per study
	Risk of case, 50.0% lower, RR 0.50, $p = 0.04$, treatment 10 of 132 (7.6%), control 28 of 185 (15.1%), NNT 13, adjusted per study, PCR+
	Risk of case, 41.0% lower, RR 0.59, $p = 0.03$, treatment 14 of 132 (10.6%), control 36 of 185 (19.5%), NNT 11, adjusted per study

Continued

Continued

[Mckinnon], 12/23/2021, Double Blind Randomized Controlled Trial, USA, peer-reviewed, trial NCT04341441 (history) (WHIP COVID-19)[170]	Risk of symptomatic case, 2.5% lower, RR 0.98, $p = 1.00$, treatment 2 of 365 (0.5%), control 1 of 178 (0.6%), NNT 7219, daily and weekly HCQ combined
	Risk of symptomatic case, no change, RR 1.00, $p = 1.00$, treatment 1 of 178 (0.6%), control 1 of 178 (0.6%), daily HCQ
	Risk of symptomatic case, 4.8% lower, RR 0.95, $p = 1.00$, treatment 1 of 187 (0.5%), control 1 of 178 (0.6%), NNT 3698, weekly HCQ
	Risk of symptomatic case, 53.3% lower, RR 0.47, $p = 1.00$, treatment 0 of 25 (0.0%), control 1 of 178 (0.6%), NNT 178, relative risk is not 0 because of continuity correction due to zero events (with reciprocal of the contrasting arm), AD patients
	Risk of case, 51.2% lower, RR 0.49, $p = 0.60$, treatment 2 of 365 (0.5%), control 2 of 178 (1.1%), NNT 174, daily and weekly HCQ combined
	Risk of case, 50.0% lower, RR 0.50, $p = 1.00$, treatment 1 of 178 (0.6%), control 2 of 178 (1.1%), NNT 178, daily HCQ
	Risk of case, 52.4% lower, RR 0.48, $p = 0.61$, treatment 1 of 187 (0.5%), control 2 of 178 (1.1%), NNT 170, weekly HCQ
	Risk of case, 69.5% lower, RR 0.30, $p = 1.00$, treatment 0 of 25 (0.0%), control 2 of 178 (1.1%), NNT 89, relative risk is not 0 because of continuity correction due to zero events (with reciprocal of the contrasting arm), AD patients
[Mitjà], 7/26/2020, randomized controlled trial, Spain, peer-reviewed[68]	Risk of death, 45.6% lower, RR 0.54, $p = 0.39$, treatment 4 of 1,196 (0.3%), control 8 of 1,301 (0.6%), NNT 357, excluding patient that did not take any study medication and had an unknown cause of death
	Risk of hospitalization, 16.8% lower, RR 0.83, $p = 0.71$, treatment 13 of 1,196 (1.1%), control 17 of 1,301 (1.3%), NNT 455, S7, excluding patient that did not take any study medication and had an unknown cause of death
	Baseline PCR—risk of cases, 32.0% lower, RR 0.68, $p = 0.27$, treatment 29 of 958 (3.0%), control 45 of 1,042 (4.3%), NNT 77
[Polat], 9/30/2020, prospective, Turkey, peer-reviewed[171]	Risk of case, 57.0% lower, RR 0.43, $p = 0.03$, treatment 12 of 138 (8.7%), control 14 of 70 (20.0%), NNT 8.8

Continued

Continued

[Shabini], 8/10/2021, prospective, Iran, peer-reviewed[172]	Risk of symptomatic case, 19.0% lower, RR 0.81, $p = 1.00$, treatment 2 of 51 (3.9%), control 3 of 62 (4.8%), NNT 109, day 7
	Risk of case, 6.4% higher, RR 1.06, $p = 1.00$, treatment 7 of 51 (13.7%), control 8 of 62 (12.9%), day 7, PCR+ and symptomatic
	Risk of case, 21.6% higher, RR 1.22, $p = 0.78$, treatment 7 of 51 (13.7%), control 7 of 62 (11.3%), day 7, PCR+ only
[Simova], 11/12/2020, retrospective, Bulgaria, peer-reviewed[173]	Risk of case, 92.7% lower, RR 0.07, $p = 0.01$, treatment 0 of 156 (0.0%), control 3 of 48 (6.2%), NNT 16, relative risk is not 0 because of continuity correction due to zero events (with reciprocal of the contrasting arm)

Source: Adapted with permission based on copyright data is in public domain HCQ for COVID-19: real-time meta-analysis of 385 studies (https://c19hcq.org/) Covid Analysis, March 2, 2023, Version 250.

REFERENCES

1. Patel A, Jernigan DB; 2019-nCoV CDC Response Team. Initial Public Health Response and Interim Clinical Guidance for the 2019 Novel Coronavirus Outbreak—United States, December 31, 2019–February 4, 2020. MMWR Morb Mortal Wkly Rep. 2020(69):140-6.
2. Guy RK, DiPaola RS, Romanelli F, Dutch RE. Rapid repurposing of drugs for COVID-19. Science. 2020;368(6493):829-30.
3. Ng YL, Salim CK, Chu JJH. Drug repurposing for COVID-19: Approaches, challenges and promising candidates. Pharmacol Ther. 2021;228:107930.
4. Ravi S, Jadhav S, Vaidya A, Ghooi R. Repurposing drugs during the COVID-19 pandemic and beyond. Pharm Pat Anal. 2021;10(1):9-12.
5. Avezum Á, Oliveira GBF, Oliveira H, Lucchetta RC, Pereira VFA, Dabarian AL, et al. Hydroxychloroquine versus placebo in the treatment of non-hospitalised patients with COVID-19 (COPE–Coalition V): A double-blind, multicentre, randomised, controlled trial. Lancet Reg Health Am. 2022;11:100243.
6. Baildya N, Ghosh NN, Chattopadhyay AP. Inhibitory activity of hydroxychloroquine on COVID-19 main protease: An insight from MD-simulation studies. J Mol Struct. 2020;1219:128595.
7. Yadav AK, Kotwal A, Ghosh S. Hydroxychloroquine/Chloroquine Prophylaxis among Health-care Workers: Was it Really Preventive?–Evidence from a Multicentric Cross-sectional Study. Indian J Community Med. 2022;47(2):202-6.
8. Yao X, Ye F, Zhang M, Cui C, Huang B, Niu P, et al. In Vitro Antiviral Activity and Projection of Optimized Dosing Design of Hydroxychloroquine for the Treatment of Severe Acute Respiratory Syndrome Coronavirus 2 (SARS-CoV-2). Clin Infect Dis. 2020;71(15):732-9.
9. Satarker S, Ahuja T, Banerjee M, Dogra S, Agarwal T, Nampoothiri M, et al. Hydroxychloroquine in COVID-19: Potential Mechanism of Action Against SARS-CoV-2. Curr Pharmacol Rep. 2020;6(5):203-11.
10. Mehra MR, Ruschitzka F, Patel AN. Retraction-Hydroxychloroquine or chloroquine with or without a macrolide for treatment of COVID-19: a multinational registry analysis. Lancet. 2020;395(10240):1820.

11. Mehra MR, Desai SS, Kuy S, Henry TD, Patel AN. Retraction: Cardiovascular Disease, Drug Therapy, and Mortality in Covid-19. N Engl J Med. 2020;382(26):2582.
12. Berry AC, Gonnering RS, Rodriguez I, Zhang Q, Berry BB. Unfavorable hydroxychloroquine COVID-19 research associated with authors having a history of political party donations. Rev Cardiovasc Med. 2021;22(1):191-8.
13. Berlivet L, Löwy I. Hydroxychloroquine Controversies: Clinical Trials, Epistemology, and the Democratization of Science. Med Anthropol Q. 2020;34(4):525-41.
14. Adam D. Who Believes in Hydroxychloroquine?. [online] Available from https://issues.org/hydroxychloroquine-hcq-controversy/. [Last accessed February, 2024].
15. Baker N, Van Noorden R, Maxmen A. Coronapod: The Surgisphere scandal that rocked coronavirus drug research. Nature. 2020.
16. Hinton DM. Re: Request for emergency use authorization for use of chloroquine phosphate or hydroxychloroquine sulfate supplied from the Strategic National Stockpile for treatment of 2019 coronavirus disease. [online] Available from www.fda.gov/media/136534/download. [Last accessed February, 2024].
17. FDA. (2022). FDA cautions against use of hydroxychloroquine or chloroquine for COVID-19 outside of the hospital setting or a clinical trial due to risk of heart rhythm problems. [online] Available from https://www.fda.gov/drugs/fda-drug-safety-podcasts/fda-cautions-against-use-hydroxychloroquine-or-chloroquine-covid-19-outside-hospital-setting-or#:~:text=Hydroxychloroquine%20and%20chloroquine%20can%20cause,the%20QT%20interval%2C%20including%20azithromycin. [Last accessed February, 2024].
18. Hatfill S, Wang W, Wertheimer AI, Marcon AR, Caulfield T. The hydroxychloroquine Twitter war: A case study examining polarization in science communication. First Monday. 2021;18(5):2811-6.
19. https://www.fda.gov/drugs/drug-safety-and-availability/fda-cautions-against-use-hydroxychloroquine-or-chloroquine-covid-19-outside-hospital-setting-or a clinical trial due to risk of heart rythm problems. Published online July 1, 2020.
20. Piller C. Former FDA leaders decry emergency authorization of malaria drugs for coronavirus Widespread use of unproven drugs could hurt clinical trials. [online] Available from https://www.science.org/content/article/former-fda-leaders-decry-emergency-authorization-malaria-drugs-coronavirus#:~:text=The%20recent%20Food%20and%20Drug,President%20Donald%20Trump%20and%20former. [Last accessed February, 2024].
21. Risch HA. Early Outpatient Treatment of Symptomatic, High-Risk COVID-19 Patients That Should Be Ramped Up Immediately as Key to the Pandemic Crisis. Am J Epidemiol. 2020;189(11):1218-26.
22. Risch HA. (2021). Hydroxychloroquine in Early Treatment of High-Risk COVID-19 Outpatients: Efficacy and Safety Evidence. [online] Available from https://earlycovidcare.org/wp-content/uploads/2021/09/Evidence-Brief-Risch-v6.pdf. [Last accessed February, 2024].
23. Waksman R. COVID-19: Leave politics out of practicing medicine. Cardiovasc Revasc Med. 2020;21(8):937-8.
24. Hatfill S. The intentional destruction of the national pandemic plan. J Am Phys Surg. 2021;26:74-6.
25. Hinton DM. (2020). FDA Emergency use authorization (EUA) of chloroquine and hydroxychloroquine. [online] Available from https://www.fda.gov/media/136534/download. [Last accessed February, 2024].
26. Todaro JM, Angell M. Gilead: Twenty-one billion reasons to discredit hydroxychloroquine. Medicine Uncensored, https://steemit.com/coronavirus/@steemsheep/gilead-twenty-one-billion-reasons-to-discredit-hydroxychloroquine

27. Kuttiatt VS, Menon RP, Kumar A. Publication ethics during the COVID times: Reflections on research integrity, authorship, peer review and editorial policies. Natl Med J India. 2022;35(3):177-9.
28. Calcaterra G, Bassareo PP, Nodari S, Di Franco A, Romeo F. An expression of concern on research during the Covid-19 pandemic. J Cardiovasc Med (Hagerstown). 2020;21(10):838-9.
29. Iacobucci G. Covid-19: Validity of key studies in doubt after leading journals issue expressions of concern. BMJ. 2020;369:m2224.
30. The Lancet Editors. Expression of concern: Hydroxychloroquine or chloroquine with or without a macrolide for treatment of COVID-19: a multinational registry analysis. Lancet. 2020;395(10240):e102.
31. S. Hrg. 116-557 — COVID-19 (Volume 2) (2024), https://www.congress.gov/event/116th-congress/senate-event/LC68949/text.pg1154,1159
32. Esper RB, da Silva RS, Teiichi F, Oikawa C, Castro MM, Razuk-Filho A, et al. (2020). Empirical treatment with hydroxychloroquine and azithromycin for suspected cases of COVID-19 followed-up by telemedicine. [online] Available from https://www.semanticscholar.org/paper/Empirical-treatment-with-hydroxychloroquine-and-for-%C3%89sper-Silva/4c9a982fb79cb3f22ee2f5c77505203e76a0abce. [Last accessed February, 2024].
33. Ip A, Ahn J, Zhou Y, Goy AH, Hansen E, Pecora AL, et al. Hydroxychloroquine in the treatment of outpatients with mildly symptomatic COVID-19: a multi-center observational study. BMC Infect Dis. 2021;21(1):1-12.
34. Million M, Lagier JC, Tissot-Dupont H, Ravaux I, Dhiver C, Tomei C, et al. Early combination therapy with hydroxychloroquine and azithromycin reduces mortality in 10,429 COVID-19 outpatients. Rev Cardiovasc Med. 2021;22(3):1063-72.
35. Gautret P, Lagier JC, Parola P, Hoang VT, Meddeb L, Mailhe M, et al. Hydroxychloroquine and azithromycin as a treatment of COVID-19: results of an open-label non-randomized clinical trial. Int J Antimicrob Agents. 2020;56(1):105949.
36. WHO Solidarity Trial Consortium; Pan H, Peto R, Henao-Restrepo AM, Preziosi MP, Sathiyamoorthy V, Karim QA, et al. Repurposed Antiviral Drugs for Covid-19—Interim WHO Solidarity Trial Results. N Engl J Med. 2021;384(6):497-511.
37. RECOVERY Collaborative Group. Effect of hydroxychloroquine in hospitalized patients with Covid-19. N Engl J Med. 2020;383(21):2030-40.
38. Borba MGS, Val FFA, Sampaio VS, Araújo Alexandre MA, Melo GC, Brito M, et al. Effect of high vs low doses of chloroquine diphosphate as adjunctive therapy for patients hospitalized with severe acute respiratory syndrome coronavirus 2 (SARS-CoV-2) infection: a randomized clinical trial. JAMA Netw Open. 2020;3(4):e208857.
39. Griffin DO, Brennan-Rieder D, Ngo B, Kory P, Confalonieri M, Shapiro L, et al. The Importance of Understanding the Stages of COVID-19 in Treatment and Trials. AIDS Rev. 2021;23(1):40-7.
40. Marik PE, Varon J, Kory P. Treatment of COVID-19 is critically phase specific. Crit Care Shock. 2020;23(5):10-2.
41. Marik PE, Iglesias J, Varon J, Kory P. A scoping review of the pathophysiology of COVID-19. Int J Immunopathol Pharmacol. 2021;35:20587384211048026.
42. McCullough PA, Alexander PE, Armstrong R Arvinte C, Bain AF, Bartlett RP et al. Multifaceted highly targeted sequential multidrug treatment of early ambulatory high-risk SARS-CoV-2 infection (COVID-19). Rev Cardiovasc Med. 2020;21(4):517-30.
43. Ngo BT, Marik P, Kory P, Shapiro L, Thomadsen R, Iglesias J, The time to offer treatments for COVID-19. Expert Opin Investig Drugs. 2021;30(5):505-18.
44. Derwand R, Scholz M, Zelenko V. COVID-19 outpatients: early risk-stratified treatment with zinc plus low-dose hydroxychloroquine and azithromycin: a retrospective case series study. Int J Antimicrob Agents. 2020;56(6):106214.

45. Berk RA. Randomized experiments as the bronze standard. J Exp Criminol. 2005;1: 417-33.
46. Fogg L, Gross D. Threats to validity in randomized clinical trials. Res Nurs Health. 2000;23(1):79-87.
47. Kostis JB, Dobrzynski JM. Limitations of randomized clinical trials. Am J Cardiol. 2020;129:109-15.
48. Yeh RW, Valsdottir LR, Yeh MW, Shen C, Kramer DB, Strom JB, et al. Parachute use to prevent death and major trauma when jumping from aircraft: randomized controlled trial. BMJ. 2018;363:k5094.
49. Anglemyer A, Horvath HT, Bero L. Healthcare outcomes assessed with observational study designs compared with those assessed in randomized trials. Cochrane Database Syst Rev. 2014;2014(4):MR000034.
50. Sinha N, Balayla G. Hydroxychloroquine and COVID-19. Postgrad Med J. 2020;96(1139):550-5.
51. Bansal P, Goyal A, Cusick A 4th, Lahan S, Dhaliwal HS, Bhyan P, et al. Hydroxychloroquine: a comprehensive review and its controversial role in coronavirus disease 2019. Ann Med. 2021;53(1):117-34.
52. Agarwal M, Ranjan P, Baitha U, Mittal A. Hydroxychloroquine as a Chemoprophylactic Agent for COVID-19: A Clinico-Pharmacological Review. Front Pharmacol. 2020;11:593099.
53. Fan J, Zhang X, Liu J, Yang Y, Zheng N, Liu Q, et al. Connecting Hydroxychloroquine In Vitro Antiviral Activity to In Vivo Concentration for Prediction of Antiviral Effect: A Critical Step in Treating Patients With Coronavirus Disease 2019. Clin Infect Dis. 2020;71(12):3232-36.
54. Fantini J, Scala CD, Chahinian H, Yahi N. Structural and molecular modelling studies reveal a new mechanism of action of chloroquine and hydroxychloroquine against SARS-CoV-2 infection. Int J Antimicrob Agents. 2020;55(5):105960.
55. Shittu MO, Afolami OI. Improving the efficacy of Chloroquine and Hydroxychloroquine against SARS-CoV-2 may require Zinc additives—A better synergy for future COVID-19 clinical trials. Infez Med. 2020;28(2):192-7.
56. Gautret P, Lagier JC, Honoré S, Hoang VT, Raoult D. Clinical efficacy and safety profile of hydroxychloroquine and azithromycin against COVID-19. Int J Antimicrob Agents. 2021;57(1):106242.
57. Lagier JC, Million M, Gautret P, Colson P, Cortaredona S, Giraud-Gatineau A, et al. Outcomes of 3,737 COVID-19 patients treated with hydroxychloroquine/azithromycin and other regimens in Marseille, France: A retrospective analysis. Travel Med Infect Dis. 2020;36:101791.
58. Rodrigues C, Freitas-Santos RS, Levi JE, Senerchia AA, Lopes ATA, Santos SR, et al. Hydroxychloroquine plus azithromycin early treatment of mild COVID-19 in an outpatient setting: a randomized, double-blinded, placebo-controlled clinical trial evaluating viral clearance. Int J Antimicrob Agents. 2021;58(5):106428.
59. Johnston C, Brown ER, Stewart J, Stankiewicz Karita HC, Kissinger PJ, Dwyer J, et al. Hydroxychloroquine with or without azithromycin for treatment of early SARS-CoV-2 infection among high-risk outpatient adults: A randomized clinical trial. EClinicalMedicine. 2021;33: 100773.
60. Omrani AS, Pathan SA, Thomas SA, Harris TRE, Coyle PV, Thomas CE, et al. Randomized double-blinded placebo-controlled trial of hydroxychloroquine with or without azithromycin for virologic cure of non-severe Covid-19. EClinicalMedicine. 2020;29:100645.
61. Schwartz I, Boesen ME, Cerchiaro G, Doram C, Edwards BD, Ganesh A, et al. Assessing the efficacy and safety of hydroxychloroquine as outpatient treatment of COVID-19: a randomized controlled trial. CMAJ Open. 2021;9(2):E693-E702.

62. Catteau L, Dauby N, Montourcy M, Bottieau E, Hautekiet J, Goetghebeur E, et al. Low-dose hydroxychloroquine therapy and mortality in hospitalised patients with COVID-19: a nationwide observational study of 8075 participants. Int J Antimicrob Agents. 2020;56(4):106144.
63. Valk CM, Swart P, Boers LS, Botta M, Bos LDJ, de Abreu MG, et al. Practice of adjunctive treatments in critically ill COVID–19 patients—rational for the multicenter observational PRoAcT-COVID study in The Netherlands. Ann Transl Med. 2021;9(9):813.
64. Skipper CP, Pastick KA, Engen NW, Bangdiwala AS, Abassi M, Lofgren SM, et al. Hydroxychloroquine in Nonhospitalized Adults With Early COVID-19 : A Randomized Trial. Ann Intern Med. 2020;173(8):623-31.
65. Pullen MF, Pastick KA, Williams DA, Nascene AA, Bangdiwala AS, Okafor EC, et al. Lessons Learned From Conducting Internet-Based Randomized Clinical Trials During a Global Pandemic. Open Forum Infect Dis. 2021;8(2):ofaa602.
66. c19early.org. COVID-19 early treatment: real-time analysis of 3,487 studies. [online] Available from https://c19early.org/. [Last accessed February, 2024].
67. Mitjà O, Corbacho-Monné M, Ubals M, Tebé C, Peñafiel J, Tobias A, et al. Hydroxychloroquine for Early Treatment of Adults With Mild Coronavirus Disease 2019: A Randomized, Controlled Trial. Clin Infect Dis. 2020;73(11):e4073-e4081.
68. Mitjà O, Corbacho-Monne M, Ubals M, Alemany A, Suñer C, Tebé C, et al. A cluster-randomized trial of hydroxychloroquine for prevention of Covid-19. N Engl J Med. 2021;384(5):417-27.
69. Cadegiani FA, Goren A, Wambier CG, McCoy J. Early COVID-19 therapy with azithromycin plus nitazoxanide, ivermectin or hydroxychloroquine in outpatient settings significantly improved COVID-19 outcomes compared to known outcomes in untreated patients. New Microbes New Infect. 2021;43:100915.
70. Fonseca SNS, Sousa A de Q, Wolkoff AG, Moreira MS, Pinto BC, Valente Takeda CF, et al. Risk of hospitalization for Covid-19 outpatients treated with various drug regimens in Brazil: Comparative analysis. Travel Med Infect Dis. 2020;38:101906.
71. Ly TDA, Zanini D, Laforge V, Arlotto S, Gentile S, Mendizabal H, et al. Pattern of SARS-CoV-2 infection among dependant elderly residents living in long-term care facilities in Marseille, France, March–June 2020. Int J Antimicrob Agents. 2020;56(6):106219.
72. Heras E, Garibaldi P, Boix M, Valero O, Castillo J, Curbelo Y, et al. COVID-19 mortality risk factors in older people in a long-term care center. Eur Geriatr Med. 2021;12(3):601-7.
73. Cangiano B, Fatti LM, Danesi L, Gazzano G, Croci M, Vitale G, et al. Mortality in an Italian nursing home during COVID-19 pandemic: correlation with gender, age, ADL, vitamin D supplementation, and limitations of the diagnostic tests. Aging. 2020;12(24): 24522-34.
74. Sulaiman T, Mohana A, Alawdah L, Mahmoud N, Hassanein M, Wani T, et al. (2020). The Effect of Early Hydroxychloroquine-based Therapy in COVID-19 Patients in Ambulatory Care Settings: A Nationwide Prospective Cohort Study. [online] Available from https://www.medrxiv.org/content/10.1101/2020.09.09.20184143v1. [Last accessed February, 2024].
75. Mokhtari M, Mohraz M, Gouya MM, Namdari Tabar H, Tabrizi JS, Tayeri K, et al. Clinical outcomes of patients with mild COVID-19 following treatment with hydroxychloroquine in an outpatient setting. Int Immunopharmacol. 2021;96:107636.
76. García-Albéniz X, del Amo J, Polo R, Morales-Asencio JM, Hernán MA. Systematic review and meta-analysis of randomized trials of hydroxychloroquine for the prevention of COVID-19. Eur J Epidemiol. 2022;37(8):789-96.
77. Abella BS, Jolkovsky EL, Biney BT, Uspal JE, Hyman MC, Frank I, et al. Efficacy and Safety of Hydroxychloroquine vs Placebo for Pre-exposure SARS-CoV-2 Prophylaxis Among Health Care Workers: A Randomized Clinical Trial. JAMA Intern Med. 2021;181(2): 195-202.

78. Agarwal M, Ranka R, Panda PK, Kumar A, Chikara G, Sharma SK, et al. (2021). Low dose hydroxychloroquine prophylaxis for COVID-19—a prospective study. [online] Available from https://www.medrxiv.org/content/10.1101/2021.09.13.21262971v1.full.pdf. [Last accessed February, 2024].
79. Ahmed AS, Alotaibi WS, Aldubayan MA, Alhowail AH, Al-Najjar AH, Chigurupati S, et al. Factors Affecting the Incidence, Progression, and Severity of COVID-19 in Type 1 Diabetes Mellitus. Biomed Res Int. 2021;2021:1676914.
80. Spila Alegiani S, Crisafulli S, Giorgi Rossi P, Mancuso P, Salvarani C, Atzeni F, et al. Risk of coronavirus disease 2019 hospitalization and mortality in rheumatic patients treated with hydroxychloroquine or other conventional disease-modifying anti-rheumatic drugs in Italy. Rheumatology (Oxford). 2021;60(SI):SI25-SI36.
81. Alzahrani ZA, Alghamdi KA, Almaqati AS. Clinical characteristics and outcome of COVID-19 in patients with rheumatic diseases. Rheumatol Int. 2021;41(6):1097-103.
82. Arleo T, Tong D, Shabto J, O'Keefe G, Khosroshahi A. Clinical course and outcomes of COVID-19 in rheumatic disease patients: a case cohort study with a diverse population. Clin Rheumatol. 2021;40(7):2633-42.
83. Dinesh B, Cs J, Kaur CP, Atiya F, Yk G, Avijit H, et al. Hydroxychloroquine for SARS-CoV-2 Prophylaxis in Healthcare Workers-A Multicentric Cohort Study Assessing Effectiveness and Safety. J Assoc Physicians India. 2021;69(6):11-2.
84. Bae S, Ghang B, Kim YJ, Lim JS, Yun SC, Kim YG, et al. Recent hydroxychloroquine use is not significantly associated with positive PCR results for SARS-CoV-2: a nationwide observational study in South Korea. Viruses. 2021;13(2):329.
85. Becetti K, Satti E, Varughese B, Rimawi YA, Saleh RS, Hadwan N, et al. Prevalence of coronavirus disease 2019 in a multiethnic cohort of patients with autoimmune rheumatic diseases in Qatar. Qatar Med J. 2022;2022(3):37.
86. Behera P, Patro BK, Singh AK, Chandanshive PD, Ravikumar SR, Pradhan SK, et al. Role of ivermectin in the prevention of SARS-CoV-2 infection among healthcare workers in India: A matched case-control study. PLoS One. 2021;16(2):1-12.
87. Belmont HM, Raabe VN, Fleming A, Samanovic MI, Lai L, Belli HM, et al. (2022). Hydroxychloroquine pre-exposure prophylaxis to prevent SARS-CoV-2 among health care workers at risk for SARS-CoV-2 exposure: A nonrandomized controlled trial. [online] Available from https://www.medrxiv.org/content/10.1101/2022.07.01.22277058v1. [Last accessed February, 2024].
88. Bhatt P, Patel V, Shah P, Parikh K. (2021). Hydroxychloroquine Prophylaxis against Coronavirus Disease-19: Practice Outcomes among Health-Care Workers. [online] Available from https://www.medrxiv.org/content/10.1101/2021.08.02.21260750v1. [Last accessed February, 2024].
89. Bhattacharya R, Chowdhury S, Nandi A. Pre-exposure hydroxychloroquine prophylaxis for COVID-19 in healthcare workers: a retrospective cohort. Int J Res Med Sci. 2020;9(1):89-96.
90. Bozzalla Cassione E, Zanframundo G, Biglia A, Codullo V, Montecucco C, Cavagna L. COVID-19 infection in a northern-Italian cohort of systemic lupus erythematosus assessed by telemedicine. Ann Rheum Dis. 2020;79(10):1382-3.
91. Chatterjee P, Anand T, Singh KJ, Rasaily R, Singh R, Das S, et al. Healthcare workers & SARS-CoV-2 infection in India: A case-control investigation in the time of COVID-19. Indian J Med Res. 2020;151(5): 459-67.
92. Cordtz R, Kristensen S, Dalgaard LPH, Westermann R, Duch K, Lindhardsen J, et al. Incidence of COVID-19 hospitalisation in patients with systemic lupus erythematosus: a nationwide cohort study from Denmark. J Clin Med. 2021;10(17):3842.
93. Cordtz R, Lindhardsen J, Soussi BG, Vela J, Uhrenholt L, Westermann R, et al. Incidence and severeness of COVID-19 hospitalization in patients with inflammatory rheumatic

disease: a nationwide cohort study from Denmark. Rheumatology (Oxford). 2020;60(SI):SI59-SI67.

94. Datta D, Ghosal S, Sinha B, Datta S, Chakraborty T, Gangopadhyay K. No role of HCQ in COVID-19 prophylaxis: a survey amongst Indian doctors. J Vaccines Vaccin. 2020;S6:002.
95. de la Iglesia JL, Fernández NC, Flores RN, Gómez MM, de Haro FJG, González MA, et al. (2020). Hydroxychloroquine for Pre-Exposure Prophylaxis for SARS-CoV-2. [online] Available from https://www.medrxiv.org/content/10.1101/2020.08.31.20185314v2. [Last accessed February, 2024].
96. Desbois AC, Marques C, Lefèvre L, Barmo S, Lorenzo C, Leclercq M, et al. Prevalence and clinical features of COVID-19 in a large cohort of 199 patients with sarcoidosis. Clin Exp Rheumatol. 2022;40(1):195-6.
97. Dev N, Meena RC, Gupta DK, Gupta N, Sankar J. Risk factors and frequency of COVID-19 among healthcare workers at a tertiary care centre in India: a case–control study. Trans R Soc Trop Med Hyg. 2021;115(5):551-6.
98. Erden A, Karakas O, Armagan B, Guven SC, Ozdemir B, Atalar E, et al. COVID-19 outcomes in patients with antiphospholipid syndrome: a retrospective cohort study. Bratisl Lek Listy. 2022;123(2):120-4.
99. Ferreira A, Oliveira-e-Silva A, Bettencourt P. Chronic treatment with hydroxychloroquine and SARS-CoV-2 infection. J Med Virol. 2021;93(2):755-9.
100. Ferri C, Giuggioli D, Raimondo V, L'Andolina M, Tavoni A, Cecchetti R, et al. COVID-19 and rheumatic autoimmune systemic diseases: report of a large Italian patients series. Clin Rheumatol. 2020;39(11):3195-204.
101. Fitzgerald KC, Mecoli CA, Douglas M, Harris S, Aravidis B, Albayda J, et al. Risk Factors for Infection and Health Impacts of the Coronavirus Disease 2019 (COVID-19) Pandemic in People With Autoimmune Diseases. Clin Infect Dis. 2021;74(3):427-36.
102. Fung KW, Baik SH, Baye F, Zheng Z, Huser V, McDonald CJ. Effect of common maintenance drugs on the risk and severity of COVID-19 in elderly patients. PLoS One. 2022;17(4):1-15.
103. Gendebien Z, von Frenckell C, Ribbens C, André B, Thys M, Gangolf M, et al. Systematic analysis of COVID-19 infection and symptoms in a systemic lupus erythematosus population: correlation with disease characteristics, hydroxychloroquine use and immunosuppressive treatments. Ann Rheum Dis. 2021;80(6):e94.
104. Gendelman O, Amital H, Bragazzi NL, Watad A, Chodick G. Continuous hydroxychloroquine or colchicine therapy does not prevent infection with SARS-CoV-2: Insights from a large healthcare database analysis. Autoimmun Rev. 2020;19(7):102566.
105. Gentry CA, Humphrey MB, Thind SK, Hendrickson SC, Kurdgelashvili G, Williams RJ II. Long-term hydroxychloroquine use in patients with rheumatic conditions and development of SARS-CoV-2 infection: a retrospective cohort study. Lancet Rheumatol. 2020;2(11):e689-e697.
106. Gianfrancesco M, Hyrich KL, Al-Adely S, Carmona L, Danila MI, Gossec L, et al. Characteristics associated with hospitalisation for COVID-19 in people with rheumatic disease: data from the COVID-19 Global Rheumatology Alliance physician-reported registry. Ann Rheum Dis. 2020;79(7):859-66.
107. Goenka MK, Afzalpurkar S, Goenka U, Das SS, Mukherjee M, Jajodia S, et al. Seroprevalence of COVID-19 amongst health care workers in a tertiary care hospital of a metropolitan city from India. J Assoc Physicians India. 2020;68(11):14-9.
108. Grau-Pujol B, Camprubí-Ferrer D, Marti-Soler H, Fernández-Pardos M, Carreras-Abad C, Andrés MV, et al. Pre-exposure prophylaxis with hydroxychloroquine for COVID-19: a double-blind, placebo-controlled randomized clinical trial. Trials. 2021;22(1):808.
109. Gönenli MG, Kayı İ, Alpay-Kanıtez N, Baydaş T, Köse M, Nalbantoğlu EA, et al. Analysis of the Prophylactic use of Hydroxychloroquine at the Beginning of the COVID-19 Pandemic Among Physicians. Infect Dis Clin Microbiol. 2022;4(4):236-43.

110. Huang M, Li M, Xiao F, Pang P, Liang J, Tang T, et al. Preliminary evidence from a multicenter prospective observational study of the safety and efficacy of chloroquine for the treatment of COVID-19. Natl Sci Rev. 2020;7(9):1428-36.
111. Huh K, Ji W, Kang M, Hong J, Bae GH, Lee R, et al. Association of prescribed medications with the risk of COVID-19 infection and severity among adults in South Korea. Int J Infect Dis. 2021;104:7-14.
112. Isnardi CA, Roberts K, Saurit V, Petkovic I, Báez RM, Quintana R, et al. Sociodemographic and clinical factors associated with poor COVID-19 outcomes in patients with rheumatic diseases: data from the SAR-COVID Registry. Clin Rheumatol. 2023;42(2):563-78.
113. Juneja S, Rana P, Chawla P, Katoch R, Singh K, Rana S, et al. Hydroxychloroquine pre-exposure prophylaxis provides no protection against COVID-19 among health care workers: a cross-sectional study in a tertiary care hospital in North India. J Basic Clin Physiol Pharmacol. 2022;33(1):103-7.
114. Jung SY, Kim MS, Kim MC, Choi SH, Chung JW, Choi ST. Effect of hydroxychloroquine pre-exposure on infection with SARS-CoV-2 in rheumatic disease patients: a population-based cohort study. Clin Microbiol Infect. 2021;27(4):611-7.
115. Kadnur HB, Aggarwal A, Soneja M, Singh K, Mittal A, Nischal N, et al. Hydroxychloroquine pre-exposure prophylaxis for COVID-19 among healthcare workers: Initial experience from India. J Family Med Prim Care. 2022;11(3):1140-5.
116. Kamstrup P, Sivapalan P, Eklöf J, Hoyer N, Ulrik CS, Pedersen L, et al. Hydroxychloroquine as a primary prophylactic agent against SARS-CoV-2 infection: A cohort study. Int J Infect Dis. 2021;108:370-6.
117. Khoubnasabjafari M, Jouyban A, Malek Mahdavi A, Namvar L, Esalatmanesh K, Hajialilo M, et al. Prevalence of COVID-19 in patients with rheumatoid arthritis (RA) already treated with hydroxychloroquine (HCQ) compared with HCQ-naive patients with RA: a multicentre cross-sectional study. Postgrad Med J. 2021;98(e2):e92-e93.
118. Khurana A, Kaushal G, Gupta R, Verma V, Sharma K, Kohli P. Prevalence and Clinical Correlates of COVID-19 Outbreak Among Health Care Workers in a Tertiary Level Hospital in Delhi. Am J Infecti Dis. 2021;17(3):107-19.
119. Konig MF, Kim AH, Scheetz MH, Graef ER, Liew JW, Simard J, et al. Baseline use of hydroxychloroquine in systemic lupus erythematosus does not preclude SARS-CoV-2 infection and severe COVID-19. Ann Rheum Dis. 2020;79(10):1386-8.
120. Korkmaz T, Şener A, Gerdan V, Kızıloglu İ. (2021). The effect of Hydroxychloroquine use due to rheumatic disease on the risk of Covid-19 infection and its course. [online] Available from https://www.authorea.com/users/417382/articles/524514-the-effect-of-hydroxychloroquine-use-due-to-rheumatic-disease-on-the-risk-of-covid-19-infection-and-its-course. [Last accessed February, 2024].
121. Küçükakkaş O, Aydın T. (2020). The effect of hydroxychloroquine against SARS-CoV-2 infection in rheumatoid arthritis patients. [online] Available from https://europepmc.org/article/ppr/ppr189744. [Last accessed February, 2024].
122. Laplana M, Yuguero O, Fibla J. Lack of protective effect of chloroquine derivatives on COVID-19 disease in a Spanish sample of chronically treated patients. PLoS One. 2020;15(12):1-8.
123. Llanos-Cuentas A, Schwalb A, Quintana JL, Delfin B, Alvarez F, Ugarte-Gil C, et al. Hydroxychloroquine to prevent SARS-CoV-2 infection among healthcare workers: early termination of a phase 3, randomised, open-label, controlled clinical trial. BMC Res Notes. 2023;16(1):22.
124. Loucera C, Carmona R, Esteban-Medina M, Bostelmann G, Muñoyerro-Muñiz D, Villegas R, et al. Real-world evidence with a retrospective cohort of 15,968 Andalusian COVID-19 hospitalized patients suggests 21 new effective treatments and one drug that increases death risk. [online] Available from https://www.medrxiv.org/content/10.1101/2022.08.14.22278751v1. [Last accessed February, 2024].

125. MacFadden DR, Brown K, Buchan SA, Chung H, Kozak R, Kwong JC, et al. Screening Large Population Health Databases for Potential Coronavirus Disease 2019 Therapeutics: A Pharmacopeia-Wide Association Study of Commonly Prescribed Medications. Open Forum Infect Dis. 2022;9(5):ofac156.
126. Macías J, González-Moreno P, Sánchez-García E, Morillo-Verdugo R, Pérez-Venegas JJ, Pinilla A, et al. Similar incidence of coronavirus disease 2019 (COVID-19) in patients with rheumatic diseases with and without hydroxychloroquine therapy. PLoS One. 2021;16(4):e0249036.
127. Mahto M, Banerjee A, Biswas B, Kumar S, Agarwal N, Singh PK. Seroprevalence of IgG against SARS-CoV-2 and its determinants among healthcare workers of a COVID-19 dedicated hospital of India. Am J Blood Res. 2021;11(1):44-52.
128. Mathai S, Behera V, Hande V. Hydroxychloroquine as pre-exposure prophylaxis against COVID-19 in health-care workers: A single-center experience. J Mar Med Soc. 2020;22(3):98-104.
129. Mathew J, Jain S, Susngi T, Naidu S, Dhir V, Sharma A, et al. Predictors of COVID-19 severity and outcomes in Indian patients with rheumatic diseases: a prospective cohort study. Rheumatol Adv Pract. 2023;7(1):rkad025.
130. Mitchell G. (2020). Markedly Lower Rates of Coronavirus Infection and Fatality in Malaria-Endemic Regions–A Clue As to Treatment? [online] Available from https://papers.ssrn.com/sol3/papers.cfm?abstract_id=3586954. [Last accessed February, 2024].
131. Nagge J, Crowther M, Hirsh J. Is Impaired Renal Function a Contraindication to the Use of Low-Molecular-Weight Heparin? Arch Intern Med. 2002;162(22):2605-9.
132. Nasri E, Fakhim H, Salahi M, Ghafel S, Pourajam S, Darakhshandeh A, et al. Efficacy of hydroxychloroquine in pre-exposure severe acute respiratory syndrome coronavirus 2 prophylaxis among high-risk healthcare workers: A multicenter study. Adv Biomed Res. 2023;12:3.
133. Obrișcă B, Vornicu A, Jurubiță R, Mocanu V, Dimofte G, Andronesi A, et al. Characteristics of SARS-CoV-2 Infection in an Actively Monitored Cohort of Patients with Lupus Nephritis. Biomedicines. 2022;10(10):2423.
134. Oku K, Kimoto Y, Horiuchi T, Yamamoto M, Kondo Y, Okamoto M, et al. Risk factors for hospitalization or mortality for COVID-19 in patients with rheumatic diseases: Results of a nationwide JCR COVID-19 registry in Japan. Mod Rheumatol. 2023;33(4):768-76.
135. Opdam MAA, Benoy S, Verhoef LM, Bijnen SV, Lamers-Karnebeek F, Traksel RAM, et al. Identification of Risk Factors for COVID-19 Hospitalization in Patients With Anti-Rheumatic Drugs: Results From a Multicenter Nested Case Control Study. Clin Pharmacol Ther. 2022;111(5):1061-5.
136. Oztas M, Bektas M, Karacan I, Aliyeva N, Dag A, Aghamuradov S, et al. Frequency and severity of COVID-19 in patients with various rheumatic diseases treated regularly with colchicine or hydroxychloroquine. J Med Virol. 2022;94(7):3431-7.
137. Patel NJ, Wang X, Fu X, Kawano Y, Cook C, Vanni KMM, et al. Factors Associated with COVID-19 Breakthrough Infection in the Pre-Omicron Era Among Vaccinated Patients with Rheumatic Diseases: A Cohort Study. Semin Arthritis Rheum. 2023;58:152108.
138. Patil A, Chanakya K, Shenoy P, Chandrashekara S, Haridas V, Kumar S, et al. A prospective longitudinal study evaluating the influence of immunosuppressives and other factors on COVID-19 in autoimmune rheumatic diseases. BMC Rheumatol. 2022;6(1):32.
139. Pham K, Torres H, Satlin MJ, Goyal P, Gulick RM. Failure of chronic hydroxychloroquine in preventing severe complications of COVID-19 in patients with rheumatic diseases. Rheumatol Adv Pract. 2021;5(1):rkab014.
140. Polo R, García-Albéniz X, Terán C, Morales M, Rial-Crestelo D, Garcinuño MA, et al. Daily tenofovir disoproxil fumarate/emtricitabine and hydroxychloroquine for pre-exposure prophylaxis of COVID-19: a double-blind placebo-controlled randomized trial in healthcare workers. Clin Microbiol Infect. 2023;29(1):85-93.

141. Rajasingham R, Bangdiwala AS, Nicol MR, Skipper CP, Pastick KA, Axelrod ML, et al. Hydroxychloroquine as Pre-exposure Prophylaxis for Coronavirus Disease 2019 (COVID-19) in Healthcare Workers: A Randomized Trial. Clin Infect Dis. 2020;72(11):e835-e843.
142. Rangel LK, Shah P, Sicco KL, Caplan AS, Femia A. Chronic hydroxychloroquine therapy and COVID-19 outcomes: A retrospective case-control analysis. J Am Acad Dermatol. 2021;84(6):1769-72.
143. Rao A, Veluswamy SK, Shankarappa BG, Reddy RM, Umesh N, John L, et al. Hydroxychloroquine as pre-exposure prophylaxis against COVID-19 infection among healthcare workers: a prospective cohort study. Expert Rev Anti Infect Ther. 2022;20(5):781-7.
144. Rentsch CT, DeVito NJ, MacKenna B, Morton CE, Bhaskaran K, Brown JP, et al. Effect of pre-exposure use of hydroxychloroquine on COVID-19 mortality: a population-based cohort study in patients with rheumatoid arthritis or systemic lupus erythematosus using the OpenSAFELY platform. Lancet Rheumatol. 2021;3(1):e19-e27.
145. Revollo B, Tebe C, Peñafiel J, Blanco I, Perez-Alvarez N, Lopez R, et al. Hydroxychloroquine pre-exposure prophylaxis for COVID-19 in healthcare workers. J Antimicrob Chemother. 2020;76(3):827-9.
146. Rojas-Serrano J, Portillo-Vásquez AM, Thirion-Romero I, et al. Hydroxychloroquine for prophylaxis of COVID-19 in health workers: A randomized clinical trial. PLoS One. 2022;17(2):e0261980.
147. Sahebari M, Mirfeizi Z, Shariati-Sarabi Z, Moghadam M, Hashemzadeh K, Firoozabadi M. Influence of biologic and conventional disease-modifying antirheumatic drugs on COVID-19 incidence among rheumatic patients during the first and second wave of the pandemic in Iran. Reumatologia. 2022;60(4):231-41.
148. Salvarani C, Mancuso P, Gradellini F, Viani N, Pandolfi P, Reta M, et al. Susceptibility to COVID-19 in Patients Treated With Antimalarials: A Population-Based Study in Emilia-Romagna, Northern Italy. Arthritis Rheumatol. 2021;73(1):48-52.
149. Samajdar SS, Mukherjee S, Mondal T, Paul J, Tripathi SK, Chakrbarty A, et al. Ivermectin and hydroxychloroquine for chemo-prophylaxis of COVID-19: a questionnaire survey of perception and prescribing practice of physicians vis-a-vis outcomes. J Assoc Physicians India. 2021;69(11):11-2.
150. Santos CS, Morales CM, Álvarez ED, Castro CÁ, Robles AL, Sandoval TP. Determinants of COVID-19 disease severity in patients with underlying rheumatic disease. Clin Rheumatol. 2020;39(9):2789-96.
151. Satti E, Ostensen M, Soha D, Hadwan N, Ashour H, AL Emadi S. Characteristics and Obstetric Outcomes in Women With Autoimmune Rheumatic Disease During the COVID-19 Pandemic in Qatar. Cureus. 2022;14(4):e24382.
152. Seet RCS, Quek AML, Ooi DSQ, Sengupta S, Lakshminarasappa SR, Koo CY, et al. Positive impact of oral hydroxychloroquine and povidone-iodine throat spray for COVID-19 prophylaxis: An open-label randomized trial. Int J Infect Dis. 2021;106:314-22.
153. Shahrin L, Mahfuz M, Rahman MW, Hossain MR, Khandaker AM, Alam MA, et al. Hospital-Based Quasi-Experimental Study on Hydroxychloroquine Pre-Exposure Prophylaxis for COVID-19 in Healthcare Providers with Its Potential Side-Effects. Life (Basel). 2022;12(12):2047.
154. Shaw KS, Yin L, Shah JK, Sally RA, Svigos KS, Adotama PU, et al. COVID-19 in Individuals Treated With Long-Term Hydroxychloroquine: A Propensity Score-Matched Analysis of Cicatricial Alopecia Patients. J Drugs Dermatol. 2021;20:914-6.
155. Shukla AK, Atal S, Banerjee A, Jhaj R, Balakrishnan S, Chugh PK, et al. An observational multi-centric COVID-19 sequelae study among health care workers. Lancet Reg Health Southeast Asia. 2023;10:100129.
156. Singer ME, Kaelber DC, Antonelli MJ. Hydroxychloroquine ineffective for COVID-19 prophylaxis in lupus and rheumatoid arthritis. Ann Rheum Dis. 2022;81(9):e161.

157. Strangfeld A, Schäfer M, Gianfrancesco MA, Lawson-Tovey S, Liew JW, Ljung L, et al. Factors associated with COVID-19-related death in people with rheumatic diseases: results from the COVID-19 Global Rheumatology Alliance physician-reported registry. Ann Rheum Dis. 2021;80(7):930-42.
158. Sukumar C, Bolanthakodi N, Venkatramanan A, Nagraj R, Vidyasagar S. The Frontline War: A Case-control study of risk factors for COVID-19 among health care workers [version 1; peer review: 1 approved, 1 not approved]. F1000Research. 2022;11:1298.
159. Syed F, Hassan M, Arif MA, Batool S, Niazi R, Laila UE, et al. Pre-exposure Prophylaxis With Various Doses of Hydroxychloroquine Among Healthcare Personnel With High-Risk Exposure to COVID-19: A Randomized Controlled Trial. Cureus. 2021;13(12):e20572.
160. Tirupakuzhi Vijayaraghavan BK, Jha V, Rajbhandari D, Myatra SN, Ghosh A, Bhattacharya A, et al. Hydroxychloroquine plus personal protective equipment versus personal protective equipment alone for the prevention of laboratory-confirmed COVID-19 infections among healthcare workers: a multicentre, parallel-group randomised controlled trial from India. BMJ Open. 2022;12(6):e059540.
161. Trefond L, Drumez E, Andre M, Costedoat-Chalumeau N, Seror R, Devaux M, et al. Effet d'un traitement par hydroxychloroquine prescrit comme traitement de fond de rhumatismes inflammatoires chroniques ou maladies auto-immunes systémiques sur les tests diagnostiques et l'évolution de l'infection à SARS-CoV-2 : étude de 871 patients. Rev Rhum Ed Fr. 2022;89(2):192-5.
162. Ugarte-Gil MF, Alarcón GS, Izadi Z, Duarte-García A, Reátegui-Sokolova C, Clarke AE, et al. Characteristics associated with poor COVID-19 outcomes in individuals with systemic lupus erythematosus: data from the COVID-19 global rheumatology alliance. Ann Rheum Dis. 2022;81(7):970-8.
163. Vivanco-Hidalgo RM, Molina I, Martinez E, Roman-Viñas R, Sánchez-Montalvá A, Fibla J, et al. Incidence of COVID-19 in patients exposed to chloroquine and hydroxychloroquine: results from a population-based prospective cohort in Catalonia, Spain, 2020. Euro Surveill. 2021;26(9):2001202.
164. Yadav RM, Pate A, Shankarkumar A, Shreyasi A, Shinde S, Bargir U. Serosurvey for health-care workers provides corroborative evidence for the effectiveness of hydroxychloroquine prophylaxis against SARS-CoV-2 infection. J Epidemiol Glob Health. 2021;11(3):283-8.
165. Zhong J, Shen G, Yang H, Huang A, Chen X, Dong Li, et al. COVID-19 in patients with rheumatic disease in Hubei province, China: a multicentre retrospective observational study. Lancet Rheumatol. 2020;2(9):e557-64.
166. Barnabas RV, Brown ER, Bershteyn A, Stankiewicz Karita HC, Johnston C, Thorpe LE, et al. Hydroxychloroquine as postexposure prophylaxis to prevent severe acute respiratory syndrome coronavirus 2 infection: a randomized trial. Ann Intern Med. 2021;174(3):344-52.
167. Boulware DR, Pullen MF, Bangdiwala AS, Pastick KA, Lofgren SM, Okafor EC, et al. A Randomized Trial of Hydroxychloroquine as Postexposure Prophylaxis for Covid-19. N Engl J Med. 2020;383(6):517-25.
168. Dhibar DP, Arora N, Chaudhary D, Prakash A, Medhi B, Singla N, et al. The 'myth of Hydroxychloroquine (HCQ) as post-exposure prophylaxis (PEP) for the prevention of COVID-19' is far from reality. Sci Rep. 2023;13(1):378.
169. Dhibar DP, Arora N, Kakkar A, Singla N, Mohindra R, Suri V, et al. Post-exposure prophylaxis with hydroxychloroquine for the prevention of COVID-19, a myth or a reality? The PEP-CQ Study. Int J Antimicrob Agents. 2020;56(6):106224.
170. McKinnon JE, Wang DD, Zervos M, Saval M, Marshall-Nightengale L, Kilgore P, et al. Safety and tolerability of hydroxychloroquine in health care workers and first responders for the prevention of COVID-19: WHIP COVID-19 Study. Int J Infect Dis. 2022;116:167-73.

171. Polat O, Korkusuz R, Berber M. Hydroxychloroquine Use on Healthcare Workers Exposed to COVID-19—A Pandemic Hospital Experience. Med J Bakirkoy. 2020;16(3):280-6.
172. Shabani M, Totonchi M, Rezaeimirghaed O, Gachkar L, Hajiesmaeili M, Khoshkar A, et al. Evaluation of the prophylactic effect of hydroxychloroquine on people in close-contact with patients with COVID-19. Pulm Pharmacol Ther. 2021;70:102069.
173. Simova I, Vekov T, Krasnaliev J, Kornovski V, Bozhinov P. Hydroxychloroquine for prophylaxis and treatment of COVID-19 in health-care workers. New Microbes New Infect. 2020;38:100813.

CHAPTER 23

Ivermectin

Colleen Aldous, Eleftherios Gkioulekas, Philip Oldfield

INTRODUCTION

Brief History of the Discovery of Ivermectin

Microbiologist Satoshi Ōmura, the 2015 Nobel Prize for Medicine winner with William Campbell, carries a picture of his wife and daughter and a small plastic specimen bag wherever he goes.[1] In 1970, he used this small specimen bag to collect NRRL 8165, the mold later named *Streptomyces avermectinius*, from the woods close to a golf course along the ocean at Kawana in Ito City in the Shizuoka region of Japan.

Ōmura worked at the Kitasato Institute (KI), a research institution in Japan recognized as a world-leading center for discovering drugs and vaccines, primarily those derived from natural sources. Founded in 1914 by Shibasaburo Kitasato, the father of serotherapy and nominated for the first Nobel Prize in 1901, the institute has a long history of investigative research and developing chemotherapeutic drugs for practical use.[1]

Researchers at the KI turned to nature to find specimens because they believed in the almost unlimited abilities of microorganisms to produce novel compounds. They deliberately selected unusual microorganisms to maximize the chances of finding new compounds.[2] They attempted to isolate microbes from every kind of natural environment, primarily from soil and later from seaweed, plant leaves, and plant roots. They believed that the source could significantly impact the type of microbe found. They also believed that nature's microbes produce metabolites offering therapeutic promise. The KI isolated extraordinary microorganisms, cultured them, and evaluated the bioactivity of potential compounds.

In 1971 Ōmura, encouraged by Professor Yukimasa Yagisawa, General Manager of the Japan Antibiotics Research Association (JARA), to exploit the possibilities for research work overseas, went to the US on a sabbatical. Professor Max Tishler had invited him to work as a Visiting Research

Professor in the newly formed Chemistry Department at Wesleyan University in the US. Tishler had recently retired as President of the Merck Sharp and Dohme Research Laboratory (MSDRL). While on sabbatical, Ōmura sought research collaborations in the US to secure funds to support research work in Tokyo after his return. He visited many major US pharmaceutical companies, presenting a proposal for a collaborative research project. Tishler approached his successor at MSDRL, Dr LH Sarett, with Ōmura's collaboration ideas. This discussion expedited the research collaboration between Ōmura and MSDRL, which began in April 1973.[2]

Ōmura and William Campbell from MSDRL collaborated to find growth-promoting antibiotics suitable for animals, enzyme inhibitors, and general-purpose antibiotics produced by microorganisms. As part of this initiative, the KI isolated extraordinary microorganisms, cultured them, and then undertook preliminary in vitro evaluation of the bioactivity of any compounds they deemed potentially interesting. The most promising specimens were then sent to MSDRL for in vivo testing in the laboratory run by his co-Nobel Prize winner, William C Campbell; among them were extracts from NRRL 8165 and thousands of other microbes collected by Ōmura and his colleagues.[2]

In Campbell's laboratory, the ivermectin precursor, avermectin, which had been extracted from NRRL 8165, was discovered as a result of an antihelminthic screening test conducted on mice infected with the nematode *Nematospiroides dubius*. The test involved using an extract that was later fractionated to reveal macrocyclic lactones as the active components responsible for eliminating the nematode infection. Among these lactones, avermectin B1a was found to have the leading activity.[1]

Ivermectin for Veterinary Use

Further research by Campbell's group revealed that avermectin B1 had superior potency and safety compared to all known antihelminthic therapies at the time. It could resolve various animal nematode (roundworm) infections.[1]

The MSDRL chemists later made a minor chemical modification to avermectin B1 to create ivermectin, marketed in 1981 for animal use. Ivermectin was effective not only against nematode infections, such as heartworm in dogs and various worm species in commercial livestock, but also against ectoparasitic insects like fleas, ticks, and botflies, which cause significant economic losses in the livestock industry.[1,2] It quickly became a "blockbuster drug" in veterinary medicine due to its efficacy, potency, and safety in treating various parasitic infections. Resistance to ivermectin began to appear, initially in small ruminants and more significantly in cattle parasites, especially *Cooperia* species. However, there have been no reports of resistance in canine heartworms or among equine *Strongyloides* parasites. Ivermectin continues to be an essential drug for livestock and other domestic animals globally.

Ivermectin for Human Use

Ivermectin has been used extensively in human health, improving billions of people's general health and well-being worldwide since it was first used in 1988 to treat onchocerciasis (river blindness), a disease caused by a parasitic worm (*Onchocerca volvulus*) and transmitted through the bites of infected blackflies. It is multipurpose, highly effective, broad-spectrum, safe, well-tolerated, and can be easily administered. Satoshi Ōmura and William Campbell were awarded the Nobel Prize in Physiology or Medicine in 2015 because their work has had a significant impact on global health, particularly in the treatment and control of debilitating diseases like onchocerciasis and lymphatic filariasis (elephantiasis), a disease caused by filarial worms (*Wuchereria bancrofti, Brugia malayi, and Brugia timori*),[3] which is transmitted to humans through mosquito bites.

Ivermectin for Onchocerciasis and Lymphatic Filariasis and the Mectizan Program

In the mid-1970s, the global community mobilized to address the major problems of neglected tropical diseases. The UN-based Special Program for Research and Training in Tropical Diseases (TDR) was established in 1975, with onchocerciasis and lymphatic filariasis among its target diseases.

Ivermectin's role in human medicine began in 1978 at the MSDRL, with William Campbell being the driving force behind investigating its potential for human use. After receiving positive results from testing ivermectin on large livestock, Campbell suggested to the MSDRL management that an avermectin could prevent the blindness associated with onchocerciasis. This hypothesis was confirmed through clinical trials led by Mohammed Aziz of Merck, which showed that a single dose of ivermectin dramatically reduced the microfilaria burden in humans, ameliorating the disease.

Ivermectin causes almost complete clearance of dermal microfilariae, the immature form of the parasite that causes onchocerciasis, within 2 days after the start of treatment, reducing the load to virtually zero within 8 days.[2] It produces long-term suppression of circulating microfilariae, making it an ideal treatment for patients with severe itching that may occur in people with onchocerciasis.

In addition to its direct effects on the disease, ivermectin has also been associated with various secondary benefits. For example, in a survey of 3,125 community members in Nigeria who had been receiving ivermectin, there was an 18.5% reduction in body itching, reduced skin rash (17.3%), and reports of 11.7% better vision.[2] The World Health Organization (WHO) has certified Colombia, Ecuador, and Mexico free of onchocerciasis. Transmission has also been halted in Guatemala. Currently, transmission has been restricted to the Amazonas region of Brazil and Venezuela. In Africa, where the disease was much more prevalent, infection rates are down fivefold. In 2014, most African countries with endemic infection moved from onchocerciasis control with annual doses of ivermectin to elimination campaigns with twice-annual dosing.

Ivermectin has also been used in elimination campaigns for lymphatic filariasis, greatly reducing the number of human cases. Ivermectin's use in treating lymphatic filariasis has a significant history. In the mid-1980s, even before ivermectin was approved for human use to treat onchocerciasis, Merck was conducting trials of ivermectin to measure its impact against lymphatic filariasis and to find optimal treatment dosages. The drug showed promise in interrupting the transmission of infection, opening up the prospect of eliminating the disease. This was made possible thanks to Glaxo Smith Kline (GSK) agreeing to donate albendazole, another anti-parasitic drug.[2]

In 1997, following advances in both diagnosis and treatment, the WHO classified lymphatic filariasis as one of six "eradicable" or "potentially eradicable" infectious diseases and requested Member States to initiate steps to eliminate lymphatic filariasis as a public health problem.[2] In late-1998, following the registration of the drug for lymphatic filariasis, Merck extended its ivermectin donation program to cover lymphatic filariasis in areas where it co-existed with Onchocerciasis.[2] Subsequently, in 1999/2000, the WHO launched the Global Program to Eliminate Lymphatic Filariasis (GPELF).[4] Ivermectin has since been used extensively to treat lymphatic filariasis, a disease that threatens over 1 billion people in over 80 countries.

The Mectizan Program

The Special Program for Research and Training in Tropical Diseases (TDR) and the Onchocerciasis Control Program (OCP) made ivermectin affordable and accessible for those most in need. Initially, Merck had indicated a price of $3 per tablet for ivermectin, which would cost a treatment dose of $6, a price beyond the reach of those most affected by the disease. TDR and OCP, recognizing the potential of ivermectin as a community-level tool to interrupt parasite transmission, campaigned to reduce the treatment cost.[5]

During the trials to test the drug's efficacy in field settings (Phase II trials starting in 1983), Merck continued to fund much of the work, with additional financial support from OCP and TDR. TDR's existing international network facilitated Merck's ability to develop workable relationships with researchers and institutions to conduct activities in Africa and South America. Thirteen community-level (Phase IV) trials were conducted between 1987 and 1989, with over 120,000 individual doses of ivermectin administered. Of the 13 community trials, TDR funded five in Liberia, Cameroon, Malawi, Guatemala, and Nigeria and spent US$2.35 million in total. Over the period, TDR spent 25–35% of its total annual budget for all filariasis work on ivermectin.

Following the registration of ivermectin for human use in 1987, Merck & Co. Inc., in an unprecedented move, donated the drug (produced under the brand name Mectizan) to treat onchocerciasis in all endemic countries for as long as it was needed. The resultant drug donation program, organized through the independent Mectizan Donation Program (MDP) established and funded by Merck, was the first, largest, longest running and most successful of all, and proved a model for all others that have followed. This decision still stands today, with Merck providing approximately 300 million doses annually of ivermectin to control and eventually eradicate onchocerciasis and lymphatic filariasis.

Despite the large-scale campaigns undertaken, human helminthic resistance to ivermectin has not yet emerged, and it remains effective for onchocerciasis and lymphatic filariasis. Today, ivermectin is being increasingly used worldwide to combat other diseases, such as strongyloidiasis (which infects some 35 million each year), scabies (mite infestation which causes 300 million cases annually), pediculosis (lice infestation), gnathostomiasis, trichuriasis, myiasis, ascariasis, cutaneous larva migrans, and filariases. New and promising properties and uses for ivermectin and other avermectin derivatives continue to be found.

Ivermectin for Other Pathologies

In addition to being used as an anti-parasitic, ivermectin has also been considered to treat several viral and other medical conditions, including asthma, *Mycobacterium* infections, and cancer. Some preclinical studies and research articles have explored the potential anti-cancer properties of ivermectin.[3] These studies are typically in vitro or animal models, and more research is needed before any definitive conclusions can be drawn about the efficacy of ivermectin in treating cancer. Studies have examined the potential effects of ivermectin on *Mycobacterium* tuberculosis, generally in preclinical settings such as in vitro experiments or animal models. These studies are exploratory. The therapeutic potential of ivermectin for tuberculosis (TB) would need to be confirmed through rigorous clinical trials to assess its efficacy and safety, specifically in treating TB.

In mid-2020, at the long-term care facility (LTCF) in France, a 66-year-old female resident with scabies was treated with *ivermectin*. Subsequently, other residents also came down with scabies. It was decided that everyone at the facility would be treated with ivermectin. During this time, the coronavirus disease 2019 (COVID-19) outbreak was rampant in the area. None of the ivermectin-treated residents or staff developed severe COVID-19 or died, while residents and staff from the other LTCF's in the area showed higher COVID-19 severity and deathrates.[6]

MECHANISM OF ACTION

It has become clear over time that ivermectin has different therapeutic uses, and many of them show different mechanisms of action of ivermectin. The mechanism of action as an antiparasite was the first to be elucidated.

Mechanism of Action as an Antiparasitic

Ivermectin targets glutamate-gated chloride ion channels (GluCls) in the invertebrates it is designed to affect.[7] These channels play fundamental roles in nematodes and insects but are not accessible in vertebrates, which is why ivermectin is safe for human and animal use.[2]

When ivermectin binds to these channels, it disrupts neurotransmission in nematodes. This disruption is believed to interfere with the ability of microfilariae (immature worms) to evade the human immune system, resulting in the host's own immune response being able to overcome and kill them.[7]

The drug has little direct effect on microfilariae when administered at pharmacologically relevant concentrations. Instead, it disrupts the fundamental host-parasite equilibrium.[8] The half-life of ivermectin in humans is 12–36 hours, while metabolites may persist for up to 3 days. As the lowest levels of dermal microfilariae occur well after this timeframe, it suggests that not all microfilariae affected by ivermectin are killed in the first few days.[8] Repeat dosing if this is appropriate.

Ivermectin is now used to treat a variety of parasitic infections, including scabies and intestinal worm infestations. While it is theoretically possible for a large die-off of parasites to lead to symptoms similar to a Herxheimer reaction, this is not commonly reported in the medical literature in the context of ivermectin use, given the low doses prescribed for parasitic infections. The Jarisch–Herxheimer reaction is most commonly associated with the treatment of bacterial infections rather than parasitic infections.

MECHANISMS OF ACTION FOR INDICATIONS OTHER THAN ANTIPARASITIC

Before the COVID-19 pandemic, in addition to being used as an antiparasitic, ivermectin had also been considered to treat several viral and other medical conditions, including asthma, Mycobacterium infections, and cancer. **Table 1** lists some of these indications and the intended mechanism of action.[9-23] The mechanism of action, if known, is described in detail in the appropriate references cited in the table.

In 2012, the discovery of inhibition of RNA helicase DDX23[24] in flaviviruses established ivermectin's potential as a drug, not just for parasites but for viruses. Consistent with this, ivermectin inhibits viral replication of several flaviviruses by blocking a viral helicase. Susceptible flaviviruses include those causing yellow fever, dengue, West Nile virus, and tick-borne encephalitis. Encouragingly, serial passage of yellow fever virus with increasing concentrations of ivermectin did not appear to select for viral resistance.

In May 2020, in a comprehensive systemic review by Heidary,[25] the antiviral effects of ivermectin were summarized, including in vitro and in

TABLE 1: Therapeutic indications of ivermectin along with purposeful mechanisms before the COVID-19 pandemic.

Indications	Actions/mechanisms	References
Viruses	By preventing the virus cargo protein from entering the nucleus, preventing viral replication	• Dengue virus[9,10] • Hendra virus[11] • Human immunodeficiency virus[9] • Venezuelan equine encephalitis virus[12,13] • Pseudorabies[14] • Human cytomegalovirus[9]
Mycobacterium infections	Not known	Tuberculosis[15]
Immunomodulatory	Reduced the production of proinflammatory cytokines	• Asthma[16] • Anti-inflammatory[17]
Cancer	Induces cell death in cancer cells	Different mechanisms cause cell death in a variety of different cancers[18,19]
Neurological disorders	Treatment of motor neuron disease by silencing excessive neuronal activity using IVERMECTIN	A variety of different motor neuron diseases[20-23]

vivo studies over the past 50 years. Several studies reported antiviral effects of ivermectin on RNA viruses such as Zika, dengue, yellow fever, West Nile, Hendra, Newcastle, Venezuelan equine encephalitis, Chikungunya, Semliki Forest, Sindbis, Avian influenza A, Porcine Reproductive and Respiratory Syndrome, human immunodeficiency virus type 1 (HIV-1), and severe acute respiratory syndrome coronavirus 2 (SARS-CoV-2). Furthermore, there are some studies showing antiviral effects of ivermectin against DNA viruses such as equine herpes type 1 (EHV-1), BK polyomavirus, pseudorabies, porcine circovirus 2 (PCV-2), and bovine herpesvirus (BoHV).[1]

In 2017, Laing et al.[24] commented that—intriguingly, ivermectin has a diverse range of effects in many different organisms, far beyond the endoparasites and ectoparasites it was developed to control. For example, ivermectin has been shown to regulate glucose and cholesterol levels in diabetic mice to suppress malignant cell proliferation in various cancers,[26] to inhibit viral replication in several flaviviruses,[27] and to reduce survival in major insect vectors of malaria and trypanosomiasis.[27,28]

The use of ivermectin in vector control in malaria has been considered for over a decade. In 2013, Chaccour et al. suggested further research into the use of endectocides, such as ivermectin, as an important potential addition to anti-malarial measures. In 2018, the Lancet published an article entitled "Ivermectin: repurposing an old drug to complement malaria vector control" by Rabinovich as one approach to solving the problem of residual transmission of malaria. Ivermectin has been shown to reduce malaria transmission by a further 44% when added to malaria prophylaxis.[29]

Possible Mechanisms of Action Against SARS-CoV-2

In the early stages of the COVID-19 pandemic, the mechanisms of action of ivermectin against SARS-CoV-2 were not widely known. A point to consider is that although ivermectin was licensed as an anti-parasitic, the additional indications shown in **Table 1** were published before the COVID-19 pandemic. Therefore, these proposed mechanisms were already known during the COVID-19 pandemic.

By May 2020, a few months into the pandemic, a laboratory study from Australia drew attention to ivermectin as a possible therapeutic. It demonstrated that ivermectin effectively inhibited replication of the SARS-CoV-2 virus by preventing it from entering the nucleus. This provided the first understanding that ivermectin could possibly be helpful in treating COVID-19. In a report by Caly et al.,[30] it was demonstrated using TaqMan reverse transcription–polymerase chain reaction (RT-PCR) that ivermectin effectively inhibited replication of the SARS-CoV-2 in vitro by blocking the ability of the host cell IMPα/β1 protein complex to bind to the SARS-CoV-2 cargo protein in the cytoplasm, thereby preventing it from going through the nuclear pore complex (NPC) and entering the nucleus. The RNA genome of SARS-CoV-2 is replicated within the nucleus of cells. The authors noted a 93–99.8% decrease in viral RNA levels for ivermectin versus control treatments at 24 hours, both in the released and cell-associated viral RNA. Likewise, they reported that by 48 hours, there was a >5,000-fold decrease of viral RNA, indicating that ivermectin treatment resulted in the effective loss of essentially all viral material by 48 hours. Consistent with this, no further reduction in viral RNA was observed at 72 hours. However, under the conditions tested,[30] the ivermectin concentration that inhibited viral replication by 50% (IC50) was determined to be approximately 2 μm. Although this concentration is greater than expected in vivo, it demonstrated that, at least theoretically, ivermectin can neutralize the SARS-CoV-2 virus.[31] This experiment was a proof-of-concept exercise and never designed to determine dosages.

As time went on, other mechanisms of action for ivermectin in treating patients with COVID-19 spanned all phases of the disease process. A 2022 review[32] documented that in addition to the effects of ivermectin on SARS-CoV-2 replication through interaction with host proteins, it can also interfere with the entry of the virus, modulate the inflammatory response, inhibit hemagglutination, and allow cardiac mitochondria to produce adenosine triphosphate (ATP) in the presence of hypoxia, thus providing benefit at all stages of the disease. In total, ivermectin has over 20 mechanisms of action including antiviral, anti-inflammatory, antithrombotic, and cardioprotective effects.[32]

Possible Mechanisms of Ivermectin during the Viral Replication Phase

During the viral replication phase of the disease, ivermectin focuses on preventing SARS-CoV-2 from entering the host cells. Ivermectin can prevent the SARS-CoV-2 virus from entering the host cell by directly interacting with the viral spike protein and binding to the angiotensin-converting enzyme 2 (ACE2) receptor. It interacted with the viral spike protein in the leucine 91 and histidine 378 regions, forming a complex between the SARS-CoV-2 spike protein and the ACE2 receptor.[33] Furthermore, ivermectin formed five H-bonds with the ACE2 receptor at Arg273, Glu398, Ser511, Arg514, and Tyr515.[34] Secondly, it is also able to prevent viral replication. As previously mentioned, Caly et al. demonstrated the potential of ivermectin to block the host cell's IMPα/β1 protein complex to bind to the SARS-CoV-2 cargo protein, effectively preventing it from going through the NPC and into the nucleus.[30] In this in vitro study, although the IC50 was determined to be 2 μm, there is a possibility that ivermectin could still have an effect since fat-soluble ivermectin would tend to accumulate in the tissue compartment. Another possible mechanism is the inhibition of SARS-CoV-2 RNA-dependent RNA polymerase (RdRP), which prevents gene translation. Studies have shown that ivermectin binds to RdRP, potentially halting virus replication and assembly within the host cell.[34,35]

During the replication phase, should SARS-CoV-2 enter the systemic circulation, this may cause red blood cell (RBC) clumping, in which the viral spike protein binds to the glycans on the RBCs. Ivermectin has been shown in vitro to disrupt the binding of SARS-CoV-2 to the RBCs, eliminating clumping.[36] However, the clinical relevance remains to be seen since, in the same in vitro study, it was demonstrated that milder variants of the disease, i.e., Omicron, produced a stronger clumping effect when compared with the Wuhan variant. Although not the same, possibly a related finding was that, using flow cytometry, there was an increase in complement activation products C3b, iC3b, C3dg, and C4d on circulating RBCs from hospitalized COVID-19 patients when compared with healthy subjects.[37] Furthermore, viral spike protein was also bound to the RBCs, linking the SARS-CoV-2 spike protein to the observed increase of complement activation products in hospitalized patients with severe COVID-19. *Ivermectin* prevents the binding of the viral spike protein to the RBCs.[37]

The SARS-CoV-2 virus has been shown to directly activate platelets, initiating the coagulation cascade process and the release of inflammatory cytokines and leukocyte-platelet aggregates (LPAs) via the viral Spike protein's binding to ACE2, primed by TMPRSS2, resulting in micro-thrombi and blood clots.[38] Ivermectin acts by blocking the interactions of the viral spike protein with ACE2 and TMPRSS2 on the surface of the platelets.

Possible Mechanisms of Ivermectin during the Hyperinflammatory Response Phase

SARS-CoV-2 directly activates the toll-like receptor 4 (TLR4) receptors, initiating the lipopolysaccharide (LPS)-mediated activation of the nuclear factor kappa B (NF-κB) pathway and mitogen-activated protein kinase 3 (MAPK3) kinases, increasing proinflammatory cytokines and chemokines responsible for cytokine storms. Ivermectin inhibits TLR4 signaling directly, preventing activation of the NF-κ pathway and MAPK3, which block the production of these proinflammatory cytokines and chemokines.[39,40]

The SARS-CoV-2 virus enhances the signal transducer and activator of transcription 3 (STAT3) pathway. STAT3 physically binds to PAK1 and increases interleukin-6 (IL-6) transcription, a major proinflammatory cytokine. Ivermectin inhibits both STAT-1 and PAK1, effectively blocking the production of IL-6.[41]

Figure 1 gives a summary of the roles ivermectin has during each phase of the disease. Although it is not an all-inclusive list, it is clear that ivermectin can be used to treat patients with COVID-19 during each phase of the disease. The mechanisms are very complex and are further discussed in the references. Although most patients recover perfectly at home, **Figure 1** illustrates the multifunctional roles ivermectin plays in treating patients with COVID-19, regardless of what stage the disease is at.

Mechanism of Action with Regard to Blood Clotting in COVID-19 Infection

The pathology observed in COVID-19 patients, particularly the crucial role of red blood cell (RBC) clumping and its subsequent ramifications, leads to an understanding of the role of spike protein in COVID-19 patients and those suffering from COVID-19 vaccination injury. Several studies have underscored that a predominant cause of pathology in COVID-19 cases is the micro-clotting of blood.[42] Most notably, RBC clumps have been consistently identified in a majority of COVID-19 patients,[42] with the rate of RBC micro-aggregates being 15 times higher in critically ill patients than in healthy controls.[43] Even among recovered COVID-19 patients who were hospitalized, there was a sixfold increase in occluded blood vessels compared to healthy individuals.[44] Of significant interest is the finding that, in nine such patients, 41% of RBCs contained traces of the SARS-CoV-2 spike protein.[37] Moreover, the presence of RBC clumps in the bloodstream appears to be at the epicenter of the most debilitating COVID-19 symptoms: from decreased oxygen saturation (SpO_2 deficits) and microvascular occlusion to myocarditis. Notably, when RBC clumping was experimentally induced in vivo using high molecular weight dextran, it resulted in these same key morbidities.[45] A notable study from a Harvard hospital drew parallels between COVID-vaccinated subjects with myocarditis and detectable spike protein (SP) in their blood.[46]

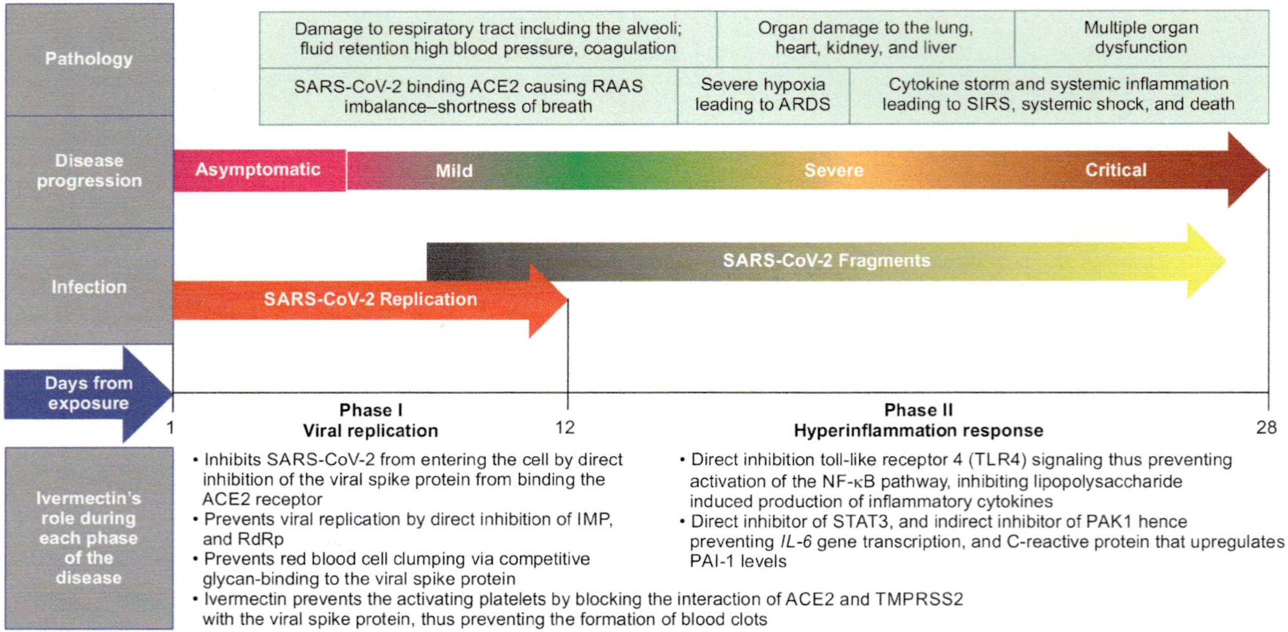

FIGURE 1: COVID-19 disease process, worst case scenario, and *ivermectin's* role in its treatment.

(ACE2: angiotensin converting enzyme 2; RAAS: renin–angiotensin–aldosterone system; ARDS: acute respiratory distress syndrome; SIRS: systemic inflammatory response syndrome; IMP: importin; RdRP: RNA-dependent RNA polymerase; NF-κ B: nuclear factor kappa B; STAT3: signal transducer and activator of transcription 3; PAK1: P21 activated kinase 1; PAI-1: plasminogen activator inhibitor-1; TMPRSS2: transmembrane protease serine 2)

Furthermore, the findings by Boschi et al. (2022) emphasize the intricate interactions between the SARS-CoV-2 SP and human RBCs. When mixed in phosphate buffer solution (PBS), these components form clumps—a reaction that can wreak havoc in a host. Ivermectin, when added to this mix, prevented RBC clumps from forming and, when added afterward, reversed this aggregation and cleared all clumps,[36] the biological mechanism being competitive binding with SARS-CoV-2 SP glycans.[47] Additionally, it is essential to appreciate the role of SA-tipped glycophorin A (GPA), densely coating the RBC surface, in these processes.[42] The ability of the virus's spike protein to latch onto human RBCs, leading to clumping and subsequently to clotting and inflammation, cannot be underestimated.

At a cellular level, the intricacies of glycan and ACE2 interactions with COVID-19 are paramount. While ACE2 serves as the virus's host target for replication, the glycan bindings of the SARS-CoV-2 spike protein predominantly dictate the virus's morbidity. Notably, blood cells have a significant density of SA-tipped glycans, though they lack ACE2. In contrast, endothelial cells exhibit a far higher concentration of SA-tipped CD147 glycan receptors than ACE2 receptors.[42]

The lungs' vulnerability, especially the alveolar septal capillaries, is a grim reminder of how SARS-CoV-2 infiltrates the bloodstream. With most severe COVID-19 patients exhibiting damaged pulmonary capillaries and hypoxemia, the evident link between these morbidities and the clumping and clotting of blood cells is undeniable.

The crucial role of RBC clumping in the pathology of COVID-19 and the interactions of the SARS-CoV-2 spike protein with glycans and its implications cannot be overlooked. As we further our understanding, refining our research methodologies will be essential.

The role of ivermectin in stopping clumping and clotting justifies its use in late-stage disease. So does its cardioprotective effect through mitochondrial support. SARS-CoV-2 has been a well-known cause for acute myocardial injury and hypoxic cardiac arrest.

In 2017, Nagai et al. demonstrated that ivermectin increased mitochondrial ATP production by inducing Cox6a2 expression. Ivermectin therefore maintains mitochondrial ATP production under hypoxic conditions and may, therefore, improve cardiac function under hypoxic conditions *https://pubmed.ncbi.nlm.nih.gov/28942281/*.

While ivermectin does have antiviral activity, it also acts at all stages of the disease in SARS-CoV-2. It has antiviral, anti-inflammatory, and immunomodulatory effects, it stops hemagglutination and is cardioprotective during hypoxia. The perception that it is reserved for early disease should be reviewed.

CLINICAL EVIDENCE

As groups across the globe started using an ivermectin regimen for the treatment of COVID-19 through 2020 due to the evidence communicated of its efficacy from several quarters, regulatory authorities were scrambling to quickly approve COVID-19 vaccines. Publications from case studies, through to observational studies and small trials emerged, and with that the cry of "insufficient evidence" from those in the regulatory and pharmaceutical industries who all had much to gain from a potentially successful vaccine. The evidence was not insufficient at the end of 2020 and through to 2021; it was just short on well-run large randomized control trials (RCTs). The emphasis on large RCTs was misplaced in the emergency of the pandemic but has a history in the indoctrination of the evidence-based medicine pyramid. The evidence-based medicine (EBM) pyramid is a concept that originated from the field of evidence-based medicine. It was developed to help healthcare professionals and researchers visualize and understand the hierarchy of evidence certainty, with the idea that the certainty of evidence increases as you move up the pyramid. The pyramid typically places systematic reviews and meta-analyses at the top, followed by RCTs, cohort studies, case-control studies, case series/reports, and animal research or in vitro studies at the bottom. The EBM pyramid is widely used in medical education and clinical decision-making. However, it is an oversimplification of evidence and mistakenly replaces "certainty" with "quality". Therefore, people are comfortable in thinking that studies that are below a RCTs are of poor quality and that RCTs epitomize good quality. Any thinking scientist knows that good quality case series have more value in the clinical setting than poorly designed RCTs, but the knee-jerk response that the lack of large RCTs in ivermectin meant insufficient evidence of "high" quality.

The evidence has continued to mount, showing the efficacy of ivermectin in case series and small studies carried out by clinicians treating COVID-19. Publication bias and information blocks in the lay and academic press and social media space since late 2020 have skewed the volume of true research data available in the public domain.

Summary of Key Clinical Trials involving Ivermectin

By October 3, 2022, there were 265 published papers on the use of ivermectin in treating COVID-19 in the PubMed database. These were classified into four types of studies:

1. Systemic studies (systematic reviews, meta-analyses, and clinical guidelines) use a structured approach to integrate, critically appraise, and filter the primary evidence.
2. Clinical studies (RCTs, cohort studies, and case–control studies) relate to all trials on live humans. This is the primary evidence/unfiltered information.
3. Mechanisms of action are research studies that did not involve humans, i.e., in-silico (computer-based), in vitro (human cells in a lab), and in vivo (live animal) studies.
4. Reviews include literature or narrative reviews, case series, case reports, and expert opinions.

These papers were reviewed to understand the researchers' conclusions regarding whether or not ivermectin was useful in treating COVID-19. This was coded on a spectrum from Yes to No:

- *Yes*: Ivermectin is useful in treating COVID-19 (or, for mechanisms of action, there is a plausible reason why ivermectin would work to treat COVID-19)
- *Promising*: There is some evidence to support its use, though more research is advised
- *Uncertain/may be*: The evidence is insufficient/conflicting; more research is required
- *Not promising*: The evidence does not support its use, though further research could identify its role, e.g., at a certain dosage, infection stage, in combination with other drugs, etc.
- *No*: Do not use ivermectin to treat COVID-19 (or, for mechanisms of action, no explanation was found about how ivermectin can treat COVID-19)

Looking at the totality of evidence, about 20% of research reports were for, and another 17% against, using ivermectin to treat COVID-19. There are two points to note, however. By mid-2022, negative RCTs far outweighed those that showed positive results in published research. It has already been mentioned that many RCTs were poorly designed and misreported, but by this time, there was a publication bias, and many positive outcome trials were unpublished. Meta-analyses that were published were selective in the articles they reviewed, with the selection and interpretation of findings being subject to bias. Comparing the Bryant *et al.* and the Popp *et al.* systematic reviews of the literature shows that higher levels of evidence in the EBM pyramid can be subject to bias.[48,49] Most papers showed positive trends in therapeutic efficacy for ivermectin but concluded indecisively, reported as "may be" in **Table 2**. Many mentioned finding no major adverse events but recommending further research to confirm findings. Mechanism

TABLE 2: Should ivermectin be used in treating COVID-19? Research findings by study type.

	Level-of-evidence	Total	Yes	No	May be
Systematic	Clinical practice guidelines	5	0	4	1
Systematic	Meta-analyses and systematic reviews	31	1	3	27
Clinical	Randomized control trials	27	6	17	4
Clinical	Cohort and case–control studies	26	8	10	8
Clinical	Case reports and case series	8	1	0	7
Reviews	Narrative reviews, expert opinion, editorials	107	6	2	99
Mechanisms	In vivo, in silico, and in vitro studies	61	31	10	20
		265	53	46	166

of action studies overwhelmingly supported the functionality of ivermectin in treating COVID-19.

An argument for looking at the totality of evidence and not just at RCTs must be made. While it is clear that there was diversity in findings in the research on ivermectin efficacy, the trends toward showing efficacy were apparent if the totality of evidence rather than in the selection of only RCTs on which to make a judgement.

Ivermectin Used for Prophylaxis Against COVID-19

A few studies indicated the potential use of ivermectin as a prophylactic treatment against COVID-19, but none were as unequivocal in their findings as the SAIVE (Study to Evaluate the Efficacy and Safety of Ivermectin in COVID-19 Prevention) trial. The SAIVE Trial (NCT05305560) offers significant contributions to the body of knowledge on the use of ivermectin for COVID-19.[50] This large, well-designed randomized control study demonstrated the efficacy of ivermectin in preventing COVID-19, showing a reduction in infection after exposure by 72%. The study was conducted among unvaccinated individuals exposed to people diagnosed with COVID-19, and it showed a much lower likelihood of contracting the illness after taking ivermectin. The study was overseen by a US-based independent Data Monitoring Committee, providing quality assurance for the study execution. The dosages used in the study were more than adequate, with daily doses of ivermectin taken orally at 200 µg/kg on Day 1, followed by 100 µg/kg daily from Day 2 to 28. The SAIVE Trial added to the growing body of evidence supporting the efficacy of ivermectin in preventing and treating COVID-19.

Safety Profile of Ivermectin

Since its introduction in 1987, ivermectin has been administered in an estimated 3.7 billion human doses, demonstrating a notable safety profile.[7,51-54] The conventional dosage for ivermectin is 200 µg/kg, commonly employed twice at weekly intervals for scabies[55] or administered one to three times annually for onchocerciasis, commonly known as river blindness.[52,56] The United States Centers for Disease Control and Prevention (CDC) endorse an oral regimen of up to 1.4 mg/kg over a 1-month period as a viable treatment option for crusted scabies.[55] This low dose averts concern regarding potential Herxheimer reactions.

Multiple studies have substantiated the drug's tolerability at elevated dosages, including a single dose of 800 µg/kg,[57] 1.6 mg/kg over a 12-week span,[58] and 1.6 mg/kg administered over 13 days.[50] Guzzo et al. in 2002 reported that ivermectin remained tolerable even when administered at a dose tenfold higher than the standard 200 µg/kg.[53] Furthermore, clinical trials employing fixed doses as high as 120 mg (up to 2,000 µg/kg) in a single administration or 180 mg (up to 3,000 µg/kg) in divided doses across 1 week have shown ivermectin to be well-tolerated, with adverse event rates comparable to placebo.[53]

A meta-analysis surveying the clinical utilization of ivermectin found negligible differences in the frequency and severity of adverse events between standard dosages and elevated doses of up to 800 µg/kg.[59] Longitudinal studies examining ivermectin use in geriatric populations at dosages as high as 400 µg/kg reported no increased mortality rates.[60,61] Crump's 2011 review further corroborates the safety of ivermectin, emphasizing its minimal side effects and suitability for administration by non-medical personnel following basic training. This has contributed to the drug's substantial positive impact on global public health.[3]

VigiAccess is the World Health Organisation's global database of reported potential side effects of medicines. In August 2023, after nearly 40 years of use in humans, a total of 7,247 adverse drug responses were recorded in VigiAccess. Of these, 26 were deaths. **Table 3** compares the safety in terms of adverse events and mortality with other drugs used during the COVID-19 pandemic.

Type I or Type II Error

Given the volume of peer-reviewed information that was available on the safety of ivermectin by 2020 as well as the emerging data on efficacy by looking at the totality of evidence, one could question whether regulatory authorities could have made a humanitarian decision based on a Type 1 error rather than dismissing ivermectin based on their definition of quality research and hearsay from other authorities and awaiting data for a Type II error decision.

A Type I error can be safely considered if there is little risk of serious adverse reactions and ivermectin has an already established safety profile. In the case of a Type I error decision, the hypothesis would have been—*ivermectin is rolled out and proven later to be ineffective.* The data showed that ivermectin is safe and effective for prophylaxis, early disease treatment, and advanced disease treatment. The costs of the drug could have been low, given that it is no longer under patent and could be produced anywhere in the

TABLE 3: Comparison of the safety in terms of ivermectin adverse events and mortality with other drugs used during the COVID-19 pandemic.

Drug	Total events	Total deaths	Reported since
Remdesivir	10,832	722	2020
Paxlovid	41,902	73	2022
Molnupiravir	2,578	16	2021
Ibuprofen	187,459	1,151	1969
Paracetamol	197,669	4,104	1983
Ivermectin	7,247	26	1999

Source: www.vigiaccess.org (Deaths reported under "General disorders and administration site conditions").

world. If it is proven ineffective at some later point, then there is a relatively small financial loss. There were unlikely to be any costs to human suffering due to the already well-established safety profile.

However, regulatory authorities decided to make a Type II error decision with the hypothesis—*ivermectin is withheld until it is shown to work in a subsequent adequately robust RCT*. At the very least, looking at the totality of evidence and the failure of the vaccines to impact the pandemic as hoped, this decision can be shown to have incurred a higher mortality rate.

CONTROVERSY AND CHALLENGES

Many controversies about evaluating the available empirical evidence for and against the use of ivermectin for the treatment of COVID-19 can be elucidated if the following basic considerations are taken into account:

- First, by now it is well-understood that the pathophysiology of COVID-19 is that it is a triphasic illness with three overlapping stages of (a) viral replication; (b) hyperinflammatory cytokine storm (COVID-19 pneumonia); (c) thrombosis, making it necessary to use multiple drugs in combination to effectively treat patients through this disease process.[62-66] Consequently, when evaluating the role of ivermectin in treating COVID-19, evidence for or against the use of ivermectin to treat one stage of the disease does not necessarily extrapolate to the same conclusion for the other two stages. Furthermore, given the complexity of the illness, it is not reasonable to anticipate that ivermectin monotherapy alone will yield satisfactory outcomes. Studies investigating the use of ivermectin in the treatment of COVID-19 should do so in the context of incorporating ivermectin in sequenced multidrug protocols.[67-71] Likewise, as was noted by Risch,[72] results on the efficacy and safety of any treatment from studies on outpatients do not extrapolate to inpatients and vice versa, and results from studies testing the efficacy of a medication as monotherapy do not extrapolate to multidrug protocols. Furthermore, results claiming lack of efficacy in a cohort of low-risk patients do not necessarily extrapolate to high-risk patients. Studies focusing on high-risk patients are advantageous because they tend to require smaller sample sizes to detect a positive efficacy signal if one is there.
- Second, the most relevant endpoints for the treatment of COVID-19 are the prevention of hospitalization and death. Negative or neutral results on soft and subjective endpoints, such as duration of disease or time to viral clearance, are not decisive considerations when dealing with a potentially lethal disease. A treatment protocol that may not reduce the duration of disease, or might even prolong it, would still be considered successful if it was shown to be effective in reducing both hospitalizations and deaths. Conversely, a treatment that may reduce the average duration or severity of the illness but has no effect or even increases hospitalizations and/or deaths would be considered unsuccessful.

- Finally, the practical question that is relevant to clinical practice is to decide whether or not particular multidrug treatment protocols that incorporate the use of ivermectin should be adopted, and ultimately, this is a yes or no question that is to be decided based on the strength of the evidence that evaluate the treatment protocols themselves as opposed to ivermectin monotherapy. The more theoretical academic question is to validate the biological mechanisms of action of ivermectin by providing convincing empirical arguments supporting the antiviral, anti-inflammatory, and anticoagulant mechanisms of action.

Interpreting the Literature

Kory et al.[73] reviewed 7 RCTs on outpatients and 6 RCTs plus 5 OCTs on inpatients, did a meta-analysis of the studies that included a mortality rate reduction endpoint and found that there is statistically significant efficacy for mortality rate reduction when these studies are combined together. The same paper also included a meta-analysis of several studies where ivermectin was used prophylactically and found a statistically significant decrease in the infection rate. The meta-analysis included the now-withdrawn Elgazzar study;[74] however, the results remain robust after removing Elgazzar from the calculation.[75] Another meta-analysis by Bryant et al.[48] confirmed the statistically significant reduction of all-cause mortality and conducted an exhaustive sensitivity analysis, showing the robustness of their conclusions. In both papers, studies of inpatients were mixed with studies of outpatients, and they should have been analyzed separately. Bryant et al.[48] considered that but observed that separating the outpatients from inpatient trials was not helpful because very few outpatient trials used mortality rate reduction as an endpoint. Consequently, the most reliable conclusion that we can draw from the Bryant et al.[48] meta-analysis is that mortality rate reduction has been shown specifically for inpatients when combining several available small studies, while it remains unclear whether the result also extends to outpatients. Several other meta-analyses of ivermectin also confirmed the existence of statistically significant mortality rate reduction efficacy.[76]

For outpatients, Procter's case series[67,68] of 869 high-risk patients, with 20 hospitalizations (2.3%) and two deaths (0.2%), who were treated through December 2020 with the combination of hydroxychloroquine, ivermectin, zinc, azithromycin or doxycycline, budesonide, foliate, thiamine, and IV fluids, is particularly compelling due to the large sample size and the high-risk status of the patients. Here, the definition of high-risk is: age ≥ 50, or comorbidities associated with high COVID-19 mortality rates, or presenting with shortness of breath. A reanalysis by Gkioulekas et al.[77] noted that during 2020, the expected mortality rate for high-risk COVID-19 patients with comorbidities or shortness of breath exceeded 5%, and the CDC estimate for the expected mortality rate for COVID-19 patients from the beginning of the pandemic through September 2021, with age ≥50 was at least 2.3%. Likewise, the probability of hospitalization for high-risk patients can be lower bounded by at least 10%.

Gkioulekas et al.[77] also introduced a new statistical technique in which the hospitalization and mortality rate lower bounds for untreated patients are compared against a corresponding 95% confidence efficacy threshold and a random selection bias threshold, calculated from the case series data. When the probability of an adverse outcome (death or hospitalization) without treatment exceeds the efficacy threshold, then the observed reduction in adverse outcomes with treatment is statistically significant with 95% confidence, and it is more likely than not that random selection bias cannot overturn this finding. When the higher random selection bias threshold is exceeded, we can have 95% confidence that random selection bias cannot overturn the finding of some statistically significant reduction in adverse outcomes with treatment. Specifically for the Procter case series, the random selection bias threshold for mortality rate reduction is 1.82%, and for hospitalization rate reduction, it is 5.2%.[77] Both are exceeded by the 2.3% mortality rate lower bound for high-risk patients and the 10% hospitalization rate lower bound for high-risk patients. Thus, there is clear and convincing evidence that the multidrug treatment protocol used by Procter,[67,68] which included the use of ivermectin and followed the principles of the McCullough protocol,[3] was effective both with respect to mortality and hospitalization rate reduction.

This leaves open the question of whether ivermectin itself is contributing in any way toward the effectiveness of outpatient multidrug protocols. As we shall explain in the following, evidence for the existence of an antiviral mechanism for ivermectin is available from the Itaji prophylaxis studies,[78,79] and evidence of benefit in hypoxic patients is available from several studies by Stone,[80] Hazan,[81] Babalola,[82-84] which implies potential benefit for both outpatients and inpatients. Additional evidence supporting the hypothesis that ivermectin contributes to both hospitalization and mortality rate reduction when used prophylactically or in treatments is given by the recently published ecological study of ivermectin use in Peru.[85]

The prospective observational prophylaxis study that was undertaken in Itajaí, Brazil[78] provides the strongest positive evidence that ivermectin has effective in vivo antiviral properties against COVID-19. The study involved a significant proportion of 159,561 out of the 223,128 citizens of Itajaí, so there is a low risk of confounding by selection bias. Between July 2020 and December 2020 the study tracked 113,845 ivermectin users who took 0.2 mg/kg of ivermectin 42 consecutive days every 15 days over a period of 150 days, and 45,716 nonusers of ivermectin, all during the same time period. From the ivermectin users, 4,311 (3.7%) were infected with 86 hospitalizations (2.0%) and 62 deaths (1.4%), and from the nonusers, 3,034 (6.6%) were infected with 99 hospitalizations (3.3%) and 79 deaths (2.6%). This corresponds to statistically significant infection risk reduction in the ivermectin users (RR 0.56; 95% CI 0.53–0.58; $p < 0.0001$). From the infected patients, without making any adjustments, both statistically significant mortality rate reduction (RR 0.55; 95% CI 0.40–0.77; $p = 0.0004$) and hospitalization rate reduction (RR 0.61; 95% CI 0.46–0.81; $p = 0.0007$) have been observed. There is a low risk of bias because the infected ivermectin users have a greater proportion of older high-risk patients than the non-users (30.3% infected ivermectin users older than 50% vs. 20.0% nonusers older than 50). Furthermore, the findings continue to hold after adjustment with propensity score matching, yielding 68% mortality rate reduction (RR 0.32; 95% CI 0.20–0.49; $p < 0.0001$) and 56% hospitalization rate reduction (RR 0.44; 95% CI 0.31– 0.63; $p < 0.0001$). Although the hospitalization and mortality rate reduction effect can be attributed to a combination of mechanisms of action, the effectiveness of the prophylactic use of ivermectin in reducing the probability of infection signals the existence of robust antiviral mechanisms by ivermectin against the SARS-CoV-2 virus itself.

A follow-up study[79] showed a stronger mortality rate reduction effect with the subgroup of ivermectin users who used the medication regularly instead of those who used it irregularly. Compared against nonusers, the mortality rate reduction for regular users of ivermectin was 92% (RR 0.08; 95% CI 0.02–0.35; $p = 0.0008$). Furthermore, among the regular users of ivermectin, the hospitalization rate was reduced 100%. The authors defined regular use as taking at least 180 mg over the study period of 150 days, and irregular use as taking less than 60 mg in total over the same time period. The dose-response effect provides additional evidence of the overall capability of ivermectin to prevent hospitalizations and death among infected COVID-19 patients when used prophylactically.

The results from the Itaji studies[78,79] confirm the findings of the SAIVE trial,[50] and are corroborated by a recently published study[85] on the state-level use of ivermectin in Peru and its effect on excess deaths, which were calculated from Peruvian national data for the age ≥60 population per each of the 25 states, where ivermectin was approved for both inpatient and outpatient treatment on May 8, 2020, until November 17, 2020, when the new president of Peru reintroduced restrictions on ivermectin use. A 14-fold reduction of excess deaths at the national level was observed after the deployment of ivermectin, which persisted until the reintroduction of restrictions on ivermectin use; at this point, a 13-fold increase in excess deaths was observed. More detailed analysis confirmed this pattern state by state, noting that there was variability in the extent and timing of the deployment of ivermectin from state to state, with the timing and magnitude of excess deaths being aligned with this state-by-state variability. Because the study was based on population-level data, there is negligible risk of selection bias, although there are other possibilities for confounding. The authors considered and ruled out possible confounding by state-by-state variability in age distribution, viral strains, compliance with social distancing recommendations, herd immunity, and population density. The authors also ruled out possible confounding by a theoretical cross-immunity with the dengue virus. One limitation of the study is that it is unclear to what extent the reduction in excess deaths can be attributed to prophylactic use of ivermectin or to use in outpatient or inpatient treatment of COVID-19 patients. Nevertheless, these results are sufficient for rejecting a null hypothesis of no benefit from ivermectin use for prophylaxis and treatment of COVID-19.

Separately from the antiviral mechanism of ivermectin, case series of severely hypoxic COVID-19 patients by Stone[80] and Hazan[81] have shown that ivermectin, when used in combination with other medications, can result in rapid recovery of SpO_2 levels, with a statistically significant normalization trend being observed within 24 hours. The Stone case series[80] consisted of 34 hypoxic COVID-19 patients presenting with room-air baseline $SpO_2 \leq 93\%$, of which 28 patients presented with $SpO_2 \leq 90\%$, who were treated between August 2020 and May 2021 in Harare, Zimbabwe, using the Siver Ivermectin Doxycycline (SID) protocol,[86] a 10-day treatment regimen with ivermectin, nanosilver, doxycycline, and zinc, and in particularly severe cases also corticosteroids and anticoagulants. The Hazan case series[81] consisted of 23 patients presenting with room-air baseline $SpO_2 \leq 90\%$, who were treated in the United States between August 2020 and February 2021 with a 10-day course of ivermectin, doxycycline, zinc, Vitamin C, and Vitamin D. The patients in the Hazan case series[81] enrolled in a clinical trial for outpatient COVID-19 treatment, but were excluded due to room-air baseline $SpO_2 \leq 90\%$ and advised to seek hospital care, but declined to be hospitalized for a variety of personal reasons, and were thus treated via telemedicine while quarantined at home. The patients in the Stone case series[80] were by necessity treated at home, via visiting nurses, or in an outpatient clinic setting due to the unavailability of hospital resources in Harare, Zimbabwe. With both case series, the outcome was zero hospitalizations and zero deaths, mediated by the rapid recovery of SpO_2 levels.

Out of 57 hypoxic patients in both case series combined, 51 patients initially presented with room-air baseline $SpO_2 \leq 90\%$, so the expected counterfactual hospitalization rate, in the absence of treatment and assuming the willingness of the patients to be hospitalized and the availability of hospital resources, should have been at least 51 out of 57. Obviously, all of these hospitalizations were successfully prevented with treatment, and the corresponding hospitalization rate reduction is statistically significant with $p = 10^{-25}$. Another case series of younger hypoxic COVID-19 patients by Babalola,[82-84] where ivermectin was used as a monotherapy over a period of 5 days, also showed a statistically significant rapid recovery in SpO_2 levels, however, the rate of recovery observed in the Hazan[81] and Stone[80] case series was more intense.

When considered together, these results show that the rapid recovery of SpO_2 levels can be attributed, in part, to ivermectin. However, using it synergistically, as part of a multidrug protocol, intensifies the effect. Because the drop in SpO_2 levels is a consequence of microscopic blood clots accumulating in the lungs, from the toxicity of the spike protein, ivermectin's anticoagulant mechanisms of action are the most likely explanation for the rapid increase in SpO_2 levels.[36,42,47] These results provide good reason to recommend the use of the SID multidrug protocol[86] for inpatients. They also point to another rationale for using ivermectin for the treatment of outpatients, separately from antiviral action; if ivermectin is capable of restoring SpO_2 levels in hypoxic patients when used in combination with nanosilver, doxycycline, and zinc, then it is a reasonable extrapolation that this combination of medications would also prevent the SpO_2 levels from dropping if given to COVID-19 patients before they develop hypoxia. Indeed, some of the empirical observations of mortality and hospitalization rate reduction for infected ivermectin users from the Itaji studies,[78,79] where ivermectin was used prophylactically, could be resulting not only from the antiviral action but also from this additional protective effect.

Trials Showing Ivermectin Failure to Treat COVID-19

Six randomized control trials published in high-impact journals have been cited as evidence against using ivermectin in treating COVID-19.[87-92] Four of these tested ivermectin monotherapy against a placebo,[89-92] so the results are irrelevant to the multidrug treatment protocols used by practicing doctors. From the remaining two studies, the COVID-OUT trial[87] is methodologically flawed because it compared a combination therapy of three consecutive days of ivermectin combined with a 14-day course of metformin against a mixed control group of patients that received only the 14-day course of metformin or a placebo. Because the trial did demonstrate some efficacy for metformin monotherapy, this comparison, as well as the underdosing of ivermectin in the study, biases the results toward the null hypothesis; therefore, a neutral result is inconclusive and cannot be reliably interpreted as evidence against the use of ivermectin.

The I-Tech study[88] is interesting because it recruited high-risk patients with age ≥50 and at least one comorbidity; the treatment group was treated with a realistic multidrug protocol combining ivermectin with corticosteroids, antibiotics, and anticoagulants with 1.2% mortality rate, the control group was treated only with corticosteroids, antibiotics, and anticoagulants, with 4.0% mortality rate. The authors claim that this was a negative result due to p-value $p = 0.09$ and also due to negative results in irrelevant soft endpoints other than hospitalization and death. Using the methodology by Gkioulekas et al.[77] on the treatment group of 241 patients with three deaths, the corresponding efficacy threshold is calculated at 3.7%. Furthermore, Gkioulekas et al.[77] noted that the expected mortality rate for untreated high-risk patients with comorbidities exceeds 5%, and even more so with the addition of the age ≥ 50 restrictions. Consequently, a comparison of the treatment group against the known historical control of untreated high-risk patients shows that it is more likely than not that there is a mortality rate reduction benefit when ivermectin is used as part of a multidrug protocol. The study allowed a 7-day window from the beginning of symptoms before initiating treatment; however, Fazio et al.[93] showed that the ideal window of opportunity for the outpatient treatment of COVID-19 is approximately 3 days from the beginning of symptoms. Thus, we can expect more robust results if the protocol used in the I-Tech study[88] is initiated within the 3-day window from the onset of symptoms.

With regards to the remaining RCTs, the Lopez-Medina[91] and ACTIV-6[89,90] trials have very low mortality rates in the control groups, so prima facie, on both arms of the trial, the patients are in the low-risk category; thus, a negative result with respect to mortality rate reduction cannot be justified by these studies. Likewise, because the treatment was monotherapy not initiated within the first three days from the onset of symptoms, these studies cannot be relied on to conclude the lack of hospitalization rate reduction benefit from early outpatient multidrug treatment protocols that incorporate the use of ivermectin. Finally, the TOGETHER trial[92] tested a 3-day ivermectin monotherapy against a placebo with negative results with respect to hospitalization and mortality rate reduction. Prima facie, the study shows that a 3-day ivermectin monotherapy where more than half of the patients initiated treatment at 4–7 days from onset of symptoms is insufficient, which can be attributed to underdosing, short duration of treatment, and given too late. More concerning is an asymmetric loss of patients in the control arm from intention-to-treat patients to per-protocol patients, compared to a negligible loss of patients in the treatment arm, indicating a possible loss of blinding. The study authors did not do a per-protocol analysis for hospitalization and mortality rate reduction and refused to release their data for independent per-protocol analysis.[94]

The totality of the evidence indicates that a combination of chemoprophylaxis using ivermectin, along with the use of multidrug protocols that incorporate the use of ivermectin, could have reduced both hospitalizations and deaths by at least one order of magnitude. The empirical evidence supports the use of ivermectin-based protocols in both outpatients and inpatients and points to the importance of initiating early outpatient treatment as soon as possible, and ideally within the first three days from the onset of symptoms. The TOGETHER trial[92] raises doubt about the efficacy of ivermectin monotherapy when given over a short 3-day period and with significant delays. Still, their findings cannot be considered settled without a per-protocol analysis of hospitalization and mortality rate reduction. They do not extrapolate to prophylactic use or to use in multidrug outpatient and inpatient treatment protocols.

Controversy Surrounding Ivermectin's Use

In spite of the available and accumulating positive evidence supporting the use of ivermectin in the treatment of COVID-19, especially in the context of prophylactic use as well as use in multidrug treatment protocols, the WHO has been cited in calls to use regulatory agencies to restrict doctors from using this medication in accordance with their better judgment.[95] Practicing physicians involved in the development of multidrug treatment protocols have faced increased levels of censorship and professional consequences. These developments may indicate a broader trend where public health measures are being leveraged to establish political authority on an international scale.

In the US, the FDA issued a statement titled, "Why You Should Not Use Ivermectin to Treat or Prevent COVID-19,"[96] and subsequently disseminated correspondence to both the Federation of State Medical Boards and the National Association of Boards of Pharmacy, urging their attention to the document's contents.

In addition to formal channels, the FDA leveraged social media platforms using the PR company Weber Shandwick, the same PR company used by Moderna, to disseminate succinct messages such as, "Ivermectin is Intended for Equine Parasitic Infections, Not COVID-19," and "Humans Are Not Livestock: The Dangers of Using Veterinary Products for Human Medical Conditions." These messages were accompanied by juxtaposing imagery of a veterinary professional embracing an equine patient and a medical doctor conducting a human patient examination. Social media platforms have international reach, particularly throughout the English-speaking world. Regulatory authorities in smaller countries mimicked the FDA in their refusal to entertain the use of ivermectin in COVID-19 treatment regimens based on the parroted call that there was "insufficient evidence". Regulatory authorities hid behind their stubborn requirement for a large randomised control trial to show efficacy. We have already pointed out above that those RCTs that were considered adequately designed were flawed.

Merck put out a statement on February 4 2021, stating that they did not believe the data available provided sufficient therapeutic and efficacy data, but alarmingly they stated there was a concerning lack of safety data in the majority of studies. The Guzzo study of 2002 had already shown the data on dosage safety levels, the WHO VigiAccess database had shown its safety, the majority of papers that were published on the use of ivermectin in COVID-19 all stated that there were few or no adverse responses and those that existed were mild and transient. This after Professor Ōmura showed enthusiasm to carry out a large randomised control trial in Japan, which they denied. Merck's response to using ivermectin for COVID-19 is anathema unless one cynically considers that they would rather have backed a product that ivermectin was in opposition to, molnupiravir perhaps? The patent to ivermectin expired years ago, and molnupiravir is a new drug. It does not take deep thinking to see which drug could be more profitable for Merck.

Misinformation and Disinformation

In looking at regulatory oversight, it is clear that many regulatory bodies discounted the potential utility of ivermectin, ostensibly due to concerns regarding the quality of supporting studies. These bodies appear to align their stances closely with guidance from globally recognized entities such as the Food and Drug Administration (FDA) and the WHO. Nevertheless, the FDA has rejected claims suggesting its influence over other regulatory institutions. This rejection came in the form of a legal brief filed by three clinicians challenging the FDA's position on ivermectin. In the document, the FDA disavowed any role in directing clinicians' off-label prescribing practices and refuted claims that it swayed other independent regulatory authorities. Additionally, the FDA contended that its social media communications were intended for informal public engagement rather than as definitive guidance.

As of August 8, 2023, the authority for physicians to prescribe ivermectin off-label has been reinstated. This development raises questions about the FDA's earlier communications, suggesting that they may have been a source of inaccurate information regarding off-label prescribing rights for ivermectin. When authoritative bodies disseminate misleading or false information, they risk undermining public trust and could potentially pose societal risks.

POTENTIAL APPLICATIONS

Since it has been shown that ivermectin has multiple mechanisms of action, it is no wonder that it has potential uses beyond being an anti-parasitic and used off-label during the COVID-19 pandemic. Ivermectin is approved as an anti-parasitic for the treatment of:

- Strongyloidiasis of the intestinal tract is due to the nematode parasite Strongyloides stercoralis and is contracted through the skin. Other organs in the body may also be affected.
- Onchocerciasis, commonly known as river blindness, is caused by the parasitic worm Onchocerca volvulus.
- Rosacea is a chronic inflammatory disorder that affects the face, and although not life-threatening, it does have a phycological effect on patients. IVERMECTIN is approved as a 1% cream used as an anti-inflammatory applied to the skin once a day.

In recent years, ivermectin has been or will be accessed in several clinical trials **(Table 1)** for various indications.

Implications for Global Health

So, here's the problem: Ivermectin is a 40-year-old anti-parasitic, off-patent medication with a long track record of being safe. Several clinical studies and real-world experience have confirmed that it is effective against several viruses. Therefore, ivermectin should also be considered for other viral infections, particularly those in which a vaccine would be useless once the infection takes hold. The following is an ideal example because this virus adversely affects the immune system.

Potential Application for Treating Patients with Ebola Hemorrhagic Fever (Ebola Virus Disease)

We do not know when or what the next pandemic will be. However, while researching for this particular section of the book, we came across another indication that, to our knowledge, has not been considered but is nonetheless important. That is the potential for ivermectin to treat people infected with the Ebola virus. Should the Ebola virus become airborne while retaining its pathogenic properties, it would make the SARS-CoV-2 pandemic seem like "a walk in the park". Ebola is a filovirus that causes hemorrhagic fever in 30–50% of cases. With the severe form of the disease, multiorgan failure occurs, and blood vessels leak their contents into the surrounding tissues. The mortality rate can be as high as 90%. A cytokine storm initiated by an excessive increase of proinflammatory cytokines and chemokines is a key feature of the disease via the activation of T-cell lymphocytes, but not before disabling the patient's innate immune system by targeting macrophages and dendritic cells.[97-99]

Before ivermectin, there was suramin, a drug dating back 100 years, used to treat river blindness and antiparasitic infections. Suramin, like ivermectin, also has antiviral and a lot more indications. It was considered that suramin had too many targets, resulting in serious adverse side effects. Therefore, suramin was replaced with ivermectin, which is safer and could be given orally. Suramin has effectively prevented the Ebola virus from entering cells and replicating in vitro.[99-101]

We already know from previous sections of this chapter that ivermectin is effective against the SARS-CoV-2 virus, which is also an RNA virus. Unlike suramin, which is highly toxic, ivermectin can be administered safely at higher dosages and is, therefore, potentially more effective than suramin, assuming that both drugs have the same mode of action for Ebola. When normal cells are damaged, they express phosphatidylserine (PS), a phospholipid on their surface, activating the innate immune system to produce proinflammatory cytokines, the normal physiological response for removing damaged or dead cells. The Ebola virus expresses PS on its surface, mimicking a damaged cell, causing a cytokine storm and disseminated intravascular coagulation.[102] The Ebola virus can also initiate a cytokine storm via TLR4 and other mechanisms similar to those of COVID-19.[98] However, the most devastating action of the virus is its ability to inactivate the immune response to the Ebola virus itself.[102] Therefore, a vaccine would be ineffective once an outbreak takes place.

From our experience with COVID-19, ivermectin would be a useful candidate to use off-label to treat patients infected with the Ebola virus and prophylactically in the geographical areas affected because of its apparent similarities to suramin. That being the case, ivermectin would be used to treat the patient during the replication and hyper-inflammation phases of the disease, as would be the case with COVID-19.[34,35,37,39,40] Any treatment should be in combination with nano-silver to prevent PS and glycoproteins on the surface of the virus from adversely modulating the immune system.[103,104]

CONCLUSION

In today's society, where information is available from many sources of varying reliability, from social media to independent or controlled press media, there is a predilection for superficial interpretations and quick categorizations of information, often favoring straightforward solutions to complex questions. There is a tendency to rely on authoritative figures and celebrities for pre-packaged opinions rather than engaging in independent, critical thinking. To genuinely understand complex issues, it is imperative to adopt an evolving thought process characterized by curiosity and critical evaluation.

Unfortunately, society generally encourages swift judgment and discourages inquisitive exploration, which fosters a climate of intellectual complacency. This inclination toward immediate, emotionally gratifying conclusions obfuscates the value of objective thought that necessitates more rigorous thinking. The act of thinking, particularly when it challenges pre-existing beliefs or the status quo, can be both cognitively demanding and emotionally uncomfortable, particularly for individuals accustomed to outsourcing their work of thinking to external authorities. It is, therefore, easy to manipulate people through controlling social media, the press, and embargoes on academic publication.

The COVID-19 pandemic provided a maelstrom of alternatives and extremes of thought. Conspiracy theories soon emerged, and with that, an almost binary approach to thinking about every measure taken to curb the disease. There were arguments about lockdowns working or not working, masks preventing disease transmission or indeed causing pneumonia, vaccines saving lives or vaccines killing numbers of people, and ivermectin working or not working. Social media and censorship tried to control the narrative, but not in an effort to balance debate. It had the effect of deepening the divide between extreme arguments. In retrospect, we will be able to see how, in certain circumstances, lockdowns were necessary but in others damaging. Vaccines certainly do have serious adverse events, and it is our duty to understand how and why they occurred, not to dismiss vaccines as ineffective or dismiss the adverse events as irrelevant. We have shown in this chapter that there was research indicating that ivermectin was effective in treating COVID-19. We need to critically reflect on why, in 2023, a Google search or a ChatGPT question will always shine a negative light on ivermectin as a potential therapeutic for COVID-19.

What We Knew in 2020 that would have Allowed a Type 1 Error Decision to Use Ivermectin?

In 2019, ivermectin's primary recognized use was as an antiparasitic drug, particularly for treating various parasitic infections in humans and animals. The drug's efficacy and safety in treating parasitic infections were well established and had been widely used for decades. However, as an antiviral agent, knowledge about ivermectin's efficacy and safety in 2019 was limited. While some studies had suggested potential antiviral effects of ivermectin against certain viruses, including some RNA viruses, the evidence was based mainly on in vitro (laboratory-based) experiments or studies in animal models. In cell culture experiments, the antiviral activity of ivermectin was mainly observed against viruses like dengue, Zika, and other flaviviruses. In these studies, ivermectin inhibited viral replication in a laboratory setting. However, translating these findings from in vitro studies to effective antiviral therapy in humans is a complex process that requires further investigation.

By 2019, few clinical trials evaluated ivermectin's potential as an antiviral in humans. Most of the available data were preclinical or based on observational studies, meaning that the drug's antiviral properties had not been thoroughly established in humans then.

It is important to emphasize that scientific knowledge evolves, and research on drugs like ivermectin continues progressing. Since 2019, there may have been new studies and clinical trials investigating the antiviral potential of ivermectin, especially in the context of the COVID-19 pandemic. It is best to consult reputable sources and medical literature to obtain the most recent information.

By the pandemic's start, ivermectin dosages for its approved anti-parasitic uses were well-established and widely known. The drug had been used for decades to treat various parasitic infections in humans and animals, and its dosing guidelines were well documented. For treating onchocerciasis (river blindness) and lymphatic filariasis, the standard oral dose of ivermectin was 150–200 μg/kg of body weight. This dose was typically administered as a single dose and repeated annually or as per the specific treatment program in regions where these diseases were prevalent. For other parasitic infections like scabies and head lice, topical formulations of ivermectin were available, and the dosages varied based on the product's concentration and the individual's age and weight.

It is important to note that the dosages for approved anti-parasitic uses were well established through extensive clinical trials and research. However, the dosing and safety profile might differ when considering using ivermectin for potential off-label purposes or as an antiviral agent. In such cases, consulting with a qualified healthcare professional who can provide appropriate guidance and monitor for potential side effects or interactions is essential.

Propaganda Against Ivermectin and the Trusted News Initiative

There have been discussions and controversies surrounding the use of ivermectin for various medical purposes, including its potential use as a treatment for COVID-19. Some of these discussions have involved accusations of misinformation, biased reporting, or propaganda on both sides. Some medical professionals, researchers, and advocates have expressed support for using ivermectin as a potential treatment for COVID-19 based on their experience and analysis of emerging literature.

Major health organizations, including the WHO, the US Food and Drug Administration (FDA), and the European Medicines Agency (EMA), have not approved ivermectin for the treatment of COVID-19. These organizations have emphasized that the available data on ivermectin's efficacy and safety as a COVID-19 treatment are insufficient and inconclusive, ignoring the totality of the evidence. They have actively warned against its use outside of approved indications or clinical trials and have highlighted potential risks associated with self-medication or inappropriate dosing. Their stance led to the off-label use of ivermectin, while legal and within the purview of a qualified doctor, being criminalized, with some doctors losing their right to practice medicine after prescribing ivermectin off-label.

In the context of COVID-19, there have been continued efforts to discredit or dismiss ivermectin and instances of misinformation and propaganda surrounding ivermectin. Several systematic reviews and meta-analyses have attempted to assess the existing evidence on ivermectin's role in COVID-19 treatment. It is essential to be critical of information from all sources. It became apparent during the pandemic that one should not rely on health regulators and every piece of scientific literature without critical thought for reliable and evidence-based information.

The Trusted News Initiative (TNI) is a partnership founded by the BBC that includes news agencies and organizations from around the globe, including Google, YouTube, Meta, Microsoft, and Twitter. TNI members work together to build audience trust and to find solutions to tackle the challenges of disinformation. However, the question remains: Who decides what is disinformation or misinformation? They have endeavored to control a global narrative by including media organizations and social media platforms. The TNI prides itself on being "...the only forum in the world of its kind designed to take on disinformation in real-time." There is a very fine line between controlling a narrative that may be false and removing journalistic freedom. Many YouTube videos covering peer-reviewed published papers were removed from the platform, and their channel owners were punished. Twitter removed tweets and tweeters from their platform if any positive scientific information on ivermectin in COVID-19 treatment was shared. The popular press would carry no story about ivermectin unless it were negative. The TNI made a central decision that any information on the efficacy of ivermectin in treating COVID-19 was mis or disinformation, and all members across the globe acted to remove ivermectin from any story. Who was the first person or group to decide to make ivermectin efficacy news mis or disinformation, regardless of the research? That is a question we may never find the answer to. There have been some of the more cynical who would say that the pharmaceutical industry influenced this decision because no vaccine could be used without the regular pre-launch research if an already existing therapeutic was available.[105]

Role of Medical Doctors in Scientific Discovery

The development of medical science must follow the scientific method, the core principle of which is that the sole judge of scientific truth is experiment, and more broadly the accumulated available empirical evidence, not the WHO, not the FDA, not the EMA, not the TNI, not the medical boards, not the news agencies, not social media companies, not governments. New fundamental discoveries often begin from a single practicing doctor formulating a hypothesis based on direct empirical observations from his efforts to save patients, combined with experience, inspiration, and insight. Article 37 of the 2013 Helsinki Declaration[106,107] codifies the ethics of the role of medical doctors in scientific discovery by stating that: *"In the treatment of an individual patient, where proven interventions do not exist or other known interventions have been ineffective, the physician, after seeking expert advice, with informed consent from the patient or a legally authorised representative, may use an unproven intervention if in the physician's judgement it offers hope of saving life, re-establishing health or alleviating suffering. This intervention should subsequently be made the object of research, designed to evaluate its safety and efficacy. In all cases, new information must be recorded and, where appropriate, made publicly available."*

New discoveries that begin with the sole practicing doctor are then investigated, developed, and published by academic scientists, and then public health agencies such as the WHO, FDA, CDC, and others periodically evaluate and conduct systematic reviews of the resulting research literature and news agencies may report the most impactful results to the general public. With scientific knowledge flowing from the practicing doctor to academics and then to the large public health agencies, it is a logical fallacy of circular reasoning for the public health agencies to accuse the practicing doctor or the academic researcher of disseminating misinformation when the latter brings forth new scientific findings that are backed by the empirical evidence that conflict with the currently accepted consensus promulgated by the agencies. Just as it is unscientific for medical boards to give higher weight to the current scientific consensus or to the opinions of public health organizations when reviewing doctors whose diverging practices are backed by the empirical outcomes of their efforts. If doctors and academic researchers are not allowed to explore, communicate, and discover, under the ethical conditions of article 37 of the 2013 Helsinki Declaration, then the scientific method of discovery itself is disrupted, at the cost of increased suffering, hospitalization, and death.

Ethics of the Dismissal of the Use of Ivermectin by Authorities

Ethical considerations are vital in ensuring that healthcare decisions consider the population's well-being. Denying a population access to a drug that could work against a disease can raise several ethical concerns, particularly in a public health crisis or when dealing with life-threatening conditions. Access to potentially life-saving treatments is considered a fundamental human right. Denying a population access to a drug that might be effective against a disease can be seen as a violation of this right, especially if limited or no alternative treatments are available. The ethical principles of beneficence (acting in the best interest of patients) and nonmaleficence (doing no harm) guide medical decision-making. If evidence suggests that a drug could be beneficial and safe, withholding it from those who may benefit could be seen as failing to uphold these principles. Ethical considerations of fairness and distributive justice come into play when deciding who gets access to potentially life-saving treatments. If individuals are aware of a drug's potential benefits and risks and are willing to take it, they should be allowed to make informed decisions about their healthcare. Denying access to a drug might limit their autonomy and right to make choices about their health.

In some cases, the denial of a drug could be justified due to a lack of robust evidence supporting an appropriate balance of safety and efficacy or due to credible evidence signaling the existence of unacceptable safety concerns. Ethical considerations involve ensuring that treatments are based on sound scientific research and that decisions are not influenced by vested interests or misinformation. In infectious diseases, denying access to a potentially effective drug could have broader public health implications. Limiting the spread of the disease and protecting vulnerable populations are critical considerations in deciding drug access. Healthcare professionals have an ethical duty to provide the best available care to their patients. If a drug is available and supported by *credible* evidence, healthcare providers may face ethical challenges in withholding it from their patients.

In the context of ivermectin in the COVID-19 pandemic, we can see that these ethics were scarce in those who actively denigrated the drug. By denying the use of the drug, people died. Their human right to make a decision on whether to take it or not was removed before they could make an informed decision. The safety data was there, and there was credible evidence at *in silico,* in vitro, in vivo, and clinical levels. The decision to make a Type II error decision shows a lack of beneficence (describes the error that occurs when one fails to reject a null hypothesis that is actually false a false negative in essence an error of omission).

Future Prospects for Ivermectin

In his Nobel acceptance speech, Professor Ōmura referred to ivermectin as a gift from the earth. History has shown this to be true. It is not only a gift to Merck to make money for the period of a patent or a gift from them to those who need it but who cannot afford it. It is a valuable medicine for the future, and we need to invest in further research into its efficacy across many pathologies. The problem is the patent no longer protects anybody's financial investment into research. An International Research Institute for Ivermectin would not be feasible as a self-funded entity. It would need to be funded from humanitarian sources, and the research products would have to be made freely available to all. As we enter the age of artificial intelligence, we will likely be able to carry out many *in-silico* experiments to find new mechanisms of action for ivermectin across all living creatures. Ivermectin could have saved many lives during the pandemic; it could have reduced the time it took for the pandemic to burn itself out. What else could it do for us in the future?

Final Thoughts and Recommendations

It is becoming increasingly clear that ivermectin is a safe and highly versatile agent with a wide variety of pharmacological targets. It has multiple modes of action, including (but not restricted to) anti-viral, anti-inflammatory, anti-thrombosis, and cardioprotective, which may act together to elicit synergistic therapeutic effects, thereby providing significant benefits to those who use it at sufficient dosage at any stage of the disease.

From research published in peer-reviewed journals, it is becoming increasingly clear that ivermectin could have saved many lives, reduced morbidity, and prevented infection during the pandemic. Who decided to prevent this information from reaching the general public? Who decided to introduce a disparaging narrative against the drug to misdirect the attention from ivermectin? There will never be a clear answer to these questions, but what is clear is that beneficence was rejected, and opportunists from industrial and political arenas made enormous financial gains.

An extended period of reflection is required for those of us who can think independently. We need to unite and plan ways to help others to think for themselves. To develop critical thinking skills. We do not want to convert people from one way of thinking to another; we want them to be genuinely able to seek reliable information and make informed decisions. We need to move away from polarized thinking that becomes binary thinking, which is not helpful. We need to find a way to protect independent journalism. While the TNI may have had noble intentions initially, their control of the narrative became an attack on freedom of information. In essence, we need to protect true democracy.

REFERENCES

1. Van Voorhis WC, Hooft van Huijsduijnen R, Wells TN. Profile of William C. Campbell, Satoshi Ōmura, and Youyou Tu, 2015 Nobel Laureates in Physiology or Medicine. Proc Natl Acad Sci U S A. 2015;112(52):15773-6.
2. Ōmura S. A splendid gift from the earth: The origins and impact of the avermectins (Nobel Lecture). Angew Chem Int Ed Engl. 2016;55(35):10190-209.
3. Crump A, Ōmura S. Ivermectin, 'Wonder drug' from Japan: the human use perspective. Proc Jpn Acad Ser B Phys Biol Sci. 2011;87(2):13-28.
4. World Health Organization. (2023). Lymphatic filariasis. [online] Available from https://www.who.int/news-room/fact-sheets/detail/lymphatic-filariasis. [Last accessed February, 2024].
5. Thylefors B. The Mectizan Donation Program (MDP). Ann Trop Med Parasitol. 2008;102 Suppl 1:39-44.
6. Bernigaud C, Guillemot D, Ahmed-Belkacem A, Grimaldi-Bensouda L, Lespine A, Berry F, et al. Oral ivermectin for a scabies outbreak in a long-term care facility: potential value in preventing COVID-19 and associated mortality. Br J Dermatol. 2021;184(6): 1207-9.
7. Crump A. Ivermectin: enigmatic multifaceted 'wonder' drug continues to surprise and exceed expectations. J Antibiot (Tokyo). 2017;70(5):495-505.
8. Moreno Y, Nabhan JF, Solomon J, Mackenzie CD, Geary TG. Ivermectin disrupts the function of the excretory-secretory apparatus in microfilariae of Brugiamalayi. Proc Natl Acad Sci U S A. 2010;107(46):20120-5.
9. Wagstaff KM, Sivakumaran H, Heaton S, Harrich DJ, Jans DA. Ivermectinis a specific inhibitor of importin a/b-mediated nuclear importable to inhibit replication of HIV-1and dengue virus. Biochem J. 2012;433:851-6.
10. Tay MY, Fraser JE, Chan WK, Moreland NJ, Rathore AP, Wang C, et al. Nuclear localization of dengue virus (DENV) 1-4 non-structural protein 5; protection against all 4DENV serotypes by the inhibitor Ivermectin. Antivir Res. 2013;99(3):301-6.
11. Atkinson S, Audsley M, Lieu K, Marsh G, Thomas DR, Heaton S, et al. Recognition by host nuclear transport proteins drives disorder-to-order transition in Hendra virus. V Sci Rep. 2018;8:23.
12. Lundberg L, Pinkhan C, Baer A, Amaya M, Narayan A, Wagstaff KM, et al. Nuclear import and export inhibitors alter capsid protein distribution in mammalian cells and reduce Venezuelan Equine Encephalitis Virus replication. Antiviral Res. 2013;100(3): 662-72.
13. Thomas DR, Lundberg L, Pinkham C, Shechter S, DeBono A, Baell J, et al. Identification of novel antivirals inhibiting recognition of Venezuelanequine encephalitis virus capsid protein by the Importin a/b1 hetero dimer through high-throughput screening. Antiviral Res. 2018;151:8-19.
14. Lv C, Liu W, Wang B, Dang R, Qiu L, Ren J, et al. Ivermectin inhibits DNA polymerase UL42 of pseudo rabies virus entrance into the nucleus and proliferation of the virus in-vitro and vivo. Antiviral Res. 2018;159:55-62.
15. Lim LE, Vilchèze C, Ng C, Jacobs WR Jr, Ramón-García S, Thompson CJ. Anthelmintic avermectins kill mycobacterium tuberculosis, including multidrug-resistant clinical strains. Antimicrob Agents Chemother. 2013;57(2):1040-6.
16. Yan S, Ci X, Chen N, Chen C, Li X, Chu X, et al. Anti-inflammatory effects of ivermectin in mouse model of allergic asthma. Inflamm Res. 2011;60(6):589-96.
17. Siddiqui K, Stein Gold L, Gill J. The efficacy, safety, and tolerability of ivermectin compared with current topical treatments for the inflammatory lesions of rosacea: a network meta-analysis. Springerplus. 2016;5(1):1151.

18. Hashimoto H, Sudo T, Maruta H, Nishimura R. The direct PAK1 inhibitor, TAT-PAK18, blocks preferentially the growth of human ovarian cancer cell lines in which PAK1 is abnormally activated by autophosphorylation at Thr 423. Drug Discov Ther. 2010;4(1): 1-4.
19. S Sharmeen S, Skrtic M, Sukhai MA, Hurren R, Gronda M, Wang X, et al. The antiparasitic agent ivermectin induces chloride-dependent membrane hyperpolarization and cell death in leukemia cells. Blood. 2010;116(18):3593-603.
20. Franklin KM, Asatryan L, Jakowec MW, Trudell JR, Bell RL, Davies DL. P2X4 receptors (P2X4Rs) represent a novel target for the development of drugs to prevent and/or treat alcohol use disorders. Front Neurosci. 2014;8:176.
21. Andries M, Van Damme P, Robberecht W, Van Den Bosch L. Ivermectin inhibits AMPA receptor-mediated excitotoxicity in cultured motor neurons and extends the life span of a transgenic mouse model of amyotrophic lateral sclerosis. Neurobiol Dis. 2007;25(1):8-16.
22. Lynagh T, Lynch JW. Ivermectin binding sites in human and invertebrate Cys-loop receptors. Trends Pharmacol Sci. 2012;33(8):432-41.
23. Estrada-Mondragon A, Lynch JW. Functional characterization of ivermectin binding sites in α1β2γ2L GABA(A) receptors. Front Mol Neurosci. 2015;8:55.
24. Laing R, Gillan V, Devaney E. Ivermectin - Old Drug, New Tricks? Trends Parasitol. 2017;33(6):463-72.
25. Heidary F, Gharebaghi R. Ivermectin: a systematic review from antiviral effects to COVID-19 complementary regimen. J Antibiot. 2020;73:593-602.
26. Chen L, Bi S, Wei Q, Zhao Z, Wang C, Xie S. Ivermectin suppresses tumour growth and metastasis through degradation of PAK1 in oesophageal squamous cell carcinoma. J Cell Mol Med. 2020;24(9):5387-401.
27. Chaccour C, Barrio ÁI, Royo AG, Urbistondo DM, Slater H, Hammann F, et al. Screening for an ivermectin slow-release formulation suitable for malaria vector control. Malar J. 2015;14(1):1-9.
28. Mastrangelo E, Pezzullo M, De Burghgraeve T, Kaptein S, Pastorino B, Dallmeier K, et al. Ivermectin is a potent inhibitor of flavivirus replication specifically targeting NS3 helicase activity: new prospects for an old drug. J Antimicrob Chemother. 2012;67(8):1884-94.
29. Rabinovich NR. Ivermectin: repurposing an old drug to complement malaria vector control. Lancet Infect Dis. 2018;18(6):584-585.
30. Caly L, Druce JD, Catton MG, Jans DA, Wagstaff KM. The FDA-approved drug ivermectin inhibits the replication of SARS-CoV-2 in-vitro. Antiviral Res. 2020;178: 104787.
31. Jans DA, Wagstaff KM. The broad spectrum host-directed agent ivermectin as an antiviral for SARS-CoV-2? Biochem Biophys Res Commun. 2021;538:163-172.
32. Zaidi AK, Dehgani-Mobaraki P. The mechanisms of action of ivermectin against SARS-CoV-2—an extensive review. J Antibiot. 2022;75:60-71.
33. Lehrer S, Rheinstein PH. Ivermectin Docks to the SARS-CoV-2 Spike Receptor-binding Domain Attached to ACE2. In Vivo. 2020;34(5):3023-6.
34. Eweas AF, Alhossary AA, Abdel-Moneim AS. Molecular Docking Reveals Ivermectin and Remdesivir as Potential Repurposed Drugs Against SARS-CoV-2. Front Microbiol. 2021;11:592908.
35. Swargiary A. (2020). Ivermectin as a promising RNA-dependent RNA polymerase inhibitor and a therapeutic drug against SARS-CoV2: Evidence from in silico studies. [online] Available from https://assets.researchsquare.com/files/rs-73308/v1/33ee098a-6891-4ab0-b93f-3d0a158fbc7b.pdf?c=1637243412. [Last accessed February, 2024].

36. Boschi C, Scheim DE, Bancod A, Militello M, Bideau ML, Colson P, et al. SARS-CoV-2 Spike Protein Induces Hemagglutination: Implications for COVID-19 Morbidities and Therapeutics and for Vaccine Adverse Effects. Int J Mol Sci. 2022;23(24):15480.
37. Lam LKM, Reilly JP, Rux AH, Murphy SJ, Kuri-Cervantes L, Weisman AR, et al. Erythrocytes identify complement activation in patients with COVID-19. Am J Physiol Lung Cell Mol Physiol. 2021;321:L485-9.
38. Zhang S, Liu Y, Wang X, Yang L, Li H, Wang Y, et al. SARS-CoV-2 binds platelet ACE2 to enhance thrombosis in COVID-19. J Hematol Oncol. 2020;13:1-22.
39. Zhang X, Song Y, Ci X, An N, Li H, Wang X, et al. Ivermectin inhibits LPS-induced production of inflammatory cytokines and improves LPS-induced survival in mice. Inflamm Res. 2008;57:524-9.
40. Jiang L, Wang P, Sun YJ, Wu YJ. Ivermectin reverses the drug resistance in cancer cells through EGFR/ERK/Akt/NF-κB pathway. J Exp Clin Cancer Res. 2019;38(1):265.
41. Matsuyama T, Kubli SP, Yoshinaga SK, Pfeffer K, Mak TW. An aberrant STAT pathway is central to COVID-19. Cell Death Differ. 2020;27(12):3209-25.
42. Scheim DE. A Deadly Embrace: Hemagglutination Mediated by SARS-CoV-2 Spike Protein at its 22 N-Glycosylation Sites, Red Blood Cell Surface Sialoglycoproteins, and Antibody. Int J Mol Sci. 2022;23:2558.
43. Favaron E, Ince C, Hilty MP, Ergin B, van der Zee P, Uz Z, et al. Capillary Leukocytes, Microaggregates, and the Response to Hypoxemia in the Microcirculation of Coronavirus Disease 2019 Patients. Crit Care Med. 2021;49:661-670.
44. Koutsiaris AG, Riri K, Boutlas S, Panagiotou TN, Kotoula M, Daniil Z, et al. COVID-19 hemodynamic and thrombotic effect on the eye microcirculation after hospitalization: A quantitative case-control study. Clin Hemorheol Microcirc. 2022;82(4):379-90.
45. Bicher HI. Blood Cell Aggregation in Thrombotic Processes. Springfield, IL: C. C. Thomas; 1972. p. 216.
46. Yonker LM, Swank Z, Bartsch YC, Burns MD, Kane A, Boribong BP, et al. Circulating Spike Protein Detected in Post-COVID-19 mRNA Vaccine Myocarditis. Circulation. 2023;147(11):867-76.
47. Aminpour M, Cannariato M, Safaeeardebili ME, Preto J, Moracchiato A, Doria D, et al. In Silico Analysis of the Multi-Targeted Mode of Action of Ivermectin and Related Compounds. Computation. 2022;10:51.
48. Bryant A, Lawrie TA, Dowswell T, Fordham EJ, Mitchell S, Hill SR, et al. Ivermectin for prevention and treatment of COVID-19 infection: a systematic review, meta-analysis, and trial sequential analysis to inform clinical guidelines. Am J Therap. 2021;28(4): e434.
49. Popp M, Stegemann M, Metzendorf M-I, Gould S, Kranke P, Meybohm P, et al. Ivermectin for preventing and treating covid-19. Cochrane Database Syst Rev. 2021;(7): CD015017.
50. Desort-Henin V, Kostova A, Babiker EA, Caramel A, Malamut R. (2023). "The SAIVE Trial, Post-Exposure use of ivermectin in Covid-19 prevention: Efficacy and Safety Results. [online] Available from https://www.medincell.com/wp-content/uploads/2023/04/Poster-SAIVE-April2023-OK3.pdf. [Last accessed February, 2024].
51. Nicolas P, Maia MF, Bassat Q, Kobylinski KC, Monteiro W, Rabinovich NR, et al. Safety of oral ivermectin during pregnancy: a systematic review and meta-analysis. Lancet Glob Health. 2020;8(1):e92-e100.
52. Lawrence J, Sodahlon YK, Ogoussan KT, Hopkins AD. Growth, Challenges, and Solutions over 25 Years of Mectizan and the Impact on Onchocerciasis Control. PLoS Negl Trop Dis. 2015;9(5):e0003507.
53. Guzzo CA, Furtek CI, Porras AG, Chen C, Tipping R, Clineschmidt CM, et al. Safety, tolerability, and pharmacokinetics of escalating high doses of ivermectin in healthy adult subjects. J Clin Pharmacol. 2002;42(10):1122-33.

54. Krolewiecki A, Lifschitz A, Moragas M, Travacio M, Valentini R, Alonso DF, et al. (2020). Antiviral effect of high-dose ivermectin in adults with COVID-19: a pilot randomised, controlled, open label, multicentre trial. [online] Available from https://papers.ssrn.com/sol3/papers.cfm?abstract_id=3714649. [Last accessed February, 2024].
55. Centers for Disease Control and Prevention (CDC). Prescription medication for the treatment of scabies. [online] Available from http://www.cdc.gov/parasites/scabies/health_professionals/meds.html. [Last accessed February, 2024].
56. Badhan R, Zakaria Z, Olafuyi O. The Repurposing of Ivermectin for Malaria: A Prospective Pharmacokinetics-Based Virtual Clinical Trials Assessment of Dosing Regimen Options. J Pharm Sci. 2018;107(8):2236-50.
57. Awadzi K, Opoku NO, Addy ET, et al. The chemotherapy of onchocerciasis. XIX: The clinical and laboratory tolerance of high dose ivermectin. Trop Med Parasitol. 1995;46(2):131-7.
58. Costa JL, Diazgranados JA. Ivermectin for spasticity in spinal-cord injury. Lancet. 1994;343(8899):739.
59. Navarro M, Camprubí D, Requena-Méndez A, Buonfrate D, Giorli G, Kamgno J, et al. Safety of high-dose ivermectin: a systematic review and meta-analysis. J Antimicrob Chemother. 2020;75(4):827-34.
60. Alexander ND, Bockarie MJ, Kastens WA, Kazura JW, Alpers MP. Absence of ivermectin-associated excess deaths. Trans R Soc Trop Med Hyg. 1998;92(3):342.
61. del Giudice P, Marty P, Gari-Toussaint M, Le Fichoux Y. Ivermectin in elderly patients. Arch Dermatol. 1999;135(3):351-2.
62. McCullough PA, Kelly RJ, Ruocco G, Lerma E, Tumlin J, Wheelan KR, et al. Pathophysiological Basis and Rationale for Early Outpatient Treatment of SARS-CoV-2 (COVID-19) Infection. Am J Med. 2020;134:16-22.
63. McCullough PA. Innovative Early Sequenced Multidrug Therapy for SARS-CoV-2 (COVID-19) Infection to Reduce Hospitalization and Death. Int J Med Sci Clin Invent. 2020;7:5139-50.
64. McCullough PA, Alexander PE, Armstrong R, Arvinte C, Bain AF, Bartlett RP, et al. Multifaceted highly targeted sequential multidrug treatment of early ambulatory high-risk SARS-CoV-2 infection (COVID-19). Rev Cardiovasc Med. 2020;21(4):517-30.
65. Palazzuoli A, Beltrami M, McCullough PA. Acute COVID-19 Management in Heart Failure Patients: A Specific Setting Requiring Detailed Inpatient and Outpatient Hospital Care. Biomedicines. 2023;11:790.
66. McCullough PA, Oskoui R. Early multidrug regimens in new potentially fatal medical problems. Rev Cardiovasc Med. 2020;21(4):507-8.
67. Procter BC, Ross C, Pickard V, Smith E, Hanson C, McCullough PA. Clinical outcomes after early ambulatory multidrug therapy for high-risk SARS-CoV-2 (COVID-19) infection. Reviews in Cardiovascular Medicine. 2021;21:611-4.
68. Procter BC, Ross C, Pickard V, Smith E, Hanson C, McCullough PA. Early Ambulatory Multidrug Therapy re-duces Hospitalization and Death in High-Risk Patients with SARS-CoV-2 (COVID-19). Int J Innov Res Med Sci. 2021;6:219-21.
69. Tyson B, Fareed G. Overcoming the Covid darkness. How two doctors successfully treated 7,000 patients. 2021.
70. Chetty S. Elucidating the pathogenesis and Rx of COVID reveals a missing element. Modern Med. 2020;45(5):28-31.
71. Borody TJ, Clancy RL. (2021). Combination therapy for COVID-19 based on ivermectin in an Australian population. [online] Available from https://www.covidmedicalnetwork.com/media/TrialSite-media-release-19.10.2021.pdf. [Last accessed February, 2024].
72. Risch HA. Early Outpatient Treatment of Symptomatic, High-Risk COVID-19 Patients that Should be Ramped-Up Immediately as Key to the Pandemic Crisis. Am J Epidemiol. 2020;189:1218-26.

73. Kory P, Meduri, Gianfranco U, Varon J, Iglesias J, Marik PE. Review of the Emerging Evidence Demonstrating the Efficacy of Ivermectin in the Prophylaxis and Treatment of COVID-19. Am J Therap. 2021;28:e299-318.
74. Elgazzar A, Eltaweel A, Youssef SA, Hany B, Hafez M, Moussa H. (2020). Efficacy and Safety of Ivermectin for Treatment and prophylaxis of COVID-19 Pandemic. [online] Available fromhttps://doi.org/10.21203/rs.3.rs-100956/v3. [Last accessed February, 2024].
75. Marik PE, Kory P. Ivermectin, A Reanalysis of the Data. Am J Ther. 2021;28(5):e579-80.
76. Santin AD, Scheim DE, McCullough PA, Yagisawa M, Borody TJ. Ivermectin: a multi-faceted drug of Nobel prize-honoured distinction with indicated efficacy against a new global scourge, COVID-19. New Microbes New Infect. 2021;43:100924.
77. Gkioulekas E, McCullough PA, Zelenko V. Statistical analysis methods applied to early outpatient COVID-19 treatment case series data. COVID. 2022;2(8):1139-82.
78. Kerr L, Cadegiani FA, Baldi F, Lobo RB, Assagra WLO, Proenca FC, et al. Ivermectin prophylaxis used for COVID-19 reduces COVID-19 infection and mortality rates: A 220,517-subject, populational-level retrospective citywide. Cureus. 2022;14(1):e21272.
79. Kerr L, Baldi F, Lobo R, Assagra WL, Proenca FC, Chamie JJ, et al. Regular Use of Ivermectin as Prophylaxis for COVID-19 Led Upto a 92% Reduction in COVID-19 Mortality Rate in a Dose-Response Manner: Results of a Prospective Observational Study of a Strictly Controlled Population of 88,012 Subjects. Cureus. 2022;14(8):e28624.
80. Stone JC, Ndarukwa P, Scheim DE, Dancis BM, Dancis J, Gill MG, et al. Changes in SpO_2 on Room Air for 34 Severe COVID-19 Patients after Ivermectin-Based Combination Treatment: 62% Normalization within 24 Hours. Biologics. 2022;2(3):196-210.
81. Hazan S, Dave S, Gunaratne AW, Dolai S, Clancy RL, McCullough PA, et al. Effectiveness of ivermectin-based multidrug therapy in severely hypoxic, ambulatory COVID-19 patients. Future Microbiology. 2022;17(5):339-50.
82. Babalola OE, Ndanusa YA, Ajayi AA, Ogedengbe JO, Thairu Y, Omede O. A Randomized Controlled Trial of Ivermectin Monotherapy versus Hydroxychloroquine, Ivermectin, and Azithromycin Combination Therapy in COVID-19 Patients in Nigeria. J Infect Dis Epidemiol. 2021;7:233.
83. Thairu Y, Babalola OE, Ajayi AA, Ndanusa Y, Ogedengbe JO, Omede O. A Comparison of Ivermectin and Non Ivermectin Based Regimen for COVID-19 in Abuja: Effects on Virus Clearance, Days-to-discharge and Mortality. J Pharm Res Int. 2022;34 (44A):1-19.
84. Babalola OE, Ajayi A, Yunusa T, Ndanusa YA, Ogedengbe J, Omede O. Ivermectinis Associated with Increase in SpO2 in Hypoxemic SARS-CoV-2 Patients: Pharmacodynamic Profile and Correlates. J Clin Chem Lab Med. 2022;5:222.
85. Chamie JJ, Hibberd JA, Scheim DE. COVID-19 Excess Deaths in Peru's 25 States in 2020: Nationwide Trends, Confounding Factors, and Correlations with the Extent of Ivermectin Treatment by State. Cureus. 2023;15(8):e43168.
86. Stone JC, Gill MG. (2020). Zimbabwe SID Protocol. [online] Available from https://www.ivermectin.africa/sid-protocol/. [Last accessed February, 2024].
87. Bramante CT, Huling JD, Tignanelli CJ, Buse JB, Liebovitz DM, Nicklas JM, et al. Randomized Trial of Metformin, Ivermectin, and Fluvoxamine for COVID-19. N Eng J Med. 2022;387:599-610.
88. Lim SCL, Hor CP, Tay KH, Jelani AM, Tan WH, Ker HB, et al. Efficacy of ivermectin treatment on disease progression among adults with mild to moderate COVID-19 and comorbidities: The I-TECH randomized clinical trial. JAMA Internal Medicine. 2022;182:426-35.
89. Naggie S, Boulware DR, Lindsell CJ, Stewart TG, Gentile N, Collins S, et al. Effect of Ivermectin vs. Placebo on Time to Sustained Recovery in Outpatients with Mild to Moderate COVID-19: A Randomized Clinical Trial. J Am Med Assoc. 2022;328:1595-603.
90. Naggie S, Boulware DR, Lindsell CJ, Stewart TG, Slandzicki AJ, Lim SC, et al. Effect of Higher-Dose Ivermectin for 6 Days vs. Placebo on Time to Sustained Recovery in

Outpatients with COVID-19: A Randomized Clinical Trial. J Am Med Assoc. 2023;329: 888-97.

91. Lopez-Medina E, Lopez P, Hurtado IC, Davalos DM, Ramirez O, Martnez E, et al. Effect of ivermectin on time to resolution of symptoms among adults with mild COVID-19: A randomized clinical trial. J Am Med Assoc. 2021;325:1426-35.
92. Reis G, Silva EASM, Silva DCM, Thabane L, Milagres AC, Ferreira TS, et al. Effect of early treatment with ivermectin among patients with COVID-19. N Eng J Med. 2022;386: 1721-31.
93. Fazio S, Bellavite P, Zanolin E, McCullough PA, Pandolfi S, Affuso F. Retrospective Study of Outcomes and Hospitalization Rates of Patients in Italy with a Confirmed Diagnosis of Early COVID-19 and Treated at Home Within 3 Days or After 3 Days of Symptom Onset with Prescribed and Non-Prescribed Treatments Between November 2020 and August 2021. Med Sci Monit. 2021;27:e935379.
94. Scheim DE, Aldous C, Osimani B, Fordham EJ, Hoy WE. When Characteristics of Clinical Trials Require Per-Protocol as Well as Intention-To-Treat Outcomes to Draw Reliable Conclusions: Three Examples. J Clin Med. 2023;12:3625.
95. Karim SSA, Devnarain N. Time to Stop Using Ineffective Covid-19 Drugs. N Eng J Med. 2022;387:654-5.
96. US FDA. "Why You Should Not Use Ivermectin to Treat or Prevent COVID-19", [online] Available from https://www.fda.gov/consumers/consumer-updates/why-you-should-not-use-ivermectin-treat-or-prevent-covid-19. [Last accessed February, 2024].
97. Wan W, Kolesnikova L, Clarke M, Koehler A, Noda T, Becker S, et al. Structure and assembly of the Ebola virus nucleocapsid. Nature. 2017;551(7680):394-7.
98. Younan P, Iampietro M, Nishida A, Ramanathan R, Santos R, Dutta M, et al. Ebola virus binding to Tim-1 on T lymphocytes induces a cytokine storm. mBio. 2017;8(5): e00845-17.
99. Falasca L, Agrati C, Petrosillo N, Di Caro A, Capobianchi M, Ippolito G, et al. Molecular mechanisms of Ebola virus pathogenesis: focus on cell death. Cell Death Differ. 2015;22(8):1250-9.
100. Wiedemar N, Hauser DA, Mäser P. 100 years of suramin. Antimicrob Agents Chemother. 2020;64(3):e01168-19.
101. Henß L, Beck S, Weidner T, Biedenkopf N, Sliva K, Weber C, et al. Suramin is a potent inhibitor of Chikungunya and Ebola virus cell entry. Virol J. 2016;13(1):149.
102. Kennedy J. Phosphatidylserine's role in Ebola's inflammatory cytokine storm and hemorrhagic consumptive coagulopathy and the therapeutic potential of annexin V. Med Hypotheses. 2020;135:109462.
103. Arjun P, Sankar B, Shankar K, Kulkarni N, Sivasankaran S, Shankar B. Silver and Silver Nanoparticles for the Potential Treatment of COVID-19: A Review. Coatings. 2022;12(11):1679.
104. Jeevanandam J, Krishnan S, Hii Y, Pan S, Chan Y, Acquah C, et al. Synthesis approach dependent antiviral properties of silver nanoparticles and nanocomposites. J Nanostructure Chem. 2022;12:809-31.
105. US FDA. Emergency Use Authorization of Medical Products and Related Authorities. [online] Available from https://www.fda.gov/regulatory-information/search-fda-guidance-documents/emergency-use-authorization-medical-products-and-related-authorities. [Last accessed February, 2024].
106. World Medical Association. World Medical Association Declaration of Helsinki: Ethical Principles for Medical Research Involving Human Subjects. J Am Med Assoc. 2013;310:2191-4.
107. World Medical Association. (2022). WMA Declaration of Helsinki: Ethical Principles for Medical Research Involving Human Subjects. [online] Available from https://www.wma.net/policies-post/wma-declaration-of-helsinki-ethical-principles-for-medical-research-involving-human-subjects/. [Last accessed February, 2024].

CHAPTER 24

Sialylated Glycan Bindings from SARS-CoV-2 Spike Protein to Blood and Endothelial Cells Govern the Severe Morbidities of COVID-19*

David E Scheim, Paola Vottero, Alessandro D Santin, Allen G Hirsh

ABSTRACT

Consistent with well-established biochemical properties of coronaviruses, sialylated glycan attachments between severe acute respiratory syndrome coronavirus 2 (SARS-CoV-2) spike protein (SP) and host cells are key to the virus's pathology. SARS-CoV-2 SP attaches to and aggregates red blood cells (RBCs), as shown in many pre-clinical and clinical studies, causing pulmonary and extrapulmonary microthrombi and hypoxia in severe COVID-19 patients. SARS-CoV-2 SP attachments to the heavily sialylated surfaces of platelets (which, like RBCs, have no ACE2) and endothelial cells (having minimal ACE2) compound this vascular damage. Notably, experimentally induced RBC aggregation in vivo causes the same key morbidities as for severe COVID-19, including microvascular occlusion, blood clots, hypoxia and myocarditis. Key risk factors for COVID-19 morbidity, including older age, diabetes and obesity, are all characterized by markedly increased propensity to RBC clumping. For mammalian species, the degree of clinical susceptibility to COVID-19 correlates to RBC aggregability with $p = 0.033$. Notably, of the five human betacoronaviruses, the two common cold strains express an enzyme that releases glycan attachments, while the deadly SARS, SARS-CoV-2 and MERS do not, although viral loads for COVID-19 and the two common cold infections are similar. These biochemical insights also explain the previously puzzling clinical efficacy of certain generics against COVID-19 and may support the development of future therapeutic strategies for COVID-19 and long COVID patients.

* Scheim DE, Vottero P, Santin AD, Hirsh AG. Sialylated glycan bindings from SARS-CoV-2 spike protein to blood and endothelial cells govern the severe morbidities of COVID-19. Int J Mol Sci. 2023;24(23):17039.

INTRODUCTION

The virus that caused COVID-19 was first named "severe acute respiratory syndrome coronavirus 2" (SARS-CoV-2) in February 2020 in recognition of the disease's pulmonary symptoms and the lung's role as its initial target organ, as with its SARS predecessor. Yet as clinical experience and histological findings accrued, the hypoxia which emerged as a key morbidity of severe COVID-19 was found in a large percentage of such patients to accompany nearly normal breathing mechanics and lung gas volume.[1-6] Although COVID-19 typically gains infectious penetration in the respiratory epithelium, microvascular occlusion is frequently observed in pulmonary septal capillaries and in other organ systems of COVID-19 patients,[7-20] accompanying morbidities such as intravascular clotting and peripheral ischemia.[2,3,8,18,21-23] Lung inflammation and other pulmonary symptoms are common with COVID-19, yet in several cases of severe disease, histological examinations have revealed microthrombi and extensively damaged endothelium in the septal capillary microvasculature adjoining relatively intact alveoli.[14,24]

Soon after the determination of SARS-CoV-2 as the viral cause of COVID-19, ACE2 was identified as the host cell receptor supporting its replication,[25-27] with neuropilin-1 its replication receptor for astrocytes and possibly certain other cell types.[28,29] Yet ACE2 is one of a variety of host cell receptors that different coronavirus strains use for replication; other receptors include DPP4 for MERS, APN for HCoV-229E, and CEACAM1 for MHV.[30] The morbidities of SARS-CoV-2, in particular, as shown below, are less dependent on its host cell replication receptor, ACE2, than on glycans having sialic acid (SA) terminal moieties found on viral spike protein (SP) and host cells. For coronaviruses, these sialylated glycans on their SP serve as the initial points of viral attachment to the host cell surface,[30-42] after which the virus can migrate to fuse with a replication receptor.[40,42-49] One clue to the centrality of glycan bindings to the morbidities of the five human betacoronaviruses is the expression by the two common cold strains, HKU1 and OC43, of hemagglutinin esterase (HE), which releases glycan bindings between viral SP and host cells.[50-54] These common cold infections are generally benign, while the SARS, SARS-CoV-2 and MERS viruses do not express HE[50-54] and are deadly, even though the viral loads for COVID-19 and these common cold infections are about the same.[55]

THE MOLECULAR COMPOSITION OF GLYCANS ON SARS-COV-2 SP AND THE RED BLOOD CELL

The arrangement and chemical composition of the SARS-CoV-2 SP glycans have been determined, with those at its 22 N-glycosylation sites having a total of nine SA terminal residues[31,48,49,56-63] and its four O-glycans having a total of three SA terminal residues.[63] This provides a basis for exploring these viral SP attachments to host cells, notably red blood cells (RBCs), platelets, leukocytes and endothelial cells.[31] RBCs and platelets have densely distributed sialoglycoproteins but no ACE2 receptors on their surfaces,[64,65] the same holds for leukocytes and most other blood cells.[66–68] Endothelial cells likewise have a heavily sialylated surface coating (glycocalyx), with about 28,000 SA-tipped CD147 receptors but only about 175 ACE2 receptors per cell.[69,70]

Of particular interest are attachments of SARS-CoV-2 SP to the RBC, the latter coated with one million SA-tipped glycophorin A (GPA) molecules and a total of 35 million SA monosaccharides per cell.[71-73] The heavily sialylated GPA strands are spaced about 14 nm apart on the RBC surface and extend out 5 nm.[71] Band 3 protein is another molecule on the RBC surface, with 1.2 million copies per RBC, which extends >10 nm from the RBC surface[71,74] and is glycosylated by poly-N-acetyllactosamine, a sialylated branched-chain glycan.[75-78] GPA and poly-N-acetyllactosamine, the two most abundant glycans on the RBC membrane,[77] have been found to mediate hemagglutination by various bacterial and viral pathogens.[78-81] The glycans attached to SARS-CoV-2 SP and those which extend from the RBC surface are depicted in **Figure 1**.

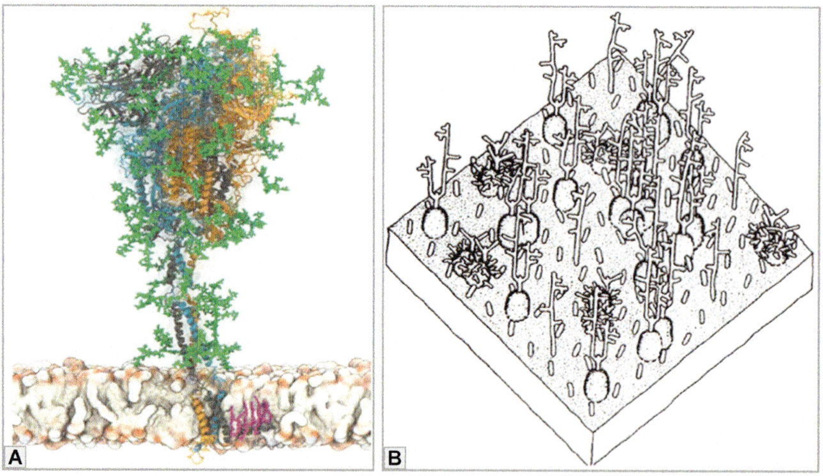

FIGURES 1A AND B: (A) Atomistic model of the full-length trimeric S protein of SARS-CoV-2 shown in cartoon representation, reproduced from Sikora et al. (2021).[90] The three monomeric chains are differentiated by color, with glycans shown in green licorice representation, and a palmitoylated cysteine residue shown in pink, anchored into the viral envelope at the bottom. (B) A representation of a 35×35 nm area of the RBC surface depicting its sialoglycoprotein coating, reproduced from Viitala et al. (1975).[71] Prominent among these sialylated glycans are GPA strands, which extend approximately 5 nm from the RBC surface, and band 3 protein, which extends > 10 nm from that surface and is glycosylated by poly-N-acetyllactosamine.

Source: Reproduced (A) under CC-BY 4.0 and (B) with permission from Elsevier.

Hemagglutination as caused by these pathogen–glycan attachments is of particular interest in view of a primal defense mounted by RBCs along with platelets against pathogens having SA terminal moieties by attaching to them and delivering them to leukocytes or conveying them to macrophages in the liver and spleen for phagocytosis.[72,82–88] Notably, GPA, one of the two most abundant glycans on the RBC surface,[77,89] has no other known physiological role other than spearheading this pathogen defense.[71,72,83,84] For severe COVID-19 infections, however, this primal defense, described as "immune adherence",[85] goes self-destructively overboard, with the total load and sizes of clumps formed exceeding the body's capacity to sequester them, as detailed below.

A clear experimental demonstration of binding between SARS-CoV-2 SP and sialylated glycans on host cells was provided using NMR spectroscopy.[34] It was found, in particular, that a site on the SP N-terminal domain (NTD) binds to α2,3 and α2,6 sialyl N-acetyllactosamine, which are components or variants thereof of the sialylated poly-N-acetyllactosamine glycans of the band 3 strands extending from the RBC surface. Intriguingly, this SP-to-glycan binding was found to be much more pronounced for α2,3 than for α2,6 SA-linked N-acetyllactosamine,[34] while α2,3 versus α2,6-linked SA is likewise much more prevalent in sialylated poly-N-acetyllactosamine of adult (vs. fetal) RBCs.[76]

Possibilities for binding are indicated as well between SARS-CoV-2 SP and/or glycans at its glycosylation sites and GPA on the RBC surface, with GPA, as noted, having no known physiological role other than this type of immune adherence. The positive electrostatic potential of SARS-CoV-2 SP[91] supports its binding to the negatively charged, densely distributed SA on the RBC surface, most on its million GPA strands.[92,93] Also, as depicted in **Figure 2**, SA in its predominant human form, Neu5Ac, is the most common terminal residue of GPA.[71,74,94] For the N- and O-glycans on SARS-CoV-2 SP, the most common terminal residues are galactose (Gal), with 27 total, and Neu5Ac (SA), with 12 total.[61-63,90] Through binding configurations proposed by Varki and Schnaar (2017)[95] and others,[34,96-98] multivalent bonds can form via α2–3 and α2–6 linkages from Neu5Ac on GPA to Gal on glycans populating SARS-CoV-2 SP glycosylation sites.

In Vitro, In Vivo and Clinical Studies Demonstrate Induction of RBC Aggregation by SARS-CoV-2 SP

Many in vitro, in vivo and clinical studies demonstrate that SARS-CoV-2 SP attaches to RBCs and induces RBC aggregation. Boschi et al. (2022) found that SARS-CoV-2 SP from each of the Wuhan, Alpha, Delta and Omicron strains induced RBC clumping (hemagglutination) when mixed with human RBCs in phosphate-buffered saline (PBS).[91] To explore whether bridging of adjacent RBCs by SARS-CoV-2 SP via glycan bonds might be the cause of this observed hemagglutination, an agent with indicated high-affinity binding

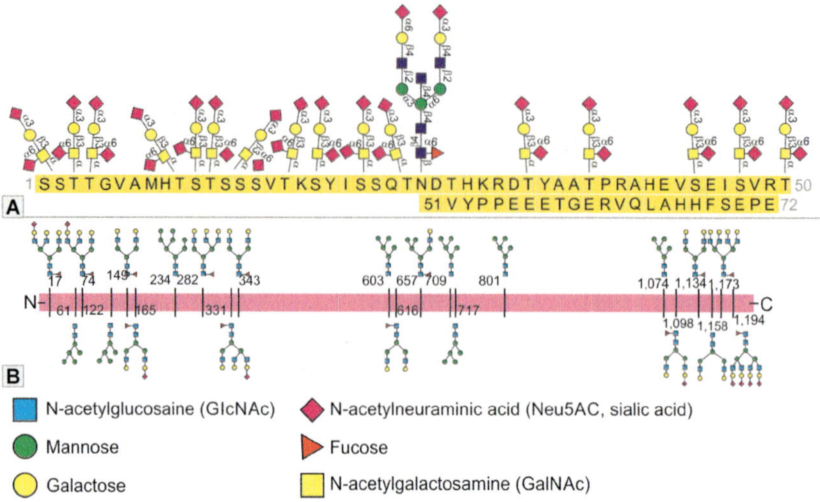

FIGURES 2A AND B: (A) Amino acid sequence of the extracellular domain (aa 1–72) of GPA with its glycan structures and attachment sites, adapted from Jaskiewicz et al. (2019).[94] (B) The terminal monosaccharides for fully populated N-glycans of a SARS-CoV-2 SP monomer, with these 22 N-glycosylation sites numbered from the N-terminal end to the C-terminal end, as adapted from Sikora et al. (2021).[90] The key to the monosaccharides shown in both (A) and (B) is at bottom of (B).

to multiple SARS-CoV-2 SP glycan-binding sites,[99] the macrocyclic lactone ivermectin (IVM), was added to the mix of SP and RBCs both before and after hemagglutination formed. IVM blocked the formation of hemagglutination when added to the initial mix and reversed hemagglutination over the course of 30 min when added after it formed.[91] In another study, SARS-CoV-2 SP added to whole blood induced clumping of RBCs, hyperactivation and clumping of platelets, and formation of anomalous fibrinogen deposits.[100]

The same SP-induced RBC clumping effect as noted above was demonstrated in zebrafish embryos, which have blood cell glycosylation patterns[101] and capillary diameters[102] similar to those of humans. When SARS-CoV-2 SP was microinjected into the common cardinal vein of a zebrafish embryo at a concentration similar to that obtained in critically ill COVID-19 patients, it caused the formation of small RBC clumps and an associated reduction in blood flow velocity within 3–5 minutes after injection, as shown in **Figure 3C**, accompanied by thrombosis in capillaries, arteries and veins.[103] When SP was coinjected with a mixture of heparan sulfate and heparin (molecular mass of each ≤30 kDa), however, with both of these glycosaminoglycans having strong binding affinity to SARS-CoV-2 SP,[103–105] the extent of thrombosis was markedly reduced.[103]

In various studies, SARS-CoV-2 SP and subunits were observed in the plasma of 64% of COVID-19 patients,[108] in the sera of 30% of hospitalized

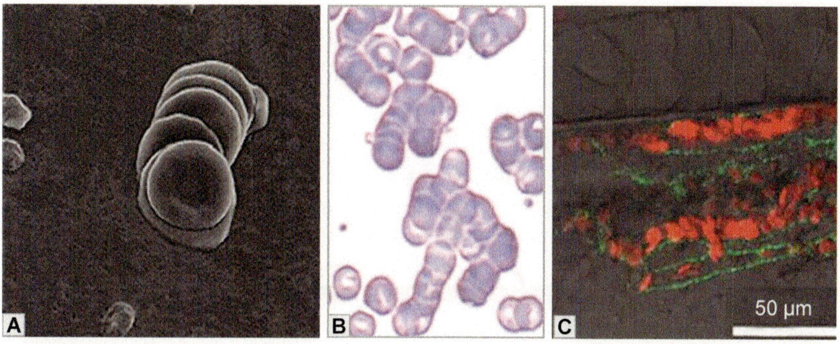

FIGURES 3A TO C: (A and B) Images of RBC rouleaux (stacked clumps) from the blood of COVID-19 patients, obtained using electron (magnification ×5,000)[106] and light (80× objective)[107] microscopy. The first study (A) found RBC clumps in all 31 patients studied, all with mild COVID-19,[106] and the second (B) found large RBC aggregates in 85% of COVID-19 patients with anemia.[107] (C) A frame from a video of RBC aggregates in capillaries of zebrafish embryos that formed within 3–5 minutes after injection of SARS-CoV-2 SP into the common cardinal vein at a similar concentration to that obtained in critically ill COVID-19 patients.[103] The velocity of blood flow in the capillaries shown in this video frame was markedly reduced from that prior to injection of SP.

COVID-19 patients[109] and in the brains of all of the 13 patients who died of this disease.[110] SP and spike S1 subunits were likewise observed over periods of months in the plasma[111-113] and monocytes,[114] respectively, of patients having post-acute sequelae of this disease (long COVID, or PASC). Leakage of SP outside of an infected host cell during SARS-CoV-2 replication has been documented in vitro and clinically[115-117] and may be the source of the SP in blood found in COVID-19 patients.

The SARS-CoV-2 SP attachments to RBCs were demonstrated directly by Lam et al. (2021) through immunofluorescence analysis of RBCs from the blood of nine hospitalized COVID-19 patients.[118] For these patients at hospital admission, the mean percentage of RBCs having SARS-CoV-2 SP traces was 41%. This finding suggests that concentrations of SARS-CoV-2 SP in blood as typically reported in other studies using plasma or serum may significantly understate actual values due to high-affinity binding to RBCs, which are removed from plasma and serum. SARS-CoV-2 SP and pseudovirus were each found to bind to nanoparticle arrays bearing SA derivatives[59] and to SA-tipped CD147 receptors, likewise detected using nanoarrays.[119] Nanoarray methods are required to detect SARS-CoV-2 SP glycan attachments, because these methods allow bindings to form multivalently, whereas univalent bindings are weak[31] and not detectable by microarray methods.[42] Studies using the latter failed to detect SARS-CoV-2 SP bindings to either SA[120] or CD147.[121] As noted above, binding of SARS-CoV-2 SP to sialylated glycans identical or closely related to those on the RBC surface was demonstrated directly using NMR spectroscopy.[34]

The presence of SARS-CoV-2 SP in the blood of COVID-19 patients and its induction of hemagglutination in vitro and in vivo would suggest that the same would occur clinically, which is indeed the case. In three publications that used scanning electron microscopy to examine blood from the cubital vein blood of patients with mild-to-moderate cases of COVID-19, all hospitalized but none requiring intensive care, a team of investigators observed blood cell clumping and other anomalies.[106,122,123] The first study found stacked RBC aggregates (rouleaux) ranging in size from 3–12 cells, as shown in **Figure 3A**, in the blood of all 31 of its COVID-19 patients, with none found in 32 matched healthy controls.[106] A follow-up publication reported the mean count of RBC aggregates in the COVID-19 patients at 3.1 to 5.5 per 1000 μm^2 scanning area, while controls had no RBC aggregates.[122] Aggregates of platelets, some with leukocytes or RBCs, were likewise found in all COVID-19 patients to significant extents, but none were found in the controls.[122]

Light microscopy examination of smears from the blood of 20 hospitalized COVID-19 patients with anemia detected large, stacked RBC clumps (rouleaux), as shown in **Figure 3B**, in 85% of those patients.[107] Another study, which examined the sublingual microcirculation of 38 COVID-19 patients in intensive care using video microscopy, found that the mean number of RBC microaggregates detected in these patients was 15 times the mean number for 33 healthy volunteers.[124] These RBC microaggregates were found in two-thirds of the COVID-19 patients versus two of the 33 healthy volunteers. A study of the blood of 172 hospitalized COVID-19 patients found that both RBC aggregability and the strength of RBC aggregates formed were significantly greater than those values for healthy controls and that this RBC hyperaggregability correlated with enhanced blood coagulation, all of these effects highly significant ($p < 0.001$).[125] The much greater degree and strength of RBC aggregation found in COVID-19 versus sepsis, with both having elevated levels of inflammation-related markers, indicate that inflammation alone cannot explain these RBC aggregation effects for COVID-19.[125]

Paralleling these studies that document RBC aggregation in severe COVID-19 are many that report microvascular occlusion. Postmortem examinations of hundreds of patients who died from COVID-19 in many studies consistently found microthrombi in the pulmonary microvasculature in most patients.[7–18] Microthrombi in alveolar capillaries were nine times as prevalent in postmortem COVID-19 patients compared to influenza patients.[10] RBC clumping and microthrombi in the lungs have been regarded as likely causes of hypoxemia in severe COVID-19 patients,[1,2,106,123] which in turn is closely associated with mortal outcomes.[126]

Microthrombi elsewhere in the body, including in the heart, kidneys and liver, were also frequently observed in autopsy examinations of COVID-19 patients, with indications that these may have contributed to multiorgan damage and failure.[7,8,20] Another indication of the widespread distribution of microthrombi throughout the body in severe COVID-19 patients, persisting even after recovery from acute illness, was provided using video capillaroscopy to examine ocular conjunctival microvessels in 17 hospitalized COVID-19 patients within 28 days after hospital discharge and 17 healthy controls.[127] The mean percentage of occluded microvessels was found to be six times as high in the hospital-discharged COVID-19 patients versus controls, while the mean rates of blood flow in the conjunctival capillaries and postcapillary venules were significantly lower.[127] Such widespread indications of microvascular occlusion in severe COVID-19 patients led cardiovascular researchers at the Johns Hopkins and Harvard University medical schools to conclude that "severe COVID-19 is a microvascular disease".[21]

Glycan Bindings from SARS-CoV-2 SP to Platelets and Endothelial Cells Cause Endothelial Damage, Inflammation and Coagulation

Attachments of SARS-CoV-2 SP to the heavily sialylated[64,65,70] surfaces of platelets and endothelial cells cause endothelial damage, platelet activation and associated coagulation which, as with the attachments to RBCs, contribute to the severe morbidities of COVID-19. Platelets, having no ACE2 receptors, like RBCs,[66,67] act with RBCs in a role that was termed "immune adherence",[85] attaching to and clearing pathogens,[87,88] and are found enmeshed with RBCs in blood cell clumps in COVID-19 patients.[122] The degree of sialylation of the endothelial cell surface is exemplified by the 28,000 SA-tipped CD147 receptors versus the 175 ACE2 receptors per endothelial cell.[69] For glomerular endothelial cells from a conditionally immortalized human cell line, the enzyme neuraminidase, which hydrolyzes SA, removed more than 50% of the cells' surface coating (glycocalyx).[70] The endothelial cell thus provides a prime target for the SARS-CoV-2 virus, and indeed, both whole virus and viral SP have been found on endothelial cells in clinical and in vivo COVID-19 infections.[10,17,24,110,128–131] Correspondingly, damaged endothelial cells have been frequently observed in severe COVID-19 patients.[21,24,132,133] Yet the importance of this direct viral attack on the endothelium in COVID-19 has been overlooked by some researchers in the belief that ACE2, which is sparse on endothelial cells, is the only host-cell binding target of interest for SARS-CoV-2.[134,135]

These SARS-CoV-2 viral or SP attachments to the endothelium can be perilous to the human host, with trillions of RBCs each flowing once per minute through the lungs and then the extrapulmonary vasculature[136] and with the cross-sectional diameter of most capillaries so small that RBCs distort their shape to squeeze through.[137] Thus, SARS-CoV-2 virus particles or SP attached to endothelial cells or RBCs could create resistance to blood flow or even potentially rip off a piece of an endothelial cell or the entire cell.[31] Indeed, one study found that serum levels of circulating endothelial cells (CECs) in mild-to-moderate COVID-19 patients were up to 100 times the levels for matched controls. The study also found that each of these CECs from the COVID-19 patients typically had several holes in their membranes approximately the size of the SARS-CoV-2 viral capsid (the viral envelope).[106] A marker of endothelial damage, von Willebrand factor (VWF), which promotes platelet activation and, in turn, coagulation,[138–140] has been found to be significantly elevated in COVID-19 patients.[21,132,141,142] These and other coagulation and proinflammatory pathways can cause blood clots or trigger a cytokine storm in the most serious cases of this infection.[21,132,133]

While these pathological pathways contribute significantly to the severe morbidities of COVID-19, the role of SARS-CoV-2 SP-induced RBC aggregation in these morbidities is nevertheless central, as demonstrated below through multiple avenues of substantiation. We show below that experimentally induced RBC clumping in vivo causes the same morbidities and the same redistribution of blood flow from smaller to larger blood vessels as for COVID-19. We further demonstrate the following: (i) key risk factors for COVID-19 morbidity are associated with markedly increased RBC aggregation; (ii) SARS-CoV-2 SP in the absence of whole virus induces microvascular occlusion in vivo and clinically; (iii) three generic drugs that have aroused widespread interest as potential COVID-19 treatments all significantly inhibit RBC aggregation; and (iv) for mammalian species, the degree of clinical susceptibility to COVID-19 correlates to aggregation propensity of RBCs with $p = 0.033$.

Experimentally Induced RBC Clumping In Vivo: Parallels to Severe COVID-19

Studies dating back to the 1940s in dogs, rabbits, mice, hamsters and other animals closely examined the effects of IV injection of high-molecular-weight dextran (HMWD), generally of molecular weight (MW, loosely equivalent to molecular mass) ≥ 100 kDa or other blood cell-agglutinating agents. In several studies, blood cell aggregation was induced within minutes to hours after IV injection of HMWD,[143–148] with molecular bridging of RBCs by HMWD molecules being a hypothesized mechanism for this effect.[149–152] After HMWD injection in vivo, small clumps of RBCs formed and then enlarged into longer stacked clumps (rouleaux) and, in some cases, into vast trees with branches of hundreds of stacked RBCs.[144,145,153] Also, the addition of low-MW dextran (LMWD, e.g., MW ≤ 40 kDa) in vivo prevented the formation of RBC aggregates when injected with HMWD[146,154] and rapidly disaggregated them with accompanying reversal of microvascular occlusion when injected after HMWD-induced clumps had formed.[148,155–158]

In vitro, the addition of HMWD to blood likewise induced RBC aggregation[159,160] and did so as well when added to RBCs in PBS.[161,162] The same RBC disaggregating effect of LMWD was observed in vitro,[163] possibly caused by competitive binding to RBCs that limited bridging between adjacent RBCs by larger molecules. Although we have focused on aggregation of RBCs, these same aggregating effects of HMWD and disaggregating effects of LMWD have been observed, both in vitro and in vivo, for platelets as well.[147,153]

Even in healthy humans or animals, RBC clumps can transiently form under conditions of slow blood flow, e.g., in deep veins of the lower limbs, but they typically disaggregate as they move into regions of faster blood flow[164-174] and are rarely problematical in healthy subjects.[148,157,175] Yet under pathological conditions in diseases such as diabetes, malignant hypertension and malaria,[154,167,175-177] these RBC aggregates can persist and grow via a positive feedback loop whereby the clumps cause decreased blood flow velocity with a concomitant reduction in shear forces that in turn causes further aggregation.[164,166-171,173,175] In mammals, a significant total mass of blood cell aggregates can lodge in a distributed network of arterioles before obstruction of blood flow reaches a critical stage.[178] Pulmonary artery tips provide a catch-trap architecture that sequesters large blood cell aggregates, which limits disseminated microvascular occlusion and mitigates resulting hypoxia and associated widespread tissue damage, including to the heart wall.[167,178]

The capability of LMWD to rapidly reverse RBC aggregation and associated microvascular occlusion caused by injection of HMWD, as noted above, distinguishes blood clumping, e.g., as induced by HMWD, from clotting, in which blood cell clumps harden into fibrin-enmeshed clots via the coagulation cascade. Indeed, several mammalian diseases are associated with increased levels of RBC aggregation and microvascular occlusion which do not typically cause blood clotting, although risks of this complication are increased.[154,175] Blood cell clumping and clotting are not completely unrelated phenomena, however, given the potential of RBC aggregation to trigger deep vein thrombosis.[179,180] and the role of fibrinogen, an essential promoter of blood clotting, in blood cell clumping as well.[164,181-183]

Induced RBC Aggregation Causes Microvascular Occlusion, Hypoxia, Blood Clots, and Redistribution of Blood Flow from Smaller to Larger Blood Vessels

When HMWD or other agglutinating agents were injected into animals at sufficient concentrations to overwhelm the host's ability to safely sequester the RBC aggregates formed, these clumps caused microvascular occlusion as detected in a variety of host tissues,[154] including the myocardium,[153,184] muscle[185] and abdominal cavity[153] of rats; the conjunctival vessels of dogs, cats and rabbits;[147,186] the cheek pouch of hamsters;[148,157] and the kidney, liver, ear chamber, bone marrow and heart tissue of rabbits, including the myocardium and pericardium.[144-146,155,156] In the myocardium of rabbits and rats, the degree of myocardial tissue damage was correlated with the observed degree of intravascular aggregation of blood cells,[144,146,153] with hypoxia resulting from vascular occlusion proposed to be the cause of tissue damage.[144,146]

Associated with the microvascular occlusion that it triggered, experimentally induced RBC aggregation caused decreased velocity of blood flow,[143,145–148,154,171,184] increased blood viscosity,[143,154,186,187] increased incidence of blood clotting[144,154,167] and decreased oxygen tension in arteries, veins and tissues, with accompanying hypoxic damage to body organs.[144,146,154,188,189] Another effect caused by induced blood cell clumping as observed in the conjunctiva of cats, dogs and rabbits and bone marrow of rabbits was a reduction in blood flow in the capillaries and other small vessels having cross-sectional diameters of about 10 μm or smaller,[147,155] indicative of a shift of blood flow into the larger vessels. A similar redistribution of blood flow from the smaller blood vessels of micrometer cross-sectional diameter to larger blood vessels was observed in patients with type 2 diabetes,[177,190] a disease characterized by an increased extent of RBC aggregation and accompanying microvascular occlusion.[167,177,191–194]

Corresponding Morbidities in Severe COVID-19

As considered above, SARS-CoV-2 SP, like HMWD dextran, induces RBC aggregation, and the same morbidities caused by experimentally induced RBC aggregation have been commonly observed for cases of severe COVID-19. These morbidities of severe COVID-19 include microvascular occlusion in the lungs and other organ systems,[7–20] hypoxia,[1,195] arterial and venous thromboembolisms,[9,15,17,18,21,196–198] disseminated intravascular coagulation[15,21,196–200] and multiorgan damage associated with these vascular aberrations and hypoxia.[7,200,201] Decreased oxygen saturation is a particularly dangerous morbidity of COVID-19, with a peripheral oxygen saturation (SpO_2) of <88% associated with a 3.7-fold increased risk of death[126] and an SpO_2 of ≤93% deemed to be a sufficient condition for classifying a COVID-19 infection as severe according to US National Institutes of Health guidelines.[202]

Redistribution of Blood Flow from Smaller to Larger Blood Microvessels in COVID-19 Patients

Another effect of experimentally induced RBC aggregation, the redistribution of blood flow from microvessels to blood vessels of larger cross-sectional diameter, as described above, is also paralleled in COVID-19. Osiaevi et al. (2023) compared videomicroscopic imaging of the sublingual microvasculature of 16 critically ill COVID-19 patients, 17 patients with long COVID and 15 healthy controls.[203] As shown in **Figure 4**, the density of functional capillaries (having flowing RBC content ≥ 50%) with cross-sectional diameter 4–10 μm was sharply reduced for active COVID-19 patients versus controls, with values for long COVID patients roughly halfway between those for active COVID-19 patients and healthy controls. The study investigators concluded from these and other measures of microvascular health that the long COVID patients had significant microvasculature impairment, lasting even 18 months after infection for some.[203]

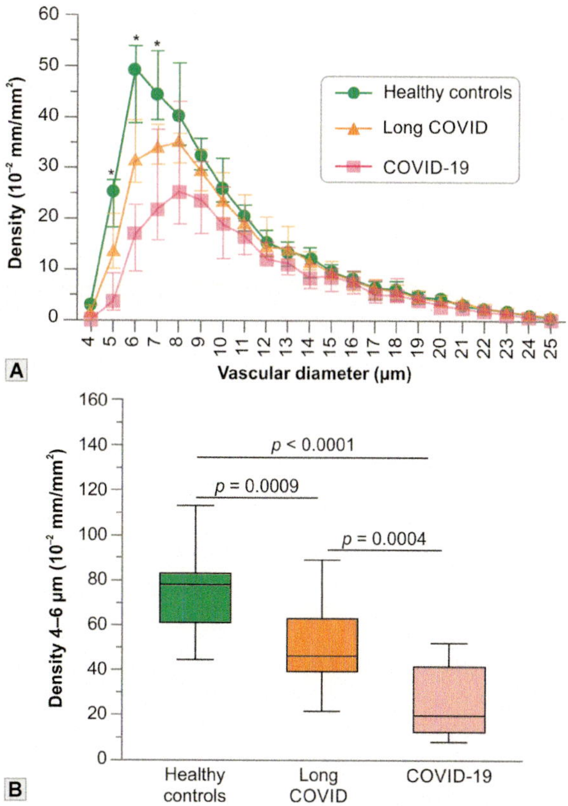

FIGURES 4A AND B: Density of functional capillaries (with flowing RBC content ≥ 50%) of cross-sectional diameter 4–25 µm in the sublingua of long and active, hospitalized COVID-19 patients and healthy controls. (A) Functional capillary density by diameter;* denotes $q < 0.05$ (q per Storey-Tibshirani). (B) Functional capillary density for capillaries of diameter 4–6 µm. Mean values for healthy controls and long and active COVID-19 patients were 77.9, 46.4 and 19.9, respectively, with $p < 0.001$ for comparisons between each pair of patient groups.
Source: Reproduced from Osiaevi et al. (2023)[203] (CC-BY 4.0).

Rovas et al. (2021) reported similar sharp reductions in densities of functional capillaries at the lower end of the 4–25 µm cross-sectional diameter range in the sublingual microvasculature of COVID-19 patients versus healthy controls.[201] The extent of reduction in density of functional capillaries of diameter 4–6 µm in the COVID-19 patients correlated with their oxygenation index (PaO_2/FiO_2) and with an index of multiorgan failure and associated mortality risk. Rovas et al. concluded from these correlations that the observed reduction in sublingual small capillary density was another manifestation of the pathological clogging of capillaries as also observed in pulmonary microthrombi at autopsies of COVID-19 patients. A similar marked shift in blood flow from smaller to larger vessels in active[204–207] and long[208] COVID-19 patients was also observed in blood vessels of larger cross-sectional diameter, 1 mm and greater, using high-resolution CT scans.

Further insights into the prevalence of microvascular occlusion in both active and long COVID-19 were provided by studies that imaged the ocular conjunctiva and retina in human subjects using noninvasive techniques. As noted previously, the percentage of occluded microvessels in the conjunctiva was found to be six times as high in hospital-discharged COVID-19 patients versus healthy controls,[209] while other studies reported that RBC aggregation in the conjunctiva correlated closely with measures of that elsewhere in the body.[158,175] Three studies of perfusion density in various retinal capillary layers found small (e.g., 3–4%) but statistically significant differences (e.g., $p = 0.011$, $p = 0.04$, $p = 0.003$) for COVID-19 patients one month after recovery[210,211] and for long COVID patients[212] versus healthy controls. Retinal capillary perfusion density was determined with optical coherence tomography angiography (OCT-A), which uses noninvasive laser imaging of RBC flow in retinal capillaries to detect perfusion aberrations.

Major Risk Factors of Age, Diabetes and Obesity for COVID-19 Severity Correlate with Increased Propensity to RBC Aggregation

The most significant risk factor for severe COVID-19 is age, with several studies showing a multifold increased risk of fatal outcomes with older age.[195,213,214] One multivariate analysis of 17 million subjects in the UK reported a sixfold increased mortality for ages 70 through 79 versus 50 through 59 years.[215] A meta-analysis of 612,000 subjects in several countries conducted in 2020 found a mortality rate of 22.8% for ages 70–79 years versus 0.3% for ages ≤29 years.[216] Note that the risk factor data considered in this section are for pre-Omicron variants of SARS-CoV-2. Since Omicron variants do not penetrate deeply into the lungs or bloodstream and cause less severe illness than prior variants, as considered in the discussion section, risk factors for Omicron infections are not necessarily the same as those for pre-Omicron variants nor is the efficacy of various therapeutics.

This multifold increase in COVID-19 mortality with older age aligns with a much greater extent of microvascular occlusion in older versus younger healthy subjects, linked to both a significantly greater propensity to RBC aggregation and slower blood flow with increased age. Microscopic examinations of the bulbar conjunctiva of healthy subjects found that 30% of those of ages 56–75 years had aggregation in the smaller venules and capillaries, as compared with a 3% rate of such aggregation of those of ages 16–35 years.[190] This tenfold increased rate of microvascular occlusion in the older subjects corresponds to much greater RBC aggregation and slower blood flow with increased age. One study that measured RBC aggregability by multiple detection methods found a statistically significant increase in this value in the blood of middle-aged versus young adults.[217] Another study found highly significant ($p < 0.001$) increases in RBC aggregability and average RBC aggregate size for subjects of ages 66–89 versus those of 20–30 years.[218] Both of these studies measured RBC aggregability in vitro using drawn blood.

As noted, RBC aggregate formation in vivo depends not only on aggregability under static conditions but also on the degree of shear forces that promote disaggregation, as associated with velocity of blood flow.[164,168-170] It is, thus, noteworthy that blood flow is slower with increased age.[219-225] Mean velocity of capillary flow under fingernail and toenails for subjects of mean age 63 years was half of that for subjects of mean age 26 years.[219] Older subjects had 23%[220] and 40%[221] diminished flow velocities versus younger subjects for capillary flow in other tissues. Arterial blood flow velocities were 26–27% lower for older versus younger subjects in two studies.[223,224] The combined effects of increased RBC aggregability and decreased blood flow velocity would appear to account for the tenfold incidence of microvascular occlusion in smaller venules and capillaries of the bulbar conjunctiva with increased age, as noted above.

In a multivariate analysis of COVID-19 risk factors for 17 million patients in the UK, mortality was increased with hazard ratios of 1.31 for diabetic patients with good glucose control, 1.95 for diabetic patients with poor glucose control and 1.92 for obesity.[215] An umbrella review of 32 high- or moderate-quality reviews reported odds ratios for mortality of 2.09 for diabetes and 2.18 for obesity.[226] A significant degree of RBC aggregation is characteristic of diabetes,[167,177,191,193,194] with this effect especially pronounced for type 1 disease[191] and for diabetic patients with poor glycemic control.[193] In studies of RBC attributes for subjects of varying body mass index (BMI), BMI correlated with RBC adhesiveness/aggregability at $p < 0.001$, while obese subjects had larger RBC aggregates ($p < 0.009$) that were more resistant to dispersion by flow.[227,228] In summary, three major risk factors for severe COVID-19—increased age, diabetes and obesity—were all characterized by increased RBC aggregability, with this correlation especially striking for age.

SARS-CoV-2 SP Unattached to Whole Virus Induces Microvascular Occlusion In Vivo

Akin to the studies noted previously demonstrating induction of RBC clumping by SARS-CoV-2 SP in vitro[91,100,229] and in vivo,[103] other studies likewise demonstrate that SARS-CoV-2 SP in the absence of whole virus caused microvascular occlusion.

Myocardial Damage as a Signal of Microvascular Occlusion

A clinical window into morbidities associated with RBC aggregation is provided by the myocardium—the heart muscle—which is among the tissues most susceptible to the damaging effects of experimentally induced RBC aggregation and ensuing microvascular occlusion. Several studies found that injection of HMWD caused myocardial damage[144,146,154,230] and/or electrocardiogram (ECG) changes[153,154,187,230] characteristic of myocarditis. In one study, 40 minutes after HMWD injection, ECG abnormalities were apparent, and HMWD induced lasting myocardial damage.[230] Both the degree of myocardial damage[144,146] and of ECG abnormalities[153] correlated with the extent of microvascular occlusion. Clinically, for hospitalized patients with coronary heart disease, the number of microthrombi per field of observation in the bulbar conjunctival microcirculation was found to be correlated with both the extent of ECG and symptomatic abnormalities.[153]

Myocardial Damage Experimentally Induced by SARS-CoV-2 SP in the Absence of Whole Virus

Induction of myocarditis by SARS-CoV-2 SP in the absence of whole virus was evidenced in two rodent studies by IV injection of BNT162b2, the Pfizer-BioNTech mRNA vaccine, an experimental system in which SP is generated by host cells, distinct from intramuscular (IM) injection used for clinically administered COVID-19 vaccinations. Clinical cases of SARS-CoV-2 SP found in endothelial cells after IV mRNA vaccination[231–233] support the possibility that SP could be generated by nucleated endothelial cells in blood vessels post-vaccination. In mice, after a second IV vaccine dose, 67% had grossly visible white patches over the visceral pericardium and all showed changes of myopericarditis, compared with only mild degenerative changes in the myocardium in the intramuscular (IM)-injection group.[234] All of the mice in the IV-injection and the IM-injection groups had myocardial WBC infiltration and cardiomyocyte degeneration and necrosis versus none in saline-injection controls. Rats given two IV doses of BNT162b2 vaccine two weeks apart in another study manifested marked blood hypercoagulability along with apoptotic cardiac muscle fibers, ECG changes and other abnormalities that reflected myocardial injury.[235]

Clinical Signs of Microvascular Occlusion and Myocarditis after Exposure to SARS-CoV-2 SP

Further insights into microvascular occlusion caused by SARS-CoV-2 SP in the absence of whole virus in a clinical setting were provided by OCT-A imaging of the retinal microvasculature. Determinations of the vascular density (VD) of flowing blood vessels in various retinal layers of human subjects, an indicator of microvascular occlusion, found that the CoronaVac vaccine, made from inactivated whole virus, caused no changes after vaccination.[236,237] The Pfizer-BioNTech mRNA vaccine caused small but statistically significant reductions in VD versus controls at three days[238] and at two and four weeks[237] after vaccination. Reductions in many of these VD values at two weeks after vaccination were statistically significant at $p < 0.001$; most of these resolved by four weeks after vaccination, but seven of these VD reductions persisted at statistically significant levels at that time.[237]

The significance of these findings derives not from the occasional ocular adverse effects that have been reported after mRNA COVID-19 vaccinations[239,240] but rather from indications that ocular microvascular occlusion mirrors a pathology elsewhere in the body.[158,175] Myocardial injury is another indicator of microvascular occlusion, as noted above, which opens another diagnostic window, PET-CT scanning, since fluorodeoxyglucose F 18 (FDG) uptake in myocardial tissue has been found to track myocardial injury.[241,242] In one study, 700 SARS-CoV-2-vaccinated and 303 nonvaccinated subjects were given PET/CT scans either to evaluate malignancies or perform other medical screenings unrelated to COVID-19 or myocarditis. In PET/CT scans taken 1–180 days after vaccination, myocardial FDG uptake was significantly higher as compared to that for unvaccinated subjects (median of 4.8 vs. 3.3, $p < 0.0001$).[243] Similar potential risks at a less than clinically overt level were indicated from cardiac test markers 2–10 weeks after COVID-19 mRNA vaccinations versus pre-vaccination values in 566 patients at a cardiac clinic, with an increase in the 5-year predicted risk of acute cardiac events from 11 to 25%.[244] Whether the clinical indicator is the rare incidence of myocarditis following COVID mRNA vaccinations [245,246] or the greater incidence of cardiac irregularities following such vaccinations, e.g., 1–7% rates of chest pains and abnormal ECG readings in two post-COVID vaccination studies in adolescents,[247,248] an association with the presence of SARS-CoV-2 SP in such adverse events is indicated. A study conducted in the US in Boston-area hospitals found that of 16 patients hospitalized for myocarditis after COVID-19 mRNA vaccinations, all had significant levels of SARS-CoV-2 SP unbound by antibodies in blood, whereas 45 asymptomatic, vaccinated subjects had no detectable SP.[249] Investigators at the same hospitals found indications that SARS-CoV-2 mRNA vaccines routinely persist up to 30 days following vaccination and are detectable in the heart.[250] SARS-CoV-2 SP was found on cardiomyocytes of 9 of 15 mRNA-vaccinated subjects with symptoms of myocarditis in another clinical series.[251]

Decreased Clinical Severity of COVID-19 by Agents that Inhibit RBC Aggregation

Analogous to the activity of LWMD (MW ≤ 40 kDa) in limiting and reversing induced RBC aggregation, as noted above, various forms of heparin and heparan sulfate, glycosaminoglycans of MW ≤ 30 kDa, have shown benefits by clinical or laboratory criteria for COVID-19 in a scattering of clinical studies. The specific agents used were subcutaneous heparin plus enoxaparin (low-MW heparin),[252] enoxaparin[122] and a low-MW mixture of 80% heparan sulfate and 20% dermatan sulfate (sulodexide).[123,253] As noted previously, both heparin and heparan sulfate bind strongly to SARS-CoV-2 SP.[103-105] Of particular interest as potential treatments for COVID-19 are three generic drugs which have been closely studied and have received wide attention.

Fluvoxamine

Fluvoxamine (FLV), a selective serotonin reuptake inhibitor (SSRI), attracted interest from prominent medical researchers[254-256] after early clinical trials indicated promising results for COVID-19 treatment.[257-260] Although rapid recovery from severe illness was not generally observed, one study showed a significant reduction in residual symptoms of COVID-19 at 14 days after start of FLV treatment versus untreated controls,[257] and another showed significant reductions in emergency room visits or hospitalizations.[259] Yet the puzzling question raised by these indications of clinical activity was by what biochemical mechanism could an SSRI used to treat depression and anxiety disorders offer therapeutic benefits against a viral disease?

A plausible biochemical mechanism is the sharp reduction by FLV in serum levels of serotonin, which is a powerful inducer of RBC and platelet aggregation. In vitro, serotonin caused marked aggregation of RBCs, platelets and leukocytes.[147] In vivo, injection of serotonin resulted in blood cell aggregates being trapped in small venules and capillaries in the ocular conjunctival vasculature.[147] In dogs, a serotonin antagonist prevented an increase in pulmonary alveolar dead space, an indication of pulmonary vascular obstruction, after hemorrhagic shock.[261]

Several studies have found that SSRIs, including FLV, sharply reduce serotonin levels in blood, with reductions in plasma serotonin levels to 20–40% of baseline values over 2–8 weeks being typical after the start of SSRI treatment.[262-268] All of these studies used high-performance liquid chromatography (HPLC) or enzyme-linked immunosorbent assay (ELISA) methodology for detection of serotonin plasma levels to avoid potential skewing of results from platelet uptake of serotonin.[256,267] For FLV in particular, mean plasma serotonin levels were reduced to 69% of the baseline value one hour after first dose of the drug.[263] A study of blood from humans and mice found that serotonin induced platelet aggregation[269] and platelet aggregation by arachidonic acid was decreased by 68% ($p = 0.00001$) in patients taking an SSRI versus controls.[270]

Hydroxychloroquine

The application of HCQ, an aminoquinoline, for treatment of COVID-19, as developed by an infectious disease team at Aix-Marseilles University in France,[271-273] has been the subject of significant controversy, a review of which is not attempted here. However, it is of note that HCQ has been found to have pronounced activity in reducing blood cell aggregation and associated microvascular occlusion. In 44 human subjects with vascular conditions including coronary artery and cerebrovascular disease, all having initial manifestations of microvascular occlusion, ocular conjunctival microvasculature was observed over a 9-month period following the start of HCQ treatment.[274] Marked reductions in the size of blood cell aggregates and the extent of microvascular occlusion were observed for most patients. Accompanying symptomatic improvements were observed in many of these subjects beginning three days after the start of HCQ treatment for some and persisting over the 9-month follow-up period.

In another human study, HCQ was administered over a 3-month period to 22 patients with rheumatoid arthritis who had signs of occlusion in the microcirculation of the ocular fundus. 20 of the 22 patients had complete normalization of the observed vasculature occlusion.[275] In mice previously injected with an RBC clumping agent, HCQ sharply reduced thrombus size and the time that thrombi persisted as compared with untreated controls.[276]

Ivermectin

To identify potential therapeutics for COVID-19, four in silico studies collectively screened over 1,000 molecules for binding to SARS-CoV-2 SP and other SARS-CoV-2 viral targets.[105,277-279] In each of these studies, the strongest or close-to-strongest binding affinity to SP was obtained for IVM, a macrocyclic lactone with multifaceted antiparasitic and antimicrobial activity, distributed in four billion doses for human diseases worldwide since 1987.[280-282] Aminpour et al. (2022) found by molecular docking computations that IVM binds with high affinity (<–7.0 kcal/mol) to seven sialoside-binding sites or other glycan-binding sites on SARS-CoV-2 S1, six on the N-terminal domain (NTD) and one on the receptor-binding domain (RBD). These binding energy values of <–7.0 kcal/mol were obtained for the RBD in both the open ("up") and closed ("down") positions.[99] As a measure of significance of this binding energy value, binding energies of <–7.0 kcal/mol predicted efficacy for a large set of HIV inhibitors with 98% sensitivity and 95% specificity in another study.[283] Additional molecular modeling studies of IVM binding to SARS-CoV-2 SP,[284-288] including one by Lehrer and Rheinstein (2020),[289] likewise found strong binding affinities for IVM.

Competitive binding by IVM to SP glycan-binding sites is thus a likely biochemical mechanism for the in vitro inhibition and reversal by IVM of aggregation of human RBCs by SARS-CoV-2 SP as noted above.[91] In early 2020, two Florida physicians, Jean-Jacques and Juliana Rajter, were intrigued by an indication of a clinical parallel to this in vitro effect—observations that several COVID-19 patients with severe respiratory impairment and SpO_2 deficits experienced normalized breathing function within 1–2 days after treatment with IVM.[290,291] Months later, Rajter et al. (2020) reported results of a propensity-matched case control study of COVID-19 patients treated with a low dose of IVM plus standard of care (SOC) at four Florida hospitals, which yielded a 40% reduction in mortality vs. controls given only SOC.[292] After that study was concluded, through mid-2021, >20 randomized controlled trials (RCTs) of IVM treatment of COVID-19 were conducted, with six of seven meta-analyses reporting notable reductions in deaths and with a mean 0.31 relative risk of mortality versus controls (a 69% reduction).[293]

By 2022, however, several other RCTs reported that IVM yielded no statistically significant benefits for COVID-19 treatment, as summarized in an August 2022 editorial which declared that it was "time to stop using ineffective COVID-19 drugs".[294] Curiously, however, the editorial prominently cited in support a June 2022 meta-analysis of 10 RCTs for IVM treatment of COVID-19 encompassing 3,472 patients[295] which actually reported as the first finding in its results section a twofold reduction in deaths in its pooled IVM treatment versus placebo groups (pooled log odds ratio of –0.67, 95% CI –1.20 to –0.13, with low heterogeneity). The mortality reduction was less (log OR –0.12) for the RCTs rated as having a low risk of bias, but included in that group, weighted to account for 63% of that pooled log OR, was a study of dubious credibility.

Coauthors of the aforementioned study, the TOGETHER trial,[296] have repeatedly refused to disclose four of their key outcome numbers, namely per protocol deaths and hospitalizations, treatment versus placebo,[297] which are of key importance given critiques of the primary outcome used in all arms of the TOGETHER trial by the US Food and Drug Administration[298] and National Institutes of Health.[299] Instead, a TOGETHER trial coauthor directed inquiring scientists to the ICODA data repository, listed as the data source in the study's data sharing statement.[297,300] After two months of futile attempts by scientists to obtain the data from ICODA, however, on 7 June 2022, an ICODA manager reported that the TOGETHER trial data were never held by that data repository and that she had instructed its authors to stop citing it as their data source.[297,301]

In another prominently cited RCT of IVM treatment of COVID-19 that reported negative conclusions,[302] IVM was substituted for placebo doses for 38 patients, a mistake caught a month later, and blinding was broken by use of sugar water as the placebo for one-third of the study's patients (liquid IVM has a bitter taste). Adverse events that are distinctive to the high IVM dose used (transient and noncritical) occurred at almost identical rates in the placebo and IVM arms, while over-the-counter sales of IVM surged in the study region during the study period.[303]

The RCT evidence for IVM-based treatments of COVID-19 is thus mixed; however, in rare cases, efficacy of a drug has been conclusively established without RCT findings when it has achieved consistent major clinical benefits in the face of an established baseline of null effect. For example, the 96% cure rate for peptic ulcers by a triple therapy achieved in a 1990 clinical trial[304] provided conclusive evidence of the therapy's efficacy, given a baseline of palliative but rarely curative results for that chronic condition.[305,306] The associated discovery of *H. pylori* as the underlying pathogen for peptic ulcers was honored with the Nobel prize for medicine in 2005.[307] For penicillin, early in vitro and mouse studies provided convincing indications of marked antibacterial activity. Alexander Fleming found in 1929 that transparent regions formed around penicillin embedded in agar plates of several species of cultured bacteria, indicating inhibition of bacterial growth.[308] In a 1940 study, almost all penicillin-treated mice survived when exposed to bacterial strains that consistently caused fatal infections in untreated control mice.[309] In the absence of RCT evidence, penicillin production was then ramped up to industrial scale, saving the lives of thousands of soldiers during World War II.[310]

For cases of moderate and severe COVID-19 in patients on room air, there is a consistent baseline of null effect in a 1–2 week timeframe: the magnitude of reductions in SpO_2 levels correlate with the extent of pulmonary damage, and neither of these normalize in that timeframe.[311-317] With that backdrop of null effect, as shown in **Figure 5**, three studies of severe COVID-19 patients on room air treated with IVM-based regimens observed sharp increases in SpO_2 after 1 day of treatment[318-321] while SpO_2 decreased during the same 1-day period in a fourth group of such patients under standard care. The two studies that used the triple therapy of IVM, doxycycline and zinc,[318,319] one of these coauthored by Thomas Borody,[319] who developed the successful triple therapy for *H. pylori*,[304] showed the most pronounced effect. For each of these three studies using IVM-based treatments, SpO_2 changes one day after treatment differed from those values for a comparison study of COVID-19

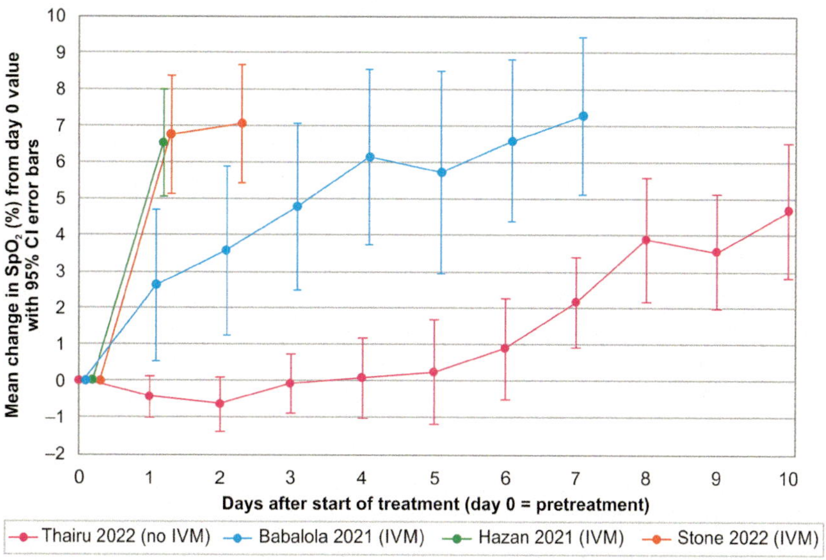

FIGURE 5: Mean changes in oxygen saturation (SpO_2) for severe COVID-19 patients following treatments including or excluding IVM. Reproduced from Stone et al. (2022)[318] (CC-BY 4.0). Patients tracked over various time periods from each regimen were those with SpO_2 values all recorded on room air, having pretreatment (day 0) values ≤ 93%. The y-axis value at day n is the mean of changes in SpO_2 values from day 0 to day n, with error bars designating 95% confidence intervals. • Thairu et al. (2022):[321,322] 26 patients, median age 45 years, treated with different combinations of lopinavir/ritonavir (Alluvia), remdesivir, azithromycin and enoxaparin as well as zinc sulfate and vitamin C. • Stone et al. (2022):[318] 34 patients, median age 56.5, treated with IVM, doxycycline and zinc. • Hazan et al. (2021):[319] 19 patients, median age 63, treated with IVM, doxycycline and zinc. • Babalola et al. (2021):[320,321] 19 patients, median age 33, treated with IVM, zinc and vitamin C, with some also given azithromycin and hydroxychloroquine.

patients on room air under standard care[321,322] with differences far outside the 95% confidence intervals for treatment versus control values.

For the Stone et al. (2022) study, taking into account some missing values for the 34 treated patients at <48 hours post-treatment, paired t-test calculations were performed for post-treatment minus pre-treatment SpO_2 values for the study patients at +12 hours, +24 hours, and +48 hours after the start of IVM administration. These paired t-test values were highly significant, with $p < 10^{-6}$ in each case. One patient in the study had an increase in SpO_2 from 79% recorded at the first IVM dose to 95% three hours later, and four other patients had increases of 12 or more in SpO_2% within 12 hours after the first IVM dose. These sharp, rapid improvements parallel the disaggregation of RBC clumps observed in vitro over the course of 30 minutes by Boschi et al. (2022) and can be explained by rapid clearance of RBC aggregates in the vasculature and corresponding increases in efficiency of oxygenation in pulmonary and extrapulmonary tissues.

In 2020, Peru provided a unique setting to track clinical efficacy of IVM-based treatment for COVID-19 with close consideration of confounding factors, using excess deaths data from its national health system, which aligned with WHO monthly summary data.[323] Treatment with IVM and adjunct agents was deployed at intensive, moderate or limited levels under semi-autonomous policies in its 25 states, enabling comparisons with reductions in excess deaths at 30 days after peak values, state by state. A Kendall tau calculation yields a two-tailed *p*-value of 0.002 for reductions in excess deaths correlated with level of IVM use in Peru's 25 states. On a national scale, during four months of IVM use in 2020, before a new president of Peru elected on November 17 restricted its use, there was a 14-fold reduction in nationwide excess deaths, and then a 13-fold increase in the two months following the restriction of IVM use.[323] This set of real-world national health data, accompanied by extensive additional data by which potential confounding influences can be tracked, provides another significant indication of efficacy of IVM treatment of COVID-19.

A Comparison of Degree of Clinical Susceptibility to COVID-19 and RBC Aggregability in Various Animal Species

Susceptibility to COVID-19 and severity of this disease have been tracked for dozens of mammalian species, as reported in a summary figure by Meekins et al. (2021).[324] RBC aggregability values and related values of blood viscosity at low shear velocity have been tracked for many mammalian species as well, as reported by Baskurt and Meiselman in 2013.[325] A correlation calculation between these two values, by species, provides a test of whether RBC aggregability is likely associated with COVID-19 morbidity.

The COVID status of mammalian species was reported by Meekins et al. using designators for viral shedding, clinical signs, mortality and transmission. We derived a composite COVID status index from the first three of these indicators (transmission was not used) with values of 0 for none of these three, 1 for viral shedding only, 2 for clinical signs and 3 for clinical signs and mortality. For RBC aggregability, an aggregation index shown in Baskurt and Meiselman for 22 mammalian species was used. They also reported values of blood viscosity under low-shear conditions for 27 mammalian species that were closely correlated with the corresponding RBC aggregation index for species having values shown in both figures. For a species tracked in Baskurt and Meiselman that reported blood viscosity but not RBC aggregability, the latter value was interpolated from the blood viscosity value. Correspondence between RBC aggregability and blood viscosity was established using the values of each for cattle and horses; these species had the minimum and maximum values of all species tracked by Baskurt and Meiselman, respectively, for both of these indices.

Table 1 shows the COVID status index and the RBC aggregability index, as described above, for the 13 species as tracked by both Meekins et al. and Baskurt and Meiselman, with the following adjustments: For the White-Tailed Deer as listed in Meekins et al., the mean of the RBC aggregation indices as interpolated from viscosity values for H. Deer, P.D. Deer and S. Deer (21.6,

TABLE 1: Indices of COVID-19 status and RBC aggregability for mammalian species.

Species	COVID index	RBC aggregation index
Domestic cat (Cat)	1 (V)	38.18
Malayan tiger (Tiger)	2 (VC)	35.10
Lion (Lion)	2 (VC)	37.58 *
Snow leopard (Leopard)	2 (C)	50.12 *
Domestic dog (Dog)	0	28.15
White-tailed deer (H. Deer, P.D. Deer, S. Deer) **	1 (V)	18.06 *
Domestic cattle (Cattle)	0	1.34
Domestic pig (Pig)	0	30.27
House mouse (Mouse)	0	0.18
Cottontail rabbit (Rabbit)	0	5.20
Common marmoset (Marmoset)	2 (C)	3.40 *
Sheep, domestic livestock (Sheep) ***	0	0.18
Goat, domestic livestock (Goat) ***	0	0.18
Kendall Tau	$\tau b = 0.52$	$p = 0.033$

* Value was interpolated from low-shear blood viscosity.

** RBC aggregation index is the mean of those for the three deer species listed.

*** COVID index values for these species were added as commonly reported in other sources.[329,330]

Note: COVID index from Meekins et al. (2021),[324] with RBC aggregation index for the matching species (listed in parentheses) from Baskurt and Meiselman 2013.[325] For COVID index, V = viral shedding, C = clinical signs; no matching species here was reported as having mortal cases.

23.5 and 9.1, respectively) reported by Baskurt and Meiselman was used. The contrast between high RBC aggregability in athletic species including horse, leopard and rhinoceros versus low RBC aggregability in sedentary species including domestic cattle, sheep and goats has been noted by several observers,[326–328] including Baskurt and Meiselman,[325] who furnished these values for all four species. The susceptibility of domestic sheep and goats, neither tracked by Meekins et al., is consistently reported to be the same (minimal[329,330]) as that for domestic cattle, and the COVID status index for these two species, 0—the same as the Meekins et al. value for domestic cattle—was, therefore, added.

Using the methodology described above to determine indices for COVID status index and RBC aggregation for 13 matching mammalian species, the Kendall tau two-tailed rank coefficient was calculated;[331] this statistical test was selected because COVID status was meaningful as a ranking rather than a numerical measure. This calculation demonstrated a moderately significant correlation ($p = 0.033$, $\tau b = 0.52$), which could be interpreted to indicate that RBC aggregation is a key determinant but not the exclusive causal factor for COVID-19 morbidity in mammals.

DISCUSSION

Consistent with coronavirus and RBC biochemistry established over past decades, the findings presented here demonstrate the central role of attachments from SARS-CoV-2 SP to sialylated glycans on RBCs and other blood cells in the severe morbidities of COVID-19. The glycans that decorate the SP of a coronavirus serve, metaphorically, as the virus's arms and legs, its appendages of initial attachment to a host cell. The RBC, with its million strands of GPA per cell, along with platelets, offers an "immune adherence" defense of pathogens which can bind to glycans.[72,82–88] The associated hemagglutination is observed for many strains of coronaviruses,[30,32,35–39,41,42] including SARS-CoV-2.[91]

Although these hemagglutinating properties of coronaviruses have been closely studied and the only known role of the GPA molecule on the RBC, the most abundant cell in the human body,[332,333] is for pathogen binding and clearance,[71,72,83,84] these glycan attachments have been largely overlooked in SARS-CoV-2 research. It is well established that RBCs, platelets and endothelial cells, which play key roles in COVID-19, are densely coated with sialylated glycans[64,65,70] but have no ACE2 (or, for endothelial cells, minimal ACE2[69]) and that the various coronavirus strains use several different host-cell receptors for replication,[30] yet ACE2 has been the exclusive host-cell target of interest in much of the research on SARS-CoV-2.

One explanation for this limited focus on the RBC and its pathogen-snagging GPA strands, one million per RBC, may be the lack of consensus on a solved structure of the extracellular domain of GPA.[334,335] Obstacles to this determination have been the extensive glycosylation of GPA, hindering the formation of a stable crystal for X-ray crystallography, and its intrinsically disordered structure[336,337] which allows a set of variable, extended and unfolded conformations.[338–340]

An overemphasis on the role of viral replication and associated viral load in the pathology of SARS-CoV-2 has led to questionable conclusions. As noted, for the five human betacoronaviruses, the two benign and three deadly strains are distinguished not by viral load, which is about the same for the two common cold strains and SARS-CoV-2,[55] but by the expression of the enzyme HE, which releases glycan attachments to viral SP, only in the common cold strains, not in SARS, SARS-CoV-2 and MERS.[50–54] For an agent for which competitive binding to SARS-CoV-2 SP glycan-binding sites has been indicated in silico,[99] IVM, one RCT tested it at a single low dose given on day 1 together with three other prophylactic regimens, each given daily for 42 days for prevention of COVID-19 infection.[341] The study concluded that IVM was ineffective because it yielded no significant reduction in viral load versus controls, yet IVM at that single dose reduced the incidence of symptomatic COVID-19 and acute respiratory distress syndrome (ARDS) each by half, with associated *p* values of 0.0034 and 0.012, respectively.[341]

Among the multifaceted demonstrations that SARS-CoV-2 SP-induced RBC aggregation and associated microvascular occlusion and hypoxia are central to severe morbidities of COVID-19, particularly informative are the countervailing effects of agents that inhibit glycan bindings of SP to RBCs. A mixture of heparan sulfate and heparin, both of which have strong binding affinity to SARS-CoV-2 SP,[103–105] markedly reduced SARS-CoV-2 SP-induced thrombosis in zebrafish.[103] As noted, the strongest or close-to-strongest binding affinity to SARS-CoV-2 SP in molecular modeling screenings of more than 1,000 total molecules was found for IVM.[105,277–279] Just as LMWD rapidly reversed HMWD- induced RBC aggregation in vitro[163] and in vivo,[148,155–158] IVM both blocked and reversed SARS-CoV-2 SP-induced hemagglutination in vitro.[91] This effect was paralleled in three clinical studies as shown in **Figure 5**, in which depressed SpO_2 values in severe COVID-19 patients on room air were sharply increased within 1–2 days[318–320] after the first IVM dose, in many cases within hours,[318] in contrast to a null effect under SOC treatment in the fourth study shown.

Neither fibrin-hardened blood clots nor the blockage of all blood flow in a small-diameter capillary by RBC clumps would be readily reversible by clump disaggregation, even if effectively achieved. Observations of the reversal of HMWD-induced blood cell clumping by LMWD, however, provide insights into how disaggregation of RBC clumps by agents that competitively bind to SARS-CoV-SP could rapidly normalize blood flow and oxygen levels in severe COVID-19 patients. In mammals, a distributed network of arterioles can hold a significant total mass of RBC clumps before obstruction of blood flow becomes critical, while a pulmonary catch-trap architecture can also sequester large blood cell aggregates.[167,178] The dynamic, reversible character of RBC clumps in vivo up to a point at which the extent of aggregation becomes critical is demonstrated in the LMWD disaggregation studies noted above. A direct in vitro parallel, as noted, is the reversal of hemagglutination induced by SARS-CoV-2 SP over the course of 30 minutes by IVM in vitro.[91] A similar effect is strikingly demonstrated in the hemagglutination assay for viruses that express an enzyme (HE or similar) that cleaves host cell glycans. An interlaced sheet of RBCs initially forms and then subsequently collapses as that enzyme breaks the glycan attachments between viral SP and RBCs.[31,32]

Although the central role of sialylated glycan bindings between SARS-CoV-2 SP and RBCs in the severe morbidities of COVID-19 has been the focus of this paper, such SP bindings to the heavily sialylated platelets and endothelial cells (which have no ACE2 and minimal ACE2, respectively) also contribute significantly to these morbidities, as noted above. Of particular interest is extensive damage to endothelial cells in severe COVID-19 patients, with an associated presence of SARS-CoV-2 virus and SP and elevated levels of VWF. As noted, an SA-cleaving enzyme was found to remove >50% of the glycocalyx of human kidney endothelial cells.[70]

This examination of attachments from SARS-CoV-2 SP to sialylated glycans of RBCs and other blood cells and endothelial cells was spurred in part by an examination of possible molecular mechanisms of IVM activity in COVID-19 treatment and prevention. This may seem curious, given a general perception that IVM is ineffective against COVID-19,[294] yet major irregularities in some of the best-known such studies with negative conclusions, as noted in section on IVM above, indicate that the RCT evidence is more accurately characterized as mixed. It was also noted that in rare cases, such as for the triple therapy for peptic ulcers and for penicillin, striking demonstrations of drug efficacy against a consistent baseline of null effect under standard care established drug efficacy without accompanying RCT evidence. The findings of four studies depicted in **Figure 5** appear to present a similar decisive demonstration of efficacy of IVM in treatment of pre-Omicron COVID infections.

The reports of distinguished scholars of scientific integrity, including current and past editors of leading scientific journals,[342-347] on the vulnerability of science to commodification[343,347] and "flagrant conflicts of interest"[342] are also useful to bear in mind as this evidence is sorted out. As one case in point, although the triple-therapy cure for *H. pylori* was rapidly deployed in Australia, preventing an estimated 18,665 deaths there between 1990 and 2015,[348] it was not widely used in the rest of the world until the late 1990s, after the patents for the two best-selling palliative drugs for that condition had expired.[349]

It is important to note, in evaluating drug treatment options for evolving COVID-19 variants, that Omicron viral strains, which became predominant in early 2022,[350] replicate less efficiently in the lung alveolar epithelium as compared with prior variants, in contrast to Omicron's faster replication in the bronchi.[351,352] The disruption of the alveolar–capillary barrier is a prime route by which SARS-CoV-2 enters the blood stream,[353] so limited replication of Omicron in alveolar tissue would limit viral loads in blood with associated reductions in RBC clumping and disease severity as caused by Omicron versus prior variants. Thus, although Boschi et al. (2022) reported a tenfold greater hemagglutinating activity of Omicron as compared with prior variants,[91] this would not appear to increase the severity of clinical infections, yet could possibly affect the incidence of adverse effects of COVID-19 booster vaccines for the Omicron variant, which have not been tested on human subjects.[354] Also, due to limited penetration by Omicron into the bloodstream, drugs that offer clinical benefits through reductions in RBC aggregation for pre-Omicron SARS-CoV-2 variants may not have significant efficacy against the less severe Omicron infections.

This has implications, for example, for evaluation of RCTs for FLV treatment of COVID-19, given that two recent such studies had substantial numbers of Omicron patients among their subjects.[355,356] On the other hand, IVM may maintain clinical efficacy against Omicron variants of SARS-CoV-2 though molecular mechanisms besides competitive inhibition of glycan bindings. For example, high-energy binding by IVM to the alpha-7 nicotinic acetylcholine receptor (α7nAChr), the main receptor activating the cholinergic anti-inflammatory pathway controlled by the vagus nerve,[99,357] was predicted in silico[99] and was confirmed experimentally in both human and animal cells.[358] Activation of the α7nAChr by IVM has been demonstrated to trigger a marked increase in Ca^{++} current evoked by acetylcholine (e.g., a 20-fold shift in the affinity of acetylcholine[358]) and, accordingly, may dramatically decrease excessive macrophage inflammation and tumor necrosis factor (TNF), which play a major role during the inflammatory phase of COVID-19 infection (i.e., the cytokine storm).[99,357,359] IVM binding to α7nAChr could also competitively inhibit viral penetration of macrophages and neuronal, endothelial and type II alveolar epithelial cells through this receptor.[99,357]

For long COVID-19 patients, the demonstrated persistent presence of SP and subunits in plasma[111-113] and monocytes,[114] respectively, and microvascular occlusion as seen in their sublingual vasculature[203] indicate an active therapeutic opportunity for drugs that limit SARS-CoV-2 SP binding to RBCs. Both OCT-A and video microscopic imaging of the sublingual microvasculature offer tools to track microvascular occlusion that typically occurs in long COVID patients and to track any improvements that may be provided by drugs, either those highlighted here or others, in clinical treatment as well as in research settings.

CONCLUSION

The central role of sialylated glycan attachments between SARS-CoV-2 SP and RBCs and other blood cells in the severe morbidities of COVID-19 is founded on well-established biochemistry of coronaviruses and RBCs and established here through multiple channels of substantiation. Many preclinical and clinical studies show that SARS-CoV-2 SP attaches to and aggregates RBCs.

Experimentally induced RBC clumping in vivo causes the same morbidities and the same redistribution of blood flow from smaller to larger blood vessels as for severe COVID-19. The key risk factors of increased age, diabetes and obesity for COVID-19 morbidity are each associated with significantly increased RBC aggregation. SARS-CoV-2 SP in the absence of whole virus as generated experimentally by IV injection of mRNA COVID vaccines in vivo, which caused SP to be generated in the absence of whole virus, induced microvascular occlusion.

Three generic agents which attracted prominent interest as COVID-19 therapeutics all yielded significant reductions in RBC aggregation. For mammalian species, the degree of clinical susceptibility to COVID-19 correlates with the aggregation propensity of RBCs with $p = 0.033$. These in vitro, in vivo and clinical findings, together, provide a convincing demonstration that RBC aggregation induced by SARS-CoV-2 SP through sialylated glycan attachments and resulting microvascular occlusion is key to the morbidities of severe COVID-19. These insights can support therapeutic and preventative strategies for evolving variants of this disease and for long COVID, while imaging of the retinal or sublingual microvasculature of active or long COVID patients can provide important support to these efforts.

Funding: This research received no external funding.

Institutional Review Board Statement: Not applicable.

Informed Consent Statement: Not applicable.

Data Availability Statement: Not applicable.

Acknowledgments: The authors are grateful to the brothers Jerome Dancis (University of Maryland) and Barry Dancis for close editing and helpful comments in developing this manuscript.

REFERENCES

1. Gattinoni L, Gattarello S, Steinberg I, Busana M, Palermo P, Lazzari S, et al. COVID-19 pneumonia: pathophysiology and management. Eur Respir Rev. 2021;30(162):210138.
2. Poor HD. Pulmonary thrombosis and thromboembolism in COVID-19. Chest. 2021;160(4):1471-80.
3. Selickman J, Vrettou CS, Mentzelopoulos SD, Marini JJ. COVID-19-related ARDS: key mechanistic features and treatments. J Clin Med. 2022;11(16):4896.
4. Halawa S, Pullamsetti SS, Bangham CRM, Stenmark KR, Dorfmüller P, Frid MG, et al. Potential long-term effects of SARS-CoV-2 infection on the pulmonary vasculature: A global perspective. Nat Rev Cardiol. 2022;19(5):314-31.
5. Couzin-Frankel J. The mystery of the pandemic's 'happy hypoxia'. Science. 2020;368(6490):455-6.
6. Marini JJ, Gattinoni L. Management of COVID-19 respiratory distress. JAMA. 2020;323(22):2329-30.
7. Li H, Deng Y, Li Z, Dorken Gallastegi A, Mantzoros CS, Frydman GH, et al. Multiphysics and multiscale modeling of microthrombosis in COVID-19. PLOS Comput Biol. 2022;18(3):e1009892.

8. Rapkiewicz AV, Mai X, Carsons SE, Pittaluga S, Kleiner DE, Berger JS, et al. Megakaryocytes and platelet-fibrin thrombi characterize multi-organ thrombosis at autopsy in COVID-19: A case series. EClinicalMedicine. 2020;24:100434.
9. Wichmann D, Sperhake JP, Lütgehetmann M, Steurer S, Edler C, Heinemann A, et al. Autopsy findings and venous thromboembolism in patients with COVID-19: a Prospective Cohort Study. Ann Intern Med. 2020;173(4):268-77.
10. Ackermann M, Verleden SE, Kuehnel M, Haverich A, Welte T, Laenger F, et al. Pulmonary vascular endothelialitis, thrombosis, and angiogenesis in COVID-19. N Engl J Med. 2020;383(2):120-8.
11. Fox SE, Akmatbekov A, Harbert JL, Li G, Quincy Brown J, Vander Heide RS. Pulmonary and cardiac pathology in African American patients with COVID-19: an autopsy series from New Orleans. Lancet Respir Med. 2020;8(7):681-6.
12. Hanff TC, Mohareb AM, Giri J, Cohen JB, Chirinos JA. Thrombosis in COVID-19. Am J Hematol. 2020;95(12):1578-89.
13. Fahmy OH, Daas FM, Salunkhe V, Petrey JL, Cosar EF, Ramirez J, et al. Is microthrombosis the main pathology in coronavirus disease 2019 severity? A Systematic Review of the Postmortem Pathologic Findings. Crit Care Explor. 2021;3(5):e0427.
14. Menter T, Haslbauer JD, Nienhold R, Savic S, Hopfer H, Deigendesch N, et al. Postmortem examination of COVID-19 patients reveals diffuse alveolar damage with severe capillary congestion and variegated findings in lungs and other organs suggesting vascular dysfunction. Histopathology. 2020;77(2):198-209.
15. McFadyen JD, Stevens H, Peter K. The emerging threat of (micro)thrombosis in COVID-19 and its therapeutic implications. Circ Res. 2020;127(4):571-87.
16. Poh KC, Jia Tay VY, Lin SH, Chee HL, Thangavelautham S. A review of COVID-19-related thrombosis and anticoagulation strategies specific to the Asian population. Singapore Med J. 2022;63(7):350-61.
17. Bussani R, Schneider E, Zentilin L, Collesi C, Ali H, Braga L, et al. Persistence of viral RNA, pneumocyte syncytia and thrombosis are hallmarks of advanced COVID-19 pathology. EBiomedicine. 2020;61:103104.
18. Overton PM, Toshner M, Mulligan C, Vora P, Nikkho S, de Backer J, et al. the PVRI Innovative Drug Development Initiative. Pulmonary thromboembolic events in COVID-19—A systematic literature review. Pulm Circ. 2022;12:e12113.
19. Tang N, Li D, Wang X, Sun Z. Abnormal coagulation parameters are associated with poor prognosis in patients with novel coronavirus pneumonia. J Thromb Haemost. 2020;18(4):844-7.
20. Pellegrini D, Kawakami R, Guagliumi G, Sakamoto A, Kawai K, Gianatti A, et al. Microthrombi as a major cause of cardiac injury in COVID-19: A pathologic study. Circulation. 2021;143(10):1031-42.
21. Lowenstein CJ, Solomon SD. Severe COVID-19 is a microvascular disease. Circulation. 2020;142(17):1609-11.
22. Price LC, McCabe C, Garfield B, Wort SJ. Thrombosis and COVID-19 pneumonia: the clot thickens! Eur Respir J. 2020;56(1):2001608.
23. Lodigiani C, Lapichino G, Carenzo L, Cecconi M, Ferrazzi P, Sebastian T, et al. Venous and arterial thromboembolic complications in COVID-19 patients admitted to an academic hospital in Milan, Italy. Thromb Res. 2020;191:9-14.
24. Magro C, Mulvey JJ, Berlin D, Nuovo G, Salvatore S, Harp J, et al. Complement associated microvascular injury and thrombosis in the pathogenesis of severe COVID-19 infection: A report of five cases. Transl Res. 2020;220:1-13.
25. Gómez J, Albaiceta GM, García-Clemente M, López-Larrea C, Amado-Rodríguez L, Lopez-Alonso I, et al. Angiotensin-converting enzymes (ACE, ACE2) gene variants and COVID-19 outcome. Gene. 2020;762:145102.

26. Aung AK, Aitken T, Teh BM, Yu C, Ofori-Asenso R, Chin KL, et al. Angiotensin converting enzyme genotypes and mortality from COVID-19: an ecological study. J Infect. 2020;81(6):961-5.
27. Abassi Z, Higazi AAR, Kinaneh S, Armaly Z, Skorecki K, Heyman SN. ACE2, COVID-19 infection, inflammation, and coagulopathy: missing pieces in the puzzle. Front Physiol. 2020;11:574753.
28. Kong W, Montano M, Corley MJ, Helmy E, Kobayashi H, Kinisu M, et al. Neuropilin-1 mediates SARS-CoV-2 infection of astrocytes in brain organoids, inducing inflammation leading to dysfunction and death of neurons. mBio. 2022;13(6):e0230822.
29. Cantuti-Castelvetri L, Ojha R, Pedro LD, Djannatian M, Franz J, Kuivanen S, et al. Neuropilin-1 facilitates SARS-CoV-2 cell entry and infectivity. Science. 2020;370(6518):856-60.
30. Hulswit RJG, de Haan CAM, Bosch BJ. Chapter 2: Coronavirus spike protein and tropism changes. In: Ziebuhr J, editor. Advances in virus research. Vol. 96. New York: Academic Press; 2016. pp. 29-57.
31. Scheim DE. A deadly embrace: hemagglutination mediated by SARS-CoV-2 spike protein at its 22 N-glycosylation sites, red blood cell surface sialoglycoproteins, and antibody. Int J Mol Sci. 2022;23(5):2558.
32. Matrosovich M, Herrler G, Klenk HD. Sialic acid receptors of viruses. In: Gerardy-Schahn R, Delannoy P, von Itzstein M, editors. SialoGlyco chemistry and biology II: tools and techniques to identify and capture sialoglycans. New York: Springer International Publishing; 2015. pp. 1-28.
33. Tortorici MA, Walls AC, Lang Y, Wang C, Li Z, Koerhuis D, et al. Structural basis for human coronavirus attachment to sialic acid receptors. Nat Struct Mol Biol. 2019;26(6):481-9.
34. Unione L, Moure MJ, Lenza MP, Oyenarte I, Ereño-Orbea J, Ardá A, et al. The SARS-CoV-2 spike glycoprotein directly binds exogeneous sialic acids: a NMR view. Angew Chem Int Ed Engl. 2022;61(18):e202201432.
35. Kapikian AZ, James HD, Jr., Kelly SJ, King LM, Vaughn AL, Chanock RM. Hemadsorption by coronavirus strain OC43. Proc Soc Exp Biol Med. 1972;139(1):179-86.
36. Agafonov AP, Gus'kov AA, Ternovoi VA, Ryabchikova EI, Durymanov AG, Vinogradov IV, et al. Primary characterization of SARS coronavirus strain Frankfurt 1. Dokl Biol Sci. 2004;394(1):58-60.
37. Vlasak R, Luytjes W, Spaan W, Palese P. Human and bovine coronaviruses recognize sialic acid-containing receptors similar to those of influenza C viruses. Proc Natl Acad Sci U S A. 1988;85(12):4526-9.
38. Storz J, Zhang XM, Rott R. Comparison of hemagglutinating, receptor-destroying, and acetylesterase activities of avirulent and virulent bovine coronavirus strains. Arch Virol. 1992;125(1-4):193-204.
39. Brian DA, Hogue BG, Kienzle TE. The coronavirus hemagglutinin esterase glycoprotein. In: Siddell SG, editor. The Coronaviridae. The viruses. Boston: Springer; 1995.
40. Qing E, Hantak M, Perlman S, Gallagher T. Distinct roles for sialoside and protein receptors in coronavirus infection. mBio. 2020;11(1):e02764-19.
41. Schultze B, Cavanagh D, Herrler G. Neuraminidase treatment of avian infectious bronchitis coronavirus reveals a hemagglutinating activity that is dependent on sialic acid-containing receptors on erythrocytes. Virology. 1992;189(2):792-4.
42. Li W, Hulswit RJG, Widjaja I, Raj VS, McBride R, Peng W, et al. Identification of sialic acid-binding function for the Middle East respiratory syndrome coronavirus spike glycoprotein. Proc Natl Acad Sci U S A. 2017;114(40):E8508-17.
43. Hulswit RJG, Lang Y, Bakkers MJG, Li W, Li Z, Schouten A, et al. Human coronaviruses OC43 and HKU1 bind to 9-O-acetylated sialic acids via a conserved receptor-binding site in spike protein domain A. Proc Natl Acad Sci U S A. 2019;116(7):2681-90.

44. Neu U, Bauer J, Stehle T. Viruses and sialic acids: rules of engagement. Curr Opin Struct Biol. 2011;21(5):610-8.
45. Huang X, Dong W, Milewska A, Golda A, Qi Y, Zhu QK, et al. Human coronavirus HKU1 spike protein uses O-acetylated sialic acid as an attachment receptor determinant and employs hemagglutinin-esterase protein as a receptor-destroying enzyme. J Virol. 2015;89(14):7202-13.
46. Park YJ, Walls AC, Wang Z, Sauer MM, Li W, Tortorici MA, et al. Structures of MERS-CoV spike glycoprotein in complex with sialoside attachment receptors. Nat Struct Mol Biol. 2019;26(12):1151-7.
47. Wielgat P, Rogowski K, Godlewska K, Car H. Coronaviruses: is sialic acid a gate to the eye of cytokine storm? From the entry to the effects. Cells. 2020;9(9):1963.
48. Koehler M, Delguste M, Sieben C, Gillet L, Alsteens D. Initial step of virus entry: Virion binding to cell-surface glycans. Annu Rev Virol. 2020;7(1):143-65.
49. Ströh LJ, Stehle T. Glycan engagement by viruses: receptor switches and specificity. Annu Rev Virol. 2014;1(1):285-306.
50. Chan JF-W, Kok KH, Zhu Z, Chu H, To KK-W, Yuan S, et al. Genomic characterization of the 2019 novel human-pathogenic coronavirus isolated from a patient with atypical pneumonia after visiting Wuhan. Emerg Microbes Infect. 2020;9(1):221-36.
51. Chen Y, Liu Q, Guo D. Emerging coronaviruses: genome structure, replication, and pathogenesis. J Med Virol. 2020;92(4):418-23.
52. Zaki AM, van Boheemen S, Bestebroer TM, Osterhaus AD, Fouchier RA. Isolation of a novel coronavirus from a man with pneumonia in Saudi Arabia. N Engl J Med. 2012;367(19):1814-20.
53. Kumar S, Nyodu R, Maurya VK, Saxena SK, Morphology, Genome Organization. Replication, and pathogenesis of severe acute respiratory syndrome coronavirus 2 (SARS-CoV-2). In: Saxena SK (Editor). In Coronavirus Disease 2019 (COVID-19): Epidemiology, Pathogenesis, Diagnosis, and Therapeutics; Saxena: Singapore 2020; pp. 23-31.
54. Yoshimoto FK. The proteins of severe acute respiratory syndrome Coronavirus-2 (SARS-CoV-2 or n-COV19), the cause of COVID-19. Protein J. 2020;39(3):198-216.
55. Jacot D, Greub G, Jaton K, Opota O. Viral load of SARS-CoV-2 across patients and compared to other respiratory viruses. Microbes Infect. 2020;22(10):617-21.
56. Shajahan A, Supekar NT, Gleinich AS, Azadi P. Deducing the N- and O-glycosylation profile of the spike protein of novel coronavirus SARS-CoV-2. Glycobiology. 2020;30(12):981-8.
57. Guo W, Lakshminarayanan H, Rodriguez-Palacios A, Salata RA, Xu K, Draz MS. Glycan nanostructures of human coronaviruses. Int J Nanomedicine. 2021;16:4813-30.
58. Choi YK, Cao Y, Frank M, Woo H, Park SJ, Yeom MS, et al. Structure, dynamics, receptor binding, and antibody binding of the fully glycosylated full-length SARS-CoV-2 spike protein in a viral membrane. J Chem Theor Comput. 2021;17(4):2479-87.
59. Baker AN, Richards SJ, Guy CS, Congdon TR, Hasan M, Zwetsloot AJ, et al. The SARS-CoV-2 spike protein binds sialic acids and enables rapid detection in a lateral flow point of care diagnostic device. ACS Cent Sci. 2020;6(11):2046-52.
60. Lardone RD, Garay YC, Parodi P, de la Fuente S, Angeloni G, Bravo EO, et al. How glycobiology can help us treat and beat the COVID-19 pandemic. J Biol Chem. 2021;296:100375.
61. Gao C, Zeng J, Jia N, Stavenhagen K, Matsumoto Y, Zhang H, et al. SARS-CoV-2 spike protein interacts with multiple innate immune receptors. bioRxiv. 2020.
62. Chen W, Hui Z, Ren X, Luo Y, Shu J, Yu H, et al. The N-glycosylation sites and Glycan-binding ability of S-protein in SARS-CoV-2 coronavirus. bioRxiv. 2020.

63. Casalino L, Gaieb Z, Goldsmith JA, Hjorth CK, Dommer AC, Harbison AM, et al. Beyond shielding: the roles of glycans in the SARS-CoV-2 spike protein. ACS Cent Sci. 2020;6(10):1722-34.
64. Hyvärinen S, Meri S, Jokiranta TS. Disturbed sialic acid recognition on endothelial cells and platelets in complement attack causes atypical hemolytic uremic syndrome. Blood. 2016;127(22):2701-10.
65. Kasinrerk W, Tokrasinwit N, Phunpae P. CD147 monoclonal antibodies induce homotypic cell aggregation of monocytic cell line U937 via LFA-1/ICAM-1 pathway. Immunology. 1999;96(2):184-92.
66. Campbell RA, Boilard E, Rondina MT. Is there a role for the ACE2 receptor in SARS-CoV-2 interactions with platelets? J Thromb Haemost. 2021;19(1):46-50.
67. Cosic I, Cosic D, Loncarevic I. RRM prediction of erythrocyte Band3 Protein as Alternative Receptor for SARS-CoV-2 Virus. Appl Sci. 2020;10(11):4053.
68. Scheim DE. From Cold to Killer: How SARS-CoV-2 Evolved without Hemagglutinin Esterase to Agglutinate, Then Clot Blood Cells in Pulmonary and Systemic Microvasculature. OSF Preprints. Available online: https://osf.io/sgdj2 [accessed on 30 October 2023].
69. Ahmetaj-Shala B, Vaja R, Atanur S, George P, Kirkby N, Mitchell J. Systemic analysis of putative SARS-CoV-2 entry and processing genes in cardiovascular tissues identifies a positive correlation of BSG with age in endothelial cells. bioRxiv. 2020.
70. Singh A, Satchell SC, Neal CR, McKenzie EA, Tooke JE, Mathieson PW. Glomerular endothelial glycocalyx constitutes a barrier to protein permeability. J Am Soc Nephrol. 2007;18(11):2885-93.
71. Viitala J, Järnefelt J. The red cell surface revisited. Trends Biochem Sci. 1985;10(10):392-5.
72. Baum J, Ward RH, Conway DJ. Natural selection on the erythrocyte surface. Mol Biol Evol. 2002;19(3):223-9.
73. Levine S, Levine M, Sharp KA, Brooks DE. Theory of the electrokinetic behavior of human erythrocytes. Biophys J. 1983;42(2):127-35.
74. Aoki T. A comprehensive review of our current understanding of red blood cell (RBC) glycoproteins. Membranes. 2017;7(4):56.
75. Zhou D. Why are glycoproteins modified by poly-N-acetyllactosamine glycoconjugates? Curr Protein Pept Sci. 2003;4(1):1-9.
76. Fukuda M, Dell A, Oates JE, Fukuda MN. Structure of branched lactosaminoglycan, the carbohydrate moiety of band 3 isolated from adult human erythrocytes. J Biol Chem. 1984;259(13):8260-73.
77. Bua RO, Messina A, Sturiale L, Barone R, Garozzo D, Palmigiano A. N-Glycomics of human erythrocytes. Int J Mol Sci. 2021;22(15):8063.
78. Liukkonen J, Haataja S, Tikkanen K, Kelm S, Finne J. Identification of N-acetylneuraminyl alpha 2-->3 poly-N-acetyllactosamine glycans as the receptors of sialic acid-binding Streptococcus suis strains. J Biol Chem. 1992;267(29):21105-11.
79. Nycholat CM, McBride R, Ekiert DC, Xu R, Rangarajan J, Peng W. et al. Recognition of sialylated poly-N-acetyllactosamine chains on N- and O-linked glycans by human and avian influenza A virus hemagglutinins|A Virus Hemagglutinins. Angew Chem Int Ed Engl. 2012;51(20):4860-3.
80. Paul RW, Lee PWK. Glycophorin is the reovirus receptor on human erythrocytes. Virology. 1987;159(1):94-101.
81. Korhonen TK, Haahtela K, Pirkola A, Parkkinen JA. A N-acetyllactosamine-specific cell-binding activity in a plant pathogen, Erwinia rhapontici. FEBS Lett. 1988;236(1):163-6.
82. Nelson DS. Immune adherence. In: Dixon FJ, Humphrey JH, (editors). Advances in Immunology Volume 3. Vol. 3. Cambridge, MA: Academic Press; 1963. pp. 131-80.
83. Anderson HL, Brodsky IE, Mangalmurti NS. The evolving erythrocyte: red blood cells as modulators of innate immunity. J Immunol. 2018;201(5):1343-51.

84. Varki A, Gagneux P. Multifarious roles of sialic acids in immunity. Ann N Y Acad Sci. 2012;1253(1):16-36.
85. Nelson RA. The immune-adherence phenomenon: an immunologically specific reaction between microorganisms and erythrocytes leading to enhanced phagocytosis. Science. 1953;118(3077):733-7.
86. De Back DZ, Kostova E, Klei T, Beuger B, van Zwieten R, Kuijpers T, et al. RBC adhesive capacity is essential for efficient 'immune adherence clearance' and provide a generic target to deplete pathogens from septic patients. Blood. 2016;128(22):1031.
87. Siegel I, Lin Liu T, Gleicher N. The red-cell immune system. Lancet. 1981;318(8246):556-9.
88. Stocker TJ, Ishikawa-Ankerhold H, Massberg S, Schulz C. Small but mighty: platelets as central effectors of host defense. Thromb Haemost. 2017;117(4):651-61.
89. Salinas ND, Tolia NH. Red cell receptors as access points for malaria infection. Curr Opin Hematol. 2016;23(3):215-23.
90. Sikora M, von Bülow S, Blanc FEC, Gecht M, Covino R, Hummer G. Computational epitope map of SARS-CoV-2 spike protein. PLOS Comput Biol. 2021;17(4):e1008790.
91. Boschi C, Scheim DE, Bancod A, Militello M, Bideau ML, Colson P, et al. SARS-CoV-2 spike protein induces hemagglutination: implications for COVID-19 morbidities and therapeutics and for vaccine adverse effects. Int J Mol Sci. 2022;23(24):15480.
92. Reid ME, Mohandas N. Red blood cell blood group antigens: structure and function. Semin Hematol. 2004;41(2):93-117.
93. Pretini V, Koenen MH, Kaestner L, Fens MHAM, Schiffelers RM, Bartels M et al. Red blood cells: chasing interactions. Front Physiol. 2019;10:945.
94. Jaskiewicz E, Jodłowska M, Kaczmarek R, Zerka A. Erythrocyte glycophorins as receptors for Plasmodium merozoites. Parasit Vectors. 2019;12(1):317.
95. Varki A, Schnaar RL, Schauer R. Chapter 15: Sialic acids and other nonulosonic acids. In: Varki A, Cummings R, Esko J (editors). Essentials of glycobiology, 3rd ed. Cold Spring Harbor, NY: Cold Spring Harbor Laboratory Press; 2017.
96. Soares CO, Grosso AS, Ereño-Orbea J, Coelho H, Marcelo F. Molecular recognition insights of sialic acid glycans by distinct receptors unveiled by NMR and molecular modeling. Front Mol Biosci. 2021;8:727847.
97. Cohen M, Varki A. Chapter 3: Modulation of glycan recognition by clustered saccharide patches. In: Jeon KW (editor). International review of cell and molecular biology. Vol. 308. Cambridge, MA: Academic Press; 2014. pp. 75-125.
98. Cohen M, Varki A. The sialome—far more than the sum of its parts. Omics. 2010;14(4):455-64.
99. Aminpour M, Cannariato M, Preto J, Safaeeardebili ME, Moracchiato A, Doria D, et al. In silico analysis of the multi-targeted mode of action of ivermectin and related compounds. Computation. 2022;10(4):51.
100. Grobbelaar LM, Venter C, Vlok M, Ngoepe M, Laubscher GJ, Lourens PJ, et al. SARS-CoV-2 spike protein S1 induces fibrin(ogen) resistant to fibrinolysis: implications for microclot formation in COVID-19. Biosci Rep. 2021;41(8).
101. Yamakawa N, Vanbeselaere J, Chang LY, Yu SY, Ducrocq L, Harduin-Lepers A, et al. Systems glycomics of adult zebrafish identifies organ-specific sialylation and glycosylation patterns. Nat Commun. 2018;9(1):4647.
102. Au SH, Storey BD, Moore JC, Tang Q, Chen YL, Javaid S, et al. Clusters of circulating tumor cells traverse capillary-sized vessels. Proc Natl Acad Sci U S A. 2016;113(18):4947-52.
103. Zheng Y, Zhao J, Li J, Guo Z, Sheng J, Ye X, et al. SARS-CoV-2 spike protein causes blood coagulation and thrombosis by competitive binding to heparan sulfate. Int J Biol Macromol. 2021;193(B):1124-9.
104. Gupta Y, Maciorowski D, Zak SE, Kulkarni CV, Herbert AS, Durvasula R, et al. Heparin: A simplistic repurposing to prevent SARS-CoV-2 transmission in light of its in-vitro nanomolar efficacy. Int J Biol Macromol. 2021;183:203-12.

105. Dayer MR. Coronavirus (SARS-CoV-2) deactivation via spike glycoprotein shielding by old drugs: molecular docking approach. J Epigenet. 2021;2:31-8.
106. Melkumyants A, Buryachkovskaya L, Lomakin N, Antonova O, Serebruany V. Mild COVID-19 and impaired blood cell–endothelial crosstalk: considering long-term use of antithrombotics? Thromb Haemost. 2022;122(1):123-30.
107. Berzuini A, Bianco C, Migliorini AC, Maggioni M, Valenti L, Prati D. Red blood cell morphology in patients with COVID-19-related anaemia. Blood Transfus. 2021;19(1):34-6.
108. Ogata AF, Maley AM, Wu C, Gilboa T, Norman M, Lazarovits R, et al. Ultra-sensitive serial profiling of SARS-CoV-2 antigens and antibodies in plasma to understand disease progression in COVID-19 patients with severe disease. Clin Chem. 2020;66(12):1562-72.
109. Perico L, Morigi M, Galbusera M, Pezzotta A, Gastoldi S, Imberti B, et al. SARS-CoV-2 spike Protein 1 activates microvascular endothelial cells and complement system leading to platelet aggregation. Front Immunol. 2022;13:827146.
110. Nuovo GJ, Magro C, Shaffer T, Awad H, Suster D, Mikhail S, et al. Endothelial cell damage is the central part of COVID-19 and a mouse model induced by injection of the S1 subunit of the spike protein. Ann Diagn Pathol. 2021;51:151682.
111. Swank Z, Senussi Y, Manickas-Hill Z, Yu XG, Li JZ, Alter G, et al. Persistent circulating SARS-CoV-2 spike Is associated with post-acute COVID-19 sequelae. Clin Infect Dis. 2022;76:e487-90.
112. Craddock V, Mahajan A, Spikes L, Krishnamachary B, Ram AK, Kumar A, et al. Persistent circulation of soluble and extracellular vesicle-linked Spike protein in individuals with postacute sequelae of COVID-19. J Med Virol. 2023;95(2):e28568.
113. Schultheiß C, Willscher E, Paschold L, Gottschick C, Klee B, Bosurgi L, et al. Liquid biomarkers of macrophage dysregulation and circulating spike protein illustrate the biological heterogeneity in patients with post-acute sequelae of COVID-19.
114. Patterson BK, Francisco EB, Yogendra R, Long E, Pise A, Rodrigues H, et al. Persistence of SARS-CoV-2 S1 protein in CD16+ monocytes in post-acute sequelae of COVID-19 (PASC) up to 15 months postinfection. Front Immunol. 2022;12:5526.
115. Rajah MM, Bernier A, Buchrieser J, Schwartz O. The mechanism and consequences of SARS-CoV-2 spike-mediated fusion and syncytia formation. J Mol Biol. 2022;434(6):167280.
116. Cattin-Ortolá J, Welch LG, Maslen SL, Papa G, James LC, Munro S. Sequences in the cytoplasmic tail of SARS-CoV-2 Spike facilitate expression at the cell surface and syncytia formation. Nat Commun. 2021;12(1):5333.
117. Duan L, Zheng Q, Zhang H, Niu Y, Lou Y, Wang H. The SARS-CoV-2 spike glycoprotein biosynthesis, structure, function, and antigenicity: implications for the design of spike-based vaccine immunogens. Front Immunol. 2020;11:576622.
118. Lam LKM, Reilly JP, Rux AH, Murphy SJ, Kuri-Cervantes L, Weisman AR, et al. Erythrocytes identify complement activation in patients with COVID-19. Am J Physiol Lung Cell Mol Physiol. 2021;321(2):L485-9.
119. Wang K, Chen W, Zhang Z, Deng Y, Lian JQ, Du P, et al. CD147-spike protein is a novel route for SARS-CoV-2 infection to host cells. Signal Transduct Target Ther. 2020;5(1):283.
120. Hao W, Ma B, Li Z, Wang X, Gao X, Li Y, et al. Binding of the SARS-CoV-2 spike protein to glycans. Sci Bull (Beijing). 2021;66(12):1205-14.
121. Shilts J, Crozier TWM, Greenwood EJD, Lehner PJ, Wright GJ. No evidence for basigin/CD147 as a direct SARS-CoV-2 spike binding receptor. Sci Rep. 2021;11(1):413.
122. Buryachkovskaya L, Lomakin N, Melkumyants A, Docenko J, Ermishkin V, Serebruany V. Enoxaparin dose impacts blood cell phenotypes during mild SARS-CoV-2 infection: the observational single-center study. Rev Cardiovasc Med. 2021;22(4):1685-91.
123. Melkumyants A, Buryachkovskaya L, Lomakin N, Antonova O, Docenko J, Ermishkin V, et al. Effect of sulodexide on circulating blood cells in patients with mild COVID-19. J Clin Med. 2022;11(7):1995.

124. Favaron E, Ince C, Hilty MP, Ergin B, van der Zee P, Uz Z, et al. Capillary leukocytes, microaggregates, and the response to hypoxemia in the microcirculation of coronavirus disease 2019 patients. Crit Care Med. 2021;49(4):661-70.
125. Nader E, Nougier C, Boisson C, Poutrel S, Catella J, Martin F, et al. Increased blood viscosity and red blood cell aggregation in patients with COVID-19. Am J Hematol. 2022;97(3):283-92.
126. Petrilli CM, Jones SA, Yang J, Rajagopalan H, O'Donnell L, Chernyak Y, et al. Factors associated with hospital admission and critical illness among 5279 people with coronavirus disease 2019 in New York City: prospective cohort study. BMJ. 2020;369:m1966.
127. Koutsiaris AG, Riri K, Boutlas S, Panagiotou TN, Kotoula M, Daniil Z et al. COVID-19 hemodynamic and thrombotic effect on the eye microcirculation after hospitalization: A quantitative case-control study. Clin Hemorheol Microcirc. 2022;82(4):379-90.
128. Ko CJ, Harigopal M, Gehlhausen JR, Bosenberg M, McNiff JM, Damsky W. Discordant anti-SARS-CoV-2 spike protein and RNA staining in cutaneous perniotic lesions suggests endothelial deposition of cleaved spike protein. J Cutan Pathol. 2021;48(1):47-52.
129. Liu F, Han K, Blair R, Kenst K, Qin Z, Upcin B, et al. SARS-CoV-2 infects endothelial cells in vivo and in vitro. Front Cell Infect Microbiol. 2021;11:701278.
130. Magro CM, Mulvey JJ, Laurence J, Seshan S, Crowson AN, Dannenberg AJ, et al. Docked severe acute respiratory syndrome coronavirus 2 proteins within the cutaneous and subcutaneous microvasculature and their role in the pathogenesis of severe coronavirus disease 2019. Hum Pathol. 2020;106:106-16.
131. Perico L, Benigni A, Remuzzi G. SARS-CoV-2 and the spike protein in endotheliopathy. Trends Microbiol. 2023.
132. Goshua G, Pine AB, Meizlish ML, Chang CH, Zhang H, Bahel P, et al. Endotheliopathy in COVID-19-associated coagulopathy: evidence from a single-centre, cross-sectional study. Lancet Haematol. 2020;7(8):e575-82.
133. Huertas A, Montani D, Savale L, Pichon J, Tu L, Parent F, et al. Endothelial cell dysfunction: A major player in SARS-CoV-2 infection (COVID-19)? Eur Respir J. 2020;56(1):2001634.
134. Muhl L, He L, Sun Y, Andaloussi Mäe M, Pietilä R, Liu J, et al. The SARS-CoV-2 receptor ACE2 is expressed in mouse pericytes but not endothelial cells: implications for COVID-19 vascular research. Stem Cell Rep. 2022;17(5):1089-104.
135. Nicosia RF, Ligresti G, Caporarello N, Akilesh S, Ribatti D. COVID-19 vasculopathy: mounting evidence for an indirect mechanism of endothelial injury. Am J Pathol. 2021;191(8):1374-84.
136. Blom JA. Monitoring of respiration and circulation. Boca Raton, FL: CRC Press; 2003. p. 27.
137. Guest MM, Bond TP, Cooper RG, Derrick JR. Red blood cells: change in shape in capillaries. Science. 1963;142(3597):1319-21.
138. Becker RC, Sexton T, Smyth SS. Translational implications of platelets as vascular first responders. Circ Res. 2018;122(3):506-22.
139. O'Sullivan JM, Gonagle DM, Ward SE, Preston RJS, O'Donnell JS. Endothelial cells orchestrate COVID-19 coagulopathy. Lancet Haematol. 2020;7(8):e553-5.
140. Turner S, Khan MA, Putrino D, Woodcock A, Kell DB, Pretorius E, et al. Long COVID: Pathophysiological factors and abnormalities of coagulation. Trends Endocrinol Metab. 2023;34(6):321-44.
141. Helms J, Tacquard C, Severac F, Leonard-Lorant I, Ohana M, Delabranche X, et al. High risk of thrombosis in patients with severe SARS-CoV-2 infection: A multicenter prospective cohort study. Intensive Care Med. 2020;46(6):1089-98.
142. Mei ZW, van Wijk XMR, Pham HP, Marin MJ. Role of von Willebrand factor in COVID-19 associated coagulopathy. J Appl Lab Med. 2021;6(5):1305-15.
143. Shoemaker WC, Brunius U, Gelin LE. Hemodynamic and microcirculatory effects of high and low viscosity dextrans. Surgery. 1965;58:518-23.

144. Stalker AL. Histological changes produced by experimental erythrocyte aggregation. J Pathol Bacteriol. 1967;93(1):203-12.
145. Stalker AL. The microcirculatory effects of dextran. J Pathol Bacteriol. 1967;93(1):191-201.
146. Fajers CM, Gelin LE. Kidney-, liver- and heart-damages from trauma and from induced intravascular aggregation of blood-cells: an experimental study. Acta Pathol Microbiol Scand. 1959;46:97-104.
147. Swank RL, Fellman JH, Hissen WW. Aggregation of blood cells by 5-hydroxytryptamine (serotonin). Circ Res. 1963;13:392-400.
148. Cullen CF, Swank RL. Intravascular aggregation and adhesiveness of the blood elements associated with alimentary lipemia and injections of large molecular substances; effect on blood-brain barrier. Circulation. 1954;9(3):335-46.
149. Pribush A, Zilberman-Kravits D, Meyerstein N. The mechanism of the dextran-induced red blood cell aggregation. Eur Biophys J. 2007;36(2):85-94.
150. Zhu R, Avsievich T, Bykov A, Popov A, Meglinski I. Influence of pulsed He–Ne laser irradiation on the red blood cell interaction studied by optical tweezers. Micromachines. 2019;10(12):853.
151. Lee K, Shirshin E, Rovnyagina N, Yaya F, Boujja Z, Priezzhev A et al. Dextran adsorption onto red blood cells revisited: single cell quantification by laser tweezers combined with microfluidics. Biomed Opt Express. 2018;9(6):2755-64.
152. Chien S, Jan Km. Ultrastructural basis of the mechanism of rouleaux formation. Microvasc Res. 1973;5(2):155-66.
153. Zhen ZY, Guo YC, Zhang ZG, Yan L, Ge PJ, Jin HM. Experimental study on microthrombi and myocardial injuries. Microvasc Res. 1996;51(1):99-107.
154. Bicher HI. Chapter II: Pathological significance of intravascular red cell aggregation. In: Blood cell aggregation in thrombotic processes. Springfield, IL: C. C. Thomas; 1972. pp. 19-46.
155. Brånemark PI. Experimental investigation of microcirculation in bone marrow. Angiology. 1961;12(7):293-305.
156. Engeset J, Stalker AL, Matheson NA. Effects of dextran 40 on red cell aggregation in rabbits. Cardiovasc Res. 1967;1(4):379-84.
157. Swank RL, Cullen CF. Circulatory changes in the Hamster's cheek pouch associated with alimentary lipemia. Proc Soc Exp Biol Med. 1953;82(3):381-4.
158. Bjoerk VO, Intonti F, Nordlund S. Correlation between sludge in the bulbar conjunctiva and the mesentery. Ann Surg. 1964;159(3):428-31.
159. Reinke W, Gaehtgens P, Johnson PC. Blood viscosity in small tubes: effect of shear rate, aggregation, and sedimentation. Am J Physiol. 1987;253(3 Pt 2):H540-7.
160. Volger E, Schmid-Schönbein H, Gosen Jv, Klose HJ, Kline KA. Microrheology and light transmission of blood. IV. The kinetics of artificial red cell aggregation induced by Dextran. Pflugers Arch. 1975;354(4):319-37.
161. Bosek M, Ziomkowska B, Pyskir J, Wybranowski T, Pyskir M, Cyrankiewicz M, et al. Relationship between red blood cell aggregation and dextran molecular mass. Sci Rep. 2022;12(1):19751.
162. Neu B, Wenby R, Meiselman HJ. Effects of dextran molecular weight on red blood cell aggregation. Biophys J. 2008;95(6):3059-65.
163. Engeset J, Stalker AL, Matheson NA. Objective measurement of the dispersing effect of dextran 40 on red cells from man, dog, and rabbit. Cardiovasc Res. 1967;1(4):385-8.
164. Baskurt OK, Meiselman HJ. Erythrocyte aggregation: basic aspects and clinical importance. Clin Hemorheol Microcirc. 2013;53(1-2):23-37.
165. Barshtein G, Wajnblum D, Yedgar S. Kinetics of linear rouleaux formation studied by visual monitoring of red cell dynamic organization. Biophys J. 2000;78:2470-4.
166. Fung Y-C Chapter 3. The flow properties of blood. In: Biomechanics: mechanical properties of living tissues. New York: Springer; 1993. pp. 66-108.

167. Bicher HI. Chapter I: Red cell aggregation in thrombotic disease, trauma and shock. In: Blood cell aggregation in thrombotic processes. Vol. I. Springfield, IL: C. C. Thomas; 1972. pp. 5-18.

168. Bicher HI Chapter III. Mechanism of red cell aggregation. In: Blood cell aggregation in thrombotic processes; C. C. Vol. III. Springfield, IL: Thomas; 1972. pp. 47-61.

169. Brooks DE, Evans EA. Rheology of blood cells. In: Chien S, Dormandy J, Ernst E, Matrai A, editors. Clinical hemorheology: applications in cardiovascular and hematological disease, diabetes, surgery and gynecology. Dordrecht, The Netherlands: Springer; 1987; pp.73-96.

170. Lowe GDO. Thrombosis and hemorheology. In: Chien S, Dormandy J, Ernst E, Matrai A, editors. Clinical hemorheology: applications in cardiovascular and hematological disease, diabetes, surgery and gynecology. Dordrecht, The Netherlands: Springer; 1987. pp. 195-226.

171. Bishop JJ, Nance PR, Popel AS, Intaglietta M, Johnson PC. Effect of erythrocyte aggregation on velocity profiles in venules. Am J Physiol Heart Circ Physiol. 2001;280(1):H222-36.

172. Chien S, Sung LA. Physicochemical basis and clinical implications of red cell aggregation. Clin Hemorheol Microcirc. 1987;7(1):71-91.

173. Maeda N, Seike M, Kon K, Shiga T. Erythrocyte aggregation as a determinant of blood flow: effect of pH, temperature and osmotic pressure. In: Mochizuki M, Honig CR, Koyama T, Goldstick TK, Bruley DF, editors. Oxygen transport to tissue. Vol. 222. Springer. New York; 1988. pp. 563-70.

174. Sakariassen KS, Orning L, Turitto VT. The impact of blood shear rate on arterial thrombus formation. Future Sci OA. 2015;1(4):FSO30.

175. Knisely MH, Bloch EH, Eliot TS, Warner L. Sludged blood. Science. 1947;106(2758):431-40.

176. Barshtein G, Ben-Ami R, Yedgar S. Role of red blood cell flow behavior in hemodynamics and hemostasis. Expert Rev Cardiovasc Ther. 2007;5(4):743-52.

177. Ditzel J, Sagild U. Morphologic and hemodynamic changes in the smaller blood vessels in diabetes mellitus. II. The degenerative and hemodynamic changes in the bulbar conjunctiva of normotensive diabetic patients. N Engl J Med. 1954;250(14):587-94.

178. Jeffords JV, Knisely MH. Concerning the geometric shapes of arteries and arterioles: A contribution to the biophysics of health, disease, and death. Angiology. 1956;7(2):105-36.

179. Yu FT, Armstrong JK, Tripette J, Meiselman HJ, Cloutier G. A local increase in red blood cell aggregation can trigger deep vein thrombosis: evidence based on quantitative cellular ultrasound imaging. J Thromb Haemost. 2011;9(3):481-8

180. Byrnes JR, Wolberg AS. Red blood cells in thrombosis. Blood. 2017;130(16):1795-9.

181. Ami RB, Barshtein G, Zeltser D, Goldberg Y, Shapira I, Roth A, et al. Parameters of red blood cell aggregation as correlates of the inflammatory state. Am J Physiol Heart Circ Physiol. 2001;280(5):H1982-8.

182. Wagner C, Steffen P, Svetina S. Aggregation of red blood cells: from rouleaux to clot formation. C R Phys. 2013;14(6):459-69.

183. Meiselman HJ. Red blood cell aggregation: 45 years being curious. Biorheology. 2009;46(1):1-19.

184. Junxiu Z, Yu F, Shaodan L, Yi L, Yin Z, Yunxia G et al. Microvascular pathological features and changes in related injury factors in a rat acute blood stasis model. J Tradit Chin Med. 2017;37(1):108-15.

185. Kim S, Popel AS, Intaglietta M, Johnson PC. Aggregate formation of erythrocytes in postcapillary venules. Am J Physiol Heart Circ Physiol. 2005;288(2):H584-90.

186. Swank RL. Suspension stability of the blood after injections of dextran. J Appl Physiol. 1958;12(1):125-8.

187. Swank RL, Escobar A. Effects of dextran injections on blood viscosity in dogs. J Appl Physiol. 1957;10(1):45-50.

188. Bicher HI, Bruley D, Knisely MH, Reneau DD. Effect of microcirculation changes on brain tissue oxygenation. J Physiol. 1971;217(3):689-707.
189. Hysi E, Saha RK, Kolios MC. Photoacoustic ultrasound spectroscopy for assessing red blood cell aggregation and oxygenation. J Biomed Opt. 2012;17(12):125006.
190. Ditzel J. Angioscopic changes in the smaller blood vessels in diabetes mellitus and their relationship to aging. Circulation. 1956;14(3):386-97.
191. Ziegler O, Guerci B, Muller S, Candiloros H, Méjean L, Donner M, et al. Increased erythrocyte aggregation in insulin-dependent diabetes mellitus and its relationship to plasma factors: A multivariate analysis. Metabolism. 1994;43(9):1182-6.
192. Chazan BI. Intravascular red cell aggregation and the chylomicron count in diabetes. Angiology. 1963;14:426-9.
193. Cho YI, Mooney MP, Cho DJ. Hemorheological disorders in diabetes mellitus. J Diabetes Sci Technol. 2008;2(6):1130-8.
194. Wautier JL, Paton RC, Wautier MP, Pintigny D, Abadie E, Passa P, et al. Increased adhesion of erythrocytes to endothelial cells in diabetes mellitus and its relation to vascular complications. N Engl J Med. 1981;305(5):237-42.
195. Mikami T, Miyashita H, Yamada T, Harrington M, Steinberg D, Dunn A, et al. Risk factors for mortality in patients with COVID-19 in New York City. J Gen Intern Med. 2021;36(1):17-26.
196. Sastry S, Cuomo F, Muthusamy J. COVID-19 and thrombosis: the role of hemodynamics. Thromb Res. 2022;212:51-7.
197. Avila J, Long B, Holladay D, Gottlieb M. Thrombotic complications of COVID-19. Am J Emerg Med. 2021;39:213-8.
198. Al-Samkari H, Karp Leaf RS, Dzik WH, Carlson JCT, Fogerty AE, Waheed A, et al. COVID-19 and coagulation: bleeding and thrombotic manifestations of SARS-CoV-2 infection. Blood. 2020;136(4):489-500.
199. Dolhnikoff M, Duarte-Neto AN, de Almeida Monteiro RA, da Silva LFF, de Oliveira EP, Saldiva PHN, et al. Pathological evidence of pulmonary thrombotic phenomena in severe COVID-19. J Thromb Haemost. 2020;18(6):1517-9.
200. Maier CL, Truong AD, Auld SC, Polly DM, Tanksley CL, Duncan A. COVID-19-associated hyperviscosity: A link between inflammation and thrombophilia? Lancet. 2020;395(10239):1758-9.
201. Rovas A, Osiaevi I, Buscher K, Sackarnd J, Tepasse PR, Fobker M, et al. Microvascular dysfunction in COVID-19: the MYSTIC study. Angiogenesis. 2021;24(1):145-57.
202. US National Institutes of Health (NIH). Clinical spectrum of SARS-CoV-2 infection; Updated March 6 2023 [cited Oct 30 2023]. Available from: https://www.covid19treatmentguidelines.nih.gov/overview/clinical-spectrum/
203. Osiaevi I, Schulze A, Evers G, Harmening K, Vink H, Kümpers P, et al. Persistent capillary rarefication in long COVID syndrome. Angiogenesis. 2023;26(1):53-61.
204. Lins M, Vandevenne J, Thillai M, Lavon BR, Lanclus M, Bonte S, et al. Assessment of small pulmonary blood vessels in COVID-19 patients using HRCT. Acad Radiol. 2020;27(10):1449-55.
205. Thillai M, Patvardhan C, Swietlik EM, McLellan T, De Backer J, Lanclus M, et al. Functional respiratory imaging identifies redistribution of pulmonary blood flow in patients with COVID-19. Thorax. 2021;76(2):182-4.
206. Morris MF, Pershad Y, Kang P, Ridenour L, Lavon B, Lanclus M, et al. Altered pulmonary blood volume distribution as a biomarker for predicting outcomes in COVID-19 disease. Eur Respir J. 2021;58(3):2004133.
207. Dierckx W, De Backer W, Lins M, De Meyer Y, Ides K, Vandevenne J, et al. CT-derived measurements of pulmonary blood volume in small vessels and the need for supplemental oxygen in COVID-19 patients. J Appl Physiol (1985). 2022;133(6):1295-9.

208. Tipre DN, Cidon M, Moats RA. Imaging pulmonary blood vessels and ventilation-perfusion mismatch in COVID-19. Mol Imaging Biol. 2022;24(4):526-36.
209. Atilgan CU, Goker YS, Hondur G, Kosekahya P, Kocer AM, Citirik M. Evaluation of the radial peripapillary capillary density in unilateral branch retinal vein occlusion and the unaffected fellow eyes. Ther Adv Ophthalmol. 2022;14:25158414221090092.
210. Erogul O, Gobeka HH, Dogan M, Akdogan M, Balci A, Kasikci M. Retinal microvascular morphology versus COVID-19: what to anticipate? Photodiagn Photodyn Ther. 2022;39:102920.
211. Savastano A, Crincoli E, Savastano MC, Younis S, Gambini G, De Vico U, et al. Peripapillary retinal vascular involvement in early post-COVID-19 patients. J Clin Med. 2020;9(9):2895.
212. Schlick S, Lucio M, Wallukat G, Bartsch A, Skornia A, Hoffmanns J, et al. Post-COVID-19 syndrome: retinal microcirculation as a potential marker for chronic fatigue. Int J Mol Sci. 2022;23(22):13683.
213. Wu R, Ai S, Cai J, Zhang S, Qian ZM, Zhang Y, et al. Predictive model and risk factors for case fatality of COVID-19: A cohort of 21,392 cases in Hubei, China. Innovation (Camb). 2020;1(2):100022.
214. Zhou F, Yu T, Du R, Fan G, Liu Y, Liu Z; et al. Clinical course and risk factors for mortality of adult inpatients with COVID-19 in Wuhan, China: A retrospective cohort study. Lancet. 2020;395(10229):1054-62.
215. Williamson EJ, Walker AJ, Bhaskaran K, Bacon S, Bates C, Morton CE, et al. OpenSAFELY: factors associated with COVID-19 death in 17 million patients. Nature. 2020;584(7821):430-6.
216. Bonanad C, García-Blas S, Tarazona-Santabalbina F, Sanchis J, Bertomeu-González V, Fácila L, et al. The effect of age on mortality in patients with COVID-19: A meta-analysis with 611,583 subjects. J Am Med Dir Assoc. 2020;21(7):915-8.
217. Manetta J, Aloulou I, Varlet-Marie E, Mercier J, Brun JF. Partially opposite hemorheological effects of aging and training at middle age. Clin Hemorheol Microcirc. 2006;35(1-2):239-44.
218. Hammi H, Perrotin P, Guillet R, Boynard M. Determination of red blood cell aggregation in young and elderly subjects evaluated by ultrasound. Clin Hemorheol Microcirc. 1994;14(1):117-26.
219. Richardson D, Schwartz R. Comparison of capillary blood flow in the nailfold circulations of young and elderly men. Age. 1985;8(3):70-5.
220. Richardson D, Shepherd S. The cutaneous microcirculation of the forearm in young and old subjects. Microvasc Res. 1991;41(1):84-91.
221. Tsuchida Y. The effect of aging and arteriosclerosis on human skin blood flow. J Dermatol Sci. 1993;5(3):175-81.
222. Ajmani RS, Rifkind JM. Hemorheological changes during human aging. Gerontology. 1998;44(2):111-20.
223. Dinenno FA, Jones PP, Seals DR, Tanaka H. Limb blood flow and vascular conductance are reduced with age in healthy humans: relation to elevations in sympathetic nerve activity and declines in oxygen demand. Circulation. 1999;100(2):164-70.
224. Krejza J, Mariak Z, Walecki J, Szydlik P, Lewko J, Ustymowicz A. Transcranial color Doppler sonography of basal cerebral arteries in 182 healthy subjects: age and sex variability and normal reference values for blood flow parameters. AJR Am J Roentgenol. 1999;172(1):213-8.
225. Ackerstaff RG, Keunen RW, van Pelt W, Montauban van Swijndregt AD, Stijnen T. Influence of biological factors on changes in mean cerebral blood flow velocity in normal ageing: A transcranial Doppler study. Neurol Res. 1990;12(3):187-91.

226. Harrison SL, Buckley BJR, Rivera-Caravaca JM, Zhang J, Lip GYH. Cardiovascular risk factors, cardiovascular disease, and COVID-19: an umbrella review of systematic reviews. Eur Heart J Qual Care Clin Outcomes. 2021;7(4):330-9.
227. Samocha-Bonet D, Ben-Ami R, Shapira I, Shenkerman G, Abu-Abeid S, Stern N, et al. Flow-resistant red blood cell aggregation in morbid obesity. Int J Obes Relat Metab Disord. 2004;28(12):1528-34.
228. Samocha-Bonet D, Lichtenberg D, Tomer A, Deutsch V, Mardi T, Goldin Y; et al. Enhanced erythrocyte adhesiveness/aggregation in obesity corresponds to low-grade inflammation. Obes Res. 2003;11(3):403-7.
229. López-Farfán D, Irigoyen N, Gómez-Díaz E. Exploring SARS-CoV-2 and Plasmodium falciparum coinfection in human erythrocytes. Front Immunol. 2023;14:1120298.
230. Bicher HI, Beemer AM. Induction of ischemic myocardial damage by red blood cell aggregation (sludge) in the rabbit. J Atheroscler Res. 1967;7(4):409-14.
231. Yamamoto M, Kase M, Sano H, Kamijima R, Sano S. Persistent varicella zoster virus infection following mRNA COVID-19 vaccination was associated with the presence of encoded spike protein in the lesion. J Cutan Immunol Allergy. 2023;6(1):18-23.
232. Sano H, Kase M, Aoyama Y, Sano S. A case of persistent, confluent maculopapular erythema following a COVID-19 mRNA vaccination is possibly associated with the intralesional spike protein expressed by vascular endothelial cells and eccrine glands in the deep dermis. J Dermatol. 2023;50(9):1208-12.
233. Mörz M. A case report: multifocal necrotizing encephalitis and myocarditis after BNT162b2 mRNA vaccination against COVID-19. Vaccines. 2022;10(10):1651.
234. Li C, Chen Y, Zhao Y, Lung DC, Ye Z, Song W, et al. Intravenous injection of coronavirus disease 2019 (COVID-19) mRNA vaccine can induce acute myopericarditis in mouse model. Clin Infect Dis. 2022;74(11):1933-50.
235. Hassan GM, Tarek M. COVID 19 m-RNA (Pfizer) vaccination impairs cardiac functions in adult male rats. Bull. Egypt. Soc. Physiol Sci. 2023;43:211-28.
236. Gedik B, Bozdogan YC, Yavuz S, Durmaz D, Erol MK. The assesment of retina and optic disc vascular structures in people who received CoronaVac vaccine. Photodiagn Photodyn Ther. 2022;38:102742.
237. Sarıtaş Ö, Yorgun MA, Gökpınar E. Effects of Sinovac-Coronavac and Pfizer-BioNTech mRNA vaccines on choroidal and retinal vascular system. Photodiagn Photodyn Ther. 2023;43:103702.
238. Gedik B, Erol MK, Suren E, Yavuz S, Kucuk MF, Bozdogan YC, et al. Evaluation of retinal and optic disc vascular structures in individuals before and after Pfizer-BioNTech vaccination. Microvasc Res. 2023;147:104500.
239. Da Silva LSCD, Finamor LPS, Andrade GC, Lima LH, Zett C, Muccioli C, et al. Vascular retinal findings after COVID-19 vaccination in 11 cases: A coincidence or consequence? Arq Bras Oftalmol. 2022;85(2):158-65.
240. Haseeb AA, Solyman O, Abushanab MM, Abo Obaia AS, Elhusseiny AM. Ocular complications following vaccination for COVID-19: A one-year retrospective. Vaccines. 2022;10(2):342.
241. Haider A, Bengs S, Schade K, Wijnen WJ, Portmann A, Etter D, et al. Myocardial 18F-FDG uptake pattern for cardiovascular risk stratification in patients undergoing oncologic PET/CT. J Clin Med. 2020;9(7):2279.
242. Yao Y, Li YM, He ZX, Civelek AC, Li XF. Likely common role of hypoxia in driving 18F-FDG uptake in cancer, myocardial ischemia, inflammation and infection. Cancer Biother Radiopharm. 2021;36(8):624-31.
243. Nakahara T, Iwabuchi Y, Miyazawa R, Tonda K, Shiga T, Strauss HW, et al. Assessment of myocardial 18F-FDG Uptake at PET/CT in Asymptomatic SARS-CoV-2-vaccinated and Nonvaccinated Patients. Radiology. 2023;308(3):e230743.

244. Gundry SR. Abstract 10712: Observational findings of PULS cardiac test findings for inflammatory markers in patients receiving mRNA vaccines. Circulation. 2021;144;Suppl 1:A10712:Abstract 10712.
245. US Centers for Disease Control and Prevention, Vaccines and Related Biological Products Advisory Committee (VRBPAC). Update on myocarditis following mRNA COVID-19 Vaccination; June 7 2022 [cited Oct 30 2023]. Available from: https://www.fda.gov/media/159007/download
246. Truong DT, Dionne A, Muniz JC, McHugh KE, Portman MA, Lambert LM, et al. Clinically suspected myocarditis temporally related to COVID-19 vaccination in adolescents and young adults: Suspected Myocarditis After COVID-19 Vaccination. Circulation. 2022;145(5):345-56.
247. Chiu SN, Chen YS, Hsu CC, Hua YC, Tseng WC, Lu CW, et al. Changes of ECG parameters after BNT162b2 vaccine in the senior high school students. Eur J Pediatr. 2023;182(3):1155-62.
248. Mansanguan S, Charunwatthana P, Piyaphanee W, Dechkhajorn W, Poolcharoen A, Mansanguan C. Cardiovascular manifestation of the BNT162b2 mRNA COVID-19 vaccine in adolescents. Trop Med Infect Dis. 2022;7(8):196.
249. Yonker LM, Swank Z, Bartsch YC, Burns MD, Kane A, Boribong BP, et al. Circulating spike protein detected in post–COVID-19 mRNA vaccine myocarditis. Circulation. 2023;147(11):867-76.
250. Krauson AJ, Casimero FVC, Siddiquee Z, Stone JR. Duration of SARS-CoV-2 mRNA vaccine persistence and factors associated with cardiac involvement in recently vaccinated patients. npj Vaccines. 2023;8(1):141.
251. Baumeier C, Aleshcheva G, Harms D, Gross U, Hamm C, Assmus B, et al. Intramyocardial inflammation after COVID-19 vaccination: an endomyocardial biopsy-proven case series. Int J Mol Sci. 2022;23(13):6940.
252. Negri EM, Piloto BM, Morinaga LK, Jardim CVP, Lamy SAE-D, Ferreira MA, et al. Heparin therapy improving hypoxia in COVID-19 patients—A case series. Front Physiol. 2020;11:573044.
253. Charfeddine S, Ibnhadjamor H, Jdidi J, Torjmen S, Kraiem S, Bahloul A, et al. Sulodexide significantly improves endothelial dysfunction and alleviates chest pain and palpitations in patients with long-COVID-19: insights from TUN-EndCOV study. Front Cardiovasc Med. 2022;9:866113.
254. Prominent Researchers Look Deeper into Fluvoxamine and See Potential as COVID-19 treatment; April 25 2021. Trialsite News [cited Oct 30 2023]. Available from: https://trialsitenews.com/prominent-researchers-look-deeper-into-fluvoxamine-see-potential-as-covid-19-treatment/
255. Johnson CK. Cheap antidepressant shows promise treating early COVID-19; October 27 2021. Yahoo News [cited Oct 30 2023]. Available from: http://News.yahoo.com/cheap-antidepressant-shows-promise-treating-223735055.html
256. Sukhatme VP, Reiersen AM, Vayttaden SJ, Sukhatme VV. Fluvoxamine: a review of its mechanism of Action and its role in COVID-19. Front Pharmacol. 2021;12:652688.
257. Seftel D, Boulware DR. Prospective cohort of fluvoxamine for early treatment of coronavirus Disease 19. Open Forum Infect Dis. 2021;8(2):ofab050.
258. Facente SN, Reiersen AM, Lenze EJ, Boulware DR, Klausner JD. Fluvoxamine for the early treatment of SARS-CoV-2 infection: a review of current evidence. Drugs. 2021;81(18):2081-9.
259. Reis G, Dos Santos Moreira-Silva EA, Silva DCM, Thabane L, Milagres AC, Ferreira TS, et al. Effect of early treatment with fluvoxamine on risk of emergency care and hospitalisation among patients with COVID-19: the TOGETHER randomised, platform clinical trial. Lancet Glob Health. 2022;10(1):e42-51.

260. Lenze EJ, Mattar C, Zorumski CF, Stevens A, Schweiger J, Nicol GE, et al. Fluvoxamine vs placebo and clinical deterioration in outpatients with symptomatic COVID-19: A randomized clinical trial. JAMA. 2020;324(22):2292-300.

261. Swank RL, Edwards MJ. Microvascular occlusion by platelet emboli after transfusion and shock. Microvasc Res. 1968;1(1):15-22.

262. Alvarez JC, Gluck N, Fallet A, Grégoire A, Chevalier JF, Advenier C, et al. Plasma serotonin level after 1 day of fluoxetine treatment: A biological predictor for antidepressant response? Psychopharmacology. 1999;143(1):97-101.

263. Celada P, Dolera M, Alvarez E, Artigas F. Effects of acute and chronic treatment with fluvoxamine on extracellular and platelet serotonin in the blood of major depressive patients. Relationship to clinical improvement. J Affect Disord. 1992;25(4): 243-9.

264. Duerschmied D, Suidan GL, Demers M, Herr N, Carbo C, Brill A, et al. Platelet serotonin promotes the recruitment of neutrophils to sites of acute inflammation in mice. Blood. 2013;121(6):1008-15.

265. Gupta M, Neavin D, Liu D, Biernacka J, Hall-Flavin D, Bobo WV, et al. TSPAN5, ERICH3 and selective serotonin reuptake inhibitors in major depressive disorder: pharmacometabolomics-informed pharmacogenomics. Mol Psychiatry. 2016;21(12): 1717-25.

266. Holck A, Wolkowitz OM, Mellon SH, Reus VI, Nelson JC, Westrin Å, et al. Plasma serotonin levels are associated with antidepressant response to SSRIs. J Affect Disord. 2019;250:65-70.

267. Kristjansdottir HL, Lewerin C, Lerner UH, Waern E, Johansson H, Sundh D, et al. High serum serotonin predicts increased risk for hip fracture and nonvertebral osteoporotic fractures: the MrOS Sweden study. J Bone Miner Res. 2018;33(9):1560-7.

268. Urbina M, Pineda S, Piñango L, Carreira I, Lima L. [3H]Paroxetine binding to human peripheral lymphocyte membranes of patients with major depression before and after treatment with fluoxetine. Int J Immunopharmacol. 1999;21(10):631-46.

269. Carneiro AM, Cook EH, Murphy DL, Blakely RD. Interactions between integrin alphaIIbbeta3 and the serotonin transporter regulate serotonin transport and platelet aggregation in mice and humans. J Clin Invest. 2008;118(4):1544-52.

270. McCloskey DJ, Postolache TT, Vittone BJ, Nghiem KL, Monsale JL, Wesley RA, et al. Selective serotonin reuptake inhibitors: measurement of effect on platelet function. Transl Res. 2008;151(3):168-72.

271. Gautret P, Lagier JC, Parola P, Hoang VT, Meddeb L, Mailhe M, et al. Hydroxychloroquine and azithromycin as a treatment of COVID-19: results of an open-label non-randomized clinical trial. Int J Antimicrob Agents. 2020;56(1):105949.

272. Gendrot M, Andreani J, Jardot P, Hutter S, Delandre O, Boxberger M, et al. In vitro antiviral activity of doxycycline against SARS-CoV-2. Molecules. 2020;25(21):5064.

273. Million M, Cortaredona S, Delorme L, Colson P, Levasseur A, Hervé T-D, et al. Early treatment with hydroxychloroquine and azithromycin: A "Real-Life" monocentric retrospective cohort study of 30,423 COVID-19 patients. medRxiv 2023.

274. Madow BP. Use of antimalarial drugs as "desludging" agents in vascular disease processes [preliminary report]. JAMA. 1960;172:1630-3.

275. Cecchi E, Ferraris F. Desludging action of hydroxychloroquine in R. A Acta Rheumatol Scand. 1962;8:214-21.

276. Edwards MH, Pierangeli S, Liu X, Barker JH, Anderson G, Harris EN. Hydroxychloroquine reverses thrombogenic properties of antiphospholipid antibodies in mice. Circulation. 1997;96(12):4380-4.

277. Nallusamy S, Mannu J, Ravikumar C, Angamuthu K, Nathan B, Nachimuthu K, et al. Exploring phytochemicals of traditional medicinal plants exhibiting inhibitory activity against main protease, spike glycoprotein, RNA-dependent RNA polymerase and

non-structural proteins of SARS-CoV-2 through virtual screening. Front Pharmacol. 2021;12:667704.

278. Kalhor H, Sadeghi S, Abolhasani H, Kalhor R, Rahimi H. Repurposing of the approved small molecule drugs in order to inhibit SARS-CoV-2 S protein and human ACE2 interaction through virtual screening approaches. J Biomol Struct Dyn. 2022;40(3): 1299-315.
279. Suravajhala R, Parashar A, Malik B, Nagaraj VA, Padmanaban G, Kavi Kishor PB, et al. Comparative docking studies on curcumin with COVID-19 proteins. Preprints. Org 2020.
280. Yagisawa M, Foster PJ, Hanaki H, Omura S. Global trends in clinical studies of ivermectin in COVID-19. Jpn J Antibiot. 2021;74:44-95.
281. Juarez M, Schcolnik-Cabrera A, Dueñas-Gonzalez A. The multitargeted drug ivermectin: from an antiparasitic agent to a repositioned cancer drug. Am J Cancer Res. 2018;8(2):317-31.
282. Campbell WC. History of avermectin and ivermectin, with notes on the history of other macrocyclic lactone antiparasitic agents. Curr Pharm Biotechnol. 2012;13(6):853-65.
283. Chang MW, Lindstrom W, Olson AJ, Belew RK. Analysis of HIV wild-type and mutant structures via in silico docking against diverse ligand libraries. J Chem Inf Model. 2007;47(3):1258-62.
284. Dasgupta J, Sen U, Bakashi A, Dasgupta A. Nsp7 and spike glycoprotein of SARS-CoV-2 are envisaged as potential targets of vitamin D and ivermectin. Preprints. Org 2020.
285. Hussien MA, Abdelaziz AEM. Molecular docking suggests repurposing of brincidofovir as a potential drug targeting SARS-CoV-2 ACE2 receptor and main protease. Netw Model Anal Health Inform Bioinform. 2020;9(1):56.
286. Kaur H, Shekhar N, Sharma S, Sarma P, Prakash A, Medhi B. Ivermectin as a potential drug for treatment of COVID-19: an in-sync review with clinical and computational attributes. Pharmacol Rep. 2021;73(3):736-49.
287. Maurya D. A combination of ivermectin and doxycycline possibly blocks the viral entry and modulate the innate immune response in COVID-19 patients. Chem Rxiv 2020.
288. Saha JK, Raihan MJ. The Binding mechanism of ivermectin and levosalbutamol with spike protein of SARS-CoV-2. Struct Chem. 2021;32(5):1985-92.
289. Lehrer S, Rheinstein PH. Ivermectin docks to the SARS-CoV-2 spike receptor-binding domain attached to ACE2. In Vivo. 2020;34(5):3023-6.
290. Rajter JJ; (Broward Health Medical Center. Fort Lauderdale, FL, USA) [Personal communication]; May 28 2020.
291. Local Doctor Tries New coronavirus drug treatment. NBC Miami News. April 14 2020. com/news/local/local-doctor-tries-new-coronavirus-drug-treatment/2219465/ [accessed on 30 October 2023].
292. Rajter JC, Sherman MS, Fatteh N, Vogel F, Sacks J, Rajter J-J. Use of ivermectin is Associated with Lower Mortality in Hospitalized Patients with COVID-19 (ICON study). Chest. 2020;159:85-92.
293. Santin AD, Scheim DE, McCullough PA, Yagisawa M, Borody TJ. Ivermectin: A multifaceted drug of Nobel Prize-honored distinction with indicated efficacy against a new global scourge, COVID-19. New Microbes New Infect. 2021;43:100924.
294. Abdool Karim SS, Devnarain N. Time to stop using ineffective COVID-19 drugs. N Engl J Med. 2022;387(7):654-5.
295. Shafiee A, Teymouri Athar MM, Kohandel Gargari O, Jafarabady K, Siahvoshi S, Mozhgani SH. Ivermectin under scrutiny: A systematic review and meta-analysis of efficacy and possible sources of controversies in COVID-19 patients. Virol J. 2022;19(1):102.
296. Reis G, Silva EASM, Silva DCM, Thabane L, Milagres AC, Ferreira TS, et al. Effect of early treatment with ivermectin among patients with COVID-19. N Engl J Med. 2022;386(18):1721-31.

297. Scheim DE, Aldous C, Osimani B, Fordham EJ, Hoy WE. When characteristics of clinical trials require per-protocol as well as intention-to-treat outcomes to draw reliable conclusions: three examples. J Clin Med. 2023;12(11):3625.
298. US Food & Drug Administration. Memorandum explaining basis for declining request for emergency use authorization of fluvoxamine maleate. Available online [cited Oct 30 2023]. Available from: https://www.accessdata.fda.gov/drugsatfda_docs/nda/2020/EUA%2520110%2520Fluvoxamine%2520Decisional%2520Memo_Redacted.pdf
299. NIH. COVID-19 treatment guidelines. Fluvoxamine Sel Clin Data Limitations Interpretation Table. December 16 2021;4c.
300. TOGETHER trial DSS and data repository screenshots. Date-Time Stamped Screenshots from Publications of the TOGETHER trial (NCT04727424). Google [cited Oct 30 2023]. Available from: https://drive.google.com/file/d/1pBZ1GihxW_ROB3Aid6tFMplqAyMYOGDl/preview
301. Email from Sarah Fullegar, sent; June 7 2022 to Edmund Fordham. Screenshot, Email Addresses Redacted [cited Oct 30 2023]. Available from: https://drive.google.com/file/d/1lUsSRf1KX-pa9T5EX4HbegdK8mYNQ_Ty/preview
302. López-Medina E, López P, Hurtado IC, Dávalos DM, Ramirez O, Martínez E, et al. Effect of ivermectin on time to resolution of symptoms among adults with mild COVID-19: A randomized clinical trial. JAMA. 2021;325(14):1426-35.
303. Scheim DE, Hibberd JA, Chamie-Quintero JJ. Protocol violations. In: López-Medina, et al., editors. Switched ivermectin (IVM) and placebo doses, failure of blinding, ubiquitous IVM use OTC in Cali, and nearly identical AEs for the IVM and control groups. Osf Preprints. Vol. 38; 2021.
304. George LL, Borody TJ, Andrews P, Devine M, Moore-Jones D, Walton M, et al. Cure of duodenal ulcer after eradication of Helicobacter pylori. Med J Aust. 1990;153(3):145-9.
305. Coghlan JG, Gilligan D, Humphries H, McKenna D, Dooley C, Sweeney E, et al. Campylobacter pylori and recurrence of duodenal ulcers—A 12-month follow-up study. Lancet. 1987;2(8568):1109-11.
306. Graham DY, Lew GM, Klein PD, Evans DG, Evans DJ, Jr., Saeed ZA, et al. Effect of treatment of Helicobacter pylori infection on the long-term recurrence of gastric or duodenal ulcer. A randomized, controlled study. Ann Intern Med. 1992;116(9):705-8.
307. Watts G. Nobel Prize is awarded to doctors who discovered H pylori. BMJ. 2005;331(7520):795.
308. Fleming A. On the antibacterial Action of Cultures of a Penicillium, with Special Reference to their Use in the Isolation of B. influenzæ. Br J Exp Pathol. 1929;10:226-36.
309. Chain E, Florey HW, Gardner AD, Heatley NG, Jennings MA, Orr-Ewing J et al. Penicillin as a chemotherapeutic agent. Lancet. 1940;236(6104):226-8.
310. Lobanovska M, Pilla G. Penicillin's discovery and antibiotic resistance: lessons for the future? Yale J Biol Med. 2017;90(1):135-45.
311. Annunziata A, Coppola A, Carannante N, Simioli F, Lanza M, Di Micco P, et al. Home management of patients with moderate or severe respiratory failure secondary to COVID-19, using remote monitoring and oxygen with or without HFNC. Pathogens. 2021;10(4):413.
312. Aoki R, Iwasawa T, Hagiwara E, Komatsu S, Utsunomiya D, Ogura T. Pulmonary vascular enlargement and lesion extent on computed tomography are correlated with COVID-19 disease severity. Jpn J Radiol. 2021;39(5):451-8.
313. Ding X, Xu J, Zhou J, Long Q. Chest CT findings of COVID-19 pneumonia by duration of symptoms. Eur J Radiol. 2020;127:109009.
314. Metwally MI, Basha MAA, Zaitoun MMA, Abdalla HM, Nofal HAE, Hendawy H, et al. Clinical and radiological imaging as prognostic predictors in COVID-19 patients. Egypt J Radiol Nucl Med. 2021;52(1):100.

315. Osman AM, Farouk S, Osman NM, Abdrabou AM. Longitudinal assessment of chest computerized tomography and oxygen saturation for patients with COVID-19. Egypt J Radiol Nucl Med. 2020;51(1):255.

316. Quispe-Cholan A, Anticona-De-La-Cruz Y, Cornejo-Cruz M, Quispe-Chirinos O, Moreno-Lazaro V, Chavez-Cruzado E. Tomographic findings in patients with COVID-19 according to evolution of the disease. Egypt J Radiol Nucl Med. 2020;51(1):215.

317. Wang Y, Dong C, Hu Y, Li C, Ren Q, Zhang X, et al. Temporal changes of CT findings in 90 patients with COVID-19 pneumonia: A longitudinal study. Radiology. 2020;296(2):E55-64.

318. Stone JC, Ndarukwa P, Scheim DE, Dancis BM, Dancis J, Gill MG et al. Changes in SpO2 on room air for 34 severe COVID-19 patients after ivermectin-based combination treatment: 62% normalization within 24 hours. Biologics. 2022;2(3):196-210.

319. Hazan S, Dave S, Gunaratne AW, Dolai S, Clancy RL, McCullough PA et al. Effectiveness of ivermectin-based multidrug therapy in severely hypoxic, ambulatory COVID-19 patients. Future Microbiol. 2022;17:339-50.

320. Babalola OE, Ndanusa Y, Adesuyi A, Ogedengbe OJ, Thairu Y, Ogu O. A randomized controlled trial of ivermectin monotherapy versus HCQ, IVM, and AZ combination therapy in COVID-19 patients in Nigeria. J Infect Dis Epidemiol. 2021;7:233.

321. Babalola OE. Bingham Univ New Karu Niger [Personal communication]; February 28 2022.

322. Thairu Y, Babalola OE, Ajayi AA, Ndanusa Y, Ogedengbe JO, Omede O. A comparison of ivermectin and Non ivermectin based regimen for COVID-19 in Abuja: Effects on Virus Clearance, Days-to-discharge and Mortality. Sq. JPRI. 2022;34:1-19.

323. Chamie JJ, Hibberd JA, Scheim DE. COVID-19 excess deaths in Peru's 25 states in 2020: nationwide trends, confounding factors, and correlations with the extent of ivermectin treatment by state. Cureus. 2023;15(8):e43168.

324. Meekins DA, Gaudreault NN, Richt JA. Natural and experimental SARS-CoV-2 infection in domestic and wild animals. Viruses. 2021;13(10):1993.

325. Baskurt OK, Meiselman HJ. Comparative hemorheology. Clin Hemorheol Microcirc. 2013;53(1-2):61-70.

326. Rampling MW, Meiselman HJ, Neu B, Baskurt OK. Influence of cell-specific factors on red blood cell aggregation. Biorheology. 2004;41(2):91-112.

327. Popel AS, Johnson PC, Kameneva MV, Wild MA. Capacity for red blood cell aggregation is higher in athletic mammalian species than in sedentary species. J Appl Physiol (1985). 1994;77(4):1790-4.

328. Weng X, Cloutier G, Pibarot P, Durand LG. Comparison and simulation of different levels of erythrocyte aggregation with pig, horse, sheep, calf, and normal human blood. Biorheology. 1996;33(4-5):365-77.

329. Wernike K, Böttcher J, Amelung S, Albrecht K, Gärtner T, Donat K, et al. Antibodies against SARS-CoV-2 suggestive of single events of spillover to cattle, Germany. Emerg Infect Dis. 2022;28(9):1916-8.

330. Bosco-Lauth AM, Walker A, Guilbert L, Porter S, Hartwig A, McVicker E, et al. Susceptibility of livestock to SARS-CoV-2 infection. Emerg Microbes Infect. 2021;10(1):2199-201.

331. Available from: Wessa.net. Free statistics software, office for research development and education. Version 1.2.1 [cited Oct 30 2023]. Available from: https://www.wessa.net/

332. Nemkov T, Reisz JA, Xia Y, Zimring JC, D'Alessandro A. Red blood cells as an organ? How deep omics characterization of the most abundant cell in the human body highlights other systemic metabolic functions beyond oxygen transport. Expert Rev Proteomics. 2018;15(11):855-64.

333. Sender R, Fuchs S, Milo R. Revised estimates for the number of human and bacteria cells in the body. PLOS Biol. 2016;14(8):e1002533.

334. Chang VT, Crispin M, Aricescu AR, Harvey DJ, Nettleship JE, Fennelly JA, et al. Glycoprotein structural genomics: solving the glycosylation problem. Structure. 2007;15(3):267-73.
335. Lee JE, Fusco ML, Saphire EO. An efficient platform for screening expression and crystallization of glycoproteins produced in human cells. Nat Protoc. 2009;4(4):592-604.
336. Dill K, Hu SH, Berman E, Pavia AA, Lacombe JM. One- and two-dimensional NMR studies of the N-terminal portion of glycophorin A at 11.7 Tesla. J Protein Chem. 1990;9(2):129-36.
337. Ekman S, Flower R, Mahler S, Gould A, Barnard RT, Hyland C, et al. In silico molecular dynamics of human glycophorin A (GPA) extracellular structure. Ann Blood. 2021;6:11.
338. Trivedi R, Nagarajaram HA. Intrinsically disordered proteins: an overview. Int J Mol Sci. 2022;23(22):14050.
339. Uversky VN, Dunker AK. Understanding protein non-folding. Biochim Biophys Acta. 2010;1804(6):1231-64.
340. Uversky VN, Gillespie JR, Fink AL. Why are "natively unfolded" proteins unstructured under physiologic conditions? Proteins. 2000;41(3):415-27.
341. Seet RCS, Quek AML, Ooi DSQ, Sengupta S, Lakshminarasappa SR, Koo CY, et al. Positive impact of oral hydroxychloroquine and povidone-iodine throat spray for COVID-19 prophylaxis: an open-label randomized trial. Int J Infect Dis. 2021;106:314-22.
342. Horton R. Offline: what is medicine's. Lancet. 2015;385(9976):P1380.
343. Ioannidis JP. Evidence-based medicine has been hijacked: A report to David Sackett. J Clin Epidemiol. 2016;73:82-6.
344. Steinbrook R, Kassirer JP, Angell M. Justifying conflicts of interest in medical journals: A very bad idea. BMJ. 2015;350:h2942.
345. Carlisle JB. False individual patient data and zombie randomised controlled trials submitted to Anaesthesia. Anaesthesia. 2021;76(4):472-9.
346. Gotzsche P. Deadly medicines and organised crime: how big pharma has corrupted healthcare. 1st ed. London, UK: CRC Press; 2013.
347. Saltelli A, Dankel DJ, Di Fiore M, Holland N, Pigeon M. Science, the endless frontier of regulatory capture. Futures. 2022;135:102860.
348. Eslick GD, Tilden D, Arora N, Torres M, Clancy RL. Clinical and economic impact of "triple therapy" for Helicobacter pylori eradication on peptic ulcer disease in Australia. Helicobacter. 2020;25(6):e12751.
349. Berndt ER, Kyle M, Ling D. The long shadow of patent expiration: generic entry and Rx-to-OTC switches. In: Feenstra RC, Shapiro MD, editors. Scanner data and price indexes. Chicago: University of Chicago Press; 2003. pp. 229-74.
350. Chatterjee S, Bhattacharya M, Nag S, Dhama K, Chakraborty C. A detailed overview of SARS-CoV-2 omicron: its sub-variants, mutations and pathophysiology, clinical characteristics, immunological landscape, immune escape, and therapies. Viruses. 2023;15(1):167.
351. Hui KPY, Ho JCW, Cheung MC, Ng KC, Ching RHH, Lai KL, et al. SARS-CoV-2 Omicron variant replication in human bronchus and lung ex vivo. Nature. 2022;603(7902):715-20.
352. Peacock TP, Brown JC, Zhou J, Thakur N, Sukhova K, Newman J, et al. The altered entry pathway and antigenic distance of the SARS-CoV-2 Omicron variant map to separate domains of spike protein. bioRxiv. 2022.
353. D'Agnillo F, Walters KA, Xiao Y, Sheng ZM, Scherler K, Park J, et al. Lung epithelial and endothelial damage, loss of tissue repair, inhibition of fibrinolysis, and cellular senescence in fatal COVID-19. Sci Transl Med. 2021;13(620):eabj7790.
354. Makary M. The real data behind the new COVID vaccines the white Houseis pushing. New York Post [cited Oct 30 2023]. Available from: https://nypost.com/2023/09/14/the-real-data-behind-the-new-covid-vaccines-the-white-house-is-pushing/; September 14 2023.

355. Bramante CT, Buse JB, Liebovitz DM, Nicklas JM, Puskarich MA, Cohen K, et al. Outpatient treatment of COVID-19 and incidence of post-COVID-19 condition over 10 months (COVID-OUT): A multicentre, randomised, quadruple-blind, parallel-group, phase 3 trial. Lancet Infect Dis. 2023;23(10):1119-29.

356. McCarthy MW, Naggie S, Boulware DR, Lindsell CJ, Stewart TG, Felker GM; et al. Effect of fluvoxamine vs placebo on time to sustained recovery in outpatients with mild to moderate COVID-19: A randomized clinical trial. JAMA. 2023;329(4):296-305.

357. Wang H, Yu M, Ochani M, Amella CA, Tanovic M, Susarla S, et al. Nicotinic acetylcholine receptor α7 subunit is an essential regulator of inflammation. Nature. 2003;421(6921):384-8.

358. Krause RM, Buisson B, Bertrand S, Corringer PJ, Galzi JL, Changeux JP, et al. Ivermectin: A positive allosteric effector of the alpha7 neuronal nicotinic acetylcholine receptor. Mol Pharmacol. 1998;53(2):283-94.

359. Fajgenbaum DC, June CH. Cytokine storm. N Engl J Med. 2020;383(23):2255-73.

CHAPTER 25

Antivirals

Priyaranjan Kata, Jose Iglesias

INTRODUCTION

Since January 2021, severe acute respiratory syndrome coronavirus 2 (SARS-CoV-2), the virus responsible for coronavirus disease-2019 (COVID-19), has caused >90 million confirmed cases worldwide and 1.9 million confirmed deaths as of January 2023.[1] This pandemic has driven the quick development of COVID-19 virus vaccines, and widespread immunization programs are still ongoing. Despite the fact that a study in Italy[2] reported that the COVID-19 vaccine can lower the mortality of COVID-19 infected individuals, other studies have found that vaccinated people can become infected with new coronavirus strains against which the original monovalent messenger ribonucleic acid (mRNA) vaccines have reduced effectiveness.[3,4]

As COVID-19 continues to mutate and future viruses pose a potential threat, finding effective treatments for the disease has become a global priority.[5,6] Researchers and pharmaceutical companies are working relentlessly to identify and develop new treatments.[7] Recently, there has been significant progress in COVID-19 research with the aim of creating simple, oral antiviral medications that can offer promising therapeutic benefits. Although remdesivir is the only antiviral drug approved by the Food and Drug Administration (FDA) for COVID-19 treatment, ritonavir-boosted nirmatrelvir (nirmatrelvir/ritonavir) and molnupiravir have received Emergency Use Authorization (EUA) from the FDA.[8-11] While remdesivir has shown good antiviral therapeutic results, it is expensive and must be administered intravenously generally in a hospital setting, which is why simpler oral medicines such as molnupiravir and nirmatrelvir/ritonavir were developed for outpatient usage.[12]

This chapter will explore the effectiveness of these drugs in clinical trials as well as their mechanism of action, and potential side effects.

ANTIVIRAL DRUGS

It is crucial that one understands the pathophysiologic stage of COVID-19 disease when evaluating and employing antiviral strategies. The viral phase when virus is actively and rapidly reproducing usually occurs during the first 5 days of infection when patient are either asymptomatic or mildly asymptomatic, then there is progression to the pulmonary phase of the disease which in some progresses to increase inflammatory state associated with worsening pulmonary infiltrates and severe respiratory failure **(Fig. 1)**.[13-16]

Thus in order to be effective it is essential that antiviral therapy be employed during the early viremic phase of the disease.

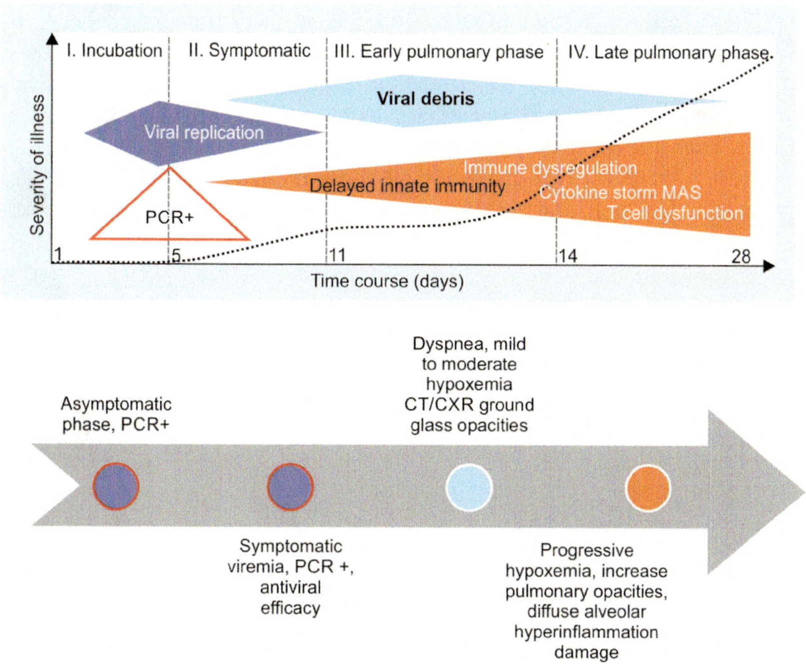

FIGURE 1: Stages of coronavirus disease-2019 (COVID-19). The incubation phase when individuals develop a symptomatic increasing viremia. The symptomatic viremic phase associated with constitutional symptoms (fever, diarrhea, malaise, cough, and myalgia). The early pulmonary phase associated with chest X-ray (CXR) and CT scan abnormalities progressive pulmonary symptoms, mild-to-moderate hypoxemia. The late pulmonary associated with hyperinflammation and diffuse alveolar damage. Of note although polymerase chain reaction (PCR) positivity may last several weeks, the degree of viremia decreases as disease progresses.[13-16]

REMDESIVIR

Remdesivir is a direct-acting antiviral prodrug that inhibits SARS-CoV-2 RNA-dependent polymerase **(Fig. 2)**.[12,17-21] Initially employed as an antiviral agent against Ebola, the agent failed in clinical trials.[12,18] Due to experimental evidence demonstrated high antiviral activity against SARS-CoV-2 in infected human airway epithelial cells and other supporting evidence the agent was repurposed for the treatment of COVID-19 disease.[12,22,23] Emergency use authjorization was granted by the FDA in May 5, 2020 after clinical trial data demonstrated in random clinical trials improved time to recovery and discharge when compared to placebo.[24] Despite being touted as a success by Anthony Fauci and others, studies demonstrated marginal effects mainly on decreased time to recovery.[24,25] The Adaptive COVID Treatment Trial-1 (ACCT-1) a National Institutes of Health (NIH) funded double-blinded randomized control trial involving 1,062 patients hospitalized with COVID-19 demonstrating a median time 5 days faster time to recovery with treatment compared to placebo, rate ratio for recovery 1.29, $p < 0.001$.[24] There was no significant difference in 29 day; mortality was 11.4% with remdesivir and 15.2% with placebo.[24] Several issues should be mentioned about the ACCT-1 trial, the greatest benefit was observed in patients treated earlier, and those with less severe disease while those on extracorporeal membrane oxygenation (ECMO), and high-flow oxygen less so.[24] In addition, the trial was

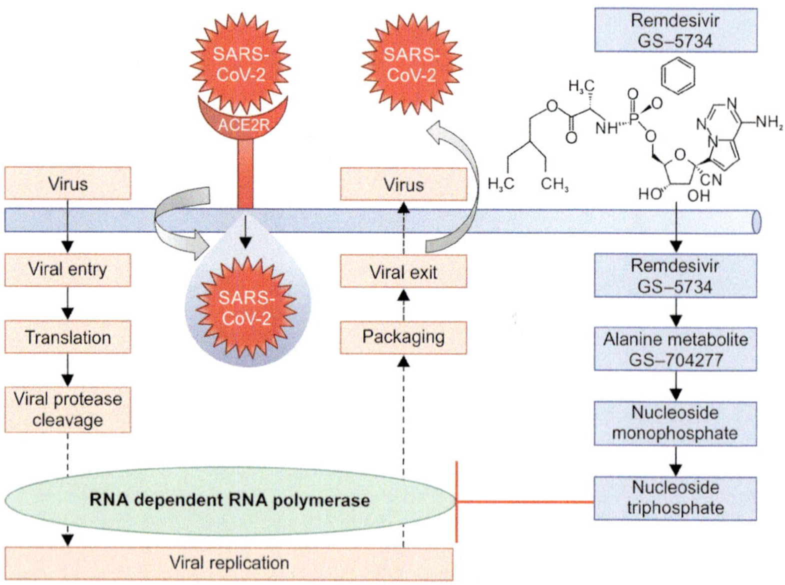

FIGURE 2: Mechanisms of action of remdesivir. The parent compound is converted intracellularly by phosphatases into the active compound which inhibits severe acute respiratory syndrome coronavirus 2 (SARS-CoV-2) ribonucleic acid (RNA)-dependent polymerase.[20]

Source: Used with permission under creative commons open use 4.0.

terminated early and placebo patients were offered treatment.[24] In contrast, interim results of the WHO solidarity trial demonstrated no clinical benefit of remdesivir, had no significant impact on mortality, need for mechanical ventilation, time to clinical improvement, and other clinically relevant outcomes.[26] This initially resulted in the WHO recommending against the use of remdesivir as effective therapy. However, the final analysis based on subgroups demonstrated that remdesivir appears to have a small benefit in terms mortality/progression to ventilation among patients who were hospitalized but not requiring mechanical ventilation.[26,27]

A Cochran meta-analysis conducted by Grundeis et al. evaluating over 11,000 patients demonstrated that remdesivir had little or no effect on mortality.[28] In addition in patients who are mechanically ventilated, there is no evidence that remdesivir improves clinical outcome.[28] There is some evidence that remdesivir may have some benefit in hospitalized patients with mild-to-moderate improvement in clinical course of the disease; however, the certainty of this finding is limited.[28] Randomized controlled trials (RCTs) with mortality, hospitalization as primary outcome of interest, and mortality as primary outcome in all RCTs are summarized in **Figures 3 and 4**.[22-24,27,29-33] Although studies have indicated that there are no significant differences in major adverse events compared control, remdesivir is a potential hepatotoxin, nephrotoxin, and may be involved in the development of multiorgan failure.[24,34,35]

MOLNUPIRAVIR

The RNA-dependent RNA polymerase (RdRp) is an essential component in the replication of SARS-CoV-2, making it an attractive target for developing COVID-19 treatments.[36] RdRp inhibitors such as remdesivir and molnupiravir have already been approved for COVID-19 treatment.[37] While there is some evidence remdesivir has been shown to reduce the progression of COVID-19 and associated clinical symptoms, as well as significantly reducing recovery time, pharmaceutical companies are struggling to develop convenient oral dosage forms for the drug.[24] On the other hand, molnupiravir has received a lot of attention due to its ability to block SARS-CoV-2 reproduction, rapidly clear the virus, and decrease the viral load, as well as its favorable pharmacokinetic profile as an oral active RdRp inhibitor.[38]

Molnupiravir (EIDD-2801/MK-4482) is a prodrug which when metabolized to the active molecule works by inhibiting RdRp of SARS-CoV-2, producing mutated RNA copies of the virus.[36] It is a prodrug that is rapidly cleaved to EIDD-1931 in plasma before distributing to different tissues and being converted into the 5′-triphosphate **(Fig. 5)**.[36] This 5'-triphosphate (MTP) molecule acts as a virally encoded RdRp substrate that induces a catastrophic replication error when incorporated into the developing RNA chain.[36] MTP competes with cytidine and uridine triphosphates and is incorporated into the emerging RNA instead, leading to an increased viral RNA mutation rate and resulting in viral inviability.[36]

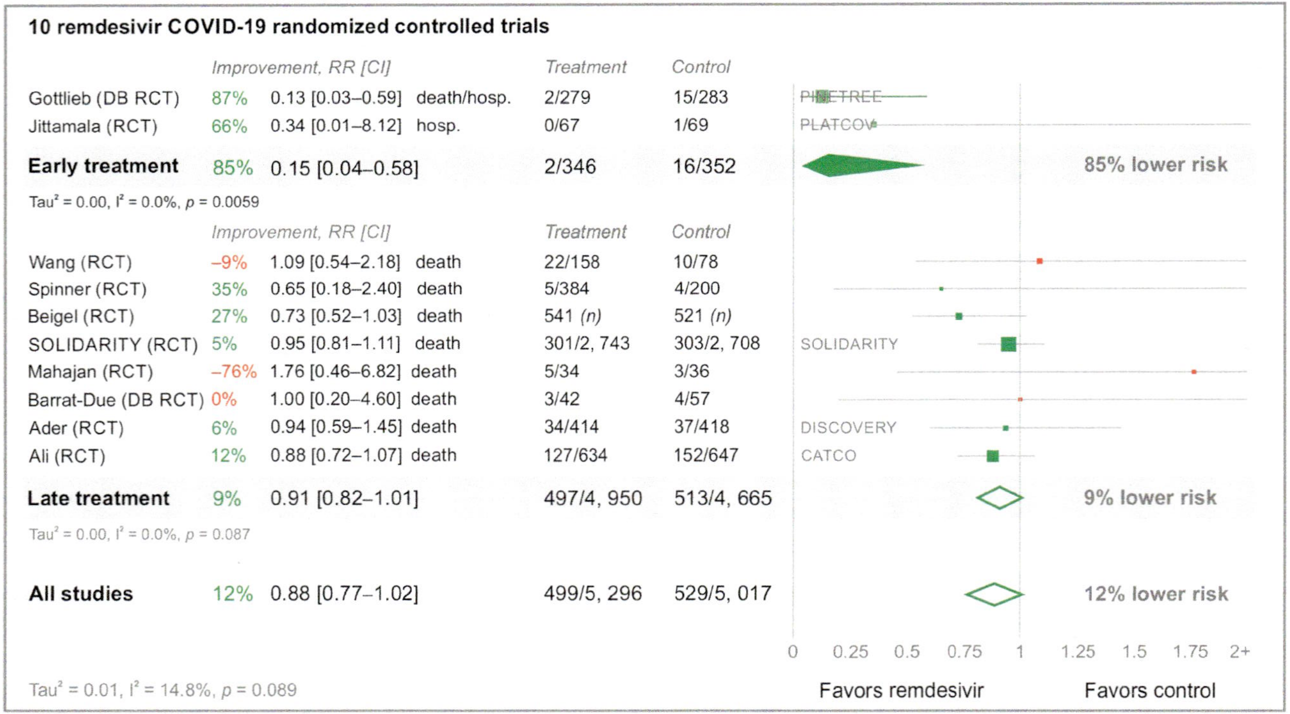

FIGURE 3: Forrest plot of meta-analysis results of randomized clinical trials that primary outcome was hospitalization and or death.[22-24,27,29-33]

Source: c19early.org. (2023). COVID-19 early treatment: real-time analysis of 3,885 studies. [online] Available from https://c19early.org/. [Last accessed February, 2024].

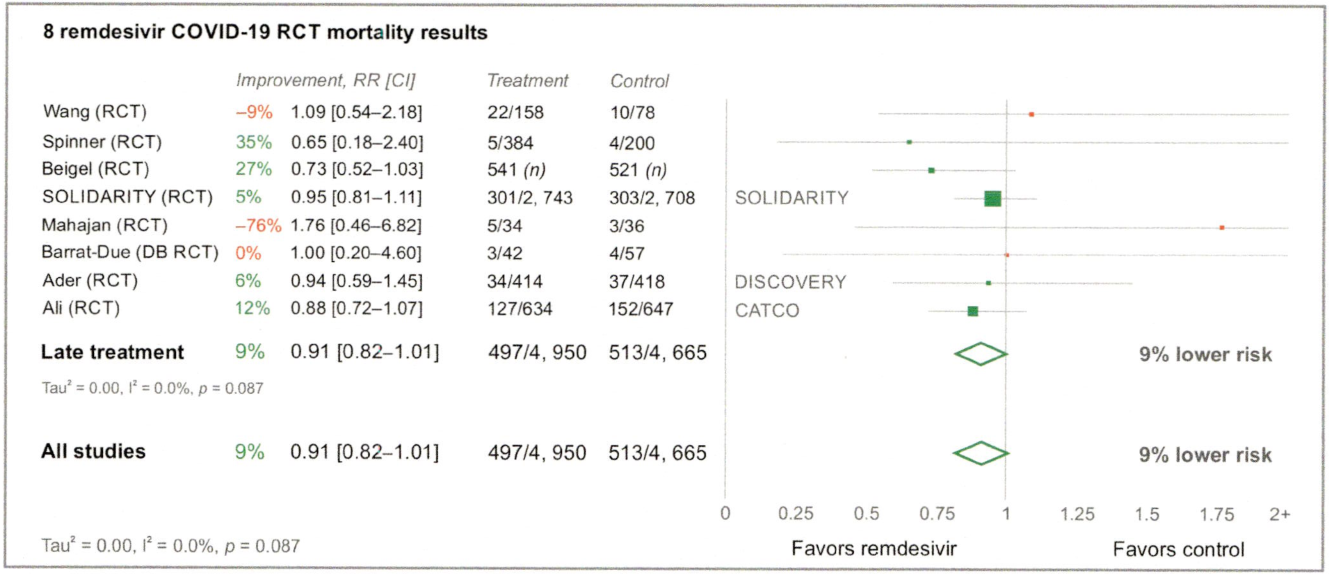

FIGURE 4: Forrest plot of meta-analysis which includes randomized control trials in which mortality was primary outcome of interest.[22-24,27,29-33]
Source: c19early.org. (2023). COVID-19 early treatment: real-time analysis of 3,885 studies. [online] Available from https://c19early.org/. [Last accessed February, 2024].

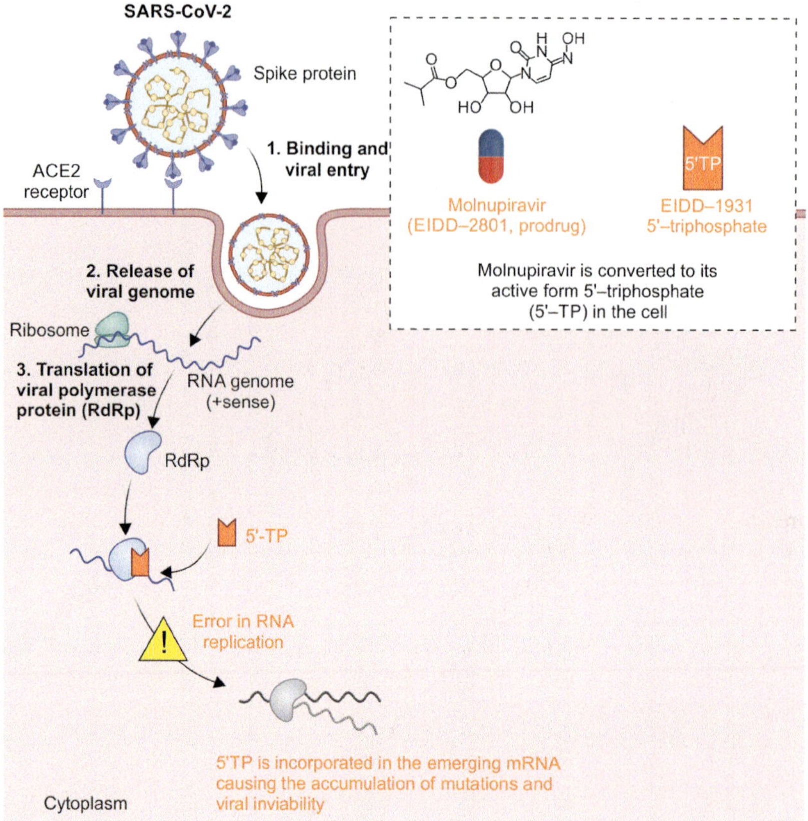

FIGURE 5: Mechanism of action of molnupiravir is prodrug that undergoes a series of intracellular metabolic transformations by host cell esterases and phosphatases into the active analogue 5'TP (EIDD-1931). EIDD-1931 has a similar structure to the natural substrates cytidine or uridine triphosphate for RdRp. As a result, EIDD-1931 triphosphate competitively inhibits RdRp and further suppresses viral replication.[36,38] "Molnupiravir" is a prodrug that undergoes hydrolysis by host cell esterase to form N4-hydroxy cytidine (NHC). The resulting alcohol analog is then phosphorylated to produce the active N4-hydroxycytidine triphosphate (EIDD-1931 triphosphate).

(mRNA: messenger ribonucleic acid; RNA: ribonucleic acid; SARS-CoV-2: severe acute respiratory syndrome coronavirus 2)

Interestingly, EUA approval for molnupiravir was based on minimal safety data, antiviral activity (more rapid decrease in viral load), and soft clinical endpoints such as improvement of symptoms and quicker decrease in viral load.[37,39-44] Sheehan et al. demonstrated that molnupiravir had potent antiviral activity against the major three pathogenic coronaviruses SARS-CoV-1, MERS-CoV, and SARS-CoV-2.[45] In addition, in vivo activity in a mouse model of SARS-CoV-2.[45] Molnupiravir was found to decrease viral replication and pathogenesis.[45] Phase 1, 2 and Phase 2/3 trials found the molecule to be safe and relatively well tolerated at therapeutic doses.[40-42,46] Corporate sponsored Phase 2/3 trials, the (MOVe-IN, n = 304) involving hospitalized patients and the other for nonhospitalized patients (MOVe-OUT, n = 1,433).[47,48] The MOVe-IN trial was terminated after interim analysis demonstrated no clinical benefits and trends for higher death rates on molnupiravir.[49] The Phase 2 stage of the MOVe-OUT trial an interim analysis resulted in a recommendation to expand recruitment to a larger trial.[49] The larger trial was stopped in October 2021 after an interim analysis of approximately 762 of the 1,433 patients showed a 50% reduction in the risk of hospitalization.[48,50] Interim analysis of the MOVe-Out trial, a randomized double-blind control comparing early treatment with molnupiravir versus placebo, demonstrated that the risk of hospitalization and all-cause 20-day mortality was lower in the molnupiravir group compared to placebo.[48,50] In general, the study population was of low-to-moderate risk as the study enrolment included only 14% of patients age >60 years of age with 86% of the subjects were ages 18–59.[48] In a subgroup analysis of patients with previous infection, those with a low viral load and diabetes this effect was attenuated and there was a trend favoring placebo.[48] In addition, efficacy was much lower in those patients infected with the delta variant.[48] This study is not without controversy as it was terminated early after 90% of subjects enrolled.[51] When final results were published, there was an overall 30% reduction in hospitalization, which was not statistically significant in a sensitivity analysis.[48,50] In the Optimus trial, a pharma funded Phase 3 RCT whose results are yet to be published in a peer review journal, results showed quicker time to polymerase chain reaction (PCR) negativity and resolution of symptoms.[49,52] Similarly, Tippabhotla et al. in a RCT involving 1,210 patient to molnupiravir or standard of care demonstrated that molnupiravir was associated with a statistically significance in clinical improvement and viral clearance.[53]

Butler et al. evaluated 26,411 patients in the Panorama trial, a RCT in the UK, demonstrated quicker recovery but no significant difference in hospitalization/death or transmission. Improved recovery may be related to the nature of the study with self-reported symptomatic data. Interestingly, viral load initially declined more quickly but was higher at 14 days.[54] Similarly, another corporate trial, the Hetero trial, initially reported an interim analysis that demonstrated evidence of a significant benefit for molnupiravir, whereas data from patients enrolled after the interim analysis showed no statistically significant benefit.[49] In an open-label RCT involving 1,218 patients with mild COVID-19, at least one risk factor for the progression of the disease, the addition of molnupiravir to the standard of care resulted in significant clinical improvement and increased rate of PCR negativity when compared to standard of care alone.[55] Butt et al., in a matched cohort design study involving 1,459 molnupiravir and matched controls, demonstrated no difference in the need for hospitalization or death within 30 days of COVID-19 diagnosis among mean platelet volume (MPV)-treated and untreated controls.[56] No benefit was observed regardless of vaccination status or age greater or <60. A subgroup analysis of asymptomatic patients demonstrated some benefit.[56] A meta-analysis of 12 corporate trials involving over 13,000 patients demonstrated significant bias, and missing data determined that molnupiravir had no apparent benefit in decreasing hospitalization.[42] In contrast, Gao et al. performed a meta-analysis of nine RCTs totaling 30,472 patients. The studies evaluated consisted mainly of outpatients with mild-to-moderate COVID-19 and a mean age ranging from 35 to 56.6 years. This meta-analysis revealed that in adult patients with mild-to-moderate COVID-19, molnupiravir likely reduced mortality [relative risk (RR), 0.43; 95% confidence interval (CI), 0.20–0.94; risk difference (RD), 0.1% fewer; moderate certainty] and the risk of hospital admission (RR, 0.67; 95% CI, 0.45–0.99; RD, 1.4% fewer; moderate certainty). Molnupiravir may also reduce time to viral clearance (mean difference, –1.81 days; 95% CI, –3.31 to –0.31; low certainty) and time to symptom resolution or clinical improvement (mean difference, –2.39 days; 95% CI, –3.71 to –1.07; low certainty). Molnupiravir is likely to increase the rate of viral clearance (RR, 3.47; 95% CI, 2.43–4.96; RD 16.1% more; moderate certainty) at 7 days (±3 days) and is unlikely to increase serious adverse events (RR, 0.84; 95% CI, 0.61–1.15; RD 0.1% fewer; moderate certainty).[57]

There is mounting evidence from real-world observational data demonstrating mixed results. The OpenSAFELY was a retrospective analysis of 75,048 outpatients in the UK, using the clone-censor-weight approach to address immortal time bias.[49] The investigators demonstrated no significant difference in combined mortality/hospitalization with molnupiravir treatment. Further analysis of the OpenSAFLEY platform cohort by Zheng et al. demonstrated that molnupiravir was associated with increased mortality and hospitalizations compared to nirmatrelvir-ritonavir.[58,59] Investigators from Italy in a large prospective observational national study investigating the Italian Medicines Agency (AIFA) database comparing all-cause mortality by day 28 of patients infected with SARS-CoV-2 and treated with molnupiravir or nirmatrelvir plus ritonavir.[60] The study included patients treated within 5 days after documentation of a PCR test-positive date and symptom onset. The registry included 17,977 outpatients treated with molnupiravir and 11,576 treated with nirmatrelvir plus ritonavir. Many of the patients were at high risk for progression to severe disease. The study found that both treatments resulted in significant mortality. However, the study also found that nirmatrelvir plus ritonavir had lower mortality compared to molnupiravir.[60]

Evans et al. retrospectively evaluated over 2,000 high-risk patients obtained from given antiviral therapy in the community by local health boards and the National Antiviral Service in Wales. Four groups were evaluated; those given molnupiravir, nirmatrelvir-ritonavir, sotrovimab, or no treatment. Patients receiving any treatment were noted to be highly vaccinated. The investigators demonstrated that treatment with any therapy resulted in a decrease in 28 days all-cause hospitalizations and death. In addition, there was no evidence of the superiority of one agent over another.[61] Inaba et al., in a retrospective study from Japan, showed that the use of molnupiravir was associated with a no statistically significant increase in all-cause hospitalization and death.[62] Bajema et al., in a large study of high-risk patients in the United States, revealed that molnupiravir was associated with a statistically significant increase in 180-day acute or long-term admissions.[63]

Goodwin et al., in a small retrospective study involving 604 outpatients in the United Kingdom, demonstrated a lower nonstatistically significant risk of hospitalization with molnupiravir treatment.[64] However, there were a few hospitalizations in all groups.

Wan et al. in a large late treatment retrospective analysis of over 30,000 patients hospitalized individuals with COVID-19, comparing those who received antiviral therapy and those who did not, demonstrated that antiviral therapy with molnupiravir or nirmatrelvir–ritonavir reduced mortality in late phase therapy regardless of vaccination status[65] In an Israeli study, retrospective analysis of 19,868 patients eligible to receive molnupiravir in which 1,069 received molnupiravir, there was a decrease in mortality in those patients age >65 years of age. Conversely, in those younger than 65 years, there was a higher mortality.[66] Najjar–Debbiny et al., in a propensity-matched study involving comparing 2,661 patients who received treatment with molnupiravir versus control found treatment to be associated with a decrease in the composite endpoint mortality and worsening of disease in older patients and those with inadequate vaccination status.[67]

This advantage positions molnupiravir as a promising drug for COVID-19 treatment, especially when compared to remdesivir, as it has a more patient-compliant oral dosage form and a straightforward chemical structure, which makes it easier to synthesize.

Thus, data suggest that molnupiravir, when employed as therapy, may have benefits in some patients. However, of significant concern regarding therapy with molnupiravir is the drug's mutagenic, genotoxic, and carcinogenic potential. In addition, the active molecule of molnupiravir N-dideoxycytidine has been found to induce mutations in SARS-CoV-2, which are resistant neutralizing antibodies.[68-70]

Administration of Molnupiravir

Who should be considered for Molnupiravir?

- Current diagnosis of mild-to-moderate COVID-19, not requiring hospitalization/supplemental oxygen[71]
- Age ≥ 18 years and weighing ≥ 40 kg
- Has risk factors for progression to severe COVID-19
- Ideally within 5 days of symptom onset

The recommended dose is 800 mg administered orally every 12 hours for 5 days.[42,48,72,73] There is no requirement for a dose adjustment for kidney or hepatic impairment.[72,73]

Adverse Effects of Molnupiravir

Further research is needed to fully understand the safety profile of molnupiravir, although current evidence suggests that it is safe and well-tolerated in the short-term.[56,71,73] The most common adverse effects of molnupiravir are diarrhea, nausea, and dizziness.[71] Recent clinical trials have not reported any serious adverse effects associated with the drug.[42,64,73] The most commonly reported adverse effects in a study by Arribas and colleagues were gastrointestinal disorders, infections, metabolic abnormalities, and respiratory problems.[38,42,55] These adverse events were also observed in COVID-19 patients who were not receiving active treatment or participating in the clinical trial.[38] As a result, it is difficult to determine if molnupiravir caused those adverse events. The available genotoxicity data and the short duration of treatment led to the conclusion that molnupiravir has a low risk for genotoxicity.[40,41,53,68,70]

Molnupiravir in Pregnancy

The FDA has advised against using molnupiravir in pregnant patients due to potential fetal toxicity, as seen in animal studies.[69-71,74] However, if other treatment options are unavailable and a pregnant individual with COVID-19 is at a high risk of developing severe disease, they may still choose to undergo molnupiravir therapy after being fully informed of the possible risks.[71] This may be a reasonable option, especially if the individual is beyond the time of embryogenesis, i.e., after the first 10 weeks of pregnancy.[71]

NIRMATRELVIR/RITONAVIR

Nirmatrelvir/ritonavir, a combination of nirmatrelvir (PF-07321332) and ritonavir, is a newer oral antiviral candidate for SARS-CoV-2 protease inhibitors released by Pfizer.[75-77] Nirmatrelvir/ritonavir is unique in that it targets the activity of the SARS-COV-2 3CL protease, which is crucial for the virus's replication **(Fig. 6)**.[78] However, nirmatrelvir cannot function independently, requiring a low dose of ritonavir to slow its metabolism.[75-77] By inhibiting cytochrome P450 (CYP) 3A4 and P-glycoprotein, ritonavir boosts the blood concentration of nirmatrelvir.[79-81] Due to its design to target the coronavirus-specific protease, nirmatrelvir/ritonavir is more specific to the virus than molnupiravir.[82,83] Although still being studied in clinical trials, nirmatrelvir/ritonavir appears to be a promising treatment for COVID-19.

Interestingly, other than encouraging results from corporate studies, there is a paucity of RCT data involving nirmatrelvir/ritonavir.[61,80, 84-87] There is, however, robust real-world data involving therapy with this agent.[87] It is of interest that Pfizer has denied access to nirmatrelvir/ritonavir for independent RCT in Africa.[88] Although real-world data results are encouraging, one must consider the issues with confounding due to immortal time bias, from confounding by contraindication and confounding by including patients in whom nirmatrelvir/ritonavir is contraindicated in the analysis.[89,90] In

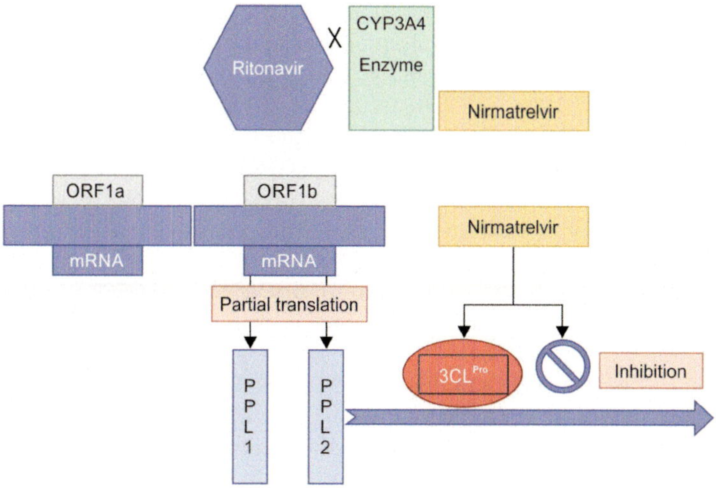

FIGURE 6: Mechanism of nirmatrelvir. In order to achieve therapeutic levels coadministration of ritonavir is needed to inhibit CYP3A4 metabolism of nirmatrelvir. It works by inhibiting the activity of the 3C-like protease ($3CL^{Pro}$) of SARS-CoV-2, which is responsible for cleaving polyproteins 1a and 1ab. Without the activity of the $3CL^{Pro}$, nonstructural proteins (including proteases) cannot be released to perform their functions, thus inhibiting viral replication and survival.[78]

(mRNA: messenger ribonucleic acid; SARS-CoV-2: severe acute respiratory syndrome coronavirus 2)

addition, real-world observational studies in many cases do not account for the different anticipated outcomes for the subsets of patients seeking and receiving early treatment.[89,91-93] For example, in a cohort study conducted by Hoertel et al. involving over 62,000 patients surveyed from 36 university hospitals in greater Paris between January 24, 2020, and November 30, 2021.[91] The objective of the study was to evaluate the individual medical contraindications for nirmatrelvir-ritonavir listed by the US FDA in a large sample of COVID-19 patients.[90] The researchers aimed to determine the proportion of patients with contraindications to nirmatrelvir-ritonavir in the sample, including those who died within 28 days of hospital admission. Of those patients who died, 50% had a contraindication to receiving nirmatrelivir/ritonavir.[90] This study provides insight into the possible challenges and considerations of using nirmatrelvir-ritonavir as a treatment.[90] This study also highlights the potential for confounding by contraindication in observational studies.[90] The most common contraindications included severe renal dysfunction and drug-drug interactions.[90]

Hammond et al., in a Phase 2/3 double-blind, RCT, the EPIC-HR RCT, enrolled 1,039 higher-risk patients who were unvaccinated treated with nirmatrelvir/ritonavir and 1,046 control patients.[80] The findings of this study demonstrated that administration of nirmatrelvir/ritonavir to symptomatic COVID-19 patients significantly reduces the risk of progression to severe COVID-19 by 89% compared to the placebo.[80] There were no apparent safety concerns with this study.[80]

The EPIC-SR clinical trial, a Phase 2/3, a multinational, double-blind RCT involving 1,145 standard risk outpatients conducted by Pfizer, did not meet its primary endpoint of self-reported, sustained alleviation of all symptoms for 4 consecutive days.[86,94-96] The treatment group exhibited a substantially reduced but nonstatistically significant mortality risk, with a 66.8% decrease compared to the control group.[86] No deaths were observed in the treatment group, whereas a single death was reported in the control group. The treatment group also demonstrated a nonstatistically significant decreased risk of intensive care unit (ICU) admission, with zero admissions recorded compared to three in the control group, out of 576 and 569 participants, respectively. There was a statistically nonsignificant decrease in risk of death or hospitalization ($p = 0.05$).[86,96]

A study by Liu et al. in a multicenter RCT examined the efficacy and safety of nirmatrelvir/ritonavir in severe adult patients with SARS-CoV-2 infection.[97] The findings demonstrated that administration of nirmatrelvir/ritonavir led to an 89.1% and 88.9% reduction in hospitalization and 28-day mortality rates.[97] Respectively, these findings were demonstrated in unvaccinated, high-risk, ambulatory COVID-19 patients.[97] However, nirmatrelvir/ritonavir did not prevent low-risk and standard-risk patients from progressing toward severe COVID-19.[97] In another retrospective study, 180,351 patients with at least one comorbidity or condition associated with high risk for severe COVID-19 were examined, and nirmatrelvir/ritonavir was shown to have a 46% risk reduction in disease progression.[98] These results suggest that nirmatrelvir/ritonavir may effectively reduce severe outcomes in high-risk COVID-19 patients but not as effectively in low-risk individuals.[97,98]

Yang et al. conducted a study on elderly COVID-19 patients with underlying conditions who were hospitalized.[99] They analyzed data from 1,281 patients and found that 91.5% recovered, 6.9% improved, and 2.6% died.[99] Some patients experienced COVID-19 rebound after initial recovery.[99] Vaccination did not have a protective effect, but nirmatrelvir/ritonavir therapy was associated with lower mortality risk.[99] Solid malignancies and neurologic disease were associated with an increase in mortality.[99]

Shao et al. conducted a study assessing the effectiveness of combined interventions on severely and critically ill COVID-19 patients.[100] The study was a Bayesian analysis of health-related quality of life (HRQoL), disability, and mortality rate of 1,082 patients.[100] A total of 139 patients (12.9%) died within the 60-day period.[100] The study's findings suggest that nirmatrelvir/ritonavir may positively impact the outcomes of severely and critically ill COVID-19 patients, with a 91.9% probability of improving survival rates by 2 months.[100] The adjusted hazard ratio (HR) of 0.71 (95% credible interval, 0.44–1.14) compared to the control group indicates that nirmatrelvir/ritonavir could be a viable treatment option for such patients.[100]

Torti et al. conducted a nationwide observational study comparing the mortality outcomes of nonhospitalized SARS-CoV-2 infected patients at risk for clinical progression who were treated with either molnupiravir or nirmatrevir/ritonavir during the omicron era in Italy.[60] The study utilized real-life data and investigated the 30-day mortality rate among the two treatment groups. Although outcomes were improved in both groups, the findings indicated that patients who received molnupiravir had a lower mortality rate than those who were treated with nirmatrevir/ritonavir.[60] This suggests that molnupiravir may be more efficacious in reducing mortality among nonhospitalized COVID-19.

A recent study by Yan et al. evaluated the effectiveness of nirmatrelvir/ritonavir as a treatment option for individuals with both SARS-CoV-2 infection and impaired kidney function during the Omicron surge.[101] The investigation specifically targeted patients with an estimated glomerular filtration rate (eGFR) of <45 mL/min/1.73 m^2 and those undergoing maintenance hemodialysis.[101] The study results were consistent with previous research, indicating that nirmatrelvir/ritonavir therapy can be beneficial in treating patients with renal impairment and SARS-CoV-2 infection.[101] Therefore, this study provides valuable insights into the effectiveness and safety of nirmatrelvir/ritonavir in patients with impaired renal function. Further studies are necessary to expand the evidence base and improve treatment strategies for individuals with renal impairment and SARS-CoV-2 infection.

Lewnard et al. conducted a recent study to assess the efficacy of nirmatrelvir/ritonavir in preventing hospitalizations and fatalities among COVID-19 patients receiving outpatient care within a large US healthcare system.[102] The study demonstrated that patients who received nirmatrelvir/ritonavir in ambulatory care settings had a significantly lower incidence of COVID-19-related emergency department visits and hospitalizations.[102] These findings suggest that nirmatrelvir/ritonavir holds the potential to be efficacious in preventing severe outcomes of COVID-19 in an outpatient environment.

In order to evaluate whether therapy with nirmatrelvir/ritonavir improved clinical outcomes in vaccinated patients, Dryden–Peterson et al. evaluated the effectiveness of nirmatrelvir/ritonavir in treating COVID-19 in a highly vaccinated cohort of over 44,000 patients age >50 years.[103] The results demonstrated nirmatrelvir/ritonavir reduced the risk of hospitalization and death in patients who received it compared to those who did not.[103] However, the results of this study may be impacted by residual confounding may exist.[103]

Evans et al. evaluated high-risk patients with COVID-19 comparing the effectiveness of three therapeutic agents molnupiravir, nirmatrelvir/ritonavir, and sotrovimab in preventing hospitalization or mortality.[61] The primary outcome measure was all-cause admission to hospital or death within 28 days of a positive test for SARS-CoV-2.[61] Molnupiravir, nirmatrelvir/ritonavir, and sotrovimab were administered to patients in a community setting.[61] The study found that patients who received any of the three drugs were less likely to be hospitalized or die than those who did not receive treatment, but did not indicate which treatment was superior.[61]

Zheng et al. evaluated the OpenSAFELY-TPP platform in order to assess the effectiveness of nirmatrelvir/ritonavir, sotrovimab, and molnupiravir in preventing severe COVID-19 outcomes among high-risk adult outpatients.[59] Patient-level electronic health record data were obtained from 24 million individuals registered with general practices in England that use TPP software.[59] Nirmatrelvir/ritonavir and sotrovimab were the primary treatment options in community settings.[59] The primary outcome evaluated was COVID-19-related hospitalization or death within 28 days of treatment initiation.[59] A total of 7,683 eligible patients were included in the study, with 4,836 treated with nirmatrelvir/ritonavir and 2,847 treated with sotrovimab. The findings showed no significant difference in the risk of severe COVID-19 outcomes between those who received nirmatrelvir/ritonavir or sotrovimab.[59] Overall, this study demonstrated that treating high-risk adult outpatients with COVID-19 with either nirmatrelvir/ritonavir or sotrovimab during routine care in England did not substantially differ in the risk of severe COVID-19 outcomes.[59]

Bajema et al. retrospectively assessed the effectiveness of nirmatrelvir/ritonavir and molnupiravir in treating COVID-19 involving over 100,000 nonhospitalized patients.[63] The findings revealed that nirmatrelvir/ritonavir reduced the likelihood of hospitalization and death within 30 days, while molnupiravir decreased mortality within 30 days and from days 31–180.[63] There was no significant difference between the two antiviral drugs regarding the risk of hospitalization or death.[63]

Schwartz et al., in a population-based study that included 177,545 patients, 8,876 (5.0%) were treated with nirmatrelvir/ritonavir, and 168,669 (95.0%) were not.[104] The results demonstrated that nirmatrelvir/ritonavir treatment can significantly reduce the risk of hospitalization and death related to COVID-19.[104] It is particularly advised for those with mild symptoms with a higher risk of serious complications.[104]

Arbel et al. evaluated the effectiveness of nirmatrelvir/ritonavir during the Delta and Omicron wave of the pandemic in 109,254 COVID-19 patients at risk for severe outcomes.[66] About 4% of the entire population received nirmatrelvir/ritonavir. Patients over 65 years who received nirmatrelvir/ritonavir had lower hospitalization and death rates.

In a propensity score weighted retrospective study involving 93,883 outpatients, of which 5,808 treated with molnupiravir and 4,921 treated with nirmatrelvir/ritonavir, Yip et al. evaluated the effectiveness of two antiviral medications, molnupiravir and nirmatrelvir/ritonavir, in nonhospitalized COVID-19 patients.[105] Nirmatrelvir/ritonavir users had a reduced risk of hospitalization compared to nonusers.[105] There was a nonstatistically significant higher hospitalization and higher combined mortality/mechanical ventilation/ICU admission with molnupiravir.[105] Neither medication was associated with a lower risk of intensive care or death.[105]

It is pertinent to note that in a certain percentage of patients, a rebound of symptomatic disease occurs after initial improvement after completion of antiviral therapy with nirmatrelvir/ritonavir and molnupiravir.[77,106,107]

A major limitation of therapy with nirmatrelvir/ritonavir is significant drug-drug interactions with common medications, which can be life-threatening.[108-110] In order to maintain adequate therapeutic levels of the antiviral nirmatrelivir/ritonavir, ritonavir, a potent rapid-acting inhibitor of cytochrome P350 3A4 (CYP3A4) metabolic pathway, is administered as a pharmacokinetic booster.[109-112] Concomitant administration of many cardiovascular medications, anticoagulants, and immunosuppressants may increase drug levels of these agents to toxic levels. Thus close therapeutic drug monitoring and even temporary cessation of these agents is required.[108,110-112]

Administration of Nirmatrelvir/Ritonavir

Who should be considered for nirmatrelvir/ritonavir?[113,114]

- Current diagnosis of mild-to-moderate COVID-19, not requiring hospitalization/supplemental oxygen
- Age ≥ 18 years or > 12 years of age and weighing ≥ 40 kg
- Has risk factors for progression to severe COVID-19
- Symptom onset within 5 days
- No history of suspected severe renal impairment (eGFR < 30 mL/min)
- No history of suspected severe hepatic impairment (Child–Pugh Class C)

Nirmatrelvir/ritonavir is prescribed at an oral dose of 300/100 mg twice daily for 5 days.[114]

Nirmatrelvir/Ritonavir in Patients with Renal and Hepatic Impairment

In patients with significant renal impairment, using ritonavir-boosted nirmatrelvir may be challenging. The FDA has approved the following dosage of ritonavir/nirmatrelvir according to eGFR, as shown in **Table 1**.[115] As nirmatrelvir/ritonavir is eliminated through the kidneys, the EUA does not recommend ritonavir-boosted nirmatrelvir for patients with an eGFR of 30 mL/min until more information is available.[114] However, some groups, such as the Ontario Renal Network (ORN), have suggested dosage adjustments for patients with an eGFR of <30 mL/min or who are on hemodialysis.[115] Due to the high incidence of severe symptomatic disease and mortality in COVID-19-positive patients with advanced chronic kidney disease (stages 4 and 5) and on dialysis, a lower dose given at a lower frequency dose has been proposed for people with estimated glomerular filtration rate (eGFR) and on dialysis **(Table 2)**.[94,115,116]

TABLE 1: Current dosing information in patients with mild and moderate renal impairment.[114]

Kidney function	Recommended dosing
eGFR ≥60–<90	300 mg nirmatrelvir + 100 mg ritonavir both twice a day for 5 days
eGFR ≥30–<60	150 mg nirmatrelvir + 100 mg ritonavir both twice a day for 5 days

(eGFR: estimated glomerular filtration rate)

Patients with mild (Child–Pugh A) or moderate (Child–Pugh B) hepatic impairment do not require dose adjustment when taking ritonavir/nirmatrelvir.[11,80,85] However, there is no data available on the safety and pharmacokinetics of nirmatrelvir/ritonavir in patients with severe hepatic impairment (Child–Pugh C), so the drug is not recommended for use in this population.[114]

Side Effects of Nirmatrelvir/Ritonavir

The most frequent side effects of nirmatrelvir/ritonavir are dysgeusia (taste disturbance), diarrhea, hypertension, myalgia, vomiting, and headache.[115]

Nirmatrelvir/ritonavir is known to have severe drug-drug interactions since ritonavir is a potent cytochrome P450 3A4 inhibitor. Ritonavir/nirmatrelvir component may raise blood concentrations of some concurrent drugs, increasing the risk of significant drug toxicity.[109-112]

Table 3 lists drugs that cannot be taken with ritonavir/nirmatrelvir and not recommended for coadministration with ritonavir/nirmatrelvir. **Table 3**

TABLE 2: Proposed dosing guidance for nirmatrelvir/ritonavir in chronic kidney disease by Ontario Renal Network (ORN).[115]

Kidney function	Proposed dosing
eGFR < 30	300 mg nirmatrelvir + 100 mg ritonavir both on day 1 then 150 mg nirmatrelvir + 100 mg ritonavir once a day for 4 more days
Dialysis	300 mg nirmatrelvir + 100 mg ritonavir both on day 1 then 150 mg nirmatrelvir + 100 mg ritonavir once a day for 4 more days, to be dosed after dialysis *If patient weight < 40 kg*: 150 mg nirmatrelvir + 100 mg ritonavir on day 1 then 150 mg nirmatrelvir + 100 mg ritonavir every 48 hours for 2 more doses, to be given after dialysis

(eGFR: estimated glomerular filtration rate)

TABLE 3: Drug interactions with ritonavir/nirmatrelvir.

Severity	Rationale	Recommendation	Drugs
Contraindicated	• Withholding drug will not mitigate interaction • Do not coadminister due to severe toxicity	• Use alternative COVID-19 treatment strategies • Do not use nirmatrelvir/ritonavir	*Anticonvulsants*: • Carbamazepine • Phenobarbital • Phenytoin • Primidone *Anti-infectives*: • Rifampin • Rifapentine

Continued

Continued

Severity	Rationale	Recommendation	Drugs
			Chemotherapeutic agents: • Apalutamide • Dabrafenib • Enzalutamide • Lorlatinib • Mitotane *Cardiovascular*: • Amiodarone • Dronedarone • Eplerenone • Flecainide • Ivabradine • Propafenone • Quinidine *Neuropsychiatric*: • Clozapine • Lurasidone • Pimozide • Risperidone *Pulmonary hypertension*: • Sildenafil • Tadalafil • Vardenafil • Bosentan *Miscellaneous*: • St John's wort • Fentanyl • Eletriptan • Tolvaptan
Do not coadminister	• Significant increase in drug concentrations • Do not coadminister due to severe toxicity	• Withhold and restart 2 days after completion of nirmatrelvir/ritonavir • Withhold for longer if the patient is an adult of advanced age	*Anticoagulants*: • Rivaroxaban *Anti-infectives/immunosuppressant*: • Glecaprevir/pibrentasvir • Tacrolimus • Cyclosporin • Sirolimus *BPH*: • Alfuzosin • Silodosin

Continued

Continued

Severity	Rationale	Recommendation	Drugs
			Cardiovascular: • Disopyramide • Dofetilide • Ticagrelor *Chemotherapeutic agents*: • Bosutinib • Cisapride • Cobimetinib • Ibrutinib • Neratinib *Erectile dysfunction*: • Vardenafil *Lipid-modifiers*: • Lomitapide • Lovastatin • Simvastatin *Migraine*: • Dihydroergotamine • Ergonovine *Neuropsychiatric*: • Clonazepam • Diazepam • Flurazepam • Midazolam (oral) • Nitrazepam • Triazolam *Respiratory*: • Salmeterol *Miscellaneous*: • Colchicine • Meperidine

is not an exhaustive list, and prescribers should always use resources like the Liverpool COVID-19 Drug Interactions to identify and manage drug-drug interactions.[116]

SUMMARY

After almost 2 years of therapeutic nihilism, antiviral therapy has finally been included in an early therapy for managing COVID-19. These agents need to be initiated within the onset of therapy. Although hard endpoints used in clinical trials, such as mortality, use in the real world has some encouraging results. However, the use of these agents has limitations, such as drug-drug interactions, breakthrough, and possibly inducing viral mutations leading to resistance.

REFERENCES

1. Abbas MM, Morland TB, Hall ES, EL-Manzalawy Y. Associations between Google Search Trends for Symptoms and COVID-19 Confirmed and Death Cases in the United States. Int J Environ Res Public Health. 2021;18(9):4560.
2. Rivasi G, Bulgaresi M, Mossello E, Buscemi P, Lorini C, Balzi D, et al. Course and lethality of SARS-CoV-2 epidemic in nursing homes after vaccination in Florence, Italy. Vaccines (Basel). 2021;9(10):1174.
3. Chia PY, Ong SWX, Chiew CJ, Ang LW, Chavatte JM, Mak TM, et al. Virological and Serological Kinetics of SARS-CoV-2 Delta Variant Vaccine-Breakthrough Infections: A Multi-Center Cohort Study. Clin Microbiol Infect. 2022;28(4):612.e1-612.e7.
4. Simon MS, Luginbuhl R, Parker RA. (2021). Reduced Incidence of Long-Covid Symptoms Related to Administration of COVID-19 Vaccines Both before COVID-19 Diagnosis and Up to 12 Weeks After. [online] Available from https://www.medrxiv.org/content/10.1101/2021.11.17.21263608v1. [Last accessed February, 2024].
5. Kanakan A, Mishra N, Vasudevan JS, Sahni S, Khan A, Sharma S, et al. Threading the Pieces Together: Integrative Perspective on SARS-CoV-2. Pathogens. 2020;9(11):912.
6. Evolutionary insight into the emergence of SARS-CoV-2 variants of concern. Nat Med. 2022;28(7):1357-8.
7. Lu R, Zhao X, Li J, Niu P, Yang B, Wu H, et al. Genomic Characterisation and Epidemiology of 2019 Novel Coronavirus: Implications for Virus Origins and Receptor Binding. Lancet. 2020;395(10224):565-74.
8. Waters L, Marra F, Pozniak A, Cockburn J, Boffito M. Ritonavir and COVID-19: pragmatic guidance is important. Lancet. 2022;399(10334):1464-5.
9. Wang L, Berger NA, Davis PB, Kaelber DC, Volkow ND, Xu R. (2022). COVID-19 Rebound after Paxlovid and Molnupiravir during January-June 2022. [online] Available from https://www.medrxiv.org/content/10.1101/2022.06.21.22276724v1. [Last accessed February, 2024].
10. Singh AK, Singh A, Singh R, Misra A. Molnupiravir in COVID-19: A systematic review of literature. Diabetes Metab Syndr. 2021;15(6):102329.
11. Marzolini C, Kuritzkes DR, Marra F, Boyle A, Gibbons S, Flexner C, et al. Recommendations for the management of drug–drug interactions between the COVID-19 antiviral nirmatrelvir/ritonavir (Paxlovid) and comedications. Clin Pharmacol Ther. 2022;112(6):1191-200.
12. Eastman RT, Roth JS, Brimacombe KR, Simeonov A, Shen M, Patnaik S, et al. Remdesivir: a review of its discovery and development leading to emergency use authorization for treatment of COVID-19. ACS Cent Sci. 2020;6(5):672-83.
13. Griffin DO, Brennan-Rieder D, Ngo B, Kory P, Confalonieri M, Shapiro L, et al. The Importance of Understanding the Stages of COVID-19 in Treatment and Trials. AIDS Rev. 2021;23(1):40-7.
14. Ngo BT, Marik P, Kory P, Shapiro L, Thomadsen R, Iglesias J, et al. The time to offer treatments for COVID-19. Expert Opin Investig Drugs. 2021;30(5):505-18.
15. Marik PE, Varon J, Kory P. Treatment of COVID-19 is critically phase specific. Crit Care Shock. 2020;23(5):10-2.
16. Marik PE, Iglesias J, Varon J, Kory P. A scoping review of the pathophysiology of COVID-19. Int J Immunopathol Pharmacol. 2021;35:20587384211048026.
17. Frediansyah A, Nainu F, Dhama K, Mudatsir M, Harapan H. Remdesivir and its Antiviral Activity Against COVID-19: A Systematic Review. Clin Epidemiol Glob Health. 2021;9:123-7.

18. Pardo J, Shukla AM, Chamarthi G, Gupte A. The journey of remdesivir: from Ebola to COVID-19. Drugs Context. 2020;9:2020-4-14.
19. Tchesnokov EP, Feng JY, Porter DP, Götte M. Mechanism of Inhibition of Ebola Virus RNA-Dependent RNA Polymerase by Remdesivir. Viruses. 2019;11(4):326.
20. Chatterjee B, Thakur SS. Remdesivir and its Combination with Repurposed Drugs as COVID-19 Therapeutics. Front Immunol. 2022;13:830990.
21. Li R, Liclican A, Xu Y, et al. Key Metabolic Enzymes Involved in Remdesivir Activation in Human Lung Cells. Antimicrob Agents Chemother. 2021;65(9):e0060221.
22. Jittamala P, Schilling WHK, Watson JA, Luvira V, Siripoon T, Ngamprasertchai T, et al. Clinical Antiviral Efficacy of Remdesivir in Coronavirus Disease 2019: An Open-Label, Randomized Controlled Adaptive Platform Trial (PLATCOV). J Infect Dis. 2023;228(10):1318-25.
23. Ali K, Azher T, Baqi M, Binnie A, Borgia S, Carrier FM, et al. Remdesivir for the treatment of patients in hospital with COVID-19 in Canada: a randomized controlled trial. CMAJ. 2022;194(7):E242-51.
24. Beigel JH, Tomashek KM, Dodd LE, Mehta AK, Zingman BS, Kalil AC, et al. Remdesivir for the Treatment of Covid-19—Final Report. N Engl J Med. 2020;383(19):1813-26.
25. Healio. (2020). Fauci on remdesivir for COVID-19: 'This will be the standard of care'. [online] Available from https://www.healio.com/news/infectious-disease/20200429/fauci-on-remdesivir-for-covid19-this-will-be-the-standard-of-care. [Last accessed February, 2024].
26. WHO Solidarity Trial Consortium; Pan H, Peto R, Henao-Restrepo AM, Preziosi MP, Sathiyamoorthy V, Karim QA, et al. Repurposed Antiviral Drugs for Covid-19—Interim WHO Solidarity Trial Results. N Engl J Med. 2021;384(6):497-511.
27. WHO Solidarity Trial Consortium. Remdesivir and three other drugs for hospitalised patients with COVID-19: final results of the WHO Solidarity randomised trial and updated meta-analyses. Lancet. 2022;399(10339):1941-53.
28. Grundeis F, Ansems K, Dahms K, Thieme V, Metzendorf MI, Skoetz N, et al. Remdesivir for the treatment of COVID-19. Cochrane Database Syst Rev. 2023;1(1):CD014962.
29. Ader F, Bouscambert-Duchamp M, Hites M, Peiffer-Smadja N, Poissy J, Belhadi D, et al. Remdesivir plus standard of care versus standard of care alone for the treatment of patients admitted to hospital with COVID-19 (DisCoVeRy): a phase 3, randomised, controlled, open-label trial. Lancet Infect Dis. 2022;22(2):209-21.
30. Barratt-Due A, Olsen IC, Nezvalova-Henriksen K, Kåsine T, Lund-Johansen F, Hoel H, et al. Evaluation of the Effects of Remdesivir and Hydroxychloroquine on Viral Clearance in COVID-19. Ann Intern Med. 2021;174(9):1261-9.
31. Spinner CD, Gottlieb RL, Criner GJ, Arribas López JR, Cattelan AM, Viladomiu AS, et al. Effect of Remdesivir vs Standard Care on Clinical Status at 11 Days in Patients with Moderate COVID-19: A Randomized Clinical Trial. JAMA. 2020;324(11):1048-57.
32. Wang Y, Zhang D, Du G, Du R, Zhao J, Jin Y, et al. Remdesivir in adults with severe COVID-19: a randomised, double-blind, placebo-controlled, multicentre trial. Lancet. 2020;395(10236):1569-78.
33. Mahajan L, Singh AP, Gifty. Clinical outcomes of using remdesivir in patients with moderate to severe COVID-19: A prospective randomised study. Indian J Anaesth. 2021;65(Suppl 1):S41-6.
34. Gholamhoseini MT, Yazdi-Feyzabadi V, Goudarzi R, Mehrolhassani MH. Safety and Efficacy of Remdesivir for the Treatment of COVID-19: A Systematic Review and Meta-Analysis. J Pharm Pharm Sci. 2021;24:237-45.
35. Zhou Y, Li J, Wang L, Zhu X, Zhang M, Zheng J. Acute Kidney Injury and Drugs Prescribed for COVID-19 in Diabetes Patients: A Real-World Disproportionality Analysis. Front Pharmacol. 2022;13:833679.

36. Chavda VP, Teli D, Balar PC, Vaghela D, Solanki KH, Vaishnav A, et al. Potential Anti-SARS-CoV-2 Prodrugs Activated by Phosphorylation and Their Role in the Aged Population. Molecules. 2023;28(5):2332.
37. Imran M, Arora MK, Asdaq SM, Khan SA, Alaqel SI, Alshammari MK, et al. Discovery, Development, and Patent Trends on Molnupiravir: A Prospective Oral Treatment for COVID-19. Molecules. 2021;26(19):5795.
38. Arribas JR, Bhagani S, Lobo SM, Khaertynova I, Mateu L, Fishchuk R, et al. Randomized Trial of Molnupiravir or Placebo in Patients Hospitalized with Covid-19. NEJM Evid. 2022;1(2):EVIDoa2100044.
39. Afni N, Suharjono S. (2022). Molnupiravir—the First Oral Antiviral for COVID-19: A Literature Review. [online] Available from https://api.semanticscholar.org/CorpusID:250098991. [Last accessed February, 2024].
40. Kaore S, Atal S. Molnupiravir in COVID-19: A scoping review. Curr Drug Res Rev. 2022;14(3):203-14.
41. Zou R, Peng L, Shu D, Zhao L, Lan J, Tan G, et al. Antiviral Efficacy and Safety of Molnupiravir Against Omicron Variant Infection: A Randomized Controlled Clinical Trial. Front Pharmacol. 2022;13:939573.
42. Fischer WA, Eron JJ, Holman W, Cohen MS, Fang L, Szewczyk LJ, et al. (2021). Molnupiravir, an Oral Antiviral Treatment for COVID-19. [online] Available from https://api.semanticscholar.org/CorpusID:235459592. [Last accessed February, 2024].
43. Khoo SH, Fitzgerald R, Fletcher T, Ewings S, Jaki T, Lyon R, et al. Optimal dose and safety of molnupiravir in patients with early SARS-CoV-2: a Phase I, open-label, dose-escalating, randomized controlled study. J Antimicrob Chemother. 2021;76(12):3286-95.
44. Khoo SH, FitzGerald R, Saunders G, Middleton C, Ahmad S, Edwards CJ, et al. Molnupiravir versus placebo in unvaccinated and vaccinated patients with early SARS-CoV-2 infection in the UK (AGILE CST-2): a randomised, placebo-controlled, double-blind, phase 2 trial. Lancet Infect Dis. 2023;23(2):183-95.
45. Sheahan TP, Sims AC, Zhou S, Graham RL, Hill CS, Leist SR, et al. (2020). An orally bioavailable broad-spectrum antiviral inhibits SARS-CoV-2 and multiple endemic, epidemic and bat coronavirus. [online] Available from https://www.biorxiv.org/content/10.1101/2020.03.19.997890v1. [Last accessed February, 2024].
46. Painter GR, Natchus MG, Cohen O, Holman W, Painter WP. Developing a direct acting, orally available antiviral agent in a pandemic: the evolution of molnupiravir as a potential treatment for COVID-19. Curr Opin Virol. 2021;50:17-22.
47. Merck M. (2021). Merck and Ridgeback Biotherapeutics Provide Update on Progress of Clinical Development Program for Molnupiravir, an Investigational Oral Therapeutic for the Treatment of Mild-to-Moderate COVID-19. [online] Available from https://www.merck.com/news/merck-and-ridgeback-biotherapeutics-provide-update-on-progress-of-clinical-development-program-for-molnupiravir-an-investigational-oral-therapeutic-for-the-treatment-of-mild-to-moderate-covid-19/. [Last accessed February, 2024].
48. Jayk Bernal A, Gomes da Silva MM, Musungaie DB, Kovalchuk E, Antonio Gonzalez 1, Reyes VD, et al. Molnupiravir for Oral Treatment of Covid-19 in Nonhospitalized Patients. N Engl J Med. 2022;386(6):509-20.
49. Lawrence JM, Mirchandani M, Hill A. Evaluation of publication bias for 12 clinical trials of molnupiravir to treat SARS-CoV-2 infection in 13694 patients with meta-analysis. J Antimicrob Chemother. 2023;78(3):613-9.
50. Guan Y, Puenpatom A, Johnson MG, Zhang Y, Zhao Y, Surber J, et al. Impact of Molnupiravir Treatment on Patient-reported Coronavirus Disease 2019 (COVID-19) Symptoms in the Phase 3 MOVe-OUT Trial: A Randomized, Placebo-Controlled Trial. Clin Infect Dis. 2023;77(11):1521-30.

51. Thorlund K, Sheldrick K, Meyerowitz-Katz G, Singh S, Hill A. Making statistical sense of the molnupiravir MOVe-OUT clinical trial. Am J Trop Med Hyg. 2022;106(5):1301-4.
52. Mali KR, Eerike M, Raj GM, Bisoi D, Priyadarshini R, Ravi G, et al. Efficacy and safety of Molnupiravir in COVID-19 patients: a systematic review. Ir J Med Sci. 2023;192(4): 1665-78.
53. Tippabhotla SK, Lahiri DS, Kandi C. (2022). Efficacy and safety of molnupiravir for the treatment of non-hospitalized adults with mild COVID-19: a randomized, open-label, parallel-group phase 3 trial. [online] Available from https://papers.ssrn.com/sol3/papers.cfm?abstract_id=4042673. [Last accessed February, 2024].
54. Butler CC, Hobbs FDR, Gbinigie OA, Rahman NM, Hayward G, Richards DB, et al. Molnupiravir plus usual care versus usual care alone as early treatment for adults with COVID-19 at increased risk of adverse outcomes (PANORAMIC): an open-label, platform-adaptive randomised controlled trial. Lancet. 2023;401(10373):281-93.
55. Sinha S, Kumarasamy N, Suram VK, Chary SS, Naik N, Singh VB, et al. Efficacy and Safety of Molnupiravir in Mild COVID-19 Patients in India. Cureus. 2022;14(11):e31508.
56. Butt AA, Yan P, Chotani RA, Shaikh OS. Mortality is not increased in SARS-CoV-2 infected persons with hepatitis C virus infection. Liver Int. 2021;41(8):1824-31.
57. Gao Y, Liu M, Li Z, Xu J, Zhang J, Tian J. Molnupiravir for treatment of adults with mild or moderate COVID-19: a systematic review and meta-analysis of randomized controlled trials. Clin Microbiol Infect. 2023;29(8):979-99.
58. The OpenSAFELY collaborative; Tazare J, Nab L, Zheng B, Hulme WJ, Green ACA, Curtis HJ, et al. (2023). Effectiveness of Sotrovimab and Molnupiravir in community settings in England across the Omicron BA.1 and BA.2 sublineages: emulated target trials using the OpenSAFELY platform. [online] Available from https://www.medrxiv.org/content/10.1101/2023.05.12.23289914v1. [Last accessed February, 2024].
59. Zheng B, Tazare J, Nab L, Mehrkar A, MacKenna B, Goldacre B, et al. (2023). Comparative effectiveness of Paxlovid versus sotrovimab and molnupiravir for preventing severe COVID-19 outcomes in non-hospitalised patients: observational cohort study using the OpenSAFELY platform. [online] Available from https://www.medrxiv.org/content/10.1101/2023.01.20.23284849v1. [Last accessed February, 2024].
60. Torti C, Olimpieri PP, Bonfanti P, Tascini C, Celant S, Tacconi D, et al. Real-life comparison of mortality in patients with SARS-CoV-2 infection at risk for clinical progression treated with molnupiravir or nirmatrelvir plus ritonavir during the Omicron era in Italy: a nationwide, cohort study. Lancet Reg Health Eur. 2023;31:100684.
61. Evans A, Qi C, Adebayo JO, Underwood J, Coulson J, Bailey R, et al. Real-world effectiveness of molnupiravir, nirmatrelvir-ritonavir, and sotrovimab on preventing hospital admission among higher-risk patients with COVID-19 in Wales: A retrospective cohort study. J Infect. 2023;86(4):352-60.
62. Inaba S, Nishioka N, Okumura H, Nakao K, Hattori Y, Futamura S, et al. (2023). Real-world data concerning the efficacy of molnupiravir in patients vaccinated against COVID-19 during the Omicron surge in Japan. [online] Available from https://assets.researchsquare.com/files/rs-2451986/v1/22de8257-5be6-4d03-b412-32edbaad34f7.pdf?c=1680610482. [Last accessed February, 2024].
63. Bajema KL, Berry K, Streja E, Rajeevan N, Li Y, Mutalik P, et al. Effectiveness of COVID-19 Treatment with Nirmatrelvir–Ritonavir or Molnupiravir among U.S. Veterans: Target Trial Emulation Studies with One-Month and Six-month Outcomes. Ann Intern Med. 2023;176(6):807-16.
64. Goodwin AT, Thompson JS, Hall IP. Evaluation of outpatient treatment for non-hospitalised patients with COVID-19: The experience of a regional centre in the UK. PLoS One. 2023;18(3):e0281915.
65. Wan EYF, Wang B, Mathur S, Chan CIY, Yan VKC, Lai FTT, et al. Molnupiravir and nirmatrelvir–ritonavir reduce mortality risk during post-acute COVID-19 phase. J Infect. 2023;86(6):622-5.

66. Arbel R, Wolff Sagy Y, Hoshen M, Battat E, Lavie G, Sergienko R, et al. Nirmatrelvir Use and Severe Covid-19 Outcomes during the Omicron Surge. N Engl J Med. 2022;387(9): 790-8.
67. Najjar-Debbiny R, Gronich N, Weber G, Khoury J, Amar M, Stein N, et al. Effectiveness of Molnupiravir in High-risk Patients: A Propensity Score Matched Analysis. Clin Infect Dis. 2023;76(3):453-60.
68. Huntsman MC. (2023). An Assessment of the Reproductive Toxicity of the Anti-COVID-19 Drug Molnupiravir using Stem Cell-Based Embryo Models. [online] Available from https://www.proquest.com/openview/33e352366023491c0a1ce1649edb7e2a/1?pq-origsite=gscholar&cbl=18750&diss=y. [Last accessed February, 2024].
69. Waters MD, Warren S, Hughes C, Lewis P, Zhang F. Human genetic risk of treatment with antiviral nucleoside analog drugs that induce lethal mutagenesis: The special case of molnupiravir. Environ Mol Mutagen. 2022;63(1):37-63.
70. Zibat A, Zhang X, Dickmanns A, Stegmann KM, Dobbelstein AW, Alachram H, et al. N4-hydroxycytidine, the active compound of Molnupiravir, promotes SARS-CoV-2 mutagenesis and escape from a neutralizing nanobody. iScience. 2023;26(10):107786.
71. National Institutes of Health. Coronavirus Disease 2019 (COVID-19) Treatment Guidelines. [online] Available from https://www.covid19treatmentguidelines.nih.gov/. [Last accessed February, 2024].
72. FDA. (2023). Fact Sheet for Healthcare Providers: Emergency Use Authorization for Lagevrio (molnupiravir) Capsules. [online] Available from https://www.fda.gov/media/155054/download. [Last accessed February, 2024].
73. Singh AK, Singh A, Singh R, Misra A. An updated practical guideline on use of molnupiravir and comparison with agents having emergency use authorization for treatment of COVID-19. Diabetes Metab Syndr. 2022;16(2):102396.
74. Pourkarim F, Pourtaghi-Anvarian S, Rezaee H. Molnupiravir: A New Candidate for COVID-19 Treatment. Pharmacol Res Perspect. 2022;10(1):e00909.
75. Niraj N, Mahajan SS, Prakash A, Sarma P, Medhi B. Paxlovid: A promising drug for the challenging treatment of SARS-COV-2 in the pandemic era. Indian J Pharmacol. 2022;54(6):452-8.
76. Hashemian SMR, Sheida A, Taghizadieh M, Memar MY, Hamblin MR, Baghi HB, et al. Paxlovid (Nirmatrelvir/Ritonavir): A new approach to Covid-19 therapy? Biomed Pharmacother. 2023;162:114367.
77. Ferrara F, Zovi A, Trama U, Vitiello A. Nirmatrelvir-remdesivir association for non-hospitalized adults with COVID-19, point of view. Inflammopharmacology. 2022;30(5):1927-31.
78. Karniadakis I, Mazonakis N, Tsioutis C, Papadakis M, Markaki I, Spernovasilis N. Oral Molnupiravir and Nirmatrelvir/Ritonavir for the Treatment of COVID-19: A Literature Review with a Focus on Real-World Evidence. Infect Dis Rep. 2023;15(6):662-78.
79. Barau C, Blouin P, Créput C, Taburet AM, Durrbach A, Furlan V. Effect of Coadministered HIV-protease Inhibitors on Tacrolimus and Sirolimus Blood Concentrations in a Kidney Transplant Recipients. Fundam Clin Pharmacol. 2009;23(4):423-5.
80. Hammond J, Leister-Tebbe H, Gardner A, Abreu P, Bao W, Wisemandle W, et al. Oral Nirmatrelvir for High-risk, Nonhospitalized Adults with Covid-19. N Engl J Med. 386(15):1397-408.
81. Sevrioukova IF, Poulos TL. Structure and Mechanism of the Complex between Cytochrome P4503A4 and Ritonavir. Proc Natl Acad Sci U S A. 2010;107(43):18422-7.
82. Wen W, Chen C, Tang J, Wang C, Zhou M, Cheng Y, et al. Efficacy and safety of three new oral antiviral treatment (molnupiravir, fluvoxamine and Paxlovid) for COVID-19: a meta-analysis. Ann Med. 2022;54(1):516-23.
83. Marzi M, Vakil MK, Bahmanyar M, Zarenezhad E. Paxlovid: Mechanism of Action, Synthesis, and in Silico Study. Biomed Res Int. 2022;2022:7341493.

84. Zheng Q, Ma P, Wang M, Cheng Y, Zhou M, Ye L, et al. Efficacy and safety of Paxlovid for COVID-19: a meta-analysis. J Infect. 2023;86(1):66-117.
85. Amani B, Amani B. Efficacy and safety of nirmatrelvir/ritonavir (Paxlovid) for COVID-19: A rapid review and meta-analysis. J Med Virol. 2023;95(2):e28441.
86. Pfizer. (2022). Pfizer Reports Additional Data on PAXLOVIDTM Supporting Upcoming New Drug Application Submission to U.S. FDA. [online] Available from https://www.pfizer.com/news/press-release/press-release-detail/pfizer-reports-additional-data-paxlovidtm-supporting#:~:text=Due%20to%20a%20very%20low,support%20the%20use%20of%20PAXLOVID. [Last accessed February, 2024].
87. Wang Y, Zhao D, Xiao W, Shi J, Chen W, Jia Q, et al. Paxlovid Reduces the Risk of Long COVID in Patients Six Months after Hospital Discharge. J Med Virol. 2023;95(8):e29014.
88. Ledford H, Maxmen A. African clinical trial denied access to key COVID drug. Nature. 2022;604(7906):412-3.
89. Aggarwal NR, Molina KC, Beaty LE, Bennett TD, Carlson NE, Mayer DA, et al. Real-world use of nirmatrelvir–ritonavir in outpatients with COVID-19 during the era of omicron variants including BA.4 and BA.5 in Colorado, USA: a retrospective cohort study. Lancet Infect Dis. 2023;23(6):696-705.
90. Hoertel N, Boulware DR, Sánchez-Rico M, Burgun A, Limosin F. Prevalence of Contraindications to Nirmatrelvir-Ritonavir among Hospitalized Patients with COVID-19 at Risk for Progression to Severe Disease. JAMA Netw Open. 2022;5(11):e2242140.
91. Kim JM, Yoo MG, Bae SJ, Kim J, Lee H. Effectiveness of Paxlovid, an Oral Antiviral Drug, Against the Omicron BA.5 Variant in Korea: Severe Progression and Death between July and November 2022. J Korean Med Sci. 2023;38(27):e211.
92. Tleyjeh IM, Kashour T, Mandrekar J, Petitti DB. Overlooked Shortcomings of Observational Studies of Interventions in Coronavirus Disease 2019: An Illustrated Review for the Clinician. Open Forum Infect Dis. 2021;8(8):ofab317.
93. Tashkin DP, Amin AN, Kerwin EM. Comparing Randomized Controlled Trials and Real-World Studies in Chronic Obstructive Pulmonary Disease Pharmacotherapy. Int J Chron Obstruct Pulmon Dis. 2020;15:1225-43.
94. Navitha Reddy G, Jogvanshi A, Naikwadi S, Sonti R. Nirmatrelvir and ritonavir combination: an antiviral therapy for COVID-19. Expert Rev Anti Infect Ther. 2023;21(9):943-55.
95. Pepperrell T, Ellis L, Wang J, Hill A. Barriers to worldwide access for Paxlovid, a new treatment for COVID-19. Open Forum Infect Dis. 2022;9(9):ofac174.
96. Harper M, Jason M. (2022). Pfizer's Paxlovid study fails to answer key questions over benefit for broader populations. [online] Available from https://www.statnews.com/2022/06/14/pfizers-paxlovid-study-fails-to-answer-key-questions-over-benefit-for-broader-populations/. [Last accessed February, 2024].
97. Liu J, Pan X, Zhang S, Li M, Ma K, Fan C, et al. Efficacy and Safety of Paxlovid in Severe Adult Patients with SARS-Cov-2 Infection: A Multicenter Randomized Controlled Study. Lancet Reg Health West Pac. 2023;33:100694.
98. Najjar-Debbiny R, Gronich N, Weber G, Khoury J, Amar M, Stein N, et al. Effectiveness of Paxlovid in Reducing Severe Coronavirus Disease 2019 and Mortality in High-Risk Patients. Clin Infect Dis. 2023;76(3):e342-9.
99. Yang D, Weng H, LI J, Ju M, Wang H, Jia YC, et al. (2023). Clinical Prognosis and Risk Factors of Death for Covid-19 Patients Complicated with Coronary Heart Disease/Diabetes/Hypertension-A Retrospective, Real-World Study. [online] Available from https://papers.ssrn.com/sol3/papers.cfm?abstract_id=4488145. [Last accessed February, 2024].
100. Shao J, Fan R, Guo C, Huang X, Guo R, Zhang F, et al. Composite Interventions on Outcomes of Severely and Critically Ill Patients with COVID-19 in Shanghai, China. Microorganisms. 2023;11(7):1859.

101. Yan J, Cai H, Wang J, Zhu M, Li P, Li P, et al. Nirmatrelvir/ritonavir for patients with SARS-CoV-2 infection and impaired kidney function during the Omicron surge. Front Pharmacol. 2023;14:1147980.
102. Lewnard JA, McLaughlin JM, Malden D, Hong V, Puzniak L, Ackerson BK, et al. Effectiveness of nirmatrelvir–ritonavir in preventing hospital admissions and deaths in people with COVID-19: a cohort study in a large US health-care system. Lancet Infect Dis. 2023;23(7):806-15.
103. Dryden-Peterson S, Kim A, Kim AY, Caniglia EC, Lennes IT, Patel R, et al. Nirmatrelvir Plus Ritonavir for Early COVID-19 in a Large U.S. Health System: A Population-Based Cohort Study. Ann Intern Med. 2023;176(1):77-84.
104. Schwartz KL, Wang J, Tadrous M, Langford BJ, Daneman N, Leung V, et al. Population-based evaluation of the effectiveness of nirmatrelvir–ritonavir for reducing hospital admissions and mortality from COVID-19. CMAJ. 2023;195(6):E220-6.
105. Yip TCF, Lui GCY, Lai MSM, Wong VWS, Tse YK, Ma BHM, et al. Impact of the Use of Oral Antiviral Agents on the Risk of Hospitalization in Community Coronavirus Disease 2019 Patients (COVID-19). Clin Infect Dis. 2023;76(3):e26-33.
106. Alshanqeeti S, Bhargava A. COVID-19 Rebound after Paxlovid Treatment: A Case Series and Review of Literature. Cureus. 2022;14(6):e26239.
107. Parums DV. Editorial: Rebound COVID-19 and Cessation of Antiviral Treatment for SARS-CoV-2 with Paxlovid and Molnupiravir. Med Sci Monit. 2022;28:e938532.
108. Bhave NM, Gluckman TJ, Wiggins BS. (2022). Drug-drug Interactions with Nirmatrelvir/Ritonavir (Paxlovid) and Select Cardiovascular Medications. [online] Available from https://www.acc.org/Latest-in-Cardiology/Articles/2022/06/17/12/17/Drug-Drug-Interactions-With-Paxlovid-and-Select-CV-Medications. [Last accessed February, 2024].
109. Igho-Osagie E, Brzozowski K, Jin H, Brown J, Williams MG, Puenpatom A. Prevalence of Potential Drug-drug Interactions with Ritonavir-containing COVID-19 Therapy in the United States: An Analysis of the National Health and Nutrition Examination Survey. Clin Ther. 2023;45(5):390-9.e4.
110. Girardin F, Manuel O, Marzolini C, Buclin T. Evaluating the risk of drug-drug interactions with pharmacokinetic boosters: the case of ritonavir-enhanced nirmatrelvir to prevent severe COVID-19. Clin Microb Infect. 2022;28(8):1044-6.
111. Focosi D, McConnell S, Shoham S, Casadevall A, Maggi F, Antonelli G. Nirmatrelvir and COVID-19: development, pharmacokinetics, clinical efficacy, resistance, relapse, and pharmacoeconomics. Int J Antimicrob Agents. 2023;61(2):106708.
112. Bae YJ. (2023). Paxlovid and Lagevrio Overview for Healthcare Professionals. [online] Available from https://qi.ipro.org/wp-content/uploads/Paxlovid-and-Lagevrio-Overview-for-Healthcare-Professionals-6-6-22-508.pdf. [Last accessed February, 2024].
113. Food and Drug Administration. (2022). Fact sheet for healthcare providers: Emergency Use Authorization for Paxlovid. [online] Available from https://www.fda.gov/media/155050/download. [Last accessed February, 2024].
114. Ontario Health. (2022). COVID-19 supplemental clinical guidance: nirmatrelvir/ritonavir (Paxlovid) use in patients with advanced chronic kidney disease and patients on dialysis with COVID-19. [online] Available from https://www.ontariohealth.ca/sites/ontariohealth/files/2022-04/PaxlovidClinicalGuide.pdf. [Last accessed February, 2024].
115. Komorowski A, Tseng A, Vandersluis S, Leung E, Ciccotelli W, Langford BJ, et al. (2022). Evidence-based recommendations on the use of nirmatrelvir/ritonavir (Paxlovid) for adults in Ontario. [online] Available from https://covid19-sciencetable.ca/sciencebrief/evidence-based-recommendations-on-the-use-of-nirmatrelvir-ritonavir-paxlovid-for-adults-in-ontario/#:~:text=Nirmatrelvir%2Fritonavir%20is%20recommended%20at,five%20days%20of%20symptom%20onset. [Last accessed February 2024].
116. University of Liverpool. (2022). COVID-19 Drug interactions. [online] Available from https://www.covid19-druginteractions.org. [Last accessed February, 2024].

CHAPTER 26

Glucocorticoids in Viral Pneumonia and COVID-19

Francesco Salton, Marco Confalonieri, Gianfranco Umberto Meduri

GLUCOCORTICOIDS IN VIRAL PNEUMONIA: EVIDENCE IN THE EARLY PHASE OF THE PANDEMIC

Glucocorticoids (GCs) are agonist compounds that bind to the GC receptor (GR-α), producing a rapid pharmacological response. Clinical efficacy depends on the magnitude and duration of exposure to GR-α; the effect is systemic, including lung tissue and circulating cells. The extraordinary research advancements of the last decade have radically reshaped our understanding of the GR-α's multi-faceted actions, the effector of GCs action. For the last half-century, we understood pro- and anti-inflammatory actions as opposite biological effects (tug of war). In the last decade, research has radically reshaped our understanding of the activated GC-GR-α's modulatory role in critical illness demonstrating (1) a complementary coregulation (dualism) between GR-α and proinflammatory transcription factors nuclear factor kappa B (NF-κB) and activator protein-1 (AP-1)-mediated pathways, and (2) GC-GR-α fine-tuning of homeostatic corrections in every temporal phase of critical illness leading to an adaptative response.[1] Consequently, GCs cannot be classified solely as anti-inflammatory or immunosuppressive.

When a massive inflammatory response occurs [e.g., during sepsis, acute respiratory distress syndrome (ARDS), or severe pneumonia], the endogenous GC-GR-α homeostatic corrections may be inadequate for the severity of the patient's critical illness [known as critical illness-related corticosteroid insufficiency (CIRCI)] due to three major pathophysiologic events—(1) dysregulation of the hypothalamic-pituitary-adrenal (HPA) axis, altered cortisol metabolism, and tissue resistance to GCs.[2] Despite the complexity involved in finalizing GC-mediated activity, it is noteworthy that the administration of exogenous GCs and other cointerventions to improve cellular responsiveness can increase the number and function of the activated GR.[1] Therefore, as reviewed in the sections below, the rationale for exogenous GC treatment in these conditions is to support the central modulatory function of GR-α.

In December 2019, pneumonia associated with the 2019 novel coronavirus (COVID-19) emerged in Wuhan, China. On March 14, 2020, the World Health Organization (WHO) declared the coronavirus outbreak a pandemic with confirmed cases in 127 countries. The WHO statement *of not recommending the routine use of corticosteroids for treatment of viral pneumonia outside clinical trials*[3] relied on incomplete evidence, and has had severe global repercussions. The dysregulated inflammation and coagulation observed in COVID-19[4] is like that of multifactorial medical ARDS where ample evidence has demonstrated the ability of prolonged GC treatment to downregulate inflammation-coagulation-fibroproliferation and accelerate disease resolution.[5] Before the pandemic, Villar et al. provided definitive evidence that prolonged GC treatment is associated with significant mortality benefits in ARDS,[6] which was concordant with previous data coming from a 2017 Cochrane meta-analysis on GC use in community-acquired pneumonia. Early clinical failure rates (defined as death from any cause, radiographic progression, or clinical instability at day 5–8) were also significantly reduced with GCs, as they were time to clinical cure, length of hospital, and intensive care unit (ICU) stays, development of respiratory failure or new onset of shock, and rates of pneumonia complications.[7] The rationale for GC treatment was previously reviewed.[8]

At the beginning of the COVID-19 pandemic, few small observational studies associated the use of GCs with a reduced admission to the ICU and with a reduced mortality.[9-11]

The WHO's brief argument to support the recommendation was mainly based on the risk of decreased viral clearance reported in one other observational study[12] and inconclusive evidence from retrospective observational studies without a predesigned study protocol and subjected to cofounding (imbalances in baseline characteristics and postbaseline time-dependent patient differences that influence the decision to prescribe corticosteroids), and hidden bias.[13] Confounding by indication is a significant bias in studies which only provided unadjusted effect estimates. We have previously commented on the unjustifiable deficiencies of the WHO's analysis.[14] The WHO and others, selectively quoted an article of critically ill patients with the Middle East respiratory syndrome to warn about the risk of decreased viral clearance with GC therapy.[12] In this study, however, those that received GC treatment for >7 days had a 50% reduction in mortality that almost reached statistical significance [OR: 0.51, 95% confidence interval (CI) 0.26–1.00; $p = 0.05$] and no impact on viral clearance (aHR: 0.94, 95% CI 0.36–2.47; $p = 0.90$).[12] This is consistent with an early observational study which associated prolonged, low dose, methylprednisolone (MP) with a dramatic mortality reduction compared to usual practice, but not with a longer time to viral shedding in severe COVID-19 pneumonia.[15,16]

Notably, the WHO ignored the positive findings of two large studies [5,327 patients with severe acute respiratory syndrome (SARS)[17] and 2,141 patients with influenza H1N1 pneumonia][18] that evaluated the impact of time, dose, and duration of GC treatment and reported a significant reduction in mortality with dosage and duration similar to the one recommended by Society of Critical Care Medicine and European Society of Intensive Care Medicine (SCCM and ESICM) Task Force.[19] In the SARS study, after adjustment for possible confounders, GC treatment was safe and decreased the risk for death by 47% (HR 0.53, 95% CI: 0.35–0.82).[17] In the H1N1 study, 1,055 patients received corticosteroids and 1,086 did not receive it. Subgroup analysis among patients with $PaO_2/FiO_2 < 300$ mm Hg (535 vs. 462), low-to-moderate-dose CST significantly reduced both 30-day mortality [aHR 0.49 (95% CI 0.32–0.77)] and 60-day mortality [aHR 0.51 (95% CI 0.33–0.7)].[18]

Finally, the dysregulated inflammation and coagulation observed in COVID-19[4] is similar to that of multifactorial medical ARDS where ample evidence has demonstrated the ability of prolonged GC treatment to downregulate inflammation-coagulation-fibroproliferation and accelerate disease resolution.[5] Additionally, the computed tomography findings of ground glass opacities[20] and the histological findings of hyaline membrane and inflammatory exudates[21] are compatible with corticosteroid-responsive inflammatory lung disease. Further, some COVID-19 patients had a cytokine elevation profile reminiscent of secondary hemophagocytic lymphohistiocytosis, a condition responsive to GC treatment.[9]

GLUCOCORTICOIDS IN COVID-19

There is currently strong evidence that GCs are beneficial in severe COVID-19 pneumonia. The UK government, *Research and Innovation News* reported that in the 9 months following the introduction of GC treatment in COVID-19, "*an inexpensive, readily available steroid, saved an estimated one million lives worldwide, including 22,000 in the UK.*"[22]

The first evidences came in spring 2020 from preliminary reports by the RECOVERY trial platform, which demonstrated that treatment with 6 mg of dexamethasone (DM) for up to 10 days reduced the risk of death at 28 days [risk ratio (RR) 0.83; 95% CI 0.75–0.93], with a higher impact among hospitalized patients who were receiving respiratory support with mechanical ventilation (MV) (RR 0.64; 95% CI 0.51–0.81) compared with oxygen therapy (RR 0.82; 95% CI 0.72–0.94). In contrast, GCs showed an increased risk of death among patients who did not require respiratory support at randomization (RR 1.19; 95% CI 0.92–1.55).[23]

Several other RCTs followed, and a large Cochrane meta-analysis reviewed the data available through early 2022.[24] 9,549 participants from 16 RCTs were included, confirming that systemic corticosteroids plus standard care compared to standard care reduce all-cause mortality at 30 days (RR 0.90, 95% CI 0.84–0.97), confirming a higher reduction in the subgroup of patients on noninvasive ventilation (NIV) or high-flow nasal cannula (HFNC) at randomization compared to low-flow oxygen only (RR 0.64; 95% CI 0.20–2.03 vs. 0.70; 95% CI 0.29–1.67) and a mortality increase in the subgroup of milder patients who were not receiving oxygen therapy (RR 1.27; 95% CI 1.00–1.61). The chance of being discharged alive at day 28 was slightly increased, while the risk of new need for invasive MV was slightly decreased (RR 0.92, 95% CI 0.84–1.01). GCs increased ventilator-free days of 2.6 days on average compared to the control group. To note, most patients received DM ($n = 3,766$).

Two RCTs investigated hydrocortisone at similar doses (150 mg daily for 7 days and 200 mg daily for 7 days followed by tapering, respectively) reporting a lower risk of mortality (RR 0.78; 95% CI 0.57–1.05), which reached even lower among the studies investigating MP (RR 0.63; 95% CI 0.26–1.54) with the exception of one randomized controlled trial (RCT) designed around a shorter and lower-dose course of MP (0.5 mg/kg/day for 5 days) that proved non superior to standard care.[25,26] This is consistent with previous literature on all-cause ARDS and with previous studies in severe COVID-19.[27,28]

Despite comparative evidence about the most effective type, dose, or timing of systemic GC remains immature, some data come from the analysis of single trial results.

Among studies that proposed a higher GC dose than 6 mg of DM, in a recent RCT 1,000 patients were randomized to receive 12 mg or 6 mg of DM once daily for 10 days in a 1:1 ratio, finding no statistically significant differences but a trend toward an increase in the number of days alive without support at 28 days in the 12 mg group.[29] Similarly, Taboada et al. found no statistically significant differences in clinical worsening at 11 days, nor in 28-day mortality and other secondary endpoints in 200 patients randomized to receive low-dose DM (6 mg once daily for 10 days) or high-dose DM with tapering (20 mg once daily for 5 days, followed by 10 mg once daily for 5 additional days).[30] A meta-analysis of four RCTs different doses, concluded that higher-dose DM may reduce all-cause mortality by 30 days compared to low-dose DM (RR 0.87, 95% CI 0.73–1.04).[31]

Possible explanations for a different effect of higher versus lower doses relies on the pharmacological principles reviewed below. In brief, GCs mainly act by binding to the GRα, but different compounds have different pharmacological properties and clinical efficacy depends on the magnitude and duration of exposure to GC.[32]

Few RCTs reported on the efficacy of MP versus DM in severe COVID-19. Ranjbar et al. randomly allocated 86 patients to either a single bolus of MP 2 mg/kg/day for 5 days tapered to 1 mg/kg/day after 5 days or DM 6 mg/day for 10 days. MP resulted in a shorter hospitalization and a lower need for MV (18.2% vs. 38.1%), but it did not reach statistical significance for all-cause mortality (RR 0.51; 95% CI 0.24–1.07).[33] Conversely, the same MP protocol was associated with a statistically significant reduction in mortality versus DM 6 mg/day for 10 days in the study by Saeed et al. ($n = 414$), in which mechanically ventilated patients were selectively included.[34] Indeed, there is strong evidence of a proportional benefit of GCs among patients who require MV rather than other lower-intensity respiratory support modalities.[23] Furthermore, patients treated with MP experienced a shorter duration of ICU stay (7.33 vs. 19.43 mean days) and a higher reduction in C-reactive protein (CRP) levels at 10 days.[34]

An Italian RCT investigated a protocol of infusive MP at a dose of 80 mg on the first day, followed by a continuous infusion of 80/day and tapering over 14 days versus DM 6 mg/day for 10 days in 690 patients requiring oxygen or noninvasive respiratory support due to COVID-19-related pneumonia, finding no significant differences in mortality (10.4% vs. 12.1%), nor in the median MV-free days. Patients in the MP group with $PaO_2:FiO_2 < 200$ mm Hg at randomization who completed the assigned treatment protocol experienced a lower rate of ICU admission and significantly higher reduction of CRP at days 7 and 14.[16] Indeed, previous data associated a faster reduction of CRP with a lower 1-year mortality after severe pneumonia and sepsis, and there is evidence that persistently elevated CRP and need for ICU admission are independent risk factors for the development of post-COVID conditions.[35,36]

Patients aged < 70 years seemed to benefit more from GCs than those aged 70 years and older across different studies. Furthermore, the few participants from a Black, Asian, or other minority ethnic group showed a larger estimated effect than the many White participants.[24]

At the currents state of things, all major guidelines suggest the use of any GC molecule, at a dose equivalent to 6 mg of DM for 7–10 days, in moderate and severe COVID-19.[37] This therapeutic schedule has proven safe and effective in several randomized clinical trials, reducing all-cause mortality without being associated with a higher incidence of complications or adverse events. Despite its unquestionable efficacy, there is likely room for refinement. Indeed, future research should be aimed at identifying not only the best standardized protocol, but also possible biomarkers which may guide titration of the dose and duration on an individual basis. Related to this, the high variability in plasma levels of GCs following administration of the same exogenous dose may relate to a certain degree of GC-resistance and explain why also noncomorbid patients can experience a severe evolution of COVID-19.[32]

The next section addresses the role that dosage, timing of initiation, mode of administration, duration, and tapering play in achieving optimal response to GC therapy according to pharmacological principles and clinical evidence.

PRINCIPLES AND EVIDENCES GUIDING GLUCOCORTICOID ADMINISTRATION

This section addresses differences among molecules and the role of dosage, timing of initiation, mode of administration, duration, and tapering play in achieving optimal response to GC therapy in ARDS. Based on pharmacological principles reviewed in reference[32] and the meta-analysis of aggregate data from randomized trials in ARDS (not associated with COVID-19),[38] the following principles may apply to COVID-19-associated ARDS. Optimal results are most likely achievable with early intervention, an initial bolus dose to achieve close to maximal GRa saturation, followed by a continuous infusion to maintain high levels of response throughout the treatment period, and slow tapering. Nevertheless, there is substantial between patient variability in plasma concentrations and intracellular response, providing the rationale for adjusting dose and duration targeting clinical and laboratory improvements (see *Factors Affecting Response Independent of the Protocol Design*). Most of the data examining the effect of timing, duration, and tapering is extrapolated from individual patient data (IPD) meta-analysis (IPDMA) of four small-to-moderate size RCTs (n = 322) investigating MP administration in early and late ARDS.[39]

Glucocorticoid Molecules

Glucocorticoid action on target tissues is determined in part by the (1) density of "nuclear" receptors and the (2) prereceptor intracellular metabolism by the two isozymes of 11 β-hydroxysteroid dehydrogenases type 1 and 2 (11β-HSD1 and 11β-HSD2). 11β-HSD1 facilitates the systemic regeneration of biologically active GCs (cortisol/hydrocortisone, corticosterone, and prednisolone) from their inactive forms (cortisone, 11-dehydrocorticosterone, and prednisone) by its oxidoreductase (11β-reductase) action. MP and DM, in contrast to hydrocortisone, are not substrates to the 11β-HSD system and thus do not have this liability of potential local activity modulation, their use may be preferable in the treatment of ARDS.

In contrast, 11β-HSD2 solely inactivates GCs. Experiments revealed insensitivity to GCs in cells that show a high 11β-HSD2 activity.[40] In ARDS, a postmortem study found high immunohistochemical expression of 11β-HSD2 in lung tissue.[41] This finding may have implications for ARDS treatment since an increased expression of 11β-HSD2 is expected to result in faster hydrocortisone breakdown in ARDS lungs. Inactivation by 11β-HSD2 instead is diminished if GC molecules are fluorinated in position 6a or 9a (e.g., in DM) or methylated at 2a or 6a (in MP).[42] This may partly explain the greater response observed with MP and DM versus hydrocortisone in ARDS.

A seminal COVID-19 transcriptomics study analyzed the changes in the gene expression, pathways, and putative mechanisms induced by SARS-CoV-2 in primary human lung epithelium, A549 cells, as well as COVID-19 lung biopsies versus their respective controls. Then used these changes to identify—among 5,694 FDA-approved drugs that could be repurposed to help COVID-19 patients with severe symptoms related to hyperinflammation. They found MP to be the drug with the most significant potential to revert the changes induced by COVID-19; five independent validation data sets confirmed the results.[43]

Several clinically oriented investigations suggest that GR-β, a natural dominant-negative inhibitor of hGR-α-induced transactivation of GC-responsive genes, is responsible for the development of tissue-specific insensitivity to GCs.[44] In experimental ARDS, lung tissue shows a significant reduction in GR-α expression[45,46] and an increase in GR-β expression,[45] leading to decreased GR-α nuclear translocation.[45] An in vitro study found that, among the GC compounds investigated in ARDS, MP, contrary to hydrocortisone and DM, was not affected by the hGR-β dominant negative-effect.[47] The suppressive effect of hGR-β on hGR-α-induced transactivation was stronger at lower concentrations of all tested GCs and blunted at higher concentrations.[47] The authors concluded that the dominant-negative effect of hGR-β on hGR-α-induced transactivation depends on both the type and the dose of the synthetic GCs in use.

There is a potential therapeutic advantage in treating pulmonary disorders with drugs that have a high penetration into affected lung tissue. Two experimental studies evaluated bronchoalveolar lavage fluid (BALF) concentrations relative to plasma for MP and prednisolone, reporting that although both drugs were rapidly distributed into the lungs, MP achieved a higher BALF exposure than prednisolone. This effect became even more pronounced over time (longer residence time), suggesting that MP persists in the BALF compartment with a slower lung clearance than that from plasma.[48,49] Greater penetration was achieved with continuous infusion vs. bolus.[48] A recent study in human volunteers evaluated the effects of DM administered as a short-term infusion pretreatment on systemic and lung inflammation following the direct instillation of endotoxin into a lung segment.[50]

Timing of Administration and Initial Dose

Early initiation (preferably within six hours of diagnosis) of GC treatment, before homeostatic corrections reach exhaustion,[1] is critical in decreasing the acute and long-term negative impact of the allostatic load imposed during vital organ support.[51-55] In the IPDMA, early (<72 hours) as compared to late (≥7 days) initiation of MP treatment—when fibroproliferation is still in the early development stage (cellular with predominant type III procollagen)—was associated with faster disease resolution, determined by time to extubation and ICU discharge, despite a lower daily MP dose (1 mg/kg/day vs. 2 mg/kg/day).[39]

An adequate initial loading bolus is necessary to achieve prompt elevation in plasma and tissue concentrations to approach maximal GR-α saturation (approximately 100 mg of MP equivalent)[56] in the cytoplasm and on the cell membrane for genomic and nongenomic actions and to overcome resistance imposed by increased GRβ.[47] A MP dose of 1 mg/kg/day in early ARDS is similar to what is commonly used in other forms of interstitial lung diseases,[57] and close to the DM dose (20 mg) used in the recent DEXA-ARDS RCT.[6] However, a larger initial dose (i.e., MP 2 mg/kg/day) may be required in (1) the sickest patients with reduction adjustment based on FiO_2 requirements and CRP levels or (2) those on MV for 5 days or longer (unresolving ARDS).

An in-vitro study provided insights on the impact that GC dosage has on inflammation downregulation. In human monocytic cells activated with graded concentrations of lipopolysaccharide (LPS) and then exposed to increasing concentrations of MP **(Fig. 1)**, the reduction in inflammatory cytokine gene [tumor necrosis factor alpha (TNF-α), Interleukin 1β (IL-1β), and IL-6] transcription (irrespective of baseline inflammation severity) was initially modest. It then reached an inflection point, followed by a rapid reduction, most likely related to achieving close to maximal drug receptor

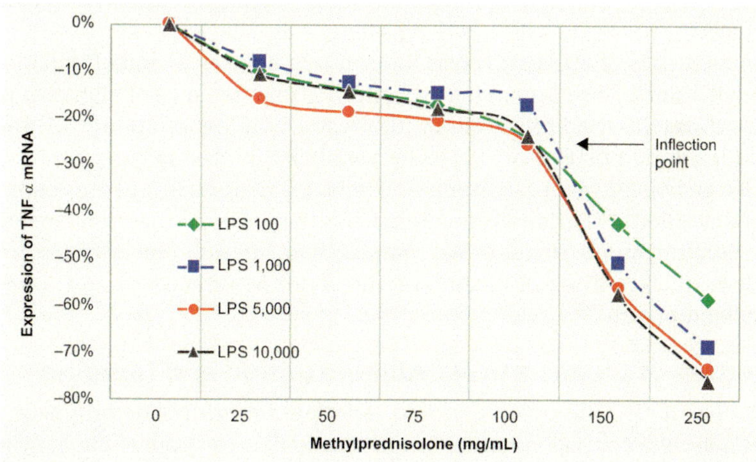

FIGURE 1: Regression of concentration of methylprednisolone on steady-state mRNA levels of tumor necrosis factor alpha (TNF-α) in U937 cells primed with graded concentrations of lipopolysaccharide (LPS).

In experimental simulation of severe inflammation, human monocytic cells (U937 cells) were activated with graded concentrations of LPS (100 ng/mL, 1.0 mg/mL, 5.0 mg/mL, or 10.0 mg/mL) for 6 hours followed by measurement of the expression of inflammatory cytokines TNF-α, IL-1β, and IL-6. Graded concentrations of LPS were followed by progressively higher inflammatory cytokine transcription for TNF-α: 185, 318, 481, and 566, respectively (not shown in figure). These cells were then exposed to graded concentrations of methylprednisolone (MP) [(mg/mL): 50, 100, 150, 200, and 250] for 6 hours followed by repeated measurement of inflammatory cytokine expression. The steady state mRNA levels of TNF-α, IL-1β, or IL-6 in LPS-activated cells were reduced by treatment with MP in a concentration-dependent manner. The percent reduction in inflammatory cytokines' transcription was initially modest. Then, after reaching an inflection point (between 100 and 150 mg/mL), a sharp drop followed (likely related to achieving maximal drug-receptor saturation). The effective dose of MP was 175 mg/mL, a value that appeared to be independent of the priming level of LPS and type of mRNA measured.[1]

saturation for a measurable genomic and nongenomic effect.[58] This finding emphasizes the relevance of adequate dose selection in achieving GR a saturation and optimal results.

Mode of Administration

The average GC plasma concentration-time profiles expressed as MP equivalents reveals substantial differences among the different GC dosing regimens with regard to exposure.[32] Indeed, infrequent dosing (with dosing intervals of 8 or 24 hours) leads to substantial periods without relevant GC serum exposure where the maintenance of GC effects in the target organs and tissues would be dependent on either persistent GC local exposure in those effects sites, or mechanisms of temporal persistence of the GC effects beyond those periods of relevant effect site exposure. Conversely, continuous administration via infusion maintains high exposure levels throughout the day.

Advantages of infusion versus intermittent boluses include (1) achievement of a stable, nonfluctuating exposure, (2) maintenance of high response levels throughout administration, (3) greater lung penetration,[48] (4) more rapid resolution of shock,[59] (5) lesser variability in plasma concentration,[60] (6) fewer hyperglycemic episodes,[61,62] and (7) decreased nursing time for administration.[63,64] Limited data from RCTs demonstrate that implementing this administration method, as compared to intermittent bolusing, may achieve quicker disease resolution with more MV-free days and a lower hospital mortality.[38]

Duration of Glucocorticoid Administration and Tapering

Duration of GC administration and tapering are critical determinants of treatment efficacy. GC treatment's role in ARDS is to support the activated GRa central homeostatic function in the acute phases of the disease and throughout the fundamental albeit underappreciated resolution phase. In COVID-19 results of RCTs demonstrated that mortality is decreased with duration of 10 days or greater.[65]

Critical care RCTs have shown that abrupt GC discontinuation after a 3-to-14 days of treatment was rapidly followed by a reconstituted systemic inflammation with severe clinical relapses in about one-third of the patients,[32] and a potential signal for increased mortality.[66] This was observed in patients receiving either an infusion or intermittent boluses.[32] In the LaSRS RCT, discontinuation of the study drug within 36 hours of successful extubation led to clinical relapse in one-quarter of MP-treated patients.[66] These patients necessitated a return to MV and did not receive a reinstitution of GC treatment. This led to poor outcomes with additional days of MV and a ninefold increased risk of 60-day mortality ($p = 0.001$) compared to patients who did not return to MV.[67]

During the Covid-19 pandemic, case reports[68,69] describe a similar experience after discontinuation of a 10-day DM treatment based on the

RECOVERY trial protocol[23] with improvements after reinstitution of GC treatment.

Monitoring during Mechanical Ventilation and Infection Surveillance

It is essential to monitor response to treatment during intervention with the daily assessment of lung [lung injury score (LIS)[70] and minute ventilation] and multiple organ function [sequential organ failure assessment (SOFA) score] along with systemic inflammation markers (i.e., CRP and ferritin). Persistent elevation in inflammatory markers portends a poor outcome, while the reduction speed correlates with time to resolution in organ dysfunction.[71,72] In response to GC treatment, rapid versus slow inflammatory cytokine reduction results in rapid versus slow physiological improvement.[73,74]

Among ARDS patients receiving a similar treatment protocol, the difference in response may be related to the great interindividual variability in (1) intracellular GR-α sensitivity during GC treatment,[75,76] and (2) achieved plasma drug concentrations.[60] Notably, lower intracellular GR-α sensitivity[75] can be overcome with progressively higher GC doses, suggesting that higher doses overcome intracellular GC resistance (see comment above). This provides the rationale for dose and duration adjustments based on clinical and laboratory response **(Fig. 2)**.

While prolonged GC treatment in ARDS has not been shown to be associated with an increased risk for infection,[38] it is essential to monitor for evidence of infection in the absence of fever during MV. In one RCT, infection surveillance using a strict protocol identified 56% of nosocomial infections in patients without fever.[77] As procalcitonin is a bacterial infection biomarker that remains unaffected by GC treatment, it is helpful for the early identification of infection.[78-81] In ARDS, MP treatment does not affect procalcitonin levels.[82] Additional infection monitoring parameters include: (1) an unexplained increase in minute ventilation (≥30%), (2) a worsening of the LIS or SOFA score, (3) a plateau or increase in CRP levels, and (4) an increase in immature neutrophils. Unless contraindicated, surveillance weekly bronchoscopic or nonbronchoscopic bronchoalveolar lavage (BAL) is helpful for early identification of ventilator-associated pneumonia and monitoring lung inflammation (neutrophilia). The need for this intervention has remarkably decreased since most ARDS patients receiving early prolonged GC treatment are ventilator-free within 7 days of treatment.[39]

Postextubation Monitoring and Treatment Adjustment

After extubation, oxygen requirements provide a simple modality to assess restoration of lung function, necessitating the continuation of GC treatment at a lower dose until the patient reaches adequate oxygenation on room air. One pharmacokinetic study reported that intestinal MP absorption is compromised for about 5 days after extubation, and that is why switching to oral administration 5 days after MV removal is a reasonable course of action.[60] **Figure 2** provides a summary of our suggested approach for MP treatment.

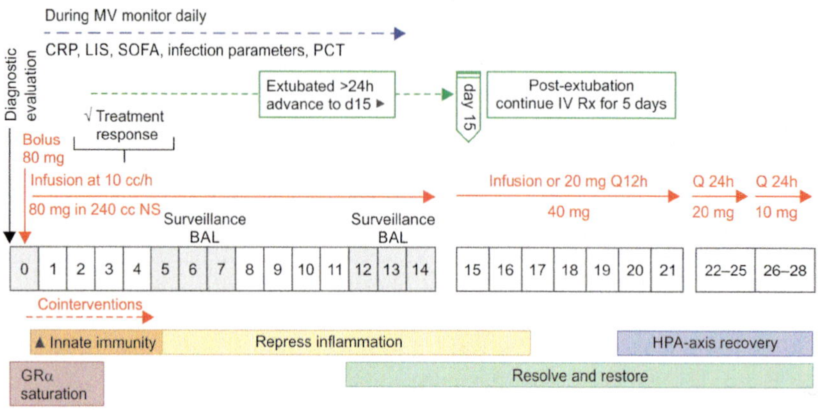

FIGURE 2: Protocol for prolonged methylprednisolone treatment in patients with early ARDS.

This protocol was recommended in the 2017 guidelines of the Multispecialty Task Force of the Society of Critical Care Medicine and the European Society of Intensive Care Medicine.[19] Vitamin supplementation was not part of the recommended protocol.

The dosage is adjusted to ideal body weight (IBW) and rounded up to the nearest 10 mg (e.g., 77 mg rounded up to 80 mg). Thereafter 80 mg is an example for a patient with an IBW of 77 kg. Day 0, intravenous bolus (80 mg in 50 cc normal saline) over 30 minutes. Day 0-to ICU discharge—infusion is done by adding the daily dosage to 240 cc of normal saline and running it at 10 cc/h. If necessary, infusion can be changed to bolus every 6 hours (one-fourth daily dose) or in the last 6 days to every 12 hours (half daily dose). If on day 3–5, there is no improvement or even worsening oxygenation indices the condition is considered "unresolving ARDS". In this case, a protocol of similar duration of treatment, but with double the daily dose of methylprednisolone (MP) (bolus followed by infusion at 160 mg/day) is initiated. If the patient is extubated before day 14, the MP infusion is advanced to day 15 of drug therapy and tapered according to schedule. Oral administration should be delayed to 5 days after extubation because enteral absorption of MP, and likely other GCs, is compromised for days after extubation. Rapid tapering can be associated with rebound systemic inflammation in the presence of suppressed adrenal function with worsening of lung physiology and an increased mortality risk.[67] If patients worsen significantly, then GC treatment should be restarted again, and after improvement followed by slow tapering, to comply with the Food and Drug Administration's package insert warnings (reference ID: 3032293).[130]

Cointerventions, vitamin supplementation based on 2022 ESPEN micronutrient guideline:[131] Thiamin 100–300 mg/day for 4 days; vitamin D, upfront bolus for rapid improvement (up to 600,000 IU) followed up with daily maintenance doses (5,000 IU orally or enterally) and personalized by 25(OH)D blood levels after a few days (which is a relatively reliable indicator and usually rapidly available); vitamin C3 g/day IV during the acute phase of inflammation (vital organ support).

(CRP: C-reactive protein; GR-α: glucocorticoids receptor alpha; HPA: hypothalamic-pituitary-adrenal; LIS: lung injury score; MV: mechanical ventilation; PCT: procalcitonin; SOFA: sequential organ failure assessment)

Factors Affecting Response Independent of the Protocol Design

As reviewed in **Box 1**, in critically ill and ARDS patients' response to endogenous GC can be affected by variables related to (1) the patient's premorbid state and (2) the critical illness. Patient-related variables include (1) cellular sensitivity[76,83], (2) comorbidities associated with GC resistance,[84,85] and less likely by GR polymorphisms.[86] Critical illness variables include (1) decreased HDL cholesterol levels (preferred lipoprotein source of the steroidogenic substrate in the adrenal gland)[87] and intracellular penetration[88], (2) prereceptor metabolism by 11β-HSD1 and 11β-HSD2, (3) GR number and isoforms (α vs. β)[89-94], (4) impact of inflammatory state (induce noncompensated GC resistance in target organs)[95-97] and oxidative stress[98-104] on multiple GR functions, and (4) impact of micronutrient deficiency on GC availability and GC-GR function.[102,103,105-110] These variables, with the exception of decreased high-density lipoprotein (HDL) cholesterol levels, may also affect response to GC treatment.

Because GC resistance is most frequently observed in critically ill patients with excessive inflammation, it remains unclear whether GC resistance is a primary phenomenon or whether the anti-inflammatory capacity of GCs is simply overwhelmed by an excessive synthesis of proinflammatory cytokines, owing to an excessive activity of various intracellular transcription factors which, in turn, may reduce the affinity of GR for its intracellular ligand.[111]

One-third of the general healthy population has significantly steroid-resistant lymphocytes, similar to the failure rate of steroid therapy across a broad range of inflammatory conditions.[112] While multiple components of the GC treatment protocol profoundly affect efficacy, interindividual variability in response to GC administration remains an unpredictable and uncontrollable factor.

Three studies call attention to an underappreciated aspect of GC treatment, the great interindividual variability in (1) intracellular GC receptor sensitivity during GC treatment,[75,76] and (2) achieved plasma drug concentrations.[60] In the first study, GC sensitivity was assessed by exposing concanavalin A stimulated lymphocytes of 40 healthy volunteers to increasing concentrations of DM. **Figures 3A and B** show great variability in inhibiting lymphocyte proliferation at every investigated dose.[75] Other studies in healthy volunteers reported a similar considerable intra-individual variation.[112,113] The second study in patients within 3 days of developing septic shock measured GC sensitivity by in vitro suppression of cytokine production from LPS-stimulated leukocytes.[76] While many septic patients showed greater sensitivity to DM, others followed the opposite trend resulting in a net increase in variance. In particular, patients with reduced GC sensitivity had evidence of greater illness severity, with higher APACHE II scores.[76] Notably, patients in the lowest quartile of measured GC sensitivity did not have a greater GR-β or 11β-HSD-2 mRNA expression than those in

BOX 1 Factors affecting response to glucocorticoid treatment.

Disease related:
- GR number and type (α vs. β)
- GR-binding capacity (Bmax)
  ▼ by inflammatory state
  ▼ by oxidative stress
- GR function
  ▼ by hypovitaminosis,* micronutrient deficiencies

Molecule related:
- Binding affinity to GR (potency)
  - Can be offset by changing magnitude of exposure

Patients related:
- Comorbid conditions associated with GC resistance†
- Between-patient wide variability in achieved GC plasma concentration
- Between-patient wide variability in cellular sensitivity to exposure of similar GC concentration

Molecule related:
- Binding affinity to GR (potency)
  - Can be offset by changing magnitude of exposure (increasing GC dosage)

Treatment-related initiation:
- GR saturation (dose-dependent)
- Timing of initiation (early vs. late)
- Dose-adjustments based on initial severity‡

Treatment related—over time:
- Optimal magnitude of exposure to GR
  - Bolus followed by continuous infusion
- Lung penetration and tissue concentration
- Dose-adjustments based on clinical response§
- Duration of treatment including tapering

Treatment related—potential complications:
- Hypothalamic-pituitary-axis suppression
  - Can be offset with slow tapering
- Failure to recognize infections in absence of fever:
  - Can be offset with infection surveillance

*Hypovitaminosis, three vitamins, (1) thiamine (vitamin B1), (2) ascorbic acid (vitamin C), and (3) vitamin D, are important for the proper functioning of the GR system and mitochondria (but their reserves are rapidly exhausted in critical illness).[129]

†Comorbidities associated with GC resistance: Obesity, chronic lung, and heart diseases, smocking, etc.[84,85]

‡A larger initial dose (i.e., methylprednisolone 2 mg/kg/day) may be required in patients requiring high oxygen levels ($FiO_2 \geq 0.8$).

§Adjustment based on C-reactive protein levels and PaO_2:FiO_2.

[▼: decreased; GR: glucocorticoid receptor; Bmax: total density (concentration) of receptors in a sample of tissue]

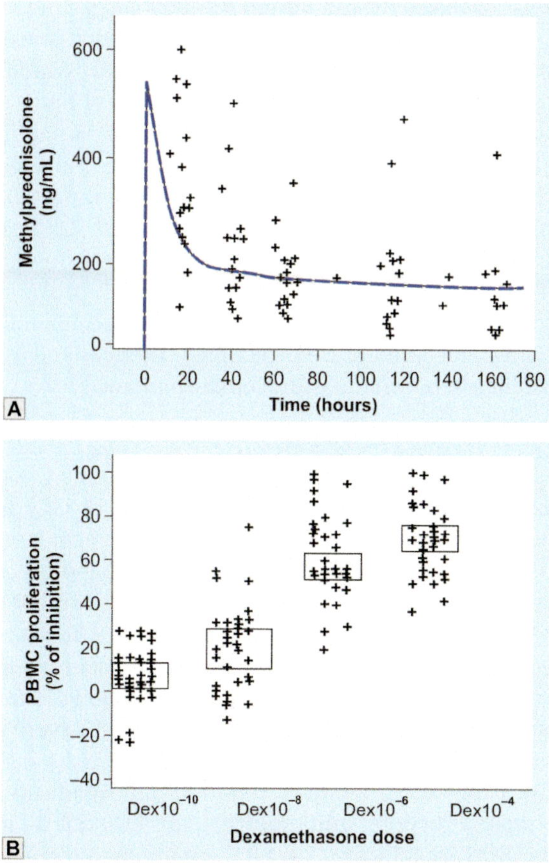

FIGURES 3A AND B: Interindividual variability in methylprednisolone plasma concentration and in intracellular anti-inflammatory response to increasing concentrations of dexamethasone. (A) Methylprednisolone plasma concentration-time profile in early ARDS patients receiving methylprednisolone 1 mg/kg loading dose, followed by a 1 mg/kg/day continuous infusion. Methylprednisolone hepatic clearance is impaired during first 48 hours and concentrations are high enough to trigger genomic and nongenomic GC effects. This most likely establishes initial control of the generalized inflammatory state.[132] Inflammatory control is at least partially established within 2 days of therapy, leading to an increased hepatic methylprednisolone clearance, secondary to re-established drug metabolizing activity. By the third day, the concentrations are maintained at a steady state exerting prolonged sustained anti-inflammatory activity. Within each period, we observe a great intraindividual variability in plasma concentration. At steady state, the mean plasma concentration is around 203 ± 147 ng/mL with a range of 50–820 ng/mL, a >10-fold variation. Plasma concentration impacts cellular concentration. Reproduced with permission from Yates et al.[60] (B) In this study, GC sensitivity was assessed by exposing concanavalin A stimulated lymphocytes of 40 healthy volunteers to increasing concentrations of dexamethasone. Great intraindividual variability in inhibiting lymphocytes proliferation is observed at every investigated dose.[75]

(ARDS: acute respiratory distress syndrome; GC: glucocorticoid)

the highest. This is consistent with others' findings suggesting a postreceptor basis for the wide variation in lymphocyte suppression sensitivity.[112] The third publication is a pharmacokinetic study of 20 ARDS patients recruited in a RCT[77] investigating MP 1 mg/kg adjusted to ideal body weight (IBW) reported concentration-time profiles with substantial variability in plasma concentrations. At a steady-state achieved during the continuous infusion, the medium MP level was 203 ± 127 ng/mL and the range 50–820 ng/mL, a greater than 10-fold variation **(Figs. 3A and B)**.[60] Clinically relevant, variability was greater after bolus and less during continuous infusion.[60] Notably, the first study[75] shows a larger response with progressively higher GC doses, suggesting that higher doses overcome intracellular GC resistance (see section Conclusion and Future Directions). There was also no difference in the GC resistance between male and female patients.[75,112]

COMPLICATIONS AND ADVERSE EVENTS

Adverse events linked to long-term administration of GCs involving the gastrointestinal, cardiovascular, endocrine, nervous, ocular, and immune systems.[114] However, these do not usually occur with the short courses of GC used in critical care. Indeed, the safety profile of GC treatment during acute conditions such as COVID-19-related pneumonia and ARDS is considerable, as benefits generally outweigh the risks.[7] The incidence and burden of complications have proved highly reproducible among dozens of RCTs investigating GC treatment in thousands of patients with severe sepsis, septic shock, ARDS, and COVID-19.

A 2017 Cochrane meta-analysis reported no significant differences between GC-treated people and controls for secondary infections or adverse events (RR 1.19; 95% CI 0.73–1.93), except for a higher incidence of hyperglycemia (RR 1.72; 95% CI 1.38–2.14).[7]

The same result was confirmed by several studies performed during the COVID-19 pandemic. In these studies, hyperglycemia was transient in response to the initial loading bolus and did not impact negatively on outcome.[16,26,115-117] Only one early study investigating hydrocortisone found a higher incidence of adverse events including superinfections and bleeding in the treatment arm versus placebo.[25] Three RCTs reported an increased incidence of hospital-acquired superinfections of these, two studies were underpowered[116,118] and the third one involved the use of high-dose, pulsed, MP.[115] Despite evidence from RCTs is lacking, some cohort studies associated a 10-days course of 6 mg daily DM with a higher incidence of pulmonary aspergillosis (CAPA), despite this was not confirmed in the multivariable model.[119]

Low-dose GC treatment has been shown not to delay viral shedding, and there is no evidence linking viral shedding to outcome in critically ill COVID-19 patients.[120,121]

More than 30% of patients receiving long-term GCs have been reported to develop adrenal insufficiency.[122] This was due to negative feedback regulation of GC production, which inhibits the HPA axis, its function requiring some time to be restored after interruption of exogenous GC administration. While this seems not to be a real concern in critical conditions requiring short courses of GCs, there is evidence relating a higher probability of returning on MV and an increase in inflammation markers after abrupt interruption of GC treatment.[123] Therefore, tapering would be advisable as already reviewed.

CONCLUSION AND FUTURE DIRECTIONS

Prolonged, low-dose GCs have shown the highest efficacy among pharmacological and nonpharmacological treatments for viral pneumonia requiring respiratory support.[124] The main body of evidence came from RCTs implemented during the COVID-19 pandemic, which was concordant with the results of former trials investigating GCs in severe pneumonia and ARDS from any cause.

The beneficial effect of GCs in viral respiratory infections is likely to depend on the timing of administration, dosage, and patient type. The best treatment protocol involves an initial bolus dose, followed by a continuous infusion for 8–14 days to maintain constant plasma levels. The optimal GC dose probably hovers around of 100 mg of MP equivalent daily, which would be better tapered to interruption instead of abruptly interrupted.[32] MP has shown the highest preclinical and clinical efficacy, mainly thanks to its higher ability to penetrate the lung.[125] The efficacy of GC treatment directly correlates with the severity of respiratory impairment.[23] Indeed, solid evidence contraindicates GCs in patients with early-stage COVID-19 who are not hospitalized.[28]

Treatment with GCs is not always effective, most likely due to the development of resistance to their effects. The mechanisms accounted for GC resistance range from individual genetic variations to molecular alterations of GC receptors,[126] which have been addressed in many studies.[127] However, it is yet unclear whether GR mutations affect GC response in COVID-19 patients. An effort is in progress to best characterize subphenotypes in ARDS,[65,128] to identify those more likely to benefit from an intervention. However, even if we improve our ability to identify responders, interindividual variability remains. The degrees of variability in patients' GC sensitivity and drug levels compounded with the variability in every aspect of the investigated protocols generates unnecessary noise. While we do not have a readily available test to identify GC resistance, a higher GC dose can overcome decreased GC sensitivity.[75] Possibly, a better approach is personalized treatment directed by combined clinical and laboratory variables; not different from what we do with MV and vasopressor support. An approach that incorporates these pharmacological principles may help to eventually personalize GC treatment protocols based on patients' individual clinical and laboratory characteristics with longitudinal adjustments directed by measurement of physiological and laboratory markers. New technologies, such as artificial intelligence-based ones, may allow for the development of dynamic algorithms aimed at integrating clinical and omics data to guide medical decisions with an individual-based, time-dependent approach.

REFERENCES

1. Meduri GU, Chrousos GP. General adaptation in critical illness: Glucocorticoid receptor-alpha master regulator of homeostatic corrections. Front Endocrinol (Lausanne). 2020;11:161.
2. Annane D, Pastores SM, Arlt W, Balk RA, Beishuizen A, Briegel J, et al. Critical illness-related corticosteroid insufficiency (CIRCI): a narrative review from a Multispecialty Task Force of the Society of Critical Care Medicine (SCCM) and the European Society of Intensive Care Medicine (ESICM). Intensive Care Med. 2017;43(12):1781-92.
3. This is the WHO emergency situational update on COVID-19, Report n.54, available at: https://www.who.int/docs/default-source/coronaviruse/situation-reports/20200314-sitrep-54-covid-19.pdf
4. Mehta P, McAuley DF, Brown M, Sanchez E, Tattersall RS, Manson JJ. COVID-19: Consider cytokine storm syndromes and immunosuppression. Lancet (London, England). 2020;395(10229):1033-4.
5. Meduri GU, Annane D, Chrousos GP, Marik PE, Sinclair SE. Activation and regulation of systemic inflammation in ARDS: Rationale for prolonged glucocorticoid therapy. Chest. 2009;136(6):1631-43.
6. Villar J, Ferrando C, Martínez D, Ambrós A, Muñoz T, Soler JA, et al. Dexamethasone treatment for the acute respiratory distress syndrome: a multicentre, randomised controlled trial. Lancet Respir Med. 2020;8(3):267-76.
7. Stern A, Skalsky K, Avni T, Carrara E, Leibovici L, Paul M; Cochrane Acute Respiratory Infections Group. Corticosteroids for pneumonia. Cochrane Database Syst Rev. 2017;2017(12):CD007720.
8. Arabi YM, Chrousos GP, Meduri GU. The ten reasons why corticosteroid therapy reduces mortality in severe COVID-19. Intensive Care Med. 2020;46(11):2067-70.
9. Huang C, Wang Y, Li X, Ren L, Zhao J, Hu Y, et al. Clinical features of patients infected with 2019 novel coronavirus in Wuhan, China. Lancet. 2020;395(10223):497-506.
10. Wu C, Chen X, Cai Y, Xia J, Zhou X, Xu S, et al. Risk factors associated with acute respiratory distress syndrome and death in patients with coronavirus disease 2019 pneumonia in Wuhan, China. JAMA Intern Med. 2020;180(7):934-43.
11. Wang D, Hu B, Hu C, Zhu F, Liu X, Zhang J, et al. Clinical characteristics of 138 hospitalized patients with 2019 novel coronavirus–infected pneumonia in Wuhan, China. JAMA. 2020;323(11):1061-9.
12. Arabi YM, Mandourah Y, Al-Hameed F, Sindi AA, Almekhlafi GA, Hussein MA, et al. Corticosteroid therapy for critically ill patients with middle east respiratory syndrome. Am J Respir Crit Care Med. 2018;197(6):757-67.
13. Delaney JW, Pinto R, Long J, Lamontagne F, Adhikari NK, Kumar A, et al. The influence of corticosteroid treatment on the outcome of influenza A(H1N1pdm09)-related critical illness. Crit Care. 2016;20:75.
14. Villar J, Confalonieri M, Pastores SM, Meduri GU. Rationale for prolonged corticosteroid treatment in the acute respiratory distress syndrome caused by coronavirus disease 2019. Crit Care Explor. 2020;2(4):e0111.

15. Salton F, Confalonieri P, Umberto Meduri G, Santus P, Harari S, Scala R, et al. Prolonged low-dose methylprednisolone in patients with severe COVID-19 pneumonia. Open forum Infect Dis. 2020;7(10):ofaa421.
16. Salton F, Confalonieri P, Centanni S, Mondoni M, Petrosillo N, Bonfanti P, et al. Prolonged higher dose methylprednisolone vs. conventional dexamethasone in COVID-19 pneumonia: A randomised controlled trial (MEDEAS). Eur Respir J. 2022;61(4):2201514.
17. Long Y, Xu Y, Wang B, Zhang L, Jia D, Xue F, et al. Clinical recommendations from an observational study on MERS: Glucocorticoids was benefit in treating SARS patients. 2016;9(5):8865-73.
18. Li H, Yang SG, Gu L, Zhang Y, Yan XX, Liang ZA, et al. Effect of low-to-moderate-dose corticosteroids on mortality of hospitalized adolescents and adults with influenza A(H1N1)pdm09 viral pneumonia. Influenza Other Respi Viruses. 2017;11(4):345-54.
19. Annane D, Pastores SM, Rochwerg B, Arlt W, Balk RA, Beishuizen A, et al. Guidelines for the diagnosis and management of critical illness-related corticosteroid insufficiency (CIRCI) in critically ill patients (Part I): Society of Critical Care Medicine (SCCM) and European Society of Intensive Care Medicine (ESICM) 2017. Crit Care Med. 2017;45(12):2078-88.
20. Tang L, Zhang X, Wang Y, Zeng X. Severe covid-19 pneumonia: Assessing inflammation burden with volume-rendered chest CT. Radiol Cardiothorac Imaging. 2020;2(2):e200044.
21. Xu Z, Shi L, Wang Y, Zhang J, Huang L, Zhang C, et al. Pathological findings of COVID-19 associated with acute respiratory distress syndrome. Lancet Respir Med. 2020;8(4): 420-2.
22. Swindon, Wiltshire E. (2022). Two years on: the COVID-19 treatment that saved millions. [online] Available from https://www.ukri.org/news/two-years-on-the-covid-19-treatment-that-saved-millions/ [Last accessed March, 2024].
23. RECOVERY Collaborative Group; Horby P, Lim WS, Emberson JR, Mafham M, Bell JL, Linsell L, et al. Dexamethasone in Hospitalized Patients with Covid-19 — Preliminary Report. N Engl J Med. 2021;384(8):693-704.
24. Wagner C, Griesel M, Mikolajewska A, Metzendorf MI, Fischer AL, Stegemann M, et al. Systemic corticosteroids for the treatment of COVID-19: Equity-related analyses and update on evidence. Cochrane Database Syst Rev. 2022;11(11):CD014963.
25. Angus DC, Derde L, Al-Beidh F, Annane D, Arabi Y, Beane A, et al. Effect of hydrocortisone on mortality and organ support in patients with severe COVID-19: The REMAP-CAP COVID-19 Corticosteroid Domain Randomized Clinical Trial. JAMA. 2020;324(13): 1317-29.
26. Dequin PF, Heming N, Meziani F, Plantefève G, Voiriot G, Badié J, et al. Effect of hydrocortisone on 21-Day mortality or respiratory support among critically ill patients with COVID-19: A Randomized Clinical Trial. JAMA. 2020;324(13):1298-306.
27. Hirano Y, Madokoro S, Kondo Y, Okamoto K, Tanaka H. Corticosteroid treatment for early acute respiratory distress syndrome: a systematic review and meta-analysis of randomized trials. J Intensive Care. 2020;8(1):1-8.
28. Wagner C, Griesel M, Mikolajewska A, Mueller A, Nothacker M, Kley K, et al. Systemic corticosteroids for the treatment of COVID-19. Cochrane Database Syst Rev. 2021;8(8): CD014963.
29. The COVID STEROID 2 Trial Group; Russell L, Uhre KR, Lindgaard ALS, Degn JF, Wetterslev M, Sivapalan P, et al. Effect of 12 mg vs 6 mg of Dexamethasone on the number of days alive without life support in adults with COVID-19 and severe hypoxemia: The COVID STEROID 2 Randomized Trial. JAMA. 2021;326(18):1807-17.
30. Taboada M, Rodríguez N, Varela PM, Rodríguez MT, Abelleira R, González A, et al. Effect of high versus low dose of dexamethasone on clinical worsening in patients hospitalised

with moderate or severe COVID-19 Pneumonia: an open-label, randomised clinical trial. Eur Respir J. 2021;60(2).

31. WHO Rapid Evidence Appraisal for COVID-19 Therapies (REACT) Working Group; Sterne JAC, Murthy S, Diaz J V, Slutsky AS, Villar J, Angus DC, et al. Association between administration of systemic corticosteroids and mortality among critically ill patients with COVID-19: A meta-analysis. JAMA. 2020;324(13):1330-41.
32. Meduri GU, Annane D, Confalonieri M, Chrousos GP, Rochwerg B, Busby A, et al. Pharmacological principles guiding prolonged glucocorticoid treatment in ARDS. Intensive Care Med. 2020;46(12):2284-96.
33. Ranjbar K, Moghadami M, Mirahmadizadeh A, Fallahi MJ, Khaloo V, Shahriarirad R, et al. Methylprednisolone or dexamethasone, which one is superior corticosteroid in the treatment of hospitalized COVID-19 patients: a triple-blinded randomized controlled trial. BMC Infect Dis. 2021;21(1):337.
34. Saeed MAM, Mohamed AH, Owaynat AH. Comparison between methylprednisolone infusion and dexamethasone in COVID-19 ARDS mechanically ventilated patients. Egypt J Intern Med. 2022;34(1):19.
35. Maamar M, Artime A, Pariente E, Fierro P, Ruiz Y, Gutiérrez S, et al. Post-COVID-19 syndrome, low-grade inflammation and inflammatory markers: a cross-sectional study. Curr Med Res Opin. 2022;38(6):901-9.
36. Mandal S, Barnett J, Brill SE, Brown JS, Denneny EK, Hare SS, et al. "Long-COVID": a cross-sectional study of persisting symptoms, biomarker and imaging abnormalities following hospitalisation for COVID-19. Thorax. 2021;76(4):396-8.
37. Agarwal A, Hunt B, Stegemann M, Rochwerg B, Lamontagne F, Siemieniuk RA, et al. A living WHO guideline on drugs for covid-19. BMJ. 2020;370:m3379.
38. Meduri GU, Confalonieri M, Chaudhuri D, Rochwerg B MB. Prolonged glucocorticoid treatment in ARDS: pathobiological rationale and pharmacological principles. In: Handbook of Stress: Stress, Immunology and Inflammation, vol. 5. Cambridge: Academic Press; 2023.
39. Meduri GU, Bridges L, Shih MC, Marik PE, Siemieniuk RAC, Kocak M. Prolonged glucocorticoid treatment is associated with improved ARDS outcomes: analysis of individual patients' data from four randomized trials and trial-level meta-analysis of the updated literature. Intensive Care Med. 2016;42(5):829-40.
40. Schreiber SN, Emter R, Hock MB, Knutti D, Cardenas J, Podvinec M, et al. The estrogen-related receptor alpha (ERRalpha) functions in PPARgamma coactivator 1alpha (PGC-1alpha)-induced mitochondrial biogenesis. Proc Natl Acad Sci U S A. 2004;101(17): 6472-7.
41. Suzuki S, Tsubochi H, Ishibashi H, Suzuki T, Kondo T, Sasano H. Increased expression of 11 beta-hydroxysteroid dehydrogenase type 2 in the lungs of patients with acute respiratory distress syndrome. Pathol Int. 2003;53(11):751-6.
42. Diederich S, Eigendorff E, Burkhardt P, Quinkler M, Bumke-Vogt C, Rochel M, et al. 11beta-hydroxysteroid dehydrogenase types 1 and 2: an important pharmacokinetic determinant for the activity of synthetic mineralo- and glucocorticoids. J Clin Endocrinol Metab. 2002;87(12):5695-701.
43. Draghici S, Nguyen TM, Sonna LA, Ziraldo C, Vanciu R, Fadel R, et al. COVID-19: disease pathways and gene expression changes predict methylprednisolone can improve outcome in severe cases. Bioinformatics. 2021;37(17):2691-8.
44. Kino T, Su YA, Chrousos GP. Human glucocorticoid receptor isoform beta: recent understanding of its potential implications in physiology and pathophysiology. Cell Mol Life Sci. 2009;66(21):3435-48.
45. Kamiyama K, Matsuda N, Yamamoto S, Takano K, Takano Y, Yamazaki H, et al. Modulation of glucocorticoid receptor expression, inflammation, and cell apoptosis in septic guinea pig lungs using methylprednisolone. Am J Physiol Lung Cell Mol Physiol. 2008;295(6).L998-1006.

46. Wang XQ, Zhou X, Zhou Y, Rong L, Gao L, Xu W. Low-dose dexamethasone alleviates lipopolysaccharide-induced acute lung injury in rats and upregulates pulmonary glucocorticoid receptors. Respirology. 2008;13(6):772-80.
47. Fruchter O, Kino T, Zoumakis E, Alesci S, De Martino M, Chrousos G, et al. The human glucocorticoid receptor (GR) isoform {beta} differentially suppresses GR{alpha}-induced transactivation stimulated by synthetic glucocorticoids. J Clin Endocrinol Metab. 2005;90(6):3505-9.
48. Vichyanond P, Irvin CG, Larsen GL, Szefler SJ, Hill MR. Penetration of corticosteroids into the lung: evidence for a difference between methylprednisolone and prednisolone. J Allergy Clin Immunol. 1989;84(6 Pt 1):867-73.
49. Greos LS, Vichyanond P, Bloedow DC, Irvin CG, Larsen GL, Szefler SJ, et al. Methylprednisolone achieves greater concentrations in the lung than prednisolone. A pharmacokinetic analysis. Am Rev Respir Dis. 1991;144(3 Pt 1):586-92.
50. Bartko J, Stiebellehner L, Derhaschnig U, Schoergenhofer C, Schwameis M, Prosch H, et al. Dissociation between systemic and pulmonary anti-inflammatory effects of dexamethasone in humans. Br J Clin Pharmacol. 2016;81(5):865-77.
51. Combes A, Costa MA, Trouillet JL, Baudot J, Mokhtari M, Gibert C, et al. Morbidity, mortality, and quality-of-life outcomes of patients requiring >or=14 days of mechanical ventilation. Crit Care Med. 2003;31(5):1373-81.
52. Wilson ME, Barwise A, Heise KJ, Loftsgard TO, Dziadzko M, Cheville A, et al. Long-term return to functional baseline after mechanical ventilation in the ICU. Crit Care Med. 2018;46(4):562-9.
53. Zilberberg MD, Nathanson BH, Ways J, Shorr AF. Characteristics, Hospital Course, and outcomes of patients requiring prolonged acute versus short-term mechanical ventilation in the united states, 2014-2018. Crit Care Med. 2020;48(11):1587-94.
54. Giordano G, Pugliese F, Bilotta F. Mechanical ventilation and long-term neurocognitive impairment after acute respiratory distress syndrome. Crit Care. 2020;24:30.
55. Straub RH, Schradin C. Chronic inflammatory systemic diseases: An evolutionary trade-off between acutely beneficial but chronically harmful programs. Evol Med Public Heal. 2016;2016(1):eow001.
56. Buttgereit F, Da Silva JPA, Boers M, Burmester GR, Cutolo M, Jacobs J, et al. Standardised nomenclature for glucocorticoid dosages and glucocorticoid treatment regimens: current questions and tentative answers in rheumatology. Ann Rheum Dis. 2002;61(8):718.
57. Jantz MA, Sahn SA. Corticosteroids in acute respiratory failure. Am J Respir Crit Care Med. 1999;160(4):1079-100.
58. Meduri GU, Kanangat S, Bronze M, Patterson DR, Meduri CU, Pak C, et al. Effects of methylprednisolone on intracellular bacterial growth. Clin Diagn Lab Immunol. 2001;8(6):1156-63.
59. Ibarra-Estrada MA, Chávez-Peña Q, Reynoso-Estrella CI, Rios-Zermeño J, Aguilera-González PE, García-Soto MA, et al. Timing, method and discontinuation of hydrocortisone administration for septic shock patients. World J Crit Care Med. 2017;6(1):65.
60. Yates CR, Vysokanov A, Mukherjee A, Ludden TM, Tolley E, Meduri GU, et al. Time-variant increase in methylprednisolone clearance in patients with acute respiratory distress syndrome: A population pharmacokinetic study. J Clin Pharmacol. 2001;41(4):415-24.
61. Weber-Carstens S, Keh D. Bolus or continuous hydrocortisone—that is the question. Crit Care. 2007;11(1):113.
62. Loisa P, Parviainen I, Tenhunen J, Hovilehto S, Ruokonen E. Effect of mode of hydrocortisone administration on glycemic control in patients with septic shock: a prospective randomized trial. Crit Care. 2007;11(1): PMC2151907.

63. Confalonieri M, Urbino R, Potena A, Piattella M, Parigi P, Puccio G, et al. Hydrocortisone infusion for severe community-acquired pneumonia: A preliminary randomized study. Am J Respir Crit Care Med. 2005;171(3):242-8.
64. Abdelsalam Rezk N, Mohamed Ibrahim A. Effects of methyl prednisolone in early ARDS. Egypt J Chest Dis Tuberc. 2013;62(1):167-72.
65. Winkler MS, Osuchowski MF, Payen D, Torres A, Dickel S, Skirecki T. Renaissance of glucocorticoids in critical care in the era of COVID-19: ten urging questions. Crit Care. 2022;26(1):1-9.
66. Steinberg KP, Hudson LD, Goodman RB, Hough CL, Lanken PN, Hyzy R, et al. Efficacy and safety of corticosteroids for persistent acute respiratory distress syndrome. N Engl J Med. 2006;354(16):1671-84.
67. Meduri GU, Bridges L, Siemieniuk RAC, Kocak M. An exploratory reanalysis of the randomized trial on efficacy of corticosteroids as rescue therapy for the late phase of acute respiratory distress syndrome. Crit Care Med. 2018;46(6):884-91.
68. Chen PH, Cheng CY, Li LF, Yu CC. Pneumonia rebound after stopping steroid in a patient with COVID-19: A case report. Respirol case reports. 2021;9(11):e0869.
69. Nguyen-Ho L. Disease progression after discontinuation of corticosteroid treatment in a COVID-19 patient with ARDS. Asian Pac J Trop Med. 2022;15(1):47.
70. Murray JF, Matthay MA, Luce JM, Flick MR. An expanded definition of the adult respiratory distress syndrome. Am Rev Respir Dis. 1988;138(3):720-3.
71. Meduri GU, Headley S, Kohler G, Stentz F, Tolley E, Umberger R, et al. Persistent elevation of inflammatory cytokines predicts a poor outcome in ARDS. Plasma IL-1 beta and IL-6 levels are consistent and efficient predictors of outcome over time. Chest. 1995;107(4):1062-73.
72. Meduri GU, Tolley EA, Chrousos GP, Stentz F. Prolonged methylprednisolone treatment suppresses systemic inflammation in patients with unresolving acute respiratory distress syndrome. 2012;165(7):983-91.
73. Umberto Meduri G, Tolley EA, Chrousos GP, Stentz F. Prolonged methylprednisolone treatment suppresses systemic inflammation in patients with unresolving acute respiratory distress syndrome: evidence for inadequate endogenous glucocorticoid secretion and inflammation-induced immune cell resistance to glucocorticoids. Am J Respir Crit Care Med. 2002;165(7):983-91.
74. Meduri GU, Headley S, Tolley E, Shelby M, Stentz F, Postlethwaite A. Plasma and BAL cytokine response to corticosteroid rescue treatment in late ARDS. Chest. 1995;108(5):1315-25.
75. Chriguer R, Elias L, da Silva I, Vieira J, Moreira A, de Castro M. Glucocorticoid sensitivity in young healthy individuals: in vitro and in vivo studies. J Clin Endocrinol Metab. 2005;90(11):5978-84.
76. Cohen J, Pretorius CJ, Ungerer JPJ, Cardinal J, Blumenthal A, Presneill J, et al. Glucocorticoid sensitivity is highly variable in critically ill patients with septic shock and is associated with disease severity. Crit Care Med. 2016;44(6):1034-41.
77. Meduri GU, Golden E, Freire AX, Taylor E, Zaman M, Carson SJ, et al. Methylprednisolone infusion in early severe ARDS: results of a randomized controlled trial. Chest. 2007;131(4):954-63.
78. Müller B, Peri G, Doni A, Perruchoud AP, Landmann R, Pasqualini F, et al. High circulating levels of the IL-1 type II decoy receptor in critically ill patients with sepsis: association of high decoy receptor levels with glucocorticoid administration. J Leukoc Biol. 2002;72(4):643-9.
79. De Kruif MD, Lemaire LC, Giebelen IA, Struck J, Morgenthaler NG, Papassotiriou J, et al. The influence of corticosteroids on the release of novel biomarkers in human endotoxemia. Intensive Care Med. 2008;34(3):518.

80. Perren A, Cerutti B, Lepori M, Senn V, Capelli B, Duchini F, et al. Influence of steroids on procalcitonin and C-reactive protein in patients with COPD and community-acquired pneumonia. Infection. 2008;36(2):163-6.
81. Rinaldi S, Adembri C, Grechi S, De Gaudio AR. Low-dose hydrocortisone during severe sepsis: effects on microalbuminuria. Crit Care Med. 2006;34(9):2334-9.
82. Seam N, Meduri GU, Wang H, Nylen ES, Sun J, Schultz MJ, et al. Effects of methylprednisolone infusion on markers of inflammation, coagulation, and angiogenesis in early acute respiratory distress syndrome. Crit Care Med. 2012;40(2):495-501.
83. Meduri GU, Yates CR. Systemic inflammation-associated glucocorticoid resistance and outcome of ARDS. Ann N Y Acad Sci. 2004;1024:24-53.
84. Wilkinson L, Verhoog NJD, Louw A. Disease- and treatment-associated acquired glucocorticoid resistance. Endocr Connect. 2018;7(12):R328.
85. Rodriguez JM, Monsalves-Alvarez M, Henriquez S, Llanos MN, Troncoso R. Glucocorticoid resistance in chronic diseases. Steroids. 2016;115:182-92.
86. Koper JW, Van Rossum EFC, Van Den Akker ELT. Glucocorticoid receptor polymorphisms and haplotypes and their expression in health and disease. Steroids. 2014;92:62-73.
87. Van Der Voort PHJ, Gerritsen RT, Bakker AJ, Boerma EC, Kuiper MA, De Heide L. HDL-cholesterol level and cortisol response to synacthen in critically ill patients. Intensive Care Med. 2003;29(12):2199-203.
88. Yates CR, Chang C, Kearbey JD, Yasuda K, Schuetz EG, et al. Structural determinants of P-glycoprotein-mediated transport of glucocorticoids. Pharm Res. 2003;20(11):1794-803.
89. Van Den Akker ELT, Koper JW, Joosten K, de Jong FH, Hazelzet JA, Lamberts SW, et al. Glucocorticoid receptor mRNA levels are selectively decreased in neutrophils of children with sepsis. Intensive Care Med. 2009;35(7):1247-54.
90. Bergquist M, Nurkkala M, Rylander C, Kristiansson E, Hedenstierna G, Lindholm C. Expression of the glucocorticoid receptor is decreased in experimental Staphylococcus aureus sepsis. J Infect. 2013;67(6):574-83.
91. Indyk JA, Candido-Vitto C, Wolf IM, Venkataraman S, Munoz R, Saladino RA, et al. Reduced glucocorticoid receptor protein expression in children with critical illness. Horm Res Paediatr. 2013;79(3):169-78.
92. Vassiliou AG, Floros G, Jahaj E, Stamogiannos G, Gennimata S, Vassiliadi DA, et al. Decreased glucocorticoid receptor expression during critical illness. Eur J Clin Invest. 2019;49(4):e13073.
93. Guerrero J, Gatica HA, Rodríguez M, Estay R, Goecke IA. Septic serum induces glucocorticoid resistance and modifies the expression of glucocorticoid isoforms receptors: a prospective cohort study and in vitro experimental assay. Crit Care. 2013;17(3):R107.
94. Park JH, Lee HK. Re-analysis of single cell transcriptome reveals that the NR3C1-CXCL8-neutrophil axis determines the severity of COVID-19. Front Immunol. 2020;11:2145.
95. Pariante CM, Pearce BD, Pisell TL, Sanchez CI, Po C, Su C, et al. The proinflammatory cytokine, interleukin-1alpha, reduces glucocorticoid receptor translocation and function. Endocrinology. 1999;140(9):4359-66.
96. Meduri GU, Muthiah MP, Carratu P, Eltorky M, Chrousos GP. Nuclear factor-kappaB- and glucocorticoid receptor alpha-mediated mechanisms in the regulation of systemic and pulmonary inflammation during sepsis and acute respiratory distress syndrome. Evidence for inflammation-induced target tissue resistance to glucocorticoids. Neuroimmunomodulation. 2005;12(6):321-38.
97. Bantel H, Schmitz ML, Raible A, Gregor M, Schulze-Osthoff K. Critical role of nuclear factor-κB and stress-activated protein kinases in steroid unresponsiveness. FASEB J. 2002;16(13):1-19.

98. Liu MY, Zhu LJ, Zhou QG. Neuronal nitric oxide synthase is an endogenous negative regulator of glucocorticoid receptor in the hippocampus. Neurol Sci. 2013;34(7):1167-72.
99. Hutchison KA, Matic G, Meshinchi S, Bresnick EH, Pratts WB. The journal of biological chemistry redox manipulation of DNA binding activity and bugr epitope reactivity of the glucocorticoid receptor. J Biol Chem. 1991;266(16):10505-9.
100. Makino Y, Okamoto K, Yoshikawa N, Aoshima M, Hirota K, Yodoi J, et al. Thioredoxin: a redox-regulating cellular cofactor for glucocorticoid hormone action. Cross talk between endocrine control of stress response and cellular antioxidant defense system. J Clin Invest. 1996;98(11):2469-77.
101. Duma D, Silva-Santos JE, Assreuy J. Inhibition of glucocorticoid receptor binding by nitric oxide in endotoxemic rats. Crit Care Med. 2004;32(11):2304-10.
102. Okamoto K, Tanaka H, Makino Y, Makino I. Restoration of the glucocorticoid receptor function by the phosphodiester compound of vitamins C and E, EPC-K1 (l-ascorbic acid 2-[3,4-dihydro-2,5,7,8-tetramethyl-2-(4,8,12-trimethyltridecyl)-2H-1-benzopyran-6-yl hydrogen phosphate] potassium salt), via a redox-dependent mechanism. Biochem Pharmacol. 1998;56(1):79-86.
103. Okamoto K, Tanaka H, Ogawa H, Makino Y, Eguchi H, Hayashi S, et al. Redox-dependent regulation of nuclear import of the glucocorticoid receptor. J Biol Chem. 1999;274(15):10363-71.
104. Hakim A, Barnes PJ, Adcock IM, Usmani OS. Importin-7 mediates glucocorticoid receptor nuclear import and is impaired by oxidative stress, leading to glucocorticoid insensitivity. FASEB J. 2013;27(11):4510-9.
105. Grimes DS. Are statins analogues of vitamin D? Lancet (London, England). 2006; 368(9529):83-6.
106. Hoepner R, Bagnoud M, Pistor M, Salmen A, Briner M, Synn H, et al. Vitamin D increases glucocorticoid efficacy via inhibition of mTORC1 in experimental models of multiple sclerosis. Acta Neuropathol. 2019;138(3):443-56.
107. Ojaimi S, Skinner NA, Strauss BJG, Sundararajan V, Woolley I, Visvanathan K. Vitamin D deficiency impacts on expression of toll-like receptor-2 and cytokine profile: a pilot study. J Transl Med. 2013;11:176.
108. Padayatty SJ, Levine M. Vitamin C physiology: the known and the unknown andGoldilocks. Oral Dis. 2016;22(6):463.
109. Patak P, Willenberg HS, Bornstein SR. Vitamin C is an important cofactor for both adrenal cortex and adrenal medulla. Endocr Res. 2004;30(4):871-5.
110. Björkhem I, Kallner A, Karlmar K-E. Effects of ascorbic acid deficiency on adrenal mitochondrial hydroxylations in guinea pigs. J Lipid Res. 1978;19(6):695-704.
111. Farrell RJ, Kelleher D. Glucocorticoid resistance in inflammatory bowel disease. J Endocrinol. 2003;178(3):339-46.
112. Hearing SD, Norman M, Smyth C, Foy C, Dayan CM. Wide variation in lymphocyte steroid sensitivity among healthy human volunteers. J Clin Endocrinol Metab. 1999;84(11):4149-54.
113. Smit P, Russcher H, De Jong FH, Brinkmann AO, Lamberts SWJ, Koper JW. Differential regulation of synthetic glucocorticoids on gene expression levels of glucocorticoid-induced leucine zipper and interleukin-2. J Clin Endocrinol Metab. 2005;90(5):2994-3000.
114. Oray M, Abu Samra K, Ebrahimiadib N, Meese H, Foster CS. Long-term side effects of glucocorticoids. Expert Opin Drug Saf. 2016;15(4):457-65.
115. Edalatifard M, Akhtari M, Salehi M, Naderi Z, Jamshidi A, Mostafaei S, et al. Intravenous methylprednisolone pulse as a treatment for hospitalised severe COVID-19 patients: results from a randomised controlled clinical trial. Eur Respir J. 2020;56(6):2002808.

116. Tang X, Feng YM, Ni JX, Zhang JY, Liu LM, Hu K, et al. Early use of corticosteroid may prolong SARS-CoV-2 shedding in non-intensive care unit patients with COVID-19 pneumonia: A Multicenter, Single-Blind, Randomized Control Trial. Respiration. 2021;100(2):116-26.
117. Tomazini BM, Maia IS, Cavalcanti AB, Berwanger O, Rosa RG, Veiga VC, et al. Effect of dexamethasone on days alive and ventilator-free in patients with moderate or severe acute respiratory distress syndrome and COVID-19: The CoDEX Randomized Clinical Trial. JAMA. 2020;324(13):1307-16.
118. Corral-Gudino L, Bahamonde A, Arnaiz-Revillas F, Gómez-Barquero J, Abadía-Otero J, García-Ibarbia C, et al. Methylprednisolone in adults hospitalized with COVID-19 pneumonia : An open-label randomized trial (GLUCOCOVID). Wien Klin Wochenschr. 2021;133(7-8):303-11.
119. Leistner R, Schroeter L, Adam T, Poddubnyy D, Stegemann M, Siegmund B, et al. Corticosteroids as risk factor for COVID-19-associated pulmonary aspergillosis in intensive care patients. Crit Care. 2022;26(1):1-11.
120. Salton F, Confalonieri P, Meduri GU, Santus P, Harari S, Scala R, et al. Prolonged low-dose methylprednisolone in patients with severe COVID-19 pneumonia. Open Forum Infect Dis. 2020;7(10);ofaa421.
121. Jeronimo CMP, Farias MEL, Val FFA, Sampaio VS, Alexandre MAA, Melo GC, et al. Methylprednisolone as adjunctive therapy for patients hospitalized with coronavirus disease 2019 (COVID-19; Metcovid): A Randomized, Double-blind, Phase IIb, Placebo-controlled Trial. Clin Infect Dis. 2021;72(9):E373-81.
122. Prete A, Bancos I. Glucocorticoid induced adrenal insufficiency. BMJ. 2021;374:n1380.
123. Nawab QUA, Golden E, Confalonieri M, Umberger R, Meduri GU. Corticosteroid treatment in severe community-acquired pneumonia: Duration of treatment affects control of systemic inflammation and clinical improvement. Intensive Care Med. 2011;37(9):1553-4.
124. Confalonieri M, Salton F, Fabiano F. Acute respiratory distress syndrome. Eur Respir Rev. 2017;26(144):160116.
125. Russo A, Davoli C, Borrazzo C, et al. Clinical characteristics and outcome of hospitalized COVID-19 patients treated with standard dose of dexamethasone or high dose of methylprednisolone. Biomed. 2022;10(7):1548.
126. Barnes P, Adcock I. Glucocorticoid resistance in inflammatory diseases. Lancet (London, England). 2009;373(9678):1905-17.
127. Bruscoli S, Puzzovio PG, Zaimi M, Tiligada K, Levi-Schaffer F, Riccardi C. Glucocorticoids and COVID-19. Pharmacol Res. 2022;185:106511.
128. Reddy K, Sinha P, O'Kane CM, Gordon AC, Calfee CS, McAuley DF. Subphenotypes in critical care: translation into clinical practice. Lancet Respir Med. 2020;8(6):631-43.
129. Amrein K, Oudemans-van Straaten HM, Berger MM. Vitamin therapy in critically ill patients: focus on thiamine, vitamin C, and vitamin D. Intensive Care Med. 2018;44(11):1940-4.
130. This in the Food and Drug Administration's package insert for methylprednisolone (Solumedrol), available at: https://www.accessdata.fda.gov/drugsatfda_docs/label/2010/011856s107lbl.pdf
131. Berger MM, Shenkin A, Schweinlin A, Amrein K, Augsburger M, Biesalski HK, et al. ESPEN Guideline ESPEN micronutrient guideline. 2022;41(6):1367-424.
132. Morgan ET. Regulation of cytochromes P450 during inflammation and infection. Drug Metab Rev. 1997;29(4):1129-88.

CHAPTER 27

Therapeutic Effects of Fluvoxamine in the Management of COVID-19

Jagan Mohan Rao Vanjarapu, Jose Iglesias

INTRODUCTION

The coronavirus disease 2019 (COVID-19) pandemic caused by the novel coronavirus resulted in unprecedented challenges to the healthcare system and accelerated the discovery of various therapeutic and prophylactic drugs for the management of COVID-19 infection. Among the people infected with COVID-19, a major proportion present with mild or moderate symptoms. However, some of them may clinically deteriorate and present with severe symptoms, resulting in increased intensive care unit (ICU) admissions and mortality. Thus, there is an increase in the need for an effective medication for the management of COVID-19 infection.

There is emerging evidence suggesting selective serotonin reuptake inhibitor (SSRI) use in early stages of infection.[1] Among them, fluvoxamine has drawn a lot of attention in the medical community. This medication is primarily used as an antidepressant and is widely used for the treatment of post-traumatic stress disorder, social anxiety disorder, and anxiety disorder.[2-4] Recently, this medication has been shown to be effective in mild-to-moderate COVID-19 infections. Recent data suggest that the use of fluvoxamine may prevent complications including intubation and improve mortality, if used in the earlier stages of the disease.[1]

POTENTIAL MECHANISMS OF ACTION

The antidepressant/anxiolytic effects of fluvoxamine are manifested by serotonin reuptake inhibition with a higher affinity for the serotonin transporter over the norepinephrine transporter.[5,6] However, the detailed mechanisms of action in COVID-19 patients still need to be explored.

The following proposed mechanisms were widely accepted:

- The acid sphingomyelinase (ASM)/ceramide system plays a major role in viral infections. Viral entry into the cell is facilitated by sphingomyelinase/

Medications such as clozapine, olanzapine, tizanidine, and theophylline should be avoided as they are metabolized by CYP 1A2 system. Also, if the patient is already on another SSRI or monoamine oxidase inhibitors (MAOIs), it should be avoided to prevent serotonin syndrome and other side effects.[20]

THERAPEUTIC EFFICACY

In November 2020, Dr Lenze et al. published a study on the potential beneficial effects of fluvoxamine in COVID-19 infected patients.[22] This study was performed among adults in an outpatient setting. Although this study was performed with a small sample size (n = 80), this triggered several studies to determine the therapeutic benefits of fluvoxamine.[22] Later, Seftel et al. reported a nonrandomized, prospective, observational cohort study in February 2021. This study was done on patients infected in the setting of a mass outbreak in California. In this study, the fluvoxamine group has lower hospitalization, lower risk for ICU admission, and lower mortality.[23]

In August 2021, a multicentered, randomized, placebo-controlled, adaptive TOGETHER trial was done on unvaccinated symptomatic adult patients with COVID-19 in Brazil. Treatment with fluvoxamine among early diagnosed COVID-19 patients in outpatient settings reduced the need for hospitalization and transfer to a tertiary care hospital. Patients treated with fluvoxamine (n = 741) versus the placebo group (n = 756) (relative risk was 0.68).[24,25] Another randomized control study by Wen et al. showed that fluvoxamine is effective in reducing the hospitalization rates and mortality in COVID-19 patients.[26]

According to a meta-analysis of 13 studies performed in real time, fluvoxamine has been shown to have several therapeutic benefits in various stages of the treatment. In this analysis, which consists of a total of 34,828 subjects, fluvoxamine showed 31% (17–43%) clinical improvement compared to controls. The mortality benefit is 37% over the controls.[27,28] Early treatment has been shown to be more effective than late treatment.[29] The ventilation rate is 22% less, hospitalization rates are 28% less, and recovery rates are 8% more compared to the controls.

Fluvoxamine has been studied in various stages for the management of COVID-19:[27]

- *Prophylaxis:* Take medications regularly to prevent infection or minimize the symptoms.[27,28] Prophylactic usage showed 27% clinical improvement.
- *Early treatment:* Start the medications immediately or soon after the symptoms are seen. Early treatment showed 56% clinical improvement.[27,28]
- *Late treatment:* Start the treatment in the later phases of the disease course. Treatment in the later phase of the disease course showed 40% improvement.[27,28]

There have been several studies that have been published recently on the therapeutic efficacy of fluvoxamine on COVID-19.

TABLE 1: Beneficial effects of fluvoxamine on COVID-19.

Study	Benefits
Fluvoxamine for outpatient management of COVID-19 to prevent hospitalization	*A systematic review and meta-analysis*: Outpatient treatment with fluvoxamine in COVID-19 patients is associated with lower hospitalization rates[30]
Fluvoxamine for the early treatment of SARS-CoV-2 infection	*A review*: Early treatment with fluvoxamine in COVID-19 patients appears to reduce COVID-19-related morbidity and mortality[31]
Fluvoxamine and amantadine	*A review*: Fluvoxamine prevents the progression of the disease when administered earlier during the disease course[32]
Fluvoxamine for COVID-19 ICU patients	*Open-label prospective cohort study*: The addition of fluvoxamine to the standard of care in COVID-19 patients admitted to the ICU could improve mortality[33]
Fluvoxamine treatment of patients with symptomatic COVID-19 in a community treatment center	*Randomized controlled study–preliminary results*: In a study of 52 participants, fluvoxamine was not effective in preventing patients with mild-to-moderate COVID-19 infection from clinical deterioration[34]
Fluvoxamine for the early treatment of SARS-CoV-2 infection: A review of current evidence	Fluvoxamine will likely reduce COVID-19-related morbidity and mortality[31]

(COVID-19: coronavirus disease 2019; ICU: intensive care unit; SARS-CoV-2: severe acute respiratory syndrome coronavirus 2)

Table 1 summarizes some of the beneficial effects of fluvoxamine on COVID-19.

EFFECT OF FLUVOXAMINE ON LONG COVID SYMPTOMS

There is an increase in evidence indicating the effect of SARS-CoV-2 virus on the central nervous system.[35,36] SARS-CoV-2 infection can result in various long-term psychiatric complications such as anxiety, depression, difficulty concentrating, cognitive impairment, and sleep problems after the infection.[37] Although the precise mechanisms underlying long COVID symptoms were not clearly understood, therapeutic use of fluvoxamine has been shown to mitigate these symptoms in COVID-19 survivors.[37]

DISCUSSION

Numerous studies have been published citing the beneficial effects of fluvoxamine on COVID-19. However, both positive and negative results are important in evaluating the efficacy of the medication. Thus, we need to evaluate the results considering the underlying strengths and biases associated with each study.

Various studies often have conflicts of interest, whereby sponsors may have an interest in outcomes being positive. However, fluvoxamine has been manufactured by various pharmaceutical companies and is available at a low price, thus minimizing the bias.

Publishing is sometimes biased toward positive results with regard to a particular medication. However, inexpensive medications or treatment modalities may not be frequently reported as they may not attract public attention. There is a general tendency to publish positive results in retrospective studies for a particular medication. However, prospective study results are published regardless of the results. There is still some ambiguity regarding the mechanism of action, the effect of medication on viral load, the inflammatory response of the host, and the dosage of the medication to deliver maximum efficacy. Thus, more prospective studies focused on these aspects are needed for a better understanding of the medication and its therapeutic effects.

SAFETY PROFILE

Fluvoxamine has been shown to be a safe medication. Numerous studies have shown the complication rates were similar to the control group.[33,26] Various postmarketing surveillance studies till date have demonstrated a good safety profile.[38] The most common side effect is reported to be nausea.[39] Other reported side effects were somnolence, headaches, and dry mouth.[39,40]

CONCLUSION

In conclusion, there is emerging evidence showing beneficial effects such as decrease in mortality and the need for hospitalization in COVID-19 patients. Fluvoxamine is known to have a favorable safety profile and is available at a low cost. It can be administered orally and is widely available, making it a great candidate for the management of COVID-19 (in underprivileged areas). This can also be used as a prophylactic mediation. Thus, fluvoxamine is a great candidate, especially in the areas where there is less access to vaccinations and medical care. However, more high-quality studies are needed to establish pharmacokinetics, efficacy, and safety profile of fluvoxamine and other SSRIs for the management of COVID-19.

REFERENCES

1. Hashimoto Y, Suzuki T, Hashimoto K. Mechanisms of action of fluvoxamine for COVID-19: A historical review. Mol Psychiatry. 2022;27(4):1898-907.
2. Asnis GM, Hameedi FA, Goddard AW, Potkin SG, Black D, Jameel M, et al. Fluvoxamine in the treatment of panic disorder: A multi-center, double-blind, placebo-controlled study in outpatients. Psychiatry Res. 2001;103(1):1-14.
3. Irons J. Fluvoxamine in the treatment of anxiety disorders. Neuropsychiatr Dis Treat. 2005;1(4):289-99.

4. Figgitt DP, McClellan KJ. Fluvoxamine. An updated review of its use in the management of adults with anxiety disorders. Drugs. 2000;60(4):925-54.
5. Racagni G, Popoli M. The pharmacological properties of antidepressants. Int Clin Psychopharmacol. 2010;25(3):117-31.
6. Stahl SM. Mechanism of action of serotonin selective reuptake inhibitors. J Affect Disord. 1998;51(3):215-35.
7. Carpinteiro A, Gripp B, Hoffmann M, Pöhlmann S, Hoertel N, Edwards MJ, et al. Inhibition of acid sphingomyelinase by ambroxol prevents SARS-CoV-2 entry into epithelial cells. J Biol Chem. 2021;296:100701.
8. Gordon DE, Hiatt J, Bouhaddou M, Rezelj VV, Ulferts S, Braberg H, et al. Comparative host-coronavirus protein interaction networks reveal pan-viral disease mechanisms. Science. 2020;370(6521) eabe9403.
9. Hashimoto Y, Suzuki T, Hashimoto K. Old drug fluvoxamine, new hope for COVID-19. Eur Arch Psychiatry Clin Neurosci. 2022;272(1):161-3.
10. Hashimoto K. Repurposing of CNS drugs to treat COVID-19 infection: Targeting the sigma-1 receptor. Eur Arch Psychiatry Clin Neurosci. 2021;271(2):249-58.
11. Hashimoto K. Activation of sigma-1 receptor chaperone in the treatment of neuropsychiatric diseases and its clinical implication. J Pharmacol Sci. 2015;127(1):6-9.
12. Narita N, Hashimoto K, Tomitaka S, Minabe Y. Interactions of selective serotonin reuptake inhibitors with subtypes of σ receptors in rat brain. Eur J Pharmacol. 1996;307(1):117-9.
13. Battinelli EM. COVID-19 concerns aggregate around platelets. Blood. 2020;136(11): 1221-3.
14. Sukhatme VP, Reiersen AM, Vayttaden SJ, Sukhatme VV. Fluvoxamine: A review of its mechanism of action and its role in COVID-19. Front Pharmacol. 2021;12:652688.
15. Anderson GM. Fluvoxamine, melatonin and COVID-19. Psychopharmacology (Berl). 2021;238(2):611.
16. Rosen DA, Seki SM, Fernández-Castañeda A, Beiter RM, Eccles JD, Woodfolk JA, et al. Modulation of the sigma-1 receptor–IRE1 pathway is beneficial in preclinical models of inflammation and sepsis. Sci Transl Med. 2019;11(478).
17. Young JJ, Bruno D, Pomara N. A review of the relationship between proinflammatory cytokines and major depressive disorder. J Affect Disord. 2014;169:15-20.
18. Laguna-Goya R, Utrero-Rico A, Talayero P, Lasa-Lazaro M, Ramirez-Fernandez A, Naranjo L,et al. IL-6–based mortality risk model for hospitalized patients with COVID-19. J Allergy Clin Immunol. 2020;146(4):799-807.
19. Herold T, Jurinovic V, Arnreich C, Lipworth BJ, Hellmuth JC, von Bergwelt-Baildon M, et al. Elevated levels of IL-6 and CRP predict the need for mechanical ventilation in COVID-19. J Allergy Clin Immunol. 2020;146(1):128-36.
20. Lenze EJ, Reiersen AM, Santosh PJ. Repurposing fluvoxamine, and other psychiatric medications, for COVID-19 and other conditions. World Psychiatry. 2022;21(2):314-5.
21. van Harten J. Overview of the Pharmacokinetics of Fluvoxamine. Clin Pharmacokinet. 1995;29(Suppl 1):1-9.
22. Lenze EJ, Mattar C, Zorumski CF, Stevens A, Schweiger J, Nicol GE, et al. Fluvoxamine vs Placebo and Clinical Deterioration in Outpatients With Symptomatic COVID-19. JAMA. 2020;324(22):2292-300.
23. Seftel D, Boulware DR. Prospective Cohort of Fluvoxamine for Early Treatment of Coronavirus Disease 19. Open Forum Infect Dis. 2021;8(2):ofab050.
24. NEJM Journal Watch. (2021). Could This Be Our First Effective, Inexpensive, Widely Available Outpatient Treatment for COVID-19? [online] Available from https://blogs.jwatch.org/hiv-id-observations/index.php/could-this-be-our-first-effective-inexpensive-widely-available-outpatient-treatment-for-covid-19/2021/08/12/ [Last accessed February, 2024].

25. Reis G, dos Santos Moreira-Silva EA, Silva DCM, Thabane L, Milagres AC, Ferreira TS, et al. Effect of early treatment with fluvoxamine on risk of emergency care and hospitalisation among patients with COVID-19: The TOGETHER randomised, platform clinical trial. Lancet Glob Health. 2022;10(1):e42-51.
26. Wen W, Chen C, Tang J, Wang C, Zhou M, Cheng Y, et al. Efficacy and safety of three new oral antiviral treatment (molnupiravir, fluvoxamine and Paxlovid) for COVID-19: A meta-analysis. Ann Med. 2022;54(1):516-23.
27. Covid Analysis. Fluvoxamine for COVID-19: Real-time meta analysis of 13 studies. [online] Available from https://c19early.org/fmeta.html#appendix_methods [Last accessed February, 2024].
28. Boretti A. Effectiveness of fluvoxamine at preventing COVID-19 infection from turning severe. Eur Neuropsychopharmacol. 2023;67:83-5.
29. Mahdi M, Hermán L, Réthelyi JM, Bálint BL. Potential Role of the Antidepressants Fluoxetine and Fluvoxamine in the Treatment of COVID-19. Int J Mol Sci. 2022;23(7):3812.
30. Lee TC, Vigod S, Bortolussi-Courval É, Hanula R, Boulware DR, Lenze EJ, et al. Fluvoxamine for Outpatient Management of COVID-19 to Prevent Hospitalization. JAMA Netw Open. 2022;5(4):e226269.
31. Facente SN, Reiersen AM, Lenze EJ, Boulware DR, Klausner JD. Fluvoxamine for the early treatment of SARS-CoV-2 infection: A review of current evidence. Drugs. 2021;81(18):2081-9.
32. Rejdak K, Grieb P. Fluvoxamine and Amantadine: Central nervous system acting drugs repositioned for COVID-19 as early intervention. Curr Neuropharmacol. 2022;20(4): 777-81.
33. Calusic M, Marcec R, Luksa L, Jurkovic I, Kovac N, Mihaljevic S, et al. Safety and efficacy of fluvoxamine in COVID-19 ICU patients: An open label, prospective cohort trial with matched controls. Br J Clin Pharmacol. 2022;88(5):2065-73.
34. Erratum: Fluvoxamine treatment of patients with symptomatic COVID-19 in a community treatment center: A preliminary result of randomized controlled trial. Infect Chemother. 2022;54(2):391.
35. Solomon IH, Normandin E, Bhattacharyya S, Mukerji SS, Keller K, Ali AS, et al. Neuropathological Features of Covid-19. N Engl J Med. 2020;383(10):989-92.
36. Puelles VG, Lütgehetmann M, Lindenmeyer MT, Sperhake JP, Wong MN, Allweiss L, et al. Multiorgan and Renal Tropism of SARS-CoV-2. N Engl J Med. 2020;383(6):590-2.
37. Hashimoto K. Overview of the potential use of fluvoxamine for COVID-19 and long COVID. Discov Ment Health. 2023;3(1):9.
38. Buchberger R, Wagner W. Fluvoxamine: safety profile in extensive post-marketing surveillance. Pharmacopsychiatry. 2002;35(3):101-8.
39. Wagner W, Zaborny BA, Gray TE. Fluvoxamine. A review of its safety profile in world-wide studies. Int Clin Psychopharmacol. 1994;9(4):223-8.
40. Altamura AC, Caldiroli A, Buoli M. Pharmacokinetic evaluation of fluvoxamine for the treatment of anxiety disorders. Expert Opin Drug Metab Toxicol. 2015;11(4):649-60.

CHAPTER 28

Randomized Placebo Controlled Trials in the COVID Era: A Question of Faith?

Marc Rendell

> ***"And the LORD said unto Satan, Hast thou considered my servant Job, that there is none like him in the earth, a perfect and an upright man, one that feareth God, and escheweth evil?***
>
> ***Then Satan answered the LORD, and said, Doth Job fear God for nought?***
>
> ***Hast not thou made an hedge about him, and about his house, and about all that he hath on every side? thou hast blessed the work of his hands, and his substance is increased in the land.***
>
> ***But put forth thine hand now, and touch all that he hath, and he will curse thee to thy face."***

PROLOGUE

Satan argued that Job's steadfast faith in God would not withstand unfavorable changes to his good life. God then allowed Satan freedom to inflict suffering on Job to challenge his faith, which was then carried out on a biblical scale, including the death of all his children, the loss of all his possessions, and incapacitating illness.

Globally, as of 6:30 PM CEST (Central European Summer Time), 16 August 2023, there have been 769,806,130 confirmed cases of coronavirus disease 2019 (COVID-19), including 6,955,497 deaths, reported to the World Health Organization. If we consider excess mortality statistics throughout the world, there have been perhaps 20 million lives lost.[1] Certainly, having endured this terrible pandemic tragedy and with so many survivors suffering residual disability, we have cause to reflect on the miseries of Job and his enduring obedience to the will of God.

ELIMINATE BIAS: THE RANDOMIZED PLACEBO CONTROLLED TRIAL

"Man must be just. We must set aside bias and prejudice. We must abandon the imitations of ancestors and forefathers. We ourselves must investigate reality and be fair in judgment."

—Abdu'l-Baha, The Promulgation of Universal Peace

The role of a doctor is to choose treatments for patients based on an individual clinical assessment. That introduces a bias that is difficult to overcome if the goal is to assess the potential value of that treatment for an entire population. Randomized controlled trials (RCTs) are designed to reduce bias by randomly selecting a group of individuals who undergo a chosen intervention and a control group taking alternative treatments or placebo which is no treatment at all. There is no better way to demonstrate a difference induced by the intervention than by comparing those who received it to those individuals, presumably alike in every way, who did not. By allocating treatments based on random chance rather than preconceived clinical beliefs, one hopefully eliminates biased selection and can determine the true effect of the intervention. As the pandemic began to take hold, the United States research establishment, personified by Dr Anthony Fauci, long time director of the National Institute of Allergy and Infectious Disease, insisted that any interventions to deal with the rapidly propagating disease had to be supported by randomized controlled trials.[2,3] In the United States and most conforming nations, randomized control trials are considered the "gold standard" to make decisions on the benefits and the risks of treatments.[3-7]

In ordinary times, the pursuit of randomized placebo controlled trials would never have been questioned. However, the COVID pandemic has been a historical event that has raised many questions, among which has come a challenge to the unwavering confidence in the randomized placebo control trial as the arbiter of treatment decisions.[8] We propose to examine the performance of RCTs during the COVID pandemic not so much to question the practice but rather to assess the practical results of the strict policy of faith in RCTs to decide on treatment.

SARS-CoV-2: AN UNUSUAL SARBECOVIRUS

Severe acute respiratory syndrome coronavirus-2 (SARS-CoV-2) belongs to the *Nidovirales*, family *Coronaviridae*, genus *Betacoronavirus*, and subgenus *Sarbecovirus*. Viruses in this family circulate freely in the population and are responsible for typical common colds which typically do not have severe repercussions and do not induce lasting immunity, with susceptibility to reinfection within a 1 year period.[9] However, unlike the typical coronavirus induced common cold, SARS-CoV-2 produces a multiphasic illness.[10] As with most coronaviruses, there is a primary viral infection, with a period of active viral replication beginning in the nasal mucosa and then affecting the upper respiratory tract. The disease manifests as an influenza like illness with sore throat, rhinorrhea, nasal congestion, headache, cough, fever, chills, myalgia, and fatigue. Loss of the sense of taste and smell is a feature which may also occur. The SARS-CoV-2 virus is so named because, in a minority of patients, this viral species infects the lungs. The severe acute lower respiratory tract pattern is not characteristic of most usual circulating coronaviruses which produce the common cold. SARS-CoV-2 is the third and most devastating of the SARS-CoVs. It is the pulmonary involvement which was a cause of death back in 2003 in the SARS-CoV-1 epidemic, with 8,000 infections and 10% mortality.[11] Then, beginning in 2012 in the Middle East, the MERS coronavirus emerged and was responsible for about 2,500 cases with approximately 35% mortality.[12]

Then came COVID-19. The SARS-CoV-2 pandemic has had severe pulmonary consequences. In SARS-CoV-2 infections, a pneumonia may ensue typically at 7–8 days after influenza like symptoms begin with worsening cough and shortness of breath, which may then deteriorate rapidly to hypoxia. By that time, the initial phase of viral replication has significantly diminished, and virus is often undetectable **(Fig. 1)**.

The pulmonary manifestations are due to a rapidly emerging excessive immune reaction to the viral spike protein, resulting in multiple clinical

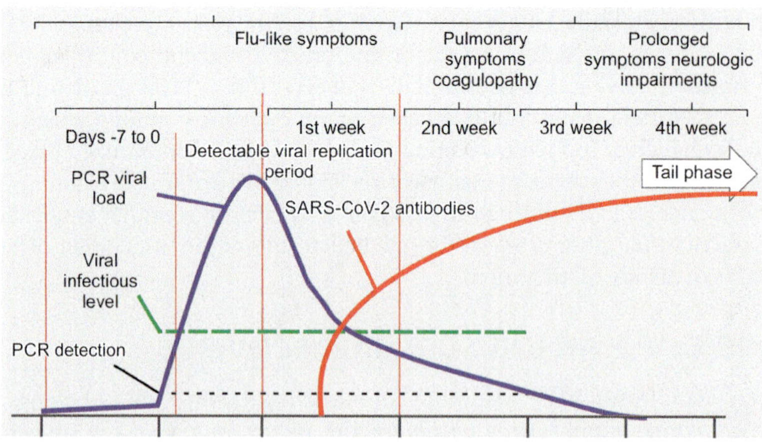

FIGURE 1: The multiphasic course of COVID-19. The first two weeks begin with viral infection, often asymptomatic. Viral replication then progresses to an influenza like syndrome. As the body mounts an antibody mediated immune response, the viral level drops, but an inflammatory phase may ensue with exaggerated cytokine response and coagulopathy. This is the dangerous phase where hypoxia can occur and necessitate external oxygenation. Patients may recover, only to enter a prolonged course which may include respiratory and neurologic impairment, the phase of "long COVID".

manifestations. It is that later phase, post the viral infection, of an immune mediated attack on the lungs with dyspnea and hypoxia, which can then progress to acute respiratory distress syndrome and additionally a hyper-coagulable syndrome, with resulting high mortality. Less well documented are serious neurologic effects of the infection, which can be a part of the long-term recovery phase of the disease, with cognitive impairments sometimes referred to as "brain fog".

Yet, the clinical severity of COVID-19 is highly variable. The disease originated in Wuhan, China in late 2019. The report on the original Wuhan epidemic documented that the illness produces mild or no symptoms in about 80% of infected individuals but, in about 20%, manifested as a pneumonia which could then progress to acute respiratory distress syndrome (ARDS) requiring mechanical ventilation in about 5% of patients.[13] A calculation based on an early outbreak among the passengers and crew of the cruise ship Diamond Princess, essentially a captive primarily elderly population, suggested a case fatality ratio of 1.3%.[14,15]

SARS-CoV-2 virus uses the angiotensin-converting enzyme (ACE) as a primary cellular receptor.[16] A unique furin cleavage site, not found in other sarbecovirus, has become a source of intense speculation as to possible manmade origin of SARS-CoV-2.[17,18] This cleavage site enables rapid membrane fusion and cellular entry into respiratory cells.[19,20]

STATISTICS: THE TRUTH SHALL BE KNOWN BY $p < 0.05$

The Math

In order to prove a positive benefit in a randomized controlled trial, the accepted criterion is that in 19 cases out of 20, an intervention must have a favorable result compared to the absence of that intervention. One can certainly argue that this criterion is arbitrary, because it is. The statistical basis for randomized control trials was established by the British geneticist and mathematician Ronald Aylmer Fisher in 1926.[21,22] To quote from his paper wherein he introduced the 5% criterion

> *"...If one in twenty does not seem high enough odds, we may, if we prefer it, draw the line at one in 50 or one in a 100. Personally, the writer prefers to set a low standard of significance at the 5% point, and ignore entirely all results which fails to reach this level. A scientific fact should be regarded as experimentally established only if a properly designed experiment rarely fails to give this level of significance..."*

> *"My interpretation of this is that the 5% standard represents the absolute minimum standard for a single study, with non-significant results only being admissible if the study falls within the context of a broader evidence base, composed of similar studies that did yield statistically significant results. So while it may be entirely reasonable to set a higher*

threshold than 5%, especially where methodological concerns raise the risk of bias, moving to a lower threshold is much more difficult to justify"

The p value criterion for assessing relevance has been a source of controversy among mathematical statisticians.[23] The key issue is magnitude of the clinical effect being observed and the reproducibility of that effect. In fact, a minority of clinical trialists argue with some justification that 9 times out of ten is good enough, because it may certainly be of clinical importance. The p value may be converted easily to the odds ratio by dividing p by 1-p to create a value between 0 and 1 with a confidence interval for that value. Here, the equivalent of the $p < 0.05$ criterion is that the upper limit of the confidence interval be < 1.

So, if the patient group receiving the active intervention has a mean value $\bar{x}_1$ for a property and the patient group receiving placebo has a mean value $\bar{x}_2$ for that property, then the formula leading to the statistical significance of the difference is:

$$t = \frac{\bar{x}_1 - \bar{x}_2}{\sqrt{\left(s^2\left(\frac{1}{n_1} + \frac{1}{n_2}\right)\right)}}$$

where t is the student's t value of a normal distribution, s^2 is the pooled standard error of the two groups, and n_1 and n_2 are the number of observations in each of the groups. The larger the value of t, the smaller the corresponding p value. The Fisher t test has been the standard for comparing two contrast groups for a century.

An alternative to the Fisher t test is Bayesian statistics. Thomas Bayes created the fundamental theorem in 1763 **(Box 1)**. Here the calculation resolves to compare the likelihood of the data set given assumptions such as, most simply, treatment A is better than placebo B.

What this means in practice is to proceed to calculate the probability that the observed dataset for a treatment cohort does not conform to a

BOX 1 Bayes theorem.

Bayes' theorem is stated mathematically as the following equation:

$$P(A \backslash B) = \frac{P(B \backslash A)P(A)}{P(B)}$$

where *A* and *B* are events and $P(B) \neq 0$

- *P(A\B) is a conditional probability*: The probability of event *A* occurring given that *B* is true. It is also called the posterior probability of *A* given *B*
- *P(B\A) is also a conditional probability*: The probability of event *B* occurring given that A is true. It can also be interpreted as the likelihood of *A* given a fixed *B* because *P(B\A) = L(A\B)*
- *P(A)* and *P(B)* are the probabilities of observing A and B respectively without any given conditions, they are known as the prior probability and marginal probability

known prior distribution, typically the normal distribution, which is the null hypothesis. The calculations must be carried out for all points of the dataset to obtain a Bayes factor BF10 which suggests to what extent the treatment differs from placebo. The computational difficulty of doing so was a significant hurdle, now overcome by the increasing speed of computer calculations. Still, the use of Bayesian methods remained confined to the statisticians who were able to handle the syntax of statistical packages: SPSS, SAS, and R, to name a few, until the revolutionary creation of JASP, a free, open source, point and click package, developed by masterful Bayesian theoreticians to democratize access to these techniques.[24]

The availability of JASP has put Bayesian statistics in reach of clinical researchers with modest programming and statistical skills and will likely lead to dominance of this approach over the Fisher t-test, which has been labeled the frequentist approach. Yet the fundamental consequences remain the same whether one adopts a frequentist or Bayesian approach.[25,26]

A comparison of the frequentist and Bayesian approach to hypothesis testing yields the following relationship for the Bayes factor:[26]

$$BF_{10} = \left[\frac{1+t^2/v}{1+t^2/\{v(1+n_\delta \sigma_\delta^2)\}} \right]^{(v+1)/2} .(1+n_\delta \sigma_\delta^2)^{-1/2}$$

The frequentist formula and the Bayesian formula are somewhat different but both finally depend on the calculation of t, even for distributions not quite normal. The real distinction between the frequentist approach and Bayesian statistics in comparing two cohorts is that the frequentist philosophy is characterized by finality: The decision comparing two groups is determined to be either positive or negative for the hypothesis whereas the Bayesian calculation suggests to what extent the results may favor the hypothesis or the null hypothesis. So Bayesian calculations may be repeated by enlarging the two comparison groups to see if the predictive value of the prior comparison holds in a larger population. This process, known as Bayesian updating, has generally not been carried out in most COVID studies to date, so that the conclusions are typically drawn from one initial comparison, again suggesting finality.

Searching for Significance

This statistical digression has large implications for clinical trials.

No Gratitude for Small Blessings

In order to have a large value for t, a big difference in $\bar{x}_1$ and $\bar{x}_2$ is the major contributor. This means that a small incremental magnitude of difference may not be provable. As a result, all randomized clinical trials for COVID-2 have really been designed ("powered" in statistical language) to look for the "game changer", a term we have heard innumerable times during the COVID era to denote a huge benefit. Yet, the importance of a clinical benefit is not simply a statistic. An improvement in mortality of 10% is not large, but it means that one life out of ten can be saved. There are many potential adjunctive agents such as Vitamin C, Vitamin D, and zinc, and quercetin which may have a small clinical benefit; yet they have not been tested due to presumed lack of a major potential effect.

Variability is Penalized

A large standard deviation decreases the value of *t*. That is clearly a problem in assessing COVID where there is such a great clinical variation running from asymptomatic viral infection to severe respiratory distress and death. So whether one chooses milestones of infection, such as hospitalizations or time for disappearance of symptoms, or definitive criteria such as mortality, there is a high variance. Cohorts with large sample sizes are required to increase the magnitude of *t*. That can be viewed as a good thing because we really want to know the effect of a given intervention on the entire population. However, in sampling restricted treatment and control groups, it is difficult to achieve the necessary sample sizes to deal with a disease as variable as COVID. As a result, many COVID RCTs, if not most, have been underpowered.

You can have Only One Choice

Treatment interventions must be well defined and most preferably solitary to implement statistical formulas. Although one may wish to compare several different treatments, such a study requires multiple groups. The sample size to achieve statistical significance in multi-arm studies grows rapidly as one adds groups.[27] For example, in a TOGETHER trial to treat COVID patients in Colombia, a 9 day course of hydroxychloroquine (HCQ) and lopinavir-ritonavir was compared to placebo.[28] A total of 214 participants were randomized to HCQ; 244—lopinavir-ritonavir; and 227—placebo. The proportion of patients hospitalized for COVID-19 was 3.7% (8 participants) in the HCQ group, 5.7% (14 participants) in the lopinavir-ritonavir group, and 4.8% (11 participants) in the placebo group. This difference did not achieve significance: HCQ hazard ratio (HR) 0.76 [95% confidence interval (CI) 0.30–1.88]; lopinavir-ritonavir: HR 1.16 (95% CI 0.53–2.56). The ostensible 24% difference favoring HCQ was ignored and the planned enrollment of 1,476 total patients was stopped, claiming futility.

A similar consideration hampers the evaluation of combination treatment. Doctors typically use combinations of agents to treat their patients. Yet RCTs are ill suited to look at such combinations due to the implication of multiple study arms. A typical example was the A-to-Z Trial.[29] That trial of zinc and ascorbic acid, popular nutritional adjuncts to treat common colds, enrolled only 214 outpatients with COVID. Patients were randomized in a 1:1:1:1 allocation ratio to receive either 10 days of zinc gluconate (50 mg), ascorbic acid (8,000 mg), both agents, or standard of care. Patients who received usual care without supplementation achieved a 50% reduction in symptoms at a mean-standard deviation (SD) of 6.7 (4.4) days compared with 5.5 (3.7) days for the ascorbic acid group, 5.9 (4.9) days for the zinc gluconate group, and

5.5 (3.4) days for the group receiving both (overall $p = 0.45$). At that point, the study was stopped, claiming futility.

Futility of Claiming Futility

The frequentist approach, used for most COVID studies to date, is to decree finality of a trial performed with a sample size calculated based on prior assumptions of potential benefit. As a result, if those assumptions fall short of the predicted benefit, the intervention is declared failed, even if the ongoing results are showing a favorable difference between the intervention and nonintervention. In the TOGETHER comparison of HCQ and lopinavir-ritonavir, it was claimed that 10,000 or more patients would be required to confirm an apparent 24% benefit of HCQ. That sample requirement was, of course, necessitated by continued inclusion of lopinavir-ritonavir which had shown no potential benefit. As we shall see, many randomized trials such as the A-to-Z trial were closed in the COVID era for alleged "futility" despite a possible benefit of intervention. The A-to-Z Trial has been cited as a particular example of methodological error, noting that a reanalysis suggested a 70% improvement with vitamin C administration.[30]

SO, WHAT IS THE QUESTION?

On July 27, 1946, in Neuilly-sur-Seine, France, Gertrude Stein, the novelist and intellectual leader of the American community in Paris, lay on her death bed surrounded by her loving friends, one of whom, her voice choking with emotion, clutched her and asked "What is the answer?". The great lady replied "What is the question?", her last words on earth. Indeed, the multiphasic nature of COVID-19 has left many unanswered questions.

Focus on Severely Ill First?

With the gravity of the beginning pandemic, the American research establishment at the National Institutes of Health (NIH) and Food and Drug Administration (FDA) decided to focus randomized controlled trials on severely ill hospitalized patients to prevent death. This is a simpler controlled setting to manage a clinical study compared to outpatient studies, which have many more confounding variables. The first agent approved was the RNA polymerase inhibitor remdesivir.[31] During the course of the study, the NIH changed the primary efficacy variable from mortality to time to improvement. A total of 1,062 patients underwent randomization (with 541 assigned to remdesivir and 521 to placebo). Those who received remdesivir had a median recovery time of 10 days (95% CI 9–11), as compared with 15 days (95% CI 13–18) among those who received placebo (rate ratio for recovery 1.29; 95% CI 1.12–1.49; $p < 0.001$), by a log-rank test. The Kaplan-Meier estimates of mortality were 6.7% with remdesivir and 11.9% with placebo by day 15 and 11.4% with remdesivir and 15.2% with placebo by day 29 (HR, 0.73; 95% CI 0.52–1.03). Yet, the 1.03 upper limit of the confidence interval of the mortality HR was viewed with great disappointment since it was viewed as a nonsignificant odds ratio. Several clinical trialists pushed to continue to increase enrollment until the elusive odds ratio <1.00 could be achieved.

Yet, in the much larger World Health Organizations Solidarity Trial, 602 (14.5%) of 4,146 patients assigned to remdesivir died versus 643 (15.6%) of 4,129 assigned to control [mortality rate ratio (RR) 0.91 (95% CI 0.82–1.02), $p = 0.12$].[32] Of those already ventilated, 151 (42.1%) of 359 assigned to remdesivir died versus 134 (38.6%) of 347 assigned to control [RR 1.13 (0.89–1.42), $p = 0.32$]. Of those not ventilated but on oxygen, 14.6% assigned to remdesivir died versus 16.3% assigned to control [RR 0.87 (0.76–0.99), $p = 0.03$]. Of 1,730 patients not on oxygen initially, 2.9% assigned to remdesivir died versus 3.8% assigned to control [RR 0.76 (0.46–1.28), $p = 0.30$]. Combining all those not ventilated initially, 11.9% assigned to remdesivir died versus 13.5% assigned to control [RR 0.86 (0.76–0.98), $p = 0.02$].

In the United States, remdesivir was approved for treatment of hospitalized patients, and the NIH pursued multiple other studies with remdesivir trying to find adjunctive treatments which would improve the elusive remdesivir mortality statistics. Those nations who conform to US leadership also adopted remdesivir for hospitalized patients whereas, in contrast, the WHO has continually recommended against the use of remdesivir for COVID inpatients.

Mortality is certainly a definitive primary efficacy variable in trials in severely ill hospitalized patients. Consistent with the excessive immune response which triggers the pulmonary inflammatory phase of COVID-19, immunomodulating drugs have demonstrated improved survival in randomized controlled studies in this relatively well defined population and are approved **(Table 1)**.

The first immunosuppressive agent to be proven effective was dexamethasone in the United Kingdom RECOVERY Trial, entirely consistent with the conventional clinical use of glucocorticoids in acute respiratory distress.[33] The observed reduction in mortality was from 25.7 to 22.9%, a small difference but which reached significance in the large intent to treat population numbering over 6,000 patients. A number of additional more recently approved immunomodulators have been authorized to treat severely ill inpatients on the basis of favorable RCTs **(Table 1)**.[31-37] These agents were all brand name drugs, currently with patent exclusivity.

But What about Those Not Yet in the Hospital?

Certainly it was important to find interventions which would lower the high mortality of patients hospitalized due to hypoxic pneumonia. However, the issue of treatment for the vast majority of SARS-CoV-2 infected patients who are ambulatory is an entirely different question. While randomized trials proceeded in 2020 on patients hospitalized due to SARS-CoV-2,

TABLE 1: The agents approved for the severe inflammatory phase of COVID.

Agent	Class	Availability as generic	Major trial	Number of patients	Mortality
Dexamethasone	Glucocorticoid	Generic for many years	RECOVERY[33]	• 2,104 dexamethasone • 4,321 usual care	(22.9%) in the dexamethasone group and (25.7%) in the usual care group died within 28 days after randomization [age-adjusted rate ratio, 0.83; 95% confidence interval (CI) 0.75–0.93; $p < 0.001$]
Remdesivir	RNA polymerase inhibitor	NO Brand Name Veklury	ACTT-1[31]	541 remdesivir 521 to placebo	11.4% with remdesivir and 15.2% with placebo by day 29 [hazard ratio (HR) 0.73; 95% CI 0.52–1.03]
			SOLIDARITY[32]	• 4,146 patients remdesivir • 4,129 control	(14.5%) assigned to remdesivir died versus (15.6%) assigned to control [mortality rate ratio (RR) 0.91 (95% CI 0.82–1.02), $p = 0.12$]
Tocilizumab	Interleukin-6 (IL-6) Receptor Inhibitors	NO Brand Name: Actemra	RECOVERY[34]	• Tocilizumab 2,022 • Usual Care 2,094	31% tocilizumab patients died compared to 35% usual care died within 28 days (rate ratio 0.85; 95% CI 0.76–0.94; $p = 0.0028$)
Baricitinib	Janus kinase inhibitor	NO Brand Name: Olumiant	COV-BARRIER[35]	• Baricitinib 764 • Placebo 761	28-day all-cause mortality 8% for baricitinib and 13% for placebo [HR 0.57 (95% CI 0.41–0.78); nominal $p = 0.0018$)
Anakinra	IL-1α/β inhibitor	NO Brand name: Kineret	SAV-MOR[36]	594 patients total	28-day mortality decreased (HR = 0.45, $p = 0.045$)
Vilobelimab	Anti-C5a monoclonal antibody	NO Brand name: Gohibic	PANAMO[37]	• Vilobelimab: 177 • Placebo 191	28-day all-cause mortality rate 32% (95% CI 25–39) in the vilobelimab group and 42% (35–49) in the placebo group (HR 0.73, 95% CI 0.50–1.06; $p = 0.094$)

ambulatory infected patients were untreated until they were sick enough to be hospitalized. Here, a schism developed between clinical researchers who adhered scrupulously to the tenet that treatment should be dictated by randomized controlled trials and physicians struggling to treat huge numbers of their sick and dying patients. Several treating physicians elected to offer patients early in the course of viral replication the use of agents which had some theoretical potential benefit, albeit with no randomized placebo controlled trial to prove that those agents were effective.[38]

So, a number of nutritional supplements, vitamins, and pharmaceutical agents with speculative beneficial immunological effects were offered to patients. Among those used were zinc, vitamin C, vitamin D, quercetin, various antimicrobial nasal sprays and mouthwashes, ivermectin, and HCQ.

HCQ has antiviral properties and is also used chronically to suppress autoimmune harm in diseases such as lupus and rheumatoid arthritis. Dr Didier Raoult, head of the Institut Hospitalo-Universitaire Méditerranée, a large and highly successful academic program for infectious disease research in Marseille, France, began treatment of large numbers of COVID-19 afflicted citizens. He combined HCQ with azithromycin in an empirical attempt to treat outpatients with COVID-19 diagnosed by PCR (polymerase chain reaction). His group was so impressed by the clinical results that they stated that a placebo controlled trial which would deny HCQ to patients was unethical and made a fateful decision not to embark on an RCT.[39]

Dr Vladimir Zelenko was a physician practicing in an Orthodox Jewish community outside New York City. Orthodox Jews often participate in large social gatherings and, hence, are particularly susceptible to rapid viral transmission. Zelenko augmented Raoult's treatment protocol with the addition of zinc sulfate, motivated by the hypothesis that HCQ increases intracellular zinc concentration, further enhancing its antiviral mechanisms of action.[40] Zelenko also introduced risk-stratification criteria to classify patients into a low-risk versus high-risk category, and noticed empirically that, for the purpose of reducing hospitalizations and deaths, it is sufficient to offer the triple drug therapy only to the high-risk patients.[41]

Over time, he introduced a quercetin-based protocol requiring no prescription for low-risk patients, with additional prescription only medications (dexamethasone, budesonide, and the anticoagulant apixaban) for the treatment of high-risk patients, for whom the triple drug therapy did not result in a typical turnaround. His results in terms of preventing hospitalization and mortality in COVID-19 infected patients were far superior to those of other physicians practicing in his area.

However, in the United States and in countries tributary to American medicine, there was insistence on randomized control clinical trials. There were two highly publicized RCTs of HCQ. Mitja et al. studied 136 HCQ treated patients with 157 in the control arm.[42] The mean age was 41.6 years (SD, 12.6), and median time from symptom onset to randomization was 3 days. It was claimed that treatment did not reduce risk of hospitalization

(7.1% control vs. 5.9% HCQ) nor shorten the time to complete resolution of symptoms (12 days, control vs. 10 days, HCQ), given the limited statistical power of these small cohorts.

In a different randomized trial with 423 patients, patients were enrolled throughout the US and received medication by express mail.[43] Of that group, 341 (81%) had laboratory-confirmed infection with SARS-CoV-2 or epidemiologically linked exposure to a person with laboratory-confirmed infection; 56% (236 of 423) were enrolled within 1 day of symptoms starting. Date of actual receipt and self-administration of medication was not precise. At 14 days, 24% (49 of 201) of participants receiving hydroxychloroquine had ongoing symptoms compared with 30% (59 of 194) receiving placebo (p = 0.21). With placebo, 10 hospitalizations occurred (2 non-COVID-19-related), including 1 hospitalized death. With hydroxychloroquine, 4 hospitalizations occurred plus 1 nonhospitalized death (p = 0.29). Again, with this limited cohort, the small suggestively favorable differences could not achieve statistical significance. There was no attempt to repeat these two trials with larger group sizes to see if a possible benefit of about 20% could be confirmed, certainly not a "game changer" but a clinical benefit. Rather than do this, in both cases, the frequentist results were simply declared to show no benefit of HCQ at all.

In an inpatient study of 497 adults hospitalized with COVID-19, treatment with HCQ compared with placebo definitely did not improve clinical status.[44] At 28 days after randomization, 25 of 241 patients (10.4%) in the hydroxychloroquine group and 25 of 236 (10.6%) in the placebo group had died [absolute difference –0.2% (95% CI –5.7 to 5.3); aOR, 1.07 (95% CI 0.54–2.09)]. Based on the failure of HCQ to demonstrate benefit in hospitalized severely ill patients, the NIH proceeded to shut down a projected outpatient trial.[45] In the United Kingdom, clinical trials of HCQ were actually banned.[46]

All nations conforming to the leadership of the United States similarly abandoned use of HCQ for COVID patients as the pandemic progressed in 2020 and adhered strictly to the belief that only treatments proven by RCTs could be used. Of course, there were no such treatments available so that meant that there was no medication for patients diagnosed with COVID until they were so sick as to be hospitalized. Physicians who used medications including HCQ and ivermectin to treat patients were denounced. Institutions, including medical schools, proceeded to remove doctors who argued for early treatment.

It is a Matter of Time

Our purpose is not to participate in the argument between clinical researchers and treating physicians as to the use of HCQ in SARS-CoV-2 infection. Rather we choose the HCQ controversy as a means to begin the analysis of bias in randomized controlled trials. Unquestionably the strength of randomized allocation to treatment is to reduce bias related to characteristics of patient selection. Yet, other sources of bias exist which do not depend on equivalence of patient selection. For example, SARS-CoV-2 infection is a rapidly changing event in time. The viral infection precedes clinical symptoms by 2–5 days. In many cases, by onset of the initial symptoms, the viral load has begun to drop. Then, by the time symptoms have encouraged patients to seek treatment, the viral load has declined substantially. The Centers for Disease Control and Prevention (CDC) now states "If you test positive for COVID-19, stay home for at least 5 days and isolate from others in your home. You are likely most infectious during these first 5 days". Day 0 of isolation is the day of symptom onset, regardless of when you tested positive. Day 1 is the first full day after the day your symptoms started".[47]

Therefore, for an antiviral agent to demonstrate benefit, it must be used early during the phase of viral replication. Similarly, for influenza B, "antiviral treatment also can be considered for any previously healthy, symptomatic outpatient not at high risk for influenza complications, who is diagnosed with confirmed or suspected influenza, on the basis of clinical judgment, if treatment can be initiated within 48 hours of illness onset".[48] The inherent bias of any randomized treatment protocol of antiviral agents is consequently related to the speed with which the antiviral agent reaches an effective concentration and the number of patients included who have already reached low viral loads. In a study of 104 consecutive COVID-19 hospitalized patients with HCQ doses ranging from 200 to 800 mg/day administered for 1 to 11 days, the median HCQ plasma concentration was 151 ng/mL. Within 72 h of HCQ initiation, only 16/104 (15.4%) COVID-19 patients had HCQ plasma levels above the in vitro half maximal effective concentration of HCQ against SARS-CoV-2 (240 ng/mL).[49]

Similarly, remdesivir given to hospitalized patients, thus late in the course of viral infection, had questionable benefit, and the WHO has recommended against its use. Yet when administered early intravenously to outpatients between 3 and 6 days of onset of symptoms, only 2 of 279 patients (0.7%) in the remdesivir group versus 15 of 283 (5.3%) in the placebo group had a COVID-19-related hospitalization by day 28.[50] No patients in either group died by day 28. Remdesivir has received an approval for use in outpatients, although the requirement for three successive days of IV infusion makes it relatively impractical for ambulatory patients.

TREATMENT AND PREVENTION

As the pandemic progressed, there were agents brought forward with initial success in randomized control trials. The first group of medications to be utilized beginning in November, 2020 were:

Monoclonal Antibodies

A series of monoclonal antibodies were developed to treat outpatients and received emergency use authorization beginning in November, 2020. These antibodies could be administered effectively in a one-time treatment by IV or intramuscularly within 3 days of symptom development and successfully decreased viral load, need for hospitalization, and death. In a review of 167,183 patients, 25, 241 patients received treatment between November 9, 2020, and June 30, 2021 with monoclonal antibodies (bamlanivimab, bamlanivimab-etesevimab, casirivimab-imdevimab, and sotrovimab[51]). Treatment was associated with lower odds of ED (Emergency Department) visits within 14 days [odds ratio (OR) 0.76; 95% CI 0.68–0.85], hospitalization within 14 days (OR, 0.52; 95% CI 0.45–0.59), and death within 30 days (OR, 0.14; 95% CI 0.10–0.20).[51] The monoclonal antibody treatment was administered rapidly within the period of viral replication; the mean (SD) time from the index date to monoclonal antibody administration was 2.4 (1.5) days. The use of these monoclonal antibodies was revoked progressively by the FDA beginning in January, 2022 as it became apparent these antibodies could not successfully neutralize the evolving SARS-CoV-2 variants. The last remaining monoclonal antibody to SARS-CoV-2 was bebtelovimab used as prophylaxis for immunocompromised patients. Its use was terminated by the FDA in December 2022.[52]

Nirmatrelvir/Ritonavir and Molnupiravir

The prime tenet of randomized control studies is that patients are assigned to treatment or to placebo control on the basis of an unselected process, be it as simple as a coin toss, or as sophisticated as a block assignment random number generator. Randomization is unmatched for validity within a given study, but when it comes to comparison between different studies, that principle breaks down. Two oral antiviral agents were developed; the SARS-CoV-2 protease inhibitor nirmatrelvir-ritonavir (Nmv/rtn) and the RNA polymerase inhibitor molnupiravir (Mpvr) were endorsed by the NIH and CDC, each one on the basis of a single randomized placebo controlled study in enriched high-risk populations infected with COVID-19.[53,54] Mortality is a hard endpoint; fortunately, despite the high death toll of COVID-19 to date, death is relatively infrequent. Globally, as of 6:30 PM CEST, 16 August 2023, there have been 769,806,130 confirmed cases of COVID-19, including 6,955,497 deaths, reported to WHO a case fatality ratio of 0.91%. From a clinical trials standpoint, that requires a very large number of subjects to assess a meaningful change in mortality due to an intervention. So given the impracticality of recruiting very large cohorts, the FDA suggested the combination of hospitalizations and deaths as a primary efficacy criterion, which, in reality, translates to hospitalizations due to the relatively low case fatality ratio.

Nirmatrelvir-ritonavir has been favored over Mpvr. In the pivotal trial of Nmv/rtn in high risk patients, estimated event rates of COVID-19-related hospitalization or death from any cause at 28 days were 0.72% and 6.53% in the nirmatrelvir and placebo groups, respectively, corresponding to a difference of −5.81 percentage points (95% CI −7.78 to −3.84; $p < 0.001$) and an 88.9% relative risk reduction.[52] In the corresponding pivotal phase

3 clinical trial, Mpvr showed approximately a 50% benefit compared to placebo in the initial interim analysis for the primary efficacy end point of all-cause hospitalization or death by day 29 [7.3% vs. 14.1%; difference, –6.8 percentage points (95% CI –11.3 to –2.4 percentage points)].[53] Then as the trial progressed to the final larger dataset, the benefit diminished to (6.8% vs. 9.7%; difference, –3.0 percentage points (CI –5.9 to –0.1 percentage points)], which was only a 37% advantage. The mean time of administration of Nmv/rtn was 2.93 ± 1.12 days from first symptom, with 67.3% of the patients receiving the drug within 3 days of onset. In contrast, in the Mpvr pivotal trial only 47.7% of the participants had onset of signs or symptoms 3 days or less before randomization. Furthermore, in comparing the placebo groups for Mpvr in the interim analysis with a 14.1% event rate to the final rate of 9.7% and then to the Nmv/rtn rate of 6.5%, it is clear that the cohorts were not similar and that hospitalization may not always represent a reliable endpoint in COVID treatment clinical trials.

It was noted in the FDA review of molnupiravir that the incidence of hospitalization or death decreased markedly in the placebo group between the first half of the study wherein most patients were recruited in South America and the second half of the study which coincided with increased proportional representation of Eastern European patients. In the MOV-2 Mpvr study, 26 sites were located in Russia and the Ukraine, comprising 27% of all sites compared to just 18% in the United States. In fact, the FDA review expressed concern that only 6% of the overall MOV-2 subjects were obtained from North America compared to 45% of the subjects in the Nmv/rtn pivotal trial. The FDA review acknowledged that there may be significant differences in the criteria for hospitalization in different geographic areas. Current NIH Covid guidelines state *"There are no fixed criteria for admitting patients with COVID-19 to the hospital; criteria may vary by region and hospital facilities."* In a multicriteria decision analysis, De Nardo et al. concluded that the most important factors assessed for possible hospital admission included PaO_2 (16.3%), followed by peripheral O_2 saturation (15.9%), chest X-ray (14.1%), Modified Early Warning Score (MEWS) (11.4%), respiratory rate (9.5%), comorbidities (6.5%), living with vulnerable people (6.4%), body mass index (BMI) (5.6%), duration of symptoms before hospital evaluation (5.4%), C-reactive protein (CRP) (5.1%), and age (3.8%).[55] So hospitalization is definitely not as firm a statistical criterion of efficacy as mortality.

Rule of Two Randomized Control Trials

It has always been conventional regulatory practice to require at least two randomized control studies with similar results to confirm value of given treatments and receive drug approval: "With regard to quantity, it has been FDA's position that Congress generally intended to require at least two adequate and well-controlled studies, each convincing on its own, to establish effectiveness".[56]

In the case of Nmv/rtn that was not done. *In the first study*, EPIC-HR (Evaluation of Protease Inhibition for Covid-19 in High-Risk Patients), for patients with at least one factor for high risk of progression of COVID, and in which those who had received SARS-CoV-2 vaccine were excluded, a total of 2,246 patients underwent randomization, 1,120 patients received Nmv/rtn), and 1,126 received placebo.[53] In the planned interim analysis of patients treated within 3 days after symptom onset (modified intention-to-treat population, comprising 774 of the 1,361 patients in the full analysis population), the incidence of COVID-19-related hospitalization or death by day 28 was 0.77% (3 of 389 patients) in the nirmatrelvir group, with 0 deaths, as compared with 7.01% (27 of 385 patients) in the placebo group. Efficacy was maintained in the final analysis involving the 1,379 patients in the modified intention-to-treat population, with a difference of –5.81 percentage points (95% CI –7.78 to –3.84; $p < 0.001$; relative risk reduction, 88.9%). All 13 deaths occurred in the placebo group. These highly favorable results were published in the New England Journal of Medicine and are the basis for the strong recommendation by FDA for Nmv/rtn in high-risk subjects.

The second study performed by the study sponsor Pfizer Inc: Evaluation of Protease Inhibition for COVID-19 in Standard-Risk Patients (EPIC-SR), ClinicalTrials.gov ID NCT05011513 focused on patients who did not have risk factors for COVID progression, and, once again, any receipt of vaccine in the past 12 months was excluded. That study began on August 25, 2021 and was stopped by Pfizer on July 25, 2022, based on the claim that placebo patients were not accruing sufficient hospitalizations and deaths to allow statistical significance. Pfizer posted the results on ClinicalTrials.gov: When the study was stopped, 632 patients had received Nmv/rtn and 618 placebo. The average age was 42, and the primary efficacy criterion was time to sustained alleviation of COVID signs and symptoms. There was not a significant difference: Nmv/rtn 12.000 (11.000–13.000) versus 13.000 (12.000–14.000). However, of the Nmv/rtn cohort, 0.765% were hospitalized compared to 1.577% of the placebo group, a small number but approximately a twofold difference which might have been a significant difference had Pfizer decided to continue on with the study rather than claiming futility. We do not know. Pfizer has not yet published this data on the study they shut down.

A third study: ClinicalTrials.gov ID NCT05047601 A Study of a Potential Oral Treatment to Prevent COVID-19 in Adults Who Are Exposed to Household Member(s) With a Confirmed Symptomatic COVID-19 Infection was performed by Pfizer beginning 2021-09-09 and terminated 2022-04-12. This was a prophylaxis study of asymptomatic household contacts, SARS-CoV-2 PCR negative, with exposure within 96 hours to a symptomatic individual who had recently tested positive for SARS-CoV-2. Patients who had received COVID vaccine or had a prior SARS-CoV-2 infection in the past 6 months were excluded. They treated 913 patients with Nmv/rtn for 5 days, 911 patients with Nmv/rtn for 10 days, and 897 with placebo. Of the 5 day cohort 2.6%

developed symptomatic PCR confirmed COVID, 2.4% of the 10 day cohort, and 3.9% of the placebo patients, declared not to have achieved $p < 0.05$. Pfizer did not extend the study to attempt to achieve statistical significance of what was perhaps a 35% difference between Nmv/rtn and placebo patients, nor has this study been published to date.

Merck carried out an inpatient study of Mvpr and terminated it with only 304 subjects when it became apparent that the antiviral was of no benefit at the post viral replication inflammatory stage of the disease: Efficacy and Safety of Molnupiravir (MK-4482) in Hospitalized Adult Participants With COVID-19 (MK-4482-001), ClinicalTrials.gov ID NCT04575584. The pivotal study in outpatients[54] which led to the FDA Emergency Use Authorization was followed by the largest study of an antiviral agent in COVID to date: the PANORAMIC randomized control trial of Mvpr in the United Kingdom.[57] Between December 8, 2021 and April 27, 2022, participants aged 50 years or older (or 18 years or older with relevant comorbidities) with COVID-19 symptoms which had begun within the previous 5 days and a positive SARS-CoV-2 test within the past 7 days were randomly assigned, 12,529 participants to use Mvpr plus usual care, and 12,525 to usual care. The mean age of the population was 56.6 years (SD 12.6), and 24,290 (94%) of 25,708 participants had received at least three doses of a SARS-CoV-2 vaccine. The primary efficacy criterion was hospitalizations or deaths, which occurred in 105 (1%) of the participants in the Mvpr plus usual care group versus 98 (1%) of those in the control care group [adjusted odds ratio 1.06 (95% Bayesian credible interval 0.81–1.41); probability of superiority 0.33]. The PANORAMIC Study was then concluded to be a failure of molnupiravir. Yet the secondary outcome of time to recovery was highly persuasive. Median time from randomization to first recovery was 9 days (IQR 5–23) in the Mvpr plus usual care group and 15 days (7–not reached) in the usual care group [estimated benefit 4.2 days (95% BCI 3.8–4.6)]; posterior probability of superiority of >0.99.

Merck also performed a prophylaxis study which they claimed futile, but results have not been posted to ClinicalTrials.gov or published.

Nirmatrelvir/ritonavir and molnupiravir were first offered to the public based on the one successful randomized control trial for each agent in December 2021, a year and a half into the pandemic. By that time, 800,000 patients had died of COVID.

COVID Vaccines

The response of the Western world to the COVID-19 pandemic was preordained to be prevention rather than to accept early treatment with agents which were unproven by RCTs. Lockdowns to block transmission of the virus by human contact was the first measure, employed more effectively in China than the United States, where freedom of behavior had been a way of life. However, from the first moments of identification of the nucleotide sequence of SARS-CoV-2, the plan was to produce a vaccine. The principle of vaccination dating back to Jenner's use of cowpox to prevent smallpox is to incite a strong prior immune reaction to a pathogen by inoculating with a surrogate antigen.[58] Vaccination has been enormously successful in dealing with a host of human diseases.[59,60]

Within 5 days of sequence release of the SARS-CoV-2 sequence by China, Moderna produced lipid-encapsulated mRNA nanoparticles expressing the SARS-CoV-2 S-2P as a transmembrane-anchored protein with the native furin cleavage site (mRNA-1273).[61] With remarkable speed, a first in human Phase 1 clinical trial commenced on March 16, 2020, 66 days after the viral sequence was released, and a Phase 2 trial began 74 days later on May 29, 2020. Pfizer-Biontech executed a similar process with their lipid-encapsulated mRNA nanoparticles almost as quickly.[62]

The pivotal phase 3 randomized control trial of the Moderna mRNA-1273 SARS-CoV-2 vaccine began in July, 2020.[63] The trial enrolled 15,209 subjects assigned to receive the mRNA-1273 vaccine, given as two doses 28 days apart and 15,206 to receive two placebo injections. The blinded portion ended in December, 2020 when an Emergency Use Authorization was granted by FDA for the vaccine.[64] At that time, placebo participants were offered vaccination with mRNA-1273. A total of only 1,076 placebo patients and 1,385 original mRNA1273 recipients achieved a 180-day follow-up which was 152 days from the second injection. Vaccine efficacy in preventing COVID-19 illness in the period of placebo controlled observation was 93.2% (95% CI 91.0–94.8), with 55 confirmed cases in the mRNA-1273 group (9.6 per 1,000 person-years; 95% CI 7.2–12.5) and 744 in the placebo group (136.6 per 1,000 person-years; 95% CI 127.0–146.8). The efficacy in preventing severe disease was 98.2% (95% CI 92.8–99.6), with 2 cases in the mRNA-1273 group and 106 in the placebo group, and the efficacy in preventing asymptomatic infection starting 14 days after the second injection was 63.0% (95% CI 56.6–68.5), with 214 cases in the mRNA-1273 group and 498 in the placebo group.

Pfizer began its study of the BNT162b2 lipid nanoparticle-formulated, nucleoside-modified RNA vaccine which encodes a prefusion stabilized, membrane-anchored SARS-CoV-2 full-length spike protein on April 20, 2020. Between July 27, 2020 and October 29, 2020, a total of 21,759 subjects were randomized in the BNT162b2 group and 21,650 in the placebo group to receive two doses 21 days apart. During the blinded period of the trial, 51% of the participants in each group had at least 4 months of follow-up after the second dose; 8% of the participants in the BNT162b2 group and 6% of those in the placebo group had 6 months of follow-up or more after the second dose.[65] COVID-19 infection with an onset of 7 days or more after the second dose was observed in 77 vaccine recipients and in 850 placebo recipients up to the data cutoff date (March 13, 2021), corresponding to a vaccine efficacy of 91.3% [95% CI 89.0–93.2]. From its peak after the second dose, observed vaccine efficacy declined. From 7 days to less than 2 months after the second dose, vaccine efficacy was 96.2% (95% CI 93.3–98.1); from

There were 19,714 subjects who received vaccine and 9,868 placebo. Over a period of 3 months, 14 cases of COVID-19 occurred among vaccine recipients and 63 among placebo recipients (vaccine efficacy, 90.4%; 95% CI 82.9–94.6; $p < 0.001$). There were ten moderate and 4 severe cases, all in placebo recipients, yielding vaccine efficacy against moderate-to-severe disease of 100% (95% CI 87.0–100). Vaccine efficacy against any variant of concern or interest was 92.6% (95% CI 83.6–96.7). The duration of placebo controlled observation was about 70 days. Unfortunately the NVX-CoV2373 vaccine authorization was significantly delayed by FDA for almost 18 months until July 13, 2022, so that vaccine has had minimal distribution compared to the two mRNA vaccines.

At this point, we should pause to highlight the extraordinary accomplishment of the randomized placebo controlled vaccine trials performed by all the manufacturers, including the extension of time in which patients agreed to remain placebo treated in several studies. These studies illustrated the power of RCTs to avoid bias in confirming a clinical benefit which was clearly observed in a relatively short duration placebo controlled period.

"NOTHING IS FOREVER EXCEPT CHANGE"

—Gautama Buddha

The March of the COVID Variants

The COVID vaccines were rapidly administered beginning with emergency authorization in late December 2020. As of August 2023, 70.5% of the world population has received at least one dose of a COVID-19 vaccine; 13.5 billion doses have been administered globally. About 676,728,782 doses have been given to the US population. The Pfizer Biontech BNT162b2 mRNA has been the most frequently administered followed by Moderna mRNA1273, but the triumph of the mRNA SARS-CoV vaccine randomized trials did not last long enough. The SARS-CoV-2 spike protein is highly mutable; a series of variants developed with greater transmissibility than the original Wuhan strain **(Table 3)**.[72]

The mRNA vaccines were modified sequences of the entire receptor binding domain of the original virus recovered in Wuhan. When the epitopes of the SARS-CoV-2 virus changed, antibodies elicited by the vaccines did not necessarily recognize the modified virus as effectively. At first, the vaccines appeared to perform well with the new variants. Then in July, 2021, only about 6 months following the rollout of the mRNA vaccines, the Delta variant appeared, described in a CDC report of a major outbreak in Barnstable County, Massachusetts.[73] There were 469 cases of COVID-19 associated with multiple summer activities. Approximately three quarters (346; 74%) of cases occurred in fully vaccinated persons. Genomic sequencing of specimens from 133 patients identified the B.1.617.2 (Delta) variant of SARS-CoV-2, the

TABLE 3: The COVID variants: Alpha to delta.

New significant SARS-CoV-2 lineage	Variant name	Variant as labeled by WHO	Country of origin	Note(s)
B.1.1.7	20I/501Y.V1	Alpha	United Kingdom	Emerging variant, CDC and WHO reported as VOC
P.1	20J/501Y.V3	Gamma	Brazil	Emerging variant, CDC and WHO declared as VOC
B.1.351	20H/501Y.V2	Beta	South Africa	Emerging variant, CDC and WHO stated as VOC
B1.427/B.1.429	Nextstrain described as 20C/5:452R	Epsilon	USA (California)	Emerging variant, CDC and WHO reported as VOI
B1.617.2	Nextstrain described as 20A/5:478K	Delta	India	Emerging variant, CDC and WHO declared as VOC
B.1525	Nextstrain described as 20C	Eta	USA (New York)	CDC and WHO stated as VOI
B.1.526	Nextstrain described as 20C	Iota	USA (New York)	CDC and WHO called as VOI

Source: Reproduced by permission from an open-access article distributed under the terms of the Creative Commons Attribution 4.0 International license.[71]

virus that causes COVID-19, in 119 (89%) and the Delta AY.3 sublineage in one (1%). Overall, 274 (79%) vaccinated patients with breakthrough infection were symptomatic, and five were hospitalized of whom four were fully vaccinated; no deaths were reported. Among fully vaccinated symptomatic persons, the median interval from ≥14 days after completion of their final vaccine dose to symptom onset was just 86 days (range = 6–178 days).

In Belgium, contact tracing studies showed that the Delta variant was associated with a demonstrable decrease in early vaccine effectiveness against transmission to 83% for BNT162b2, but there then followed a further time dependent decrease down to 63% for BNT162b2 (Delta, 150–200 days after vaccination).[74]

A systematic analysis by Lin et al. compared the disease severity and clinical outcomes of the Alpha, Beta, Gamma, and Delta SARS-CoV-2 variants with respect to hospitalization, ICU admission, and mortality.[75] The alpha variant was associated with more severe disease than the original Wuhan virus as was the beta variant **(Figs. 2 and 3)**.

Then the delta variant manifested with more severe disease outcomes than the prior variants **(Fig. 4)**.

In November, 2021, the Delta variant was succeeded by the Omicron variant, first detected in South Africa. The Omicron variant had many more

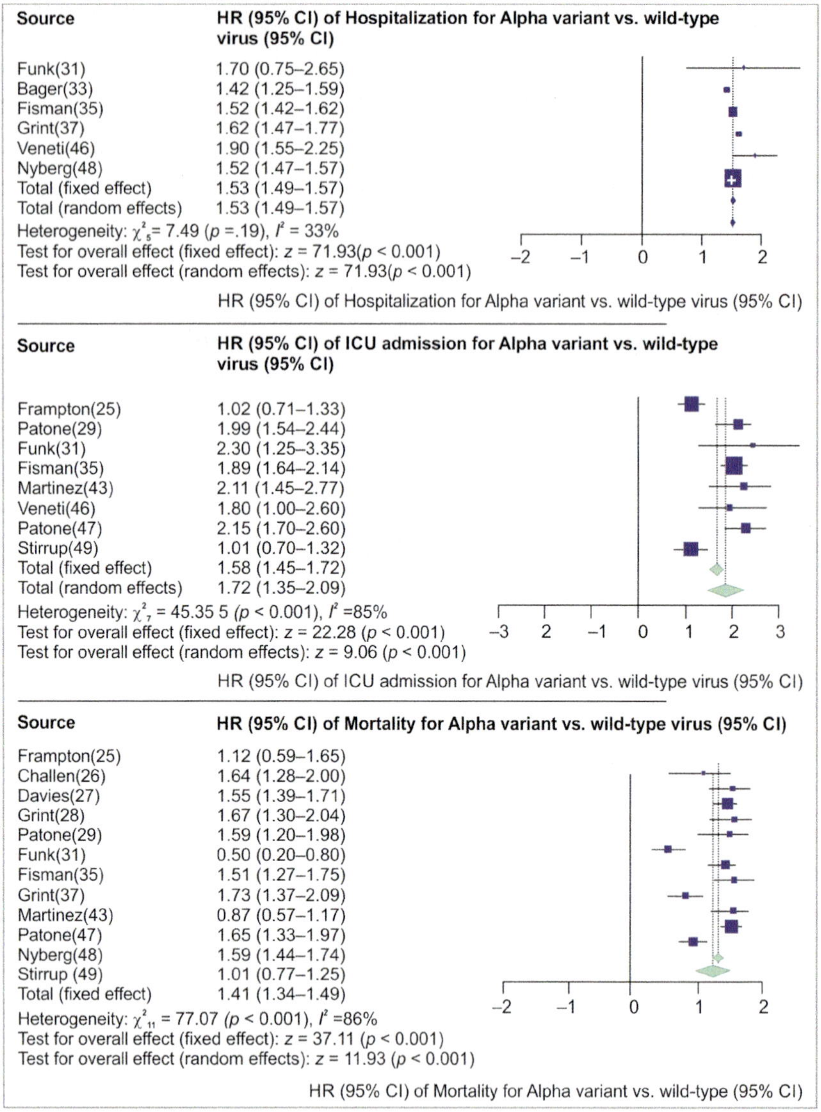

FIGURE 2: Comparative severity of alpha variant.

Source: Reproduced by permission from an open-access article distributed under the terms of the Creative Commons Attribution 4.0 International license.[74] The rate of hospitalizations, ICU admissions, and mortality taken from multiple publications are noted.

mutations than preceding variants, and the mutational activity rapidly diverged to create many subvariants **(Fig. 5)**.[76]

The Omicron variant precipitated a much larger surge in infections than any of the prior variants; yet the severity of illness was not as high due to a lesser tendency of the Omicron variants to attack the lower respiratory tract.

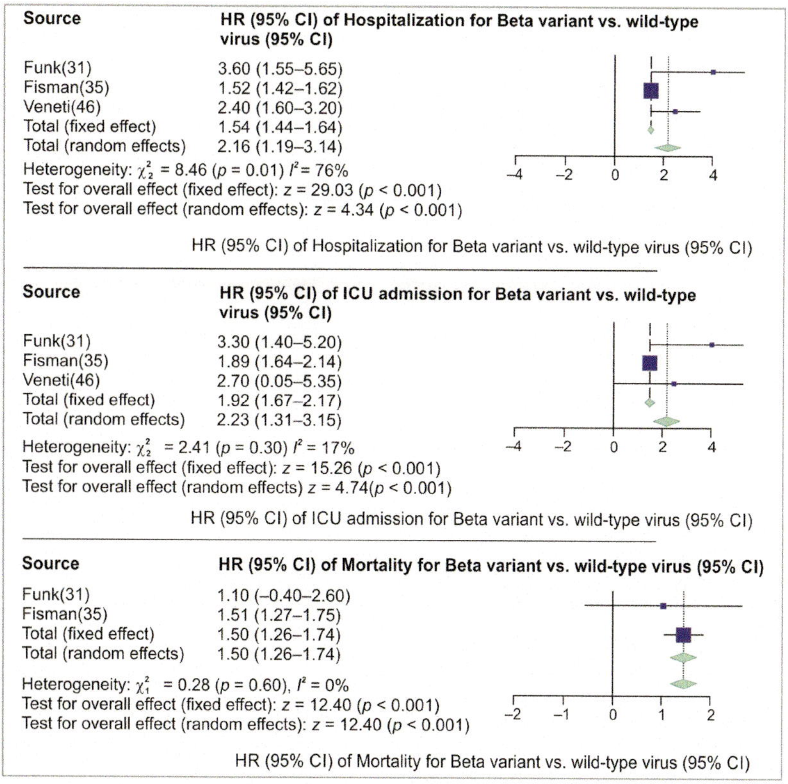

FIGURE 3: Comparative severity of beta variant relative to Wuhan original virus.
Source: Reproduced by permission under Creative Commons License.[74]

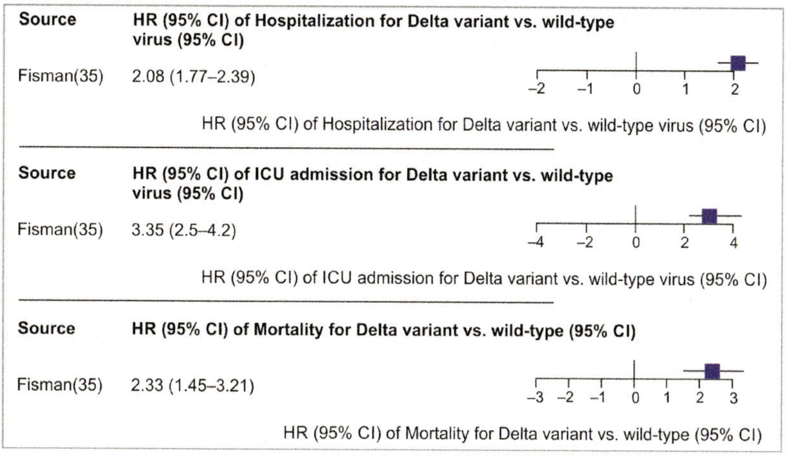

FIGURE 4: Comparative severity of delta variant.
Source: Reproduced by permission under Creative Commons License.[74] Only one publication provided the data for this figure.

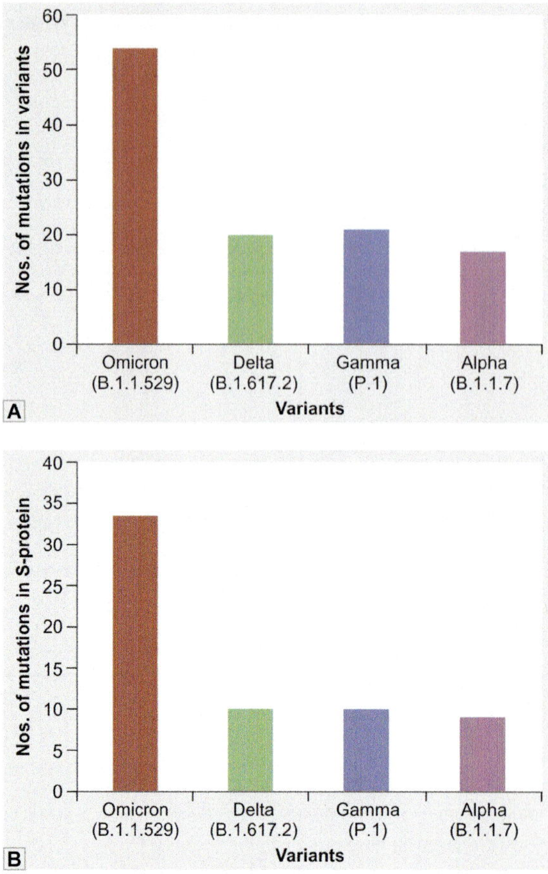

FIGURES 5A AND B: Mutational burden of the variants. The number of total mutations in each variant and the number of mutations in the S-protein are given, demonstrating the much higher number in the Omicron variant.

Source: Reproduced by permission under Creative Commons License.[76]

Yet, there was a large peak mortality, approaching that of the preceding variants, but, in relation to the more massive case load, the case fatality ratio was significantly lower **(Fig. 6)**.

"Big Data" will Give Us the Answer

The surge of Delta infections and the much larger surge of Omicron infections triggered a rapid campaign of booster shots using the original Moderna and Pfizer products. Clearly it was very difficult to design randomized control trials in previously vaccinated, previously infected populations. There were too many confounding variables to isolate. As a result, the current standard of evidence for benefit of preventive measures or treatment of COVID-19 shifted away from RCTs toward large scale population studies based on

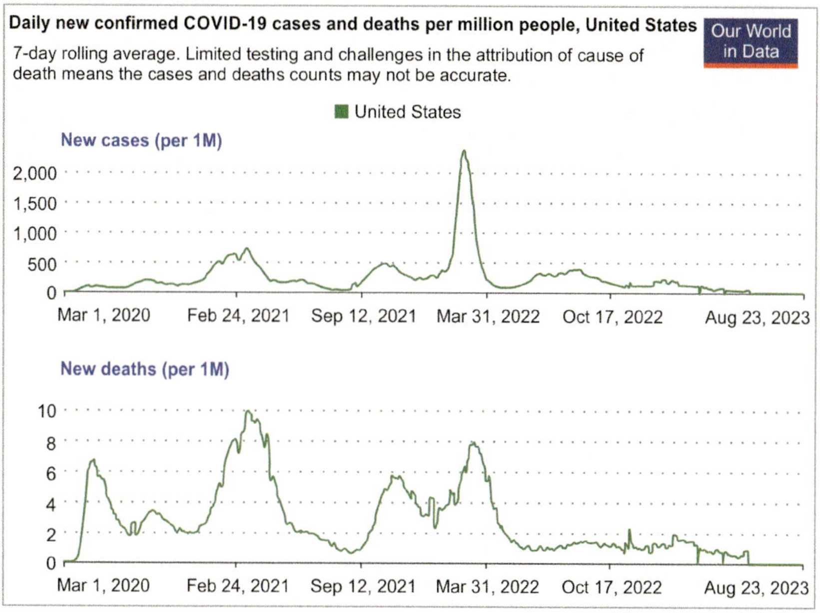

FIGURE 6: Daily confirmed COVID cases and deaths in the United States. The number of deaths actually exceeded the delta wave, but the number of cases was threefold higher.
Source: Reproduced by permission from Our World in Data under Creative Commons Licenses.

mining of massive clinical databases. So, the current recommendations for mRNA SARS-CoV-2 vaccination are based on observation of results primarily in the Israeli and British populations where their well-integrated National Health Systems afford comprehensive homogeneous data.[77,78] The goal here was to eliminate bias by contrasting vaccinated to unvaccinated patients in a significant subfraction of the entire population. Of course, there still exist many confounding variables. The technique of propensity score matching has been used to attempt to assemble contrast cohorts which match on a large number of characteristics.[79-81] There has been recent enthusiasm for carrying the process further to use large database information to emulate randomized clinical trials.[82]

Truth by Association

With the ability to mine large databases, the assumption has been made that evidence gathered would provide validity by virtue of approaching the size of the entire population. After all, what we want to know is the effect of treatment on the whole population. However, that does truly require full and equal participation of all.

The COVID vaccine trials in Israel: The success of the Pfizer BNT162b2 mRNA vaccine was documented by a well-executed series of observational analyses in the integrated healthcare system in Israel. Israel has national health insurance for all citizens administered through four separate healthcare plans with identical benefits. All data is comprehensively digitized and analyzable.[83]

Pfizer participated with Israeli investigators to thoroughly analyze the response to their vaccine in the Israeli health system, and the Pfizer BNT162b2 mRNA vaccine was the only COVID vaccine with any significant utilization in Israel. Israel led the rapid rollout of Pfizer vaccine in the world and has had perhaps the greatest impact on understanding the COVID vaccine response, far out of proportion to the small Israeli population.[84-86] Israel was first to report the early success of a nationwide vaccination program. 20% of the Israeli population received the first dose of the vaccines' two dose regimen in the span of three weeks.[78] The results were extremely favorable, in accordance with the Pfizer multinational randomized placebo controlled trial which led to approval of the BNT162b2 mRNA COVID-19 vaccine.[78,87-91] Pregnant women received the BNT162b2 mRNA vaccine with apparent favorable results in neonates and infants.[92-94] The first reports of waning of vaccine effectiveness and breakthrough infections came from Israel.[95-101] Facing the reality of increasing COVID infections, the Israeli government rapidly made the decision to administer a repeat BNT162b2 vaccine booster dose with apparent benefit.[102-106] That practice begun in Israel was then endorsed in the US and many countries in the world.

But the Israeli reports were not based on RCTs: Given the major well publicized findings of their research on the effects of the Pfizer vaccine on their pandemic, Israel has been portrayed as a highly vaccinated nation. That is not entirely true. Israel was certainly first out of the gate, but not ultimately among the most highly vaccinated population. Actually the fraction of the Israeli population achieving full COVID vaccination was no greater than in the United States and far less than in the most highly vaccinated nations such as Japan or Cuba **(Fig. 7)**.

The surprising magnitude of the "healthy vaccinee" effect: Despite a highly centralized healthcare delivery system, Israel has a diverse population wherein individuals make decisions on their own healthcare.[107] Unlike the United States, Israel never adopted vaccine mandates. People made their own choices. In order to demonstrate the effectiveness of the successive immunizations with the BNT162b2 vaccine, comparison with the relatively large population of unvaccinated Israelis was performed. These comparisons utilized propensity scoring methods to assemble ostensibly well matched populations, but that was not an RCT. On the contrary, the individuals who were compared self selected themselves to either choose to be vaccinated or to decline vaccination. In a small Israeli online survey performed in the early months of the pandemic, although half of the respondents reported they had not received influenza vaccine last year, 40% of them intended to receive influenza vaccine in the coming winter, and 66% of them intended to receive COVID-19 vaccine.[108]

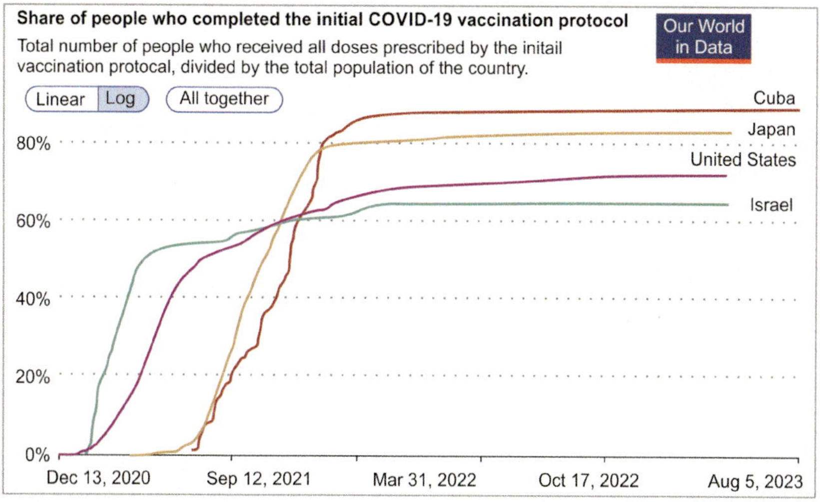

FIGURE 7: Percentage of total population who completed the initial vaccine series in Israel, the United States, Japan, and Cuba.

Source: Reproduced by permission from Our World in Data under Creative Commons License.

In the first paper describing safety findings of the Pfizer vaccine, it was notable that there were substantially lower incidences of acute renal failure and of intracranial hemorrhage in the vaccinated population compared to the unvaccinated.[109] Although the authors claimed that this was due to a benefit of the vaccine, it was pointed out it was more likely that other factors were in play such as uncontrolled diabetes or hypertension among the unvaccinated. The question was raised in a letter to the New England Journal of Medicine whether the unvaccinated Israelis were less health conscious than their vaccinated counterparts? Did they visit their clinics less often? Did they forget to take prescribed medications?

The journal refused to publish that letter back then. Now several years later, a startling new analysis of the benefit of the Pfizer booster vaccine on overall mortality in Israel was published in the New England Journal of Medicine by Hoeg, Durisetti, and Prasad.[110] They pointed out that the booster study found 65 COVID-19-associated deaths (reported as 0.16 per 100,000 persons per day) among patients who received the BNT162b2 booster shot compared to 2.98 per 100,000 among those in the nonbooster group—a 94.6% difference. Arbel et al. had stated that there were 441 deaths not related to COVID-19 in the booster group and 963 deaths not related to COVID-19 in the nonbooster group.[111] Hoeg et al. then used these figures to calculate a 94.8% lower mortality *not* related to COVID-19 among participants in the booster group thus indicating a markedly lower incidence of non-COVID adverse health outcomes in the booster group. They concluded that:

> *"Underlying health plays a substantial role in COVID-19-related mortality. The unadjusted differences in mortality related to COVID-19 and mortality not related to COVID-19, according to vaccination status, were essentially the same in the 2021 study by Arbel and colleagues. These findings arouse strong concern regarding unadjusted confounding. The adjusted 90% lower mortality due to COVID-19 reported among the participants who received a booster cannot, with certainty, be attributed to boosting. 'Healthy vaccinee bias' in this population may have also led to overestimates of vaccine effectiveness in similar studies from Clalit Health Services. Inclusion of mortality not related to COVID-19 in all observational COVID-19 vaccine studies would provide important context."*

This challenge to the original paper demonstrating benefit of the BNT162b2 vaccine booster incited a response from Arbel et al. who performed an analysis using Cox proportional-hazards regression model with time-dependent covariates to estimate vaccine efficacy. They adjusted for confounding variables such as congestive heart failure and chronic renal disease and confirmed that the HR for mortality not due to COVID in their original report was 0.23. They pointed out that "The policy in Israel prioritized the administration of boosters to persons in the community setting who were at the highest risk. However, boosters were generally not administered to hospitalized patients who were at high risk for death from any cause". Therefore, they further adjusted their calculations for hospitalization and found "the estimated association between receipt of the booster and mortality not related to COVID-19 (HR for death among participants who received the booster, 0.27; 95% CI 0.24–0.31)" thereby confirming the premise that the apparent strong benefit of booster vaccination was in large part due to a bias of health conscious individuals to take the booster vaccine.

This exchange in the New England Journal of Medicine clearly demonstrated at least a threefold "Healthy Vaccinee" bias in the Israeli findings of decreased COVID mortality attributable to their booster vaccination campaign. So despite the power of large numbers to provide answers to major questions of benefit of healthcare interventions in populations, the lack of randomization introduced enormous potential for misinterpretation of the value of the booster campaign.

This error in using observational data rather than randomized control data has persisted in multiple test negative control studies. The assumption is that those who test positive for COVID and are unvaccinated are well matched controls to those who test positive and are vaccinated. One recent example was a Pfizer sponsored study in the Kaiser Permanente health system showing that children aged 6 months to 5 years who had received BNT162b2 vaccine had a lower frequency of emergency room visits for COVID than those who were unvaccinated. Compared with unvaccinated children, the adjusted odds ratio for children who received 2 or 3 doses of BNT162b2 was 0.70 (95% CI 0.52–0.93) for a COVID-19-related emergency room or urgent care encounter, 0.60 (95% CI 0.39–0.92) for outpatient visits.[112]

Clearly, confounding for social, economic, and prior good health self-care is an ongoing reminder of the power of the randomized control study to eliminate bias.

BIAS OF NONRANDOMIZED TRIALS

In Bias of Having a Good Doctor

"Medicines cure diseases, but only doctors can cure patients>"

—Carl Jung

There are several effects which work against results obtained by attempting a match to inclusion and exclusion criteria designed for a randomized control trial, despite propensity score matches.[113] The first is that randomized control trials truly restrict clinical discretion of the investigator to make decisions based on prior knowledge and experience. In the COVID era, therein lies the genesis of the inherent conflict between the clinicians and the clinical researchers. That is why we, as patients, constantly search for "a good doctor" whose real world abilities transcend the constraints of research protocols. For example, the Hong Kong experience with Nmv/rtn and Mvpr illustrates the strength of real world evaluation of treatment effects.[114] In a large cohort survey in Hong Kong nursing homes they studied 14,617 patients [mean (SD) age, 84.8 (10.2) years]. Of these patients, 8,939 (61.2%) did not use oral antivirals, 5,195 (35.5%) used Mvpr, and 483 (3.3%) used Nmv/rtn. Compared with patients who did not use oral antivirals, those who used Mvpr and Nmv/rtn were more likely to be female and less likely to have comorbid illnesses and hospitalization in the past year. At a median (IQR) follow-up of 30 (30-30) days, 6,223 patients (42.6%) were hospitalized and 2,307 patients (15.8%) experienced inpatient disease progression. After propensity score weighting, Mvpr was associated with a reduced risk of hospitalization, WHR [weighted hazard ratio (WHR), 0.46; 95% CI 0.37–0.57; $p<0.001$ as was Nmv/rtn WHR, 0.46; 95% CI 0.32–0.65; $p<0.001$] and inpatient disease progression (Mvpr, WHR, 0.35; 95% CI 0.23–0.51; $p<0.001$; Nmv/rtn, WHR, 0.17; 95% CI 0.06–0.44; $p<0.001$). So, strong benefit shown, although realizing the potential bias in clinical selection.

In an electronic health records (EHRs) search of 92 million patients using TriNetX Advanced Analytics Platform, a multicenter and nationwide database in the US, 11,270 outpatients treated with Nmv/rtn were compared to 2,374 Mvpr treated individuals.[115] Once again, Mvpr patients were older with more comorbidities. After propensity score matching, the 30 day rate of hospitalization of the Mvpr patients (1.39%) did not differ significantly from that for Nmv/rtn (1.21%). Again, clinical selection was source of potential bias.

It is quite clear that one must consider clinical selection of treatment which is based on the acumen and beliefs of the treating physician and thus introduces significant bias. Of course, clinical bias is statistically undesirable, but may be highly beneficial for the patients.

Bias of Good Health Behavior

The second challenge to large population studies is "good health behavior" which encompasses "activities undertaken to maintain good health, to prevent ill health, as well as dealing with any departure from a good state of health".[116] These activities include overt behavioral patterns, actions and habits that relate to health maintenance, health restoration, and to health improvement. A variety of behaviors fall within such a definition including smoking, alcohol use, diet, physical activity, sexual behavior, physician visits, medication adherence, screening exams for health problems, and, yes, seeking out vaccination.

This means that people self-select themselves for activities which they believe are beneficial for their health.[117]

BUT THERE IS ALSO BIAS IN RANDOMIZED CONTROL TRIALS

"You are what you believe in.
You become that which you believe you can become."
—Bhagavad Gita

Bias of Benefit Over Risk

Randomized control trials were developed to confirm evidence of benefit of an intervention. The corresponding analysis of safety is not performed in the same rigorous analytic framework. In order to proceed to a randomized control trial in humans, an intervention must show preliminary evidence of benefit and lack of outstanding safety concerns, and benefit is the focus of the trial. If safety concerns were to appear, either in animal or initial Phase 1 or Phase 2 human studies, an intervention will not advance to the stage of a pivotal RCT. This means that a calculation of *t* for a benefit is expected to be large, but, if one were to calculate a difference in incidence of adverse events between an intervention cohort and the control cohort, the value would be expected to be small.

$$t = \frac{\bar{x}_1 - \bar{x}_2}{\sqrt{\left(s^2\left(\frac{1}{n_1} + \frac{1}{n_2}\right)\right)}}$$

In practice in RCTs, there is not a formal comparison of safety events. Adverse events are collected and catalogued and compared in an observational sense with the contrast cohort, but it is understood that a relatively low level of significant events may not appear in a randomized sample that is quite small in relation to the overall population.[118,119] Furthermore, inclusion exclusion criteria in RCTs usually restrict patient selection in order to avoid potential adverse events. Yet what we really want to know is the risk benefit ratio in the entire population.

In the COVID era, the most prominent safety issue of an intervention was the possible risk from the vaccines. In the United States three vaccines initially received approval: the Moderna and Pfizer mRNA vaccines and the Janssen viral vector vaccine. In the European Union, an Astra Zeneca viral vector agent also received emergency use authorization. In a large survey in the European Union, Adults (age ≥18 years) who received at least one dose of a COVID-19 vaccine [ChAdOx1-S (Oxford-AstraZeneca), BNT162b2 (Pfizer-BioNTech), mRNA-1273 (Moderna), or Ad26.COV2.S (Janssen/Johnson and Johnson)], from December 2020 to mid-2021 were evaluated for the risk of thromboembolic events.[120]

Overall, 1,332,719 first dose ChAdOx1-S recipients were matched to 2,124,339 BNT162b2 recipients from Germany and the UK. Additionally, 762,517 people receiving Ad26.COV2.S were matched to 2.851.976 receiving BNT162b2 in Germany, Spain, and the US. All 628,164 Ad26.COV2S recipients from the US were matched to 2,230,157 mRNA-1273 recipients. A total of 862 thrombocytopenia events were observed in the matched first dose ChAdOx1-S recipients from Germany and the UK, and 520 events after a first dose of BNT162b2. Comparing ChAdOx1-S with a first dose of BNT162b2 revealed an increased risk of thrombocytopenia [pooled calibrated incidence rate ratio 1.33 (95% CI 1.18–1.50) and calibrated incidence rate difference of 1.18 (0.57–1.8) per 1,000 person-years]. Additionally, a pooled calibrated incidence rate ratio of 2.26 (0.93–5.52) for venous thrombosis with thrombocytopenia syndrome was seen with Ad26.COV2S compared with BNT162b2.

As a result of these rare events not noted in the pivotal RCTs, the Janssen vaccine has been withdrawn from use in the United States. The Astra Zeneca vaccine never received authorization in the US and has been paused in the European Union.

Risk of Myocarditis

Another lingering concern has been myocarditis post-SARS-CoV-2 vaccination. In the pivotal RCT Trials for the Pfizer and Moderna mRNA products, myocarditis was not noticed. The collection of adverse events during those trials was focused on the typical initial symptoms of immune reactogenicity which characterize injection of foreign antigens, local injection site reactions, and fever, typically lasting 2–3 days. Shortly after the vaccination campaign began in December 2020, reports of myocarditis following the mRNA vaccinations began to emerge. Many reports were submitted to the US Vaccine Adverse Events Reporting System (VAERS),

(95% CI 1.28–1.92), and 1.72 (95% CI 1.33–2.22), respectively] but was lower than the risks after a positive SARS-CoV-2 test before or after vaccination [11.14 (95% CI 8.64–14.36) and 5.97 (95% CI 4.54–7.87), respectively]. However, in men younger than 40 years old, the number of excess myocarditis events per million people was higher after a second dose of mRNA-1273 than after a positive SARS-CoV-2 test [97 (95% CI 91–99) vs. 16 (95% CI 12–18)]. In women younger than 40 years, the number of excess events per million was similar after a second dose of mRNA-1273 and a positive test [7 (95% CI 1–9) vs. 8 (95% CI 6–8)].

The equivalence of risk of myocarditis after second dose of the mRNA-1273 vaccine to that of risk of SARS-CoV-2 infection in the younger than age 40 group is concerning. These findings and other similar epidemiologic studies have led to a pause in the use of Moderna's COVID-19 vaccine in Sweden, Denmark, Finland, and Iceland for use in young people.[129] If we consider that there have been 103 million cases of COVID documented to date in the United States and 676 million doses of mRNA COVID vaccine, administered,[130] that amounts to a ratio of about 6 doses of vaccine administered to actual COVID infections. If we then postulate that the duration of protection from infection is approximately 6 months, that means that a 6-month schedule of periodic vaccination is likely to produce a progressively increasing number of cases of myocarditis in young men exceeding the myocarditis cases due to COVID infection. With the findings that the CoronaVac inactivated virus vaccine has a much lower incidence of myocarditis than the SARS-CoV-2 mRNA vaccines, a randomized control trial comparing level of protection and adverse consequences with alternative vaccines is needed, allocating subjects randomly to one or more vaccines. Given the surprising demonstration by Hoeg et al. of a healthy vaccinee effect, such a study should include both mRNA and conventional protein subunit vaccines and should be done on a whole population basis so as to collect meaningful data on low frequency safety events such as myocarditis.

Bias of "Intention to Treat" versus "Per Protocol"

Randomizing patient selection protects against clinical selection and self-selection, but does not eliminate inherent bias resulting from study design. When performing a randomized control study, it is essential to account for all randomized subjects. However, all subjects may not complete the protocol. Therefore results are often presented as "intent to treat" to include all randomized subjects. However, if there are a large number of subjects who do not complete the protocol as originally designed, there is a strong bias introduced in interpretation. That bias was presented in the TOGETHER trials of fluvoxamine and ivermectin. The TOGETHER investigators presented their intent to treat data but did not offer the per protocol data, resulting in questions as to the interpretation of the results.[131]

Good Timing is Everything

"Lose no time to do good deeds before you are caught up in an ailment which may damage your health."

—Imam At-Tirmidhi

COVID is a dynamic viral illness with rapid transition from an asymptomatic viral infection, to symptomatic viral replication, to a subsequent phase of immunologic reaction to the viral infection, to, in a relative minority of patients, an excessive immune mediated inflammatory phase with ongoing coagulopathy. Randomized trials to date have focused primarily on the late inflammatory phase and in the viral phase, many days following onset. The successful antiviral trials of the monoclonal antibodies, nirmatrelvir-ritonavir, and molnupiravir were all designed to dose in patients who had less than a 5-day history of symptoms, and, in fact, less than 3 days. However, there have been relatively very few trials attempting immediate prophylaxis in exposed individuals prior to onset of viral replication and disease. Hydroxychloroquine studies were the first, but HCQ takes significant time to reach pharmacokinetic stable levels.[49]

Boulware et al. enrolled 821 asymptomatic participants, 719 of which reported a high-risk exposure to a confirmed COVID-19 contact within the prior 4 days.[132] HCQ was then express mailed to patients, with incipient delay. The result was that 49 of 414 (11.8%) receiving HCQ versus 58 of 407 (14.3%) developed symptoms compatible with COVID-19, the absolute difference was –2.4 percentage points (95% CI –7.0–2.2; $p = 0.35$). Once again, the lack of a p value <0.05 was deemed conclusive of no HCQ benefit, and there was no attempt to increase the recruitment to arrive at adequate statistical power.

A second HCQ prevention study was carried out in Spain. They enrolled 2,250 patients with exposure to a COVID patient within the past 7 days.[133] However, they included 304 patients who were already PCR COVID positive with symptoms at baseline. That group should have been excluded since the primary efficacy criterion was, in fact, PCR positivity with symptoms. That left 1,031 control patients who did not receive HCQ of whom 45 (4.4%) developed PCR positive symptomatic COVID and 915 patients who received HCQ of whom 28 (3.0%) developed PCR positive symptomatic COVID. Once again, an odds ratio >1.0 was cited as evidence that the 32% decrease in COVID infections was not potentially significant, and there was no attempt to increase recruitment, still another instance of the futility of pursuit of futility.

The Bulgarian Connection

The most successful randomized placebo controlled COVID prevention trial was performed in Bulgaria, one of the poorest nations in Europe with the worst record of COVID infection and excess mortality. In Bulgaria from January 3, 2020 to August 16, 2023 there have been 1,299,201 confirmed cases of COVID-19 and 38,397 deaths reported **(Fig. 8)**. Bulgaria is one of the nations with the lowest rate of COVID vaccination in the world with 68 injections per 100 inhabitants compared to 390 injections per 100 in Cuba and 202 per 100 in the United States.

A small French company named Medincell, which has developed a technology to create long duration injectable administration of various agents, elected to perform in Bulgaria a double blind, placebo controlled study of daily administration of ivermectin tablets to unvaccinated individuals with recent close exposure to individuals infected with COVID. This was a proof of concept trial to show that a 28-day ivermectin course administered at a modest dosage to produce continuous serum levels similar to what could be obtained with a long duration injection could prevent COVID transmission. This study, named the SAIVE Trial, was registered as NCT05305560 on ClinicalTrials.gov and performed during the Omicron period March to October of 2022.[134]

Main inclusion criterion was confirmed contact within 5 days with a positive COVID-19 case (assessed by RT-PCR). Participants were randomized in a 1/1 ratio to a modest dose of ivermectin (200 μg/kg on day 1 then 100 μg/kg/day up to day 28) or matching placebo. By day 28, there were 30 PCR positive infections in 200 ivermectin recipients and 105 infections in 199 placebo patients (RR 0.28; 95% CI 0.20–0.41). Of the 30 PCR positive ivermectin patients, 4 showed a high viral load compared to 99 placebo patients. Fortunately, no patient developed severe symptoms, and there were no hospitalizations.

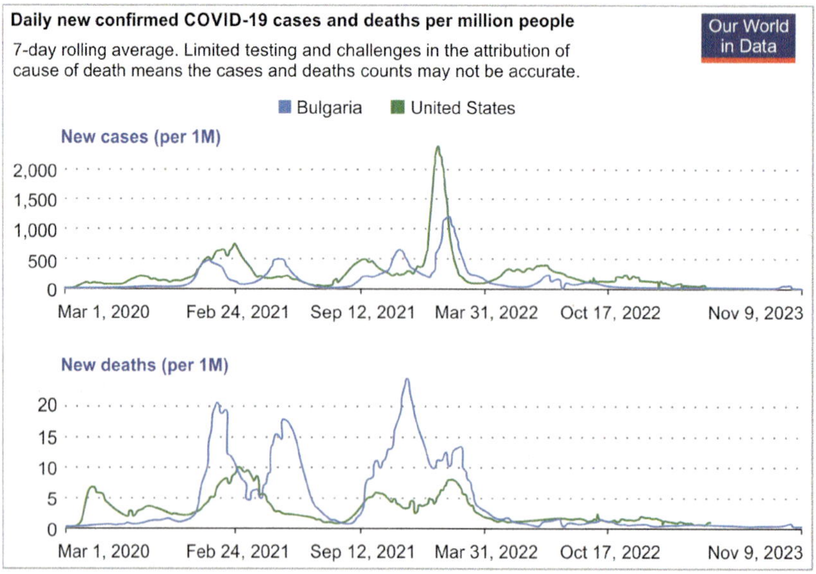

FIGURE 8: COVID cases and deaths compared United States and Bulgaria.
Source: Reproduced by permission from Our World in Data Creative Commons.

These highly positive findings of the SAIVE Trial stood in contrast to several studies including the ACTIV6 and TOGETHER trials which offered ivermectin tablets to patients with duration of established symptomatic COVID infections up to 7 days. The NIH ACTIV6 trial added to this prolonged duration of symptoms the time to receive ivermectin by mail, adding to the time lost since the original viral infection. The SAIVE Trial showed that exposed patients, not yet symptomatic, were likely to manifest symptoms about 7 days after their initial contact with an infected person. During that period of time, ivermectin levels could build up, notably in repository tissues, including fat stores.

The findings of the SAIVE Trial lent support to two observational analyses. The Itajai program offered ivermectin prophylaxis to the 100,000 plus inhabitants of the Brazilian city of Itajai.[135] The program consisted of inviting the entire population of Itajaí, in the absence of contraindications, ivermectin tablets as an optional treatment to be taken for two consecutive days every 15 days at a dose of 0.2 mg/kg/day. Of the 223,128 citizens of Itajaí considered for the study, a total of 159,561 subjects were included in the analysis: 113,845 (71.3%) regular ivermectin users and 45,716 (23.3%) nonusers. Of these, 4,311 ivermectin users were infected (3.7% infection rate), and 3,034 nonivermectin users were infected (6.6% infection rate), with a 44% reduction in COVID-19 infection rate [risk ratio (RR) 0.56; 95% CI 0.53–0.58; $p < 0.0001$]. Using propensity score matching, two cohorts of 3,034 subjects suffering from COVID-19 infection were compared. The regular use of ivermectin led to a 68% reduction in COVID-19 mortality [25 (0.8%) vs. 79 (2.6%) among ivermectin nonusers; RR 0.32; 95% CI 0.20–0.49; $p < 0.0001$]. There was a 56% reduction in hospitalization rate (44 versus 99 hospitalizations among ivermectin users and nonusers, respectively; RR 0.44; 95% CI 0.31–0.63; $p < 0.0001$). Furthermore, in those patients who had good compliance and regular use of ivermectin, mortality rate was 92% lower in regular users than nonusers (RR 0.08; 95% CI 0.02–0.35; $p = 0.0008$) and 84% lower than irregular users (RR 0.16; 95% CI 0.04–0.71; $p = 0.016$), while irregular users had a 37% lower mortality rate reduction than nonusers (RR 0.67; 95% CI 0.40–0.99; $p = 0.049$).[136] Of course, Itajai was not a randomized control study; selection bias of individuals who chose to use ivermectin as a result of health conscious decisions may have played a significant role, and those people may have had better health just as the Israeli vaccinated population.

All the People

So, unless one can compare an entire population, it is very difficult to avoid selection bias. A recent publication offers us a glimpse of a whole population approach as the second observational study of ivermectin. In Peru, there exist 25 semiautonomous states. On May 8, 2020, the Peruvian Health Ministry authorized a nationwide program of ivermectin distribution, contingent on participation by each state. Following the authorization, each of the 25 states of Peru implemented inpatient and outpatient treatments with ivermectin to different extents and in different time frames.[137] In 10 states, ivermectin was distributed on a mass scale through a national program led by the Ministry of Defense, Mega-Operación Tayta (MOT). There was a marked reduction in excess deaths correlating with inception of distribution in each state, eventually amounting to a 14-fold decrease in overall mortality. In November 2020, a new president took office and terminated the distribution programs. With the end of ivermectin use in November 2020, excess mortality rose sharply amounting to a 13-fold increase. Clearly this was no RCT, but, in terms of assessing benefit of an intervention in an entire population, after all the goal, a most interesting finding.

Where the Money Was!

William Francis (aka Willie) Sutton (1901–1980) was an accomplished bank robber.[138] He spent his life planning elaborate heists, which often did lead to his arrest and incarceration, from which he several times escaped only to return to his favored profession of bank robbery. Toward the end of his life, he was interviewed and was questioned "Willie, why did you rob banks?" to which the famous felon replied without hesitation "That is where the money was!

The devastation caused by the COVID onslaught led to a major response by the nations of the world. In the United States, according to the Committee for a Responsible Federal Budget, federal government expenditures for development of COVID vaccines and treatments have totaled about 52 billion dollars.[139] The bulk of the payments have been directed to large drug manufacturers for new investigational agents **(Table 4)**.

It can be seen that the largest fraction of payments went for vaccines with almost half the disbursements going to Pfizer, and an additional 11 billion dollars to Moderna. With the extension of American vaccines and therapeutics to conforming countries in Europe and Japan, the big pharmaceutical companies had enormous profits relative to their prepandemic finances.

Pfizer annual gross profit for 2020 was $33.167B, a 0.96% increase from 2019. Pfizer annual gross profit for 2021 was $50.467B, a 52.16% increase from 2020. Pfizer annual gross profit for 2022 was $65.986B, a 30.75% increase from 2021. Moderna annual gross profit for 2020 was $0.795B, a 1225% increase from 2019. Moderna annual gross profit for 2021 was $15.854B, a 1894.21% increase from 2020. Moderna annual gross profit for 2022 was $13.847B, a 12.66% decline from 2021. The NIH also expended further additional funds to test the new agents.

There was comparatively little expenditure on agents which were not new but could have had potential benefit. One striking example was the failure to engage in randomized controlled trials of the Gilead antiviral tenofovir, a highly successful agent used extensively to combat HIV and hepatitis B.

TABLE 4: US expenditures for vaccines and other COVID therapeutics.	
Development of vaccines and treatment	$52.3 billion
Pfizer vaccine and therapeutic	$24.6 billion
Moderna vaccine	$11.4 billion
Regeneron therapeutic	$3.26 billion
Johnson and Johnson (J&J) vaccine and therapeutic	$2.18 billion
AstraZeneca vaccine and therapeutic	$2.11 billion
GlaxoSmithKline vaccine	$2.07 billion
J&J vaccine	$2.03 billion
Eli Lilly and company therapeutic	$2.02 billion
Novavax vaccine	$1.60 billion
Merck vaccine and therapeutic	$662 million
J&J therapeutic	$152 million
SAb Biotherapeutics therapeutic	$111 million
Genentech therapeutic	$22.6 million
Emergent BioSolutions therapeutic	$15.5 million
Grifols therapeutic	$12.6 million
Purchasing other monoclonal antibodies	$4.70 billion

Tenofovir has been past patent lifetime for several years. There have been few outside challenges to the course of study and endorsement of new, expensive investigational agents by the mainstream consisting of the NIH, FDA, CDC, and mega-pharmaceutical companies. So, it is rare that one sees criticism of the official approach of the public health authorities and their relationship with the large for profit pharmaceutical manufacturers, but a unique article appeared in the prestigious Annals of Internal medicine sharply criticizing the NIH and the US. Pharmaceutical Industry for focusing on remdesivir and other new investigational agents and ignoring tenofovir.[140] The authors cited several observational trials showing benefit of ongoing tenofovir treatment for COVID in large cohorts of HIV patients and one attempted large randomized trial of prophylaxis in healthcare workers that was stopped after the advent of vaccines at the beginning of 2021. That one tenofovir randomized study included an additional hydroxychloroquine arm, thus two potentially active agents and two separate placebo groups. Given four contrast groups, it is not surprising that the observed positive trend could not achieve statistical significance, with early termination at only 25% enrollment, yet still suggested a 30% reduction in relative risk of COVID infection.

The authors noted that only anti-COVID interventions with significant financial gain have been brought forward by public health authorities. In fact,

Poor shall be with You Always

"And he looked up, and saw the rich men casting their gifts into the treasury. And he saw also a certain poor widow casting in thither two mites. And he said, Of a truth I say unto you, that this poor widow hath cast in more than they all: for all these have of their abundance cast in unto the offerings of God: but she of her penury hath cast in all the living that she had."

—Luke 21:1-4

Governmental funds have been spent primarily supporting the efforts of large pharmaceutical companies to combat COVID. NIH studies under the ACTIV Program were primarily directed at new investigational agents brought forward by these corporations which already enjoyed the resources needed to carry out the preclinical and clinical programs to find preventive and treatment agents for COVID. Yet, we take note of efforts by small resource limited entities to fight the pandemic.

MedinCell Story

The successful Bulgarian study of ivermectin prophylaxis was carried out by this small French company with a market capitalization of $201 million dollars, clearly less than Pfizer Inc (192 billion dollars), Moderna Inc (41.3 billion dollars), and GlaxoSmithKline, the company which offers remdesivir (74.4 billion dollars), or Merck (273.6 billion dollars). Yet with the aid of a small grant from the Gates Foundation, MedinCell was able to carry out a clean randomized placebo controlled clinical trial in Bulgaria with results showing a strong preventive effect of ivermectin on COVID infection.[134] That feat has not been accomplished either by Pfizer for nirmatrelvir/ritonavir nor Merck for molnupiravir.

What We may Learn from Cuba?

Cuba is a small island nation of 11 million people. According to a 2022 report from the Cuban Human Rights Observatory (OCDH), 72% of Cubans live below the poverty line.[155] Yet Cuba under Fidel Castro universalized free healthcare and committed substantial resources to biomedical research, disproportionate to the financial state of their economy. The most successful program of COVID vaccination in the world actually came from Cuba where they have developed multiple endogenously produced protein subunit vaccines. The level of vaccination of their population with their endogenous vaccines approaches 90%, perhaps the highest percentage in the world. The population acceptance of the vaccines appears to have been entirely voluntary. One study including 1,355,638 persons [mean age 49.5 years (SD 18.2)] showed an estimated vaccine efficacy of their Abdala COVID protein subunit vaccine against severe illness of 98.2% (95% CI 97.9–98.5) and against death 98.7% in fully vaccinated persons.[156] We note that self-selection bias in this study was substantially reduced since almost the entire Cuban population is vaccinated.

Nitric Oxide Effect

SARS-CoV-2 begins viral replication in the nasal cavity. There have been a number of nasal sprays including diluted iodide suggested to reduce COVID infections at the nasal source.[157] SaNOtize, a Canadian company so small that it was not possible to obtain a figure for its market capitalization, has developed a nasal spray of a long lasting formulation which releases nitric oxide, which is virucidal. They carried out two placebo controlled RCTs. In an initial randomized, double-blind, placebo-controlled trial, they evaluated their nitric oxide spray in early treatment of 80 confirmed cases of COVID-19 in the United Kingdom.[158] Use of their spray 5–6 times daily for 9 days significantly reduced participants' levels of SARS-CoV-2. The average viral load reduction in the first 24 hours was 95%, and within 72 hours, the viral load dropped by more than 99%. Similar results were obtained in a larger multicenter study in India.[159] Patients (18–70 years) with mild symptomatic PCR positive COVID-19 were randomized, 153 to the nitric oxide spray and 153 to placebo. Complete viral clearance occurred a median of 4 days earlier in nitric oxide treated patients.

Bias in Deed

"Believers, let not a group (of men) scoff at another group, it may well be that the latter (at whom they scoff) are better than they. And do not taunt one another, nor revile one another by nicknames."

—Surah Hujurat Ayat 11 (49:11 Quran)

The pandemic was a public health emergency. Hospital beds were full. Deaths were overwhelming mortuaries. It is not surprising that health authorities exhorted the public to take actions to counter the virus. Lockdowns and mask mandates were considered necessary and clearly unpopular in populations accustomed to freedom. With the rollout of the mRNA vaccines, the government made strong efforts to encourage people to be vaccinated, including mandates. These efforts were clearly understandable, although a CDC payment of 50 million dollars to Weber Shandwick, a major public relations firm representing Pfizer and Moderna, to operate officially within the CDC for media support has been called into question.[160]

The NIH, FDA, CDC Doth Protest Too Much Methinks

Even more concerning was governmental action to strongly criticize the use of agents not as yet supported by positive RCTs deemed acceptable by the NIH and FDA. The most glaring examples have been strenuous efforts to suppress clinical use of ivermectin by individuals and doctors to combat COVID. Kory and McCarthy published a book detailing the efforts of public health authorities to oppose the use of ivermectin including broad based media censorship.[161] These efforts were successful and inflicted considerable personal damage on the physicians and investigators who supported the use of ivermectin. To be sure, a large number of studies supported the use

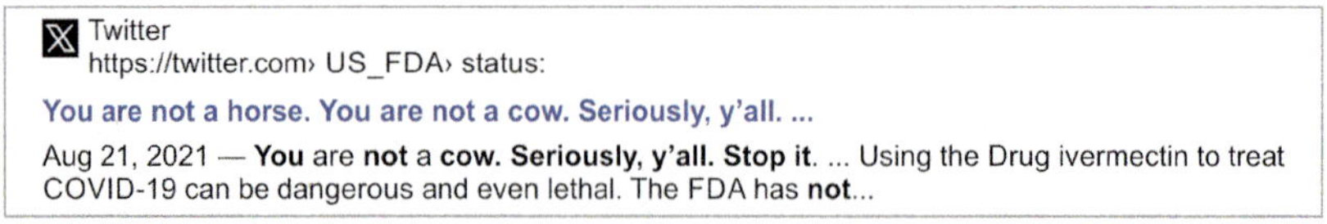

Twitter
https://twitter.com› US_FDA› status:

You are not a horse. You are not a cow. Seriously, y'all. ...

Aug 21, 2021 — **You** are **not** a **cow. Seriously, y'all. Stop it**. ... Using the Drug ivermectin to treat COVID-19 can be dangerous and even lethal. The FDA has **not**...

FIGURE 9: You are not a horse. You are not a cow.

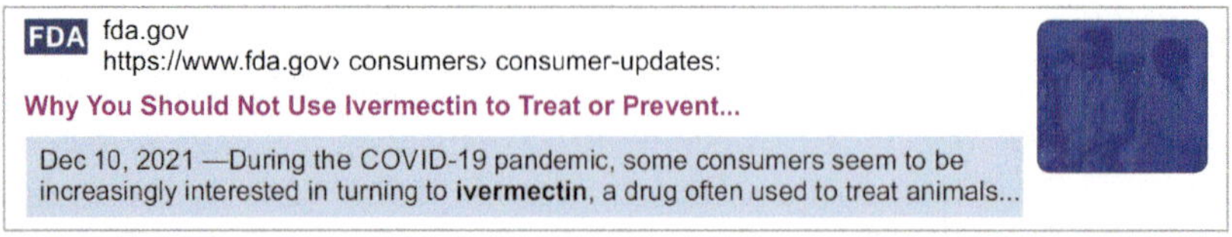

FDA fda.gov
https://www.fda.gov› consumers› consumer-updates:

Why You Should Not Use Ivermectin to Treat or Prevent...

Dec 10, 2021 —During the COVID-19 pandemic, some consumers seem to be increasingly interested in turning to **ivermectin**, a drug often used to treat animals...

FIGURE 10: Why you should not use ivermectin.

of ivermectin in COVID.[162] However, none of these studies were accepted by the FDA, CDC, and NIH. Ivermectin is a powerful preventive agent against parasites in animals. Clearly the dose administered to a 500 kg horse can be as much as 1,200 mg, whereas for humans doses 100 times less are safe. The FDA and CDC ran ads opposing the use of ivermectin ignoring that important distinction **(Figs. 9 and 10)**.

Even more important than the ads was encouragement by the public health authorities to medical licensing boards, hospitals, and insurance companies, to punish doctors who were prescribing ivermectin for COVID patients. In a recent Appeals Court ruling, a three judge panel suggested that the FDA cannot run advertisements directly stating that ivermectin, an approved human treatment, should not be used off label to treat and prevent COVID.[163]

EPILOGUE

Job clung to his faith in God despite the loss of his seven daughters and three sons, all his material possessions, and painful illness. Three friends came to him engaging in a long discussion to attempt to understand his misfortunes and to explore the basis for his constant belief in the goodness of God. Job resolutely deflected his friends. He even had to tolerate his wife who, less diplomatic than his friends, told him to *"Curse God and die".* In the end, Job's wife died and was buried. God then intervened to reward Job for his faith, reversed his misfortunes and cured his illness, provided him a new wife Dinah, daughter of Jacob, who gave him once again seven daughters and three sons, and he returned to his previous prosperity and more. Thus the Book of Job reassures us that faith in God helps us to endure the miseries we may encounter in life. Yet, the Book of Job and our own life experience still leaves us to ask an enduring question: If God is all powerful and manifests infinite kindness *"Why do bad things happen to good people?"* That question is left to the reader.

Now, of course, we must return to our questions regarding the role of the RCT to determine the treatments to be offered to the people of the world suffering the tragedy of COVID. The randomized control trial is a powerful tool to combat clinical and self-selection bias. However, there are many other sources of bias which clearly exist and may interfere with evaluation of treatment modalities. Remdesivir was the first agent to achieve a modestly successful NIH inpatient trial and was rapidly approved in the United States. The larger World Health Organization Solidarity randomized controlled trial then did not confirm the value of remdesivir in hospitalized patients. However, a number of immunomodulatory agents were approved after showing benefit in RCTs in the severe inflammatory stage of COVID in ill hospitalized patients. The Pfizer and Moderna mRNA vaccines had remarkably successful initial randomized trials to prevent COVID infection and were administered to billions of people. Despite two successful randomized trials of the Novovax conventional protein antigen vaccine, a long delay in approval by the FDA came too late for that vaccine to have a major impact or to allow comparison to the two officially favored mRNA vaccines. The monoclonal antibodies had successful RCTs and were approved in succession, but as the SARS-CoV-2 variants mutations evolved and overcame the immunological protection afforded by the antibodies, these agents eventually disappeared. There are currently no monoclonal antibodies available to combat COVID. The same process of viral evolution impacted on the duration of protection of the vaccines, both mRNA and the CoronaVac inactivated vaccine used in China, so that breakthrough infections led to ongoing repeated vaccinations. The coming of the Omicron variants brought about a revision of the existing vaccines which hopefully might improve protection. However, the use of the mRNA vaccines in large populations led to the recognition of possible harm in large non-randomized observational studies. Myocarditis resulting from mRNA vaccination has led to a pause in vaccination campaigns in many countries for the younger population who may be more susceptible to mRNA vaccine induced myocarditis. In fact, only in the United States is COVID vaccination recommended for ages as young as 6 months.

Pfizer had one successful randomized placebo controlled trial showing significant benefit of nirmatrelvir-ritonavir administered within 3 days in a cohort at high risk of severe COVID outcomes, and that study led to approval for use in the adult population. Follow-up RCTs in patients at average risk and in a prevention trial were deemed unsuccessful by Pfizer and stopped prematurely before statistical significance could be achieved. Again and again, similar studies showing potential benefit of various agents have been stopped for alleged futility with insufficient numbers due to lack of a desired "gamechanger" result. These attempts to decree the level of benefit which is clinically significant with a single agent are not acceptable. It must be remembered that doctors typically use multiple agents to combat serious conditions. Since when do we treat hypertensive patients with only one drug?

It is essential to quantitate clinical benefit, even if relatively small, because combinations of small benefits may be large.

Merck ran a less homogeneous high-risk study population for their one pivotal RCT of molnupiravir than did Pfizer and showed benefit, ostensibly less than that of nirmatrelvir-ritonavir. Whereas Pfizer closed its follow-up studies of nirmatrelvir-ritonavir in standard risk patients and as prophylaxis in exposed controls, Merck carried out the adequately powered large-scale PANORAMIC Study of molnupiravir in the United Kingdom. That study has been proclaimed a failure due to no difference in hospitalization or death compared to the control cohort, but, at the time PANORAMIC was performed, the frequency of severe COVID leading to hospitalization had diminished significantly due to lower pathogenicity of the Omicron variant. In the PANORAMIC RCT, there was a convincing improvement of 4 days in time to recovery with molnupiravir.

The ACTIV6 trials of so-called "repurposed" off patent agents have led to negative recommendations for their use to combat COVID, but other trials such as the TOGETHER series strongly suggest that further well designed RCTs using lambda interferon and combined fluvoxamine and inhaled steroids should proceed to confirm those results. Now the very unambiguous favorable outcome of ivermectin as a preventive agent in the randomized controlled Medincell SAIVE Trial must be followed by further confirmatory RCT studies, and that should now be a priority for the public health establishment, given lack of other oral proven preventive agents. Public health authorities should devote funds to support RCTs for agents emanating from resource-limited organizations rather than concentrating on the already well financed mega-pharmaceutical companies.

One of the greatest opportunities which now exists, given that there are several mRNA and other protein subunit COVID vaccines deemed safe and effective is to proceed with large scale vaccine comparison studies in the entire population. Although there are clear intrusions of bias in vaccine observational studies, randomized selection could provide a powerful tool to compare benefit and adverse health consequences of the mRNA and the protein subunit based vaccines, including those developed in Cuba. There is clearly a need to investigate the issue of SARS-CoV-2 vaccine induced myocarditis. Randomized distribution of different vaccines to the entire population could allow analysis of both benefit and even low frequency adverse events resulting from the various vaccines.

So, in the end, it is clear that the efforts to deal with the COVID pandemic have proven the value of the randomized control trial to overcome clinical and patient self-selection bias in assessing benefits of interventions. Of course, there are many other sources of bias which have intervened. As in the Book of Job, we return to a somewhat different question. Practicing clinicians attempted many treatments and preventive measures to deal with COVID. Public health authorities successfully opposed interventions with no prior proof of benefit via randomized control trials. Many possible agents, ranging from vitamins to HCQ, and ivermectin, were deemed useless and blocked. Now, of course, in light of all that has been learned, we are left to ponder whether the insistence on successful RCT confirmation prior to allowing use of treatments by doctors was the best course during the tragedy that has been COVID. That question is left to the reader.

REFERENCES

1. Giattino C, Ritchie H, Ortiz-Ospina E, Hasell J, Rodés-Guirao L, Roser M. (2020). Excess mortality during the Coronavirus pandemic (COVID-19). [online] Available from https://ourworldindata.org/excess-mortality-covid [Last accessed March, 2024].
2. Kalil AC. Treating COVID-19—Off-label drug use, compassionate use, and randomized clinical trials during pandemics. JAMA. 2020;323:1897-8.
3. Fauci A. (2020). Dr. Fauci Hydroxychloroquine Statement Transcript: House Coronavirus Hearing July 31. [online] Available from https ://www.rev.com/blog/transcripts/dr-fauci-hydroxychloroquine-statement-transcript-house-coronavirus-hearing-july-31. [Last accessed March, 2024].
4. Bothwell LE, Podolsky SH. The emergence of the randomized, controlled trial. N Engl J Med. 2016;375:501-4.
5. Sibbald B, Roland M. Understanding controlled trials: Why are randomized controlled trials important? BMJ. 1998;316:201.
6. Hariton E, Locascio JJ. Randomised controlled trials – the gold standard for effectiveness research: Study design: randomised controlled trials. BJOG. 2018;125:1716.
7. Jones DS, Podolsky SH. The history and fate of the gold standard. Lancet. 2015;385(9977):1502-3.
8. Doroshow D, Podolsky S, Barr J. Biomedical research in times of emergency: Lessons from history. Ann Intern Med. 2020;173:297-9.
9. Edridge AWD, Kaczorowska J, Hoste ACR, Bakker M, Klein M, Loens K, et al. Seasonal coronavirus protective immunity is short-lasting. Nat Med. 2020;26,1691-3.
10. Griffin DO, Brennan-Rieder D, Ngo B, Kory P, Confalonieri M, Shapiro L, et al. The importance of understanding the stages of Covid-19 in treatment and trials. AIDS Rev. 2021;23:40-7.
11. LeDuc JW, Barry MA. SARS, the first pandemic of the 21st century. Emerg Infect Dis. 2004;10:e26.
12. Arabi YM, Balkhy HH, Hayden FG, Bouchama A, Luke T, Baillie JK, et al. Middle East respiratory syndrome. N Engl J Med. 2017;376:584-94.
13. Wu Z, McGoogan JM. Characteristics of and important lessons from the coronavirus disease 2019 (COVID-19) outbreak in China. Summary of a report of 72 314 cases from the Chinese Center for Disease Control and Prevention. JAMA. 2020;323:1239-42.
14. Rajgor DD, Har Lee M, Archuleta, S, Bagdasarian N, Quek SC. The many estimates of the COVID-19 case fatality rate. Lancet Infect Dis. 2020 ;20 :776-7.
15. Russell TW, Hellewell J, Jarvis CI, van Zandvoort K, Abbott S, Ratnayake R, et al.; CMMID COVID-19 working group. Estimating the infection and case fatality ratio for coronavirus disease (COVID-19) using age-adjusted data from the outbreak on the Diamond Princess cruise ship, February 2020. Euro Surveill. 2020;25:2000256.
16. Davidson AM, Wysocki J, Batlle D. Interaction of SARS-CoV-2 and other coronavirus with ACE (angiotensin-converting enzyme)-2 as their main receptor: therapeutic implications. Hypertension. 2020;76:1339-49.
17. Wu Y, Zhao S. Furin cleavage sites naturally occur in coronaviruses. Stem Cell Res. 2020;50:102115.

18. Berche P. Gain-of-function and origin of Covid19. Presse Med. 2023;52:104167.
19. Xia S, Lan Q, Su S, Wang X, Xu W, Liu Z, et al. The role of furin cleavage site in SARS-CoV-2 spike protein-mediated membrane fusion in the presence or absence of trypsin. Sig Transduct Target Ther. 2020;5:92.
20. Jackson CB, Farzan M, Chen B, Choe H. Mechanisms of SARS-CoV-2 entry into cells. Nat Rev Mol Cell Biol. 2022;23:3-20.
21. Fisher RA. The arrangement of field experiments. J Ministry Agriculture Great Britain. 1926;33:503-13.
22. Besley JD. Origin of the 5% p value threshold. Rapid response to interpreting and reporting clinical trials with results of borderline significance. BMJ. 2011;343: d3340.
23. Wasserstein RL, Lazar NA. The ASA's Statement on p -Values: Context, process, and purpose. The American Statistician. 2016;70:129-33.
24. JASP. A Fresh Way to Do Statistics JASP. [online] Available from https://jasp-stats.org. [Last accessed March, 2024].
25. Kelter R. Bayesian and frequentist testing for differences between two groups with parametric and nonparametric two-sample tests. WIREs Comput Stat. 2021;13: e1523.
26. Gönen M, Johnson WO, Lu Y. The Bayesian two-sample t Test. The American Statistician. 2005;59:252-7.
27. Wason J, Magirr D, Law M, Jaki T. Some recommendations for multi-arm multi-stage trials. Stat Methods Med Res. 2016;25:716-27.
28. Reis G, Moreira Silva EADS, Medeiros Silva DC, Thabane L, Singh G, Park JJH, et al. Effect of early treatment with hydroxychloroquine or lopinavir and ritonavir on risk of hospitalization among patients with COVID-19: The TOGETHER randomized clinical trial. JAMA Netw Open. 2021;4:e216468.
29. Thomas S, Patel D, Bittel B, Medeiros Silva DC, Thabane L, Singh G, et al.; TOGETHER Investigators. Effect of high-dose zinc and ascorbic acid supplementation vs usual care on symptom length and reduction among ambulatory patients with SARS-CoV-2 infection: The COVID A to Z randomized clinical trial. JAMA Netw Open. 2021;4(2):e210369.
30. Hemilä H, Carr A, Chalker E. Vitamin C may increase the recovery rate of outpatient cases of SARS-CoV-2 Infection by 70%: Reanalysis of the COVID A to Z randomized clinical trial. Front Immunol. 2021;12:674681.
31. Beigel JH, Tomashek KM, Dodd LE, Mehta AK, Zingman BS, Kalil AC, et al.; ACTT-1 Study Group Members. Remdesivir for the Treatment of Covid-19 - Final Report. N Engl J Med. 2020;383:1813-26.
32. WHO Solidarity Trial Consortium. Remdesivir and three other drugs for hospitalised patients with COVID-19: final results of the WHO Solidarity randomised trial and updated meta-analyses. Lancet. 2022;399(10339):1941-53.
33. The RECOVERY Collaborative Group. Dexamethasone in hospitalized patients with Covid-19. N Engl J Med. 2021;384:693-704.
34. RECOVERY Collaborative Group. Tocilizumab in patients admitted to hospital with COVID-19 (RECOVERY): a randomised, controlled, open-label, platform trial. Lancet. 2021;397(10285):1637-45.
35. Marconi VC, Ramanan AV, de Bono S, Kartman CE, Krishnan V, Liao R, et al.; COV-BARRIER Study Group. Efficacy and safety of baricitinib for the treatment of hospitalised adults with COVID-19 (COV-BARRIER): a randomised, double-blind, parallel-group, placebo-controlled phase 3 trial. Lancet Respir Med. 2021;9:1407-18.
36. Kyriazopoulou E, Poulakou G, Milionis H, Metallidis S, Adamis G, Tsiakos K, et al. Early treatment of COVID-19 with anakinra guided by soluble urokinase plasminogen receptor plasma levels: a double-blind, randomized controlled phase 3 trial. Nat Med. 2021;27(10):1752-60.

37. Vlaar APJ, Witzenrath M, van Paassen P, Heunks LMA, Mourvillier B, de Bruin S, et al.; PANAMO study group. Anti-C5a antibody (vilobelimab) therapy for critically ill, invasively mechanically ventilated patients with COVID-19 (PANAMO): a multicentre, double-blind, randomised, placebo-controlled, phase 3 trial. Lancet Respir Med. 2022;10:1137-46.
38. McCullough PA, Kelly RJ, Ruocco G, Lerma E, Tumlin J, Wheelan KR, et al. Pathophysiological basis and rationale for early outpatient treatment of SARS-CoV-2 (COVID-19) infection. Am J Med. 2021;134:16-22.
39. Gautret P, Lagier JC, Parola P, Hoang VT, Meddeb L, Mailhe M, et al. Hydroxychloroquine and azithromycin as a treatment of COVID-19: results of an open-label non-randomized clinical trial. Int J Antimicrob Agents. 2020;56:105949.
40. Kavanagh ON, Bhattacharya S, Marchetti L, Elmes R, O'Sullivan F, Farragher JP, et al. Hydroxychloroquine does not function as a direct zinc ionophore. Pharmaceutics. 2022;14:899.
41. Derwand R, Scholz M, Zelenko V. COVID-19 outpatients: early risk-stratified treatment with zinc plus low-dose hydroxychloroquine and azithromycin: a retrospective case series study. Int J Antimicrob Agents. 2020;56:106214.
42. Mitjà O, Corbacho-Monné M, Ubals M, Tebé C, Peñafiel J, Tobias A, et al. Hydroxychloroquine for early treatment of adults with mild coronavirus disease 2019: A randomized, controlled trial. Clin Infect Dis. 2021;73:e4073-81.
43. Skipper CP, Pastick KA, Engen NW, Bangdiwala AS, Abassi M, Lofgren SM, et al. Hydroxychloroquine in nonhospitalized adults with early COVID-19: A randomized trial. Ann Intern Med. 2020;173:623-31.
44. Self WH, Semler MW, Leither LM, Casey JD, Angus DC, Brower RG, et al.; National Heart, Lung, and Blood Institute PETAL Clinical Trials Network. Effect of hydroxychloroquine on clinical status at 14 days in hospitalized patients with COVID-19: A randomized clinical trial. JAMA. 2020;324:2165-76.
45. National Institutes of Health. (2020). NIH halts clinical trial of hydroxychloroquine. [online] Available from https://www.nih.gov/news-events/news-releases/nih-halts-clinical-trial-hydroxychloroquine. [Last accessed March, 2024].
46. https://www.reuters.com/article/us-health-coronavirus-hydroxychloroquine/uk-halts-trial-of-hydroxychloroquine-as-useless-for-covid-19-patients- June 6, 2020 accessed 12 Oct 2022
47. Centers for Disease Control and Prevention. (2023). Isolation and Precautions for People with COVID-19.[online] Available from https://www.cdc.gov/coronavirus/2019-ncov/your-health/isolation.html [Last accessed March, 2023].
48. Centers for Disease Control and Prevention. (2023). Influenza Antiviral Medications: Summary for Clinicians. [online] Available https://www.cdc.gov/flu/professionals/antivirals/summary-clinicians.htm#summary. [Last accessed March, 2024].
49. Zahr N, Urien S, Llopis B, Pourcher V, Paccoud O, Bleibtreu A, et al. Pharmacokinetics and pharmacodynamics of hydroxychloroquine in hospitalized patients with COVID-19. Therapie. 2021;76:285-95.
50. Gottlieb RL, Vaca CE, Paredes R, Mera J, Webb BJ, Perez G, et al Early remdesivir to prevent progression to severe Covid-19 in outpatients. N Engl J Med. 2022;386:305-15.
51. McCreary EK, Escobar ZK, Justo JA. Monoclonal antibodies for the treatment of COVID-19—Every day you fight like you're running out of time. JAMA Netw Open. 2023;6:e239702.
52. Ambrose N, Amin A, Anderson B, Barrera-Oro J, Bertagnolli M, Campion F, et al. Neutralizing monoclonal antibody use and COVID-19 infection outcomes. JAMA Netw Open. 2023;6:e239694.
53. Hammond J, Leister-Tebbe H, Gardner A, Abreu P, Bao W, Wisemandle W, et al. Oral nirmatrelvir for high-risk, nonhospitalized adults with Covid-19. N Engl J Med. 2022;386:1397-408.

54. Jayk Bernal A, Gomes da Silva MM, Musungaie DB, Kovalchuk E, Gonzalez A, Delos Reyes V, et al.; MOVe-OUT Study Group. Molnupiravir for oral treatment of Covid-19 in nonhospitalized patients. N Engl J Med. 2022;386:509-20.
55. De Nardo P, Gentilotti E, Mazzaferri F, Cremonini E, Hansen P, Goossens H, et al. Multi-criteria decision analysis to prioritize hospital admission of patients affected by COVID-19 in low-resource settings with hospital-bed shortage. Int J Infect Dis. 2020;98:494-500.
56. https://www.fda.gov/files/drugs/published/Providing-Clinical-Evidence-of-Effectiveness-for-Human-Drug-and-Biological-Products.pdf accessed 08/24/2023
57. Butler CC, Hobbs FDR, Gbinigie OA, Rahman NM, Hayward G, Richards DB, et al.; PANORAMIC Trial Collaborative Group. Molnupiravir plus usual care versus usual care alone as early treatment for adults with COVID-19 at increased risk of adverse outcomes (PANORAMIC): an open-label, platform-adaptive randomised controlled trial. Lancet. 2023;401(10373):281-93.
58. Plotkin S. History of vaccination. Proc Natl Acad Sci U S A. 2014;111(34):12283-7.
59. Orenstein WA, Ahmed R. Simply put: Vaccination saves lives. Proc Natl Acad Sci U S A. 2017;114:4031-3.
60. Amanna IJ, Slifka MK. Successful vaccines. Curr Top Microbiol Immunol. 2020;428:1-30.
61. Corbett KS, Edwards DK, Leist SR, Abiona OM, Boyoglu-Barnum S, Gillespie RA, et al. SARS-CoV-2 mRNA vaccine design enabled by prototype pathogen preparedness. Nature. 2020;586(7830):567-71.
62. Thorn CR, Sharma D, Combs R, Bhujbal S, Romine J, Zheng X, et al. The journey of a lifetime - development of Pfizer's COVID-19 vaccine. Curr Opin Biotechnol. 2022;78:102803.
63. Baden LR, El Sahly HM, Essink B, Kotloff K, Frey S, Novak R, et al.; COVE Study Group. Efficacy and safety of the mRNA-1273 SARS-CoV-2 vaccine. N Engl J Med. 2021;384: 403-16.
64. El Sahly HM, Baden LR, Essink B, Doblecki-Lewis S, Martin JM, Anderson EJ, et al.; COVE Study Group. Efficacy of the mRNA-1273 SARS-CoV-2 vaccine at completion of blinded phase. N Engl J Med. 2021;385:1774-85.
65. Thomas SJ, Moreira ED Jr, Kitchin N, Absalon J, Gurtman A, Lockhart S, et al.; C4591001 Clinical Trial Group. Safety and efficacy of the BNT162b2 mRNA Covid-19 vaccine through 6 months. N Engl J Med. 2021;385:1761-73.
66. Sadoff J, Gray G, Vandebosch A, Cárdenas V, Shukarev G, Grinsztejn B, et al.; ENSEMBLE Study Group. Final analysis of efficacy and safety of single-dose Ad26.COV2.S. N Engl J Med. 2022;386:847-60.
67. Falsey AR, Sobieszczyk ME, Hirsch I, Sproule S, Robb ML, Corey L, et al.; AstraZeneca AZD1222 Clinical Study Group. Phase 3 safety and efficacy of AZD1222 (ChAdOx1 nCoV-19) Covid-19 vaccine. N Engl J Med. 2021;385:2348-60.
68. Jin L, Li Z, Zhang X, Li J, Zhu F. CoronaVac: A review of efficacy, safety, and immunogenicity of the inactivated vaccine against SARS-CoV-2. Hum Vaccin Immunother. 2022;18:2096970.
69. Heath PT, Galiza EP, Baxter DN, Boffito M, Browne D, Burns F, et al. Safety and efficacy of NVX-CoV2373 COVID-19 vaccine. N Engl J Med. 2021;385:1172-83.
70. Heath PT, Galiza EP, Baxter DN, Boffito M, Browne D, Burns F, et al. Safety and efficacy of the NVX-CoV2373 Coronavirus Disease 2019 Vaccine at completion of the placebo-controlled phase of a randomized controlled trial. Clin Infect Dis. 2023;76:398-407.
71. Dunkle LM, Kotloff KL, Gay CL, Áñez G, Adelglass JM, Hernández AQB, et al. Efficacy and safety of NVX-CoV2373 in adults in the United States and Mexico. N Engl J Med. 2022;386:531-43.

72. Chakraborty C, Sharma AR, Bhattacharya M, Agoramoorthy G, Lee SS. Evolution, mode of transmission, and mutational landscape of newly emerging SARS-CoV-2 variants. mBio. 2021;12:e0114021.
73. Brown CM, Vostok J, Johnson H, Burns M, Gharpure R, Sami S, et al. Outbreak of SARS-CoV-2 infections, including COVID-19 vaccine breakthrough infections, associated with large public gatherings — Barnstable County, Massachusetts, July 2021. MMWR Morb Mortal Wkly Rep. 2021;70:1059-62.
74. Lin L, Liu Y, Tang X, He D. The disease severity and clinical outcomes of the SARS-CoV-2 variants of concern. Front Public Health. 2021;9:775224.
75. Braeye T, Catteau L, Brondeel R, van Loenhout JAF, Proesmans K, Cornelissen L, et al. Vaccine effectiveness against onward transmission of SARS-CoV-2-infection by variant of concern and time since vaccination, Belgian contact tracing, 2021. Vaccine. 2022;40:3027-37.
76. Chakraborty C, Bhattachary M, Sharma AR, Mallik B. Omicron (B.1.1.529) - A new heavily mutated variant: Mapped location and probable properties of its mutations with an emphasis on S-glycoprotein. Int J Biol Macromol. 2022;219:980-9.
77. Lopez Bernal J, Andrews N, Gower C, Robertson C, Stowe J, Tessier E, et al. Effectiveness of the Pfizer-BioNTech and Oxford-AstraZeneca vaccines on covid-19 related symptoms, hospital admissions, and mortality in older adults in England: test negative case-control study. BMJ. 2021;373:n1088.
78. Dagan N, Barda N, Kepten E, Miron O, Perchik S, Katz MA, et al. BNT162b2 mRNA Covid-19 vaccine in a nationwide mass vaccination setting. N Engl J Med. 2021;384(15): 1412-23.
79. Austin PC. Optimal caliper widths for propensity-score matching when estimating differences in means and differences in proportions in observational studies. Pharm Stat. 2011;10(2):150-61.
80. Li Y, Li L. Propensity score analysis with local balance. Stat Med. 2023;42:2637-60.
81. Wang J. To use or not to use propensity score matching? Pharm Stat. 2021;20(1):15-24.
82. Wang SV, Schneeweiss S, RCT-DUPLICATE Initiative. Emulation of randomized clinical trials with nonrandomized database analyses: results of 32 clinical trials. JAMA. 2023;329:1376-85.
83. Balicer RD, Afek A. Digital health nation: Israel's global big data innovation hub. The Lancet. 2017;389(10088):2451-3.
84. Rosen B, Davidovitch N, Chodick G, Israeli A. The role of Israeli researchers in the scientific literature regarding COVID-19 vaccines. Isr J Health Policy Res. 2022;11:39.
85. Rosen B, Waitzberg R, Israeli A. Israel's rapid rollout of vaccinations for COVID-19. Isr J Health Policy Res. 2021;10:6.
86. Haas EJ, Angulo FJ, McLaughlin JM, Anis E, Singer SR, Khan F, et al. Impact and effectiveness of mRNA BNT162b2 vaccine against SARS-CoV-2 infections and COVID-19 cases, hospitalisations, and deaths following a nationwide vaccination campaign in Israel: an observational study using national surveillance data. Lancet. 2021;397(10287):1819-29.
87. Rossman H, Shilo S, Meir T, Gorfine M, Shalit U, Segal E. COVID-19 dynamics after a national immunization program in Israel. Nat Med. 2021;27(6):1055.
88. Angel Y, Spitzer A, Henig O, Saiag E, Sprecher E, Padova H, et al. Association between vaccination with BNT162b2 and incidence of symptomatic and asymptomatic SARS-CoV-2 infections among health care workers. JAMA. 2021;325(24):2457-65.
89. Prunas O, Warren JL, Crawford FW, Gazit S, Patalon T, Weinberger DM, et al. Vaccination with BNT162b2 reduces transmission of SARS-CoV-2 to household contacts in Israel. Science. 2022;375(6585):1151.

90. Milman O, Yelin I, Aharony N, Katz R, Herzel E, Ben-Tov A, et al. Community-level evidence for SARS-CoV-2 vaccine protection of unvaccinated individuals. Nat Med. 2021;27:1367.
91. Chodick G, Tene L, Rotem RS, Patalon T, Gazit S, Ben-Tov A, et al. The effectiveness of the two-dose BNT162b2 vaccine: analysis of real-world data. Clin Infect Dis. 2022;74: 472-8.
92. Goldshtein I, Steinberg DM, Kuint J, Chodick G, Segal Y, Shapiro Ben David S, et al. Association of BNT162b2 COVID-19 vaccination during pregnancy with neonatal and early infant outcomes. JAMA Pediatr. 2022;176:470-7.
93. Goldshtein I, Nevo D, Steinberg DM, Rotem RS, Gorfine M, Chodick G, et al. Association between BNT162b2 vaccination and incidence of SARS-CoV-2 infection in pregnant women. JAMA. 2021;326:728-35.
94. Dagan N, Barda N, Biron-Shental T, Makov-Assif M, Key C, Kohane IS, et al. Effectiveness of the BNT162b2 mRNA COVID-19 vaccine in pregnancy. Nat Med. 2021;27:1693.
95. Brosh-Nissimov T, Orenbuch-Harroch E, Chowers M, Elbaz M, Nesher L, Stein M, et al. BNT162b2 vaccine breakthrough: clinical characteristics of 152 fully vaccinated hospitalized COVID-19 patients in Israel. Clin Microbiol Infect. 2021;27:1652-7.
96. Mizrahi B, Lotan R, Kalkstein N, Peretz A, Perez G, Ben-Tov A, et al. Correlation of SARS-CoV-2-breakthrough infections to time-from-vaccine. Nat Commun. 2021;12:6379.
97. Feikin DR, Higdon MM, Abu-Raddad LJ, Andrews N, Araos R, Goldberg Y, et al. Duration of effectiveness of vaccines against SARS-CoV-2 infection and COVID-19 disease: results of a systematic review and meta-regression. Lancet. 2022;399(10328):924-44.
98. Israel A, Shenhar Y, Green I, Merzon E, Golan-Cohen A, Schäffer AA, et al. Large-scale study of antibody titer decay following BNT162b2 mRNA vaccine or SARS-CoV-2 infection. Vaccines. 2022;10:64.
99. Lustig Y, Zuckerman N, Nemet I, Atari N, Kliker L, Regev-Yochay G, et al. Neutralising capacity against Delta (B.1.617.2) and other variants of concern following Comirnaty (BNT162b2, BioNTech/Pfizer) vaccination in health care workers, Israel. Eurosurveillance. 2021;26:0557.
100. Levine-Tiefenbrun M, Yelin I, Alapi H, Katz R, Herzel E, Kuint J, et al. Viral loads of Delta-variant SARS-CoV-2 breakthrough infections after vaccination and booster with BNT162b2. Nat Med. 2021;27:2108.
101. Kustin T, Harel N, Finkel U, Perchik Shah, Harari S, Tahor M, et al. Evidence for increased breakthrough rates of SARS-CoV-2 variants of concern in BNT162b2-mRNA-vaccinated individuals. Nat Med. 2021;27:1379.
102. Spitzer A, Angel Y, Marudi O, Zeltser D, Saiag E, Goldshmidt H, et al. Association of a third dose of BNT162b2 vaccine with incidence of SARS-CoV-2 infection among health care workers in Israel. JAMA. 2022;327:341-9.
103. Barda N, Dagan N, Cohen C, Hernán MA, Lipsitch M, Kohaane IS, et al. Effectiveness of a third dose of the BNT162b2 mRNA COVID-19 vaccine for preventing severe outcomes in Israel: an observational study. Lancet. 2021;398(10316):2093-100.
104. Patalon T, Gazit S, Pitzer VE, Prunas O, Warren JL, Weinberger DM. Odds of testing positive for SARS-CoV-2 following receipt of 3 vs 2 doses of the BNT162b2 mRNA vaccine. JAMA Intern Med. 2022;182:179-84.
105. Bar-On YM, Goldberg Y, Mandel M, Bodenheimer O, Freedman L, Alroy-Preis S, et al. Protection against Covid-19 by BNT162b2 booster across age groups. N Engl J Med. 2021;385:2421-30.
106. Arbel R, Hammerman A, Sergienko R, Friger M, Peretz A, Netzer D, et al. BNT162b2 vaccine booster and mortality due to Covid-19. N Engl J Med. 2021;385:2413-20.
107. Green MS, Abdullah R, Vered S, Nitzan D. A study of ethnic, gender and educational differences in attitudes toward COVID-19 vaccines in Israel—implications for vaccination implementation policies. Isr J Health Policy Res. 2021;10(1):26.

108. Shmueli L. Predicting intention to receive COVID-19 vaccine among the general population using the health belief model and the theory of planned behavior model. BMC Public Health. 2021;21:804.
109. Barda N, Dagan N, Ben-Shlomo Y, Kepten E, Waxman J, Ohana R, et al. Safety of the BNT162b2 mRNA Covid-19 vaccine in a nationwide setting. N Engl J Med. 2021;385:1078-90.
110. Høeg TB, Duriseti R, Prasad V. Potential "Healthy Vaccinee Bias" in a Study of BNT162b2 Vaccine against Covid-19. N Engl J Med. 2023;389:284-5.
111. Arbel R, Sergienko R, Hammerman A. BNT162b2 Vaccine booster and Covid-19 mortality. Reply. N Engl J Med. 2022;386:1000-1.
112. Tartof SY, Frankland TB, Slezak JM, Puzniak L, Ackerson BK, Jodar L, et al. Receipt of BNT162b2 Vaccine and COVID-19 ambulatory visits in US children younger than 5 Years. JAMA. 2023;330(13):1282-4.
113. Reiffel JA. Propensity score matching: the 'devil is in the details' where more may be hidden than you know. Am J Med. 2020;133:178-81.
114. Ma BH, Yip TC, Lui GC, Lai MS, Hui E, Wong VW, et al. Clinical outcomes following treatment for COVID-19 with Nirmatrelvir/Ritonavir and Molnupiravir among patients living in nursing homes. JAMA Netw Open. 2023;6(4):e2310887.
115. Wang L, Berger NA, Davis PB, Kaelber DC, Volkow ND, Xu R. COVID-19 rebound after Paxlovid and Molnupiravir during January-June 2022. medRxiv [Preprint]. 2022:2022.06.21.22276724.
116. MacKian S; University of Manchester, Manchester. (2003). A review of health seeking behaviour: problems and prospects. [online] Available from https://assets.publishing.service.gov.uk/media/57a08d1de5274a27b200163d/05-03_health_seeking_behaviour.pdf. [Last accessed March, 2024].
117. Conner M, Norman P. Health behaviour: Current issues and challenges. Psychol Health. 2017;32:895-906.
118. Ioannidis JP, Lau J. Improving safety reporting from randomized trials. Drug Saf. 2002;25:77-84.
119. Papanikolaou PN, Christidi GD, Ioannidis JPA. Comparison of evidence on harms of medical interventions in randomized and nonrandomized studies. CMAJ. 2006;174:635-41.
120. Li X, Burn E, Duarte-Salles T, Yin C, Reich C, Delmestri A, et al. Comparative risk of thrombosis with thrombocytopenia syndrome or thromboembolic events associated with different covid-19 vaccines: international network cohort study from five European countries and the US. BMJ. 2022;379:e071594.
121. Klein NP, Lewis N, Goddard K, Fireman B, Zerbo O, Hanson KE, et al. Surveillance for adverse events after COVID-19 mRNA vaccination. JAMA. 2021;326(14):1390-9.
122. Goddard K, Lewis N, Fireman B, Weintraub E, Shimabukuro T, Zerbo O, et al. Risk of myocarditis and pericarditis following BNT162b2 and mRNA-1273 COVID-19 vaccination. Vaccine. 2022;40:5153-9.
123. Sharff KA, Dancoes DM, Longueil JL, Lewis PF, Johnson ES. Myopericarditis after COVID-19 booster dose vaccination. Am J Cardiol. 2022;172:165-6.
124. Mevorach D, Anis E, Cedar N, Bromberg M, Haas EJ, Nadir E, et al. Myocarditis after BNT162b2 mRNA Vaccine against Covid-19 in Israel. N Engl J Med. 2021;385:2140-9.
125. Cho JY, Kim KH, Lee N, Cho SH, Kim SY, Kim EK, et al. COVID-19 vaccination-related myocarditis: a Korean nationwide study. Euro Heart J. 2023;44:2234-43.
126. Bozkurt B, Kamat I, Hotez PJ. Myocarditis with COVID-19 mRNA vaccines. Circulation. 2021;144:471-84.
127. Fan M, Lai FTT, Cheng FWT, Tsie NTY, Li X, Wan EYF, et al. Risk of carditis after three doses of vaccination with mRNA (BNT162b2) or inactivated (CoronaVac) Covid-19

vaccination: a self-controlled cases series and a case-control study. Lancet Reg Health West Pac. 2023;35:100745.

128. Patone M, Mei XW, Handunnetthi L, Dixon S, Zaccardi F, Shankar-Hari M, et al. Risk of myocarditis after sequential doses of COVID-19 vaccine and SARS-CoV-2 infection by age and sex. Circulation. 2022;146:743-54.
129. Lahto E. (2021). Finland joins Sweden and Denmark in limiting Moderna COVID-19 vaccine. [online] Available from https://www.reuters.com/world/europe/finland-pauses-use-moderna-covid-19-vaccine-young-men-2021-10-07/ [Last accessed March, 2024].
130. USA Facts. US Coronavirus vaccine tracker. [online] Available from https://usafacts.org/visualizations/covid-vaccine-tracker-states/. [Last accessed March, 2024].
131. Scheim DE, Aldous C, Osimani B, Fordham EJ, Hoy WE. When characteristics of clinical trials require per-protocol as well as intention-to-treat outcomes to draw reliable conclusions: three examples. J Clin Med. 2023;12:3625.
132. Boulware DR, Pullen MF, Bangdiwala As, Pastick KA, Lofgren SM, Okafor EC, et al. A randomized trial of hydroxychloroquine as postexposure prophylaxis for Covid-19. N Engl J Med. 2020;383:517-25.
133. Mitjà O, Corbacho-Monné M, Ubals M, Alemany A, Suñer C, Tebé C, et al.; BCN-PEP-CoV2 Research Group. A cluster-randomized trial of hydroxychloroquine for prevention of Covid-19. N Engl J Med. 2021;384:417-27.
134. Desort-Henin V, Kostova Anna, Babiker EA, Caramel A, Malamut R. (2023). The SAIVE trial, post-exposure use of ivermectin in Covid-19 prevention: Efficacy and safety results. [online] Available from https://www.medincell.com/wp-content/uploads/2023/04/Poster-SAIVE-April2023-OK3.pdf [Last accessed March, 2024].
135. Kerr L, Cadegiani FA, Baldi F, Lobo RB, Assagra WLO, Proença FC, et al. Ivermectin prophylaxis used for COVID-19: A citywide, prospective, observational study of 223,128 subjects using propensity score matching. Cureus. 2022;14:e21272.
136. Kerr L, Baldi F, Lobo R, Assagra WL, Proença FC, Chamie JJ, et al. Regular use of ivermectin as prophylaxis for COVID-19 led up to a 92% reduction in COVID-19 mortality rate in a dose-response manner: results of a prospective observational study of a strictly controlled population of 88,012 subjects. Cureus. 2022;14:e28624.
137. Chamie J, Hibberd JA, Scheim DE. COVID-19 excess deaths in Peru's 25 states in 2020: Nationwide trends, confounding factors, and correlations with the extent of ivermectin treatment by state. 2023;15(8):e43168.
138. Reynolds Q. I, Willie Sutton: The Personal Story of The Most Daring Bank Robber and Jail Breaker of Our Time. New York: Farrar, Straus, & Young; 1953.
139. Committee for a Responsible Federal Budget. (2020). Welcome to the new COVID money tracker. [online] Available from https://www.crfb.org/blogs/welcome-new-covid-money-tracker [Last accessed March, 2024].
140. Hernán MA, del Amo J. Drug repurposing and observational studies: the case of antivirals for the treatment of COVID-19. Ann Intern Med. 2023;76:556-60.
141. The Pharma Letter. (1996). U.S.A. clears ivermectin for human use. [online] Available from https://www.thepharmaletter.com/article/usa-clears-ivermectin-for-human-use. [Last accessed March, 2024].
142. MERCK. (2021). Merck statement on ivermectin use during the COVID-19 pandemic. [online] Available from https://www.merck.com/news/merck-statement-on-ivermectin-use-during-the-covid-19-pandemic. [Last accessed March, 2024].
143. National Institutes of Health. (2023). COVID-19 therapeutics prioritized for testing in clinical trials. [online] Available from https://www.nih.gov/research-training/medical-research-initiatives/activ/covid-19-therapeutics-prioritized-testing-clinical-trials#ongoing-trials. [Last accessed March, 2024].

144. Reis G, Dos Santos Moreira-Silva EA, Silva DCM; TOGETHER investigators. Effect of early treatment with fluvoxamine on risk of emergency care and hospitalisation among patients with COVID-19: the TOGETHER randomised, platform clinical trial. Lancet Glob Health. 2022;10:e42-51.
145. Bramante CT, Huling JD, Tignanelli CJ; COVID-OUT Trial Team. Randomized trial of metformin, ivermectin, and fluvoxamine for Covid-19. N Engl J Med. 2022;387:599-610.
146. Yu LM, Bafadhel M, Dorward J; PRINCIPLE Trial Collaborative Group. Inhaled budesonide for COVID-19 in people at high risk of complications in the community in the UK (PRINCIPLE): a randomised, controlled, open-label, adaptive platform trial. Lancet. 2021;398(10303):843-55.
147. Song JY, Yoon JG, Seo YB, Lee J, Eom JS, Lee JS, et al. Ciclesonide inhaler treatment for mild-to-moderate COVID-19: A randomized, open-label, phase 2 trial. J Clin Med. 2021;10(16):3545.
148. Kuo KC, Chen CH, Wang CJ, Wu JC, Chung HP, Chen YT, et al. Clinical benefits of inhaled ciclesonide for hospitalized patients with COVID-19 infection: a retrospective study. BMC Pulm Med. 2022;22(1):368.
149. Clemency BM, Varughese R, Gonzalez-Rojas Y, Morse CG, Phipatanakul W, Koster DJ, et al. Efficacy of inhaled ciclesonide for outpatient treatment of adolescents and adults with symptomatic COVID-19: A randomized clinical trial. JAMA Intern Med. 2022;182:42-9.
150. Griesel M, Wagner C, Mikolajewska A, Stegemann M, Fichtner F, Metzendorf MI, et al. Inhaled corticosteroids for the treatment of COVID-19. Cochrane Database Syst Rev. 2022;(3):CD015125.
151. Boulware DR, Lindsell CJ, Stewart TG, Hernandez AF, Collins S, McCarthy MW, et al.; ACTIV-6 Study Group and Investigators. Inhaled fluticasone furoate for outpatient treatment of Covid-19. N Engl J Med. 2023;389:1085-95.
152. Reis G, dos Santos Moreira Silva EA, Medeiros Silva DC, Thabane L, de Souza Campos VH, Ferreira TS, et al.; TOGETHER Investigators. Oral fluvoxamine with inhaled budesonide for treatment of early-onset COVID-19: A randomized platform trial. Ann Intern Med. 2023;176:667-75.
153. Donnelly RP, Kotenko SV. Interferon-lambda: a new addition to an old family. J Interferon Cytokine Res. 2010;30:555-64.
154. Reis G, Moreira Silva EAS, Medeiros Silva DC, Thabane L, Campos VHS, Ferreira TS, et al.; TOGETHER Investigators. Early treatment with pegylated interferon lambda for Covid-19. N Engl J Med. 2023;388:518-28.
155. The Borgen project. (2023). Being poor in Cuba. [online] Available from https://borgenproject.org/tag/cuban-observatory-for-human-rights-ocdh/. [Last accessed March, 2024].
156. Más-Bermejo PI, Dickinson-Meneses FO, Almenares-Rodríguez K, Sánchez-Valdés L, Guinovart-Díaz R, Vidal-Ledo M, et al. Cuban Abdala vaccine: Effectiveness in preventing severe disease and death from COVID-19 in Havana, Cuba; A cohort study. Lancet Reg Health Am. 2022;16:100366.
157. Chavda VP, Baviskar KP, Vaghela DA, Raut SS, Bedse AP. Nasal sprays for treating COVID-19: a scientific note. Pharmacol Rep. 2023;75:249-65.
158. Winchester S, John S, Jabbar K, John I. Clinical efficacy of nitric oxide nasal spray (NONS) for the treatment of mild COVID-19 infection. J Infect. 2021;83:237-79.
159. Tandon M, Wu W, Moore K, Winchester S, Tu YP, Miller C, et al.; Study Group. SARS-CoV-2 accelerated clearance using a novel nitric oxide nasal spray (NONS) treatment: A randomized trial. Lancet Reg Health Southeast Asia. 2022;3:100036.
160. Dailymail.com. (2022). PR firm that represents Moderna sits on CDC vaccine division. [online] Available from https://www.dailymail.co.uk/health/article-11303017. [Last accessed March, 2024].

161. Kory P, McCarthy J. War on Ivermectin: The Medicine That Saved Millions and Could Have Ended the Pandemic. New York: Skyhorse Publishing; 2021.
162. Kory P, Meduri GU, Varon J, Iglesias J, Marik PE. Review of the emerging evidence demonstrating the efficacy of ivermectin in the prophylaxis and treatment of COVID-19. Am J Ther. 2021;28:e299-318.
163. Langford C. (2023). Fifth Circuit sides with ivermectin-prescribing doctors in their quarrel with the FDA. [online] Available from https://www.courthousenews.com/fifth-circuit-sides-with-ivermectin-prescribing-doctors-in-their-quarrel-with-the-fda/ [Last accessed March, 2024].

5

SECTION

Complications

CHAPTER 29

An Update on the Relationship between SARS-CoV-2 (COVID-19) and its Neurological Manifestations

Ruchi S Raval, Nihal Sriramaneni, Sumul N Raval

INTRODUCTION: A BRIEF UNDERSTANDING OF THE CURRENT COVID-19 SITUATION

In the years since December 2019 and the emergence of the now recognized SARS-CoV-2 (COVID-19) novel coronavirus, the medical and public health landscapes have altered drastically.[1] With an estimated R_0 of 1.5–3.5, SARS-CoV-2 is considered to be a highly infectious agent.[2] Transmissible mainly through inhalation or via contact with infected droplets, COVID-19 is responsible for a series of symptoms that range from mild to deadly. The most common symptoms are fever, shortness of breath, cough, loss of smell/taste, and fatigue.[2] In some, the disease may progress to pneumonia, ARDS (acute respiratory distress syndrome), and even multiorgan dysfunction.[3] Commonly, the elderly and/or those with comorbidities are most susceptible to catastrophic progression of the disease. Though many individuals experience symptoms, there are also COVID-19 patients that present with no symptoms. These asymptomatic individuals can also contribute to the spread of COVID-19.[3]

With a total of 767,364,883 confirmed global cases including 6,938,353 deaths as reported by the World Health Organization (WHO), the RNA virus COVID-19 has evoked considerable international comradery toward developing a solution.[4] In perhaps the most groundbreaking research campaign of the century, two major vaccinations for COVID-19 have been developed and distributed to date. As of May 5, 2023, 668,168,096 vaccine doses have been administered to the general public with the United States accounting for over ⅔ of the population with at least one dose.[4]

Now, post-COVID syndrome or long-COVID, where COVID-19 symptoms persist or develop beyond 3 months of COVID-19 onset, poses a significant threat to those who suffered COVID-19.[5] An often debilitating illness, long-COVID has been shown to impact at least 10% of those who had identified COVID-19 infections.[6] Though the disease is still not entirely understood, the literature suggests that it affects COVID-19 survivors at varying levels of severity.[5] Along with providing an update on the relationship between COVID-19 and its neurological manifestations, this chapter will bring forth a discussion on long-COVID and neurological symptoms that persist or develop in the months following initial onset, which pose a significant threat to the global healthcare landscape.[7]

COVID-19 AND THE NERVOUS SYSTEM

Though the most common symptoms of COVID-19 are related to respiratory illness, there are also several others that suggest involvement of the nervous system. Neurological complications of SARS-CoV-2 include confusion, ataxia, hypogeusia, hyposmia, neuralgia, and seizures.[8] The existence of these symptoms allows for several questions. What are both the short- and long-term neurological manifestations of COVID-19, when in COVID-19 disease progression do neurological symptoms manifest, and how long do they last? While some, like Nalbandian et al., in the journal Nature note that lingering or permanent neurological deficits of COVID-19 fall under the umbrella post-acute COVID-19, wherein persistent complications exist beyond 4 weeks from onset of COVID-19 related symptoms, others state neurological complications appear concurrently with other symptoms.[9] **Figure 1** depicts the postulated timeline for postacute COVID-19 along with related symptoms.[10]

Understanding the timeline underlying COVID-19-related neurological manifestations further delineates whether the relationship between the two is causal. In other words, does COVID-19 directly cause neurological manifestations or are they simply a byproduct. As will be discussed, research indicates that it seems to be a combination. Since December 2019, a robust amalgam of evidence has arisen that confirms the relationship between COVID-19 and nervous system involvement. Having recognized the types of symptoms and when they occur, the various potential mechanisms that allow the SARS-CoV-2 virus to infiltrate the nervous system producing neurological symptoms will also be discussed. Furthermore, the coming sections will also take a dive into post-COVID syndrome or long-COVID, which has since been defined as COVID-19 symptoms that persist or develop beyond 3 months of COVID-19 onset.

COVID-19-RELATED NEUROLOGICAL SYMPTOMS

Neurological manifestations related to SARS-CoV-2 or COVID-19 have been shown to begin as early as disease onset. As more and more literature related to COVID-19 has been amassed in the years since December 2019, patterns indicate that the neurological manifestations can emerge in many different ways. Importantly, the literature suggests that neurological symptoms can develop long after initial COVID-19 diagnosis, as part of the recently coined post-COVID syndrome.

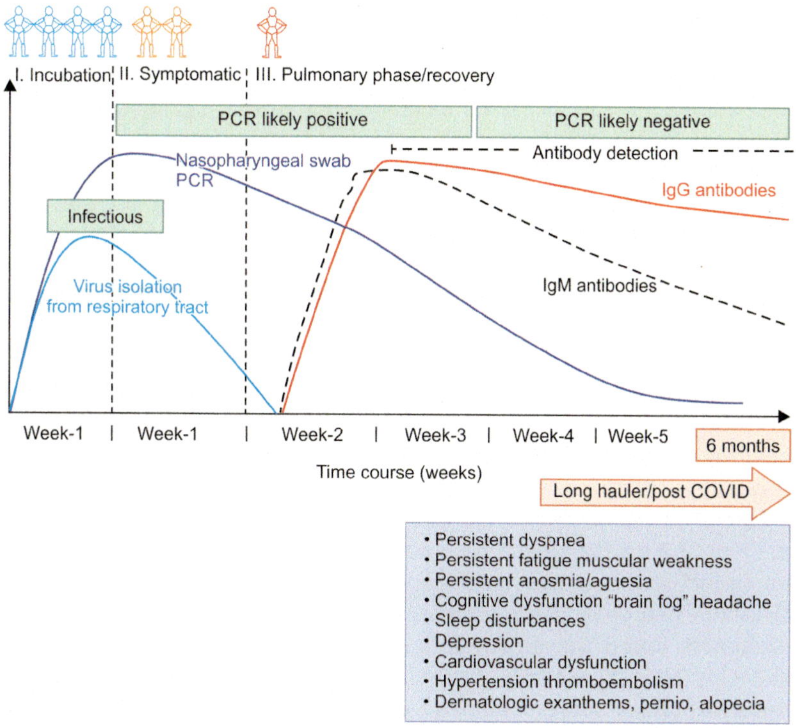

FIGURE 1: Timeline for postacute COVID-19 defined as chronic complications beyond 4 weeks of symptom onset.
Courtesy: Permission granted by Paul Marik MD.

While the manifestations can be neurological complications of the systemic disease, they can also be direct effects of the virus on the nervous system, parainfectious, or postinfectious immune-related disease.[11] Examples of parainfectious diseases include: Guillain–Barré syndrome (GBS), transverse myelitis, and acute disseminated encephalomyelitis.[10] Regardless of the mechanism, however, emergent studies demonstrate that the most frequent neurological symptoms are short term like cephalalgia, muscle aches, dizziness, anosmia, and ageusia. In severe cases, other, more direct manifestations of the virus in the central nervous system (CNS) can also occur.[8]

In one study, involving 214 patients, neurological manifestations occurred in 36.4% of individuals. The investigation indicated that those with more severe COVID-19 demonstrated increasing severity of neurological symptoms including acute cerebrovascular diseases, depressed levels of consciousness, and skeletal muscle injury.[12]

A retrospective study of a large database containing 81 million patients of which 237,379 were diagnosed with COVID-19, 33.6% developed new-onset neuropsychiatric symptoms in the 6 months after the onset of the disease.[13]

Interestingly, of the COVID-19 patients that were admitted to intensive care units, 46.42% diagnosed with neurological manifestations and 62.34% with encephalopathy, indicating that the more severe COVID-19 cases were, in fact, coupled with an increased incidence of neurological manifestations.[13] In the cohort of COVID-19 patients that were admitted to the ICU, the estimated incidences were as follows: 2.66% for intracranial hemorrhage, 6.92% for ischemic stroke, 0.26% for parkinsonism, 1.74% for dementia, 19.15% (17.90–20.48) for anxiety disorder, and 2.77% for psychotic disorder[13] **(Fig. 2)**.

Another study systematically reviewed 13,480 patients, with a mean age of 50.3 years.[14] This article affirmed that the most common neurological manifestations of acute COVID-19 infection include myalgia, taste impairment, smell impairment, headache, dizziness, and encephalopathy.[14] This study found that myalgia, elevated creatinine kinase (CK), lactate dehydrogenase (LDH), and acute cerebrovascular disease (CVD) were more prevalent in severe causes of COVID-19.[14]

One prospective study, seeking to evaluate the neurological symptoms of inpatient COVID-19 patients, including those in the intensive care unit (ICU) found that when mapping hospitalized COVID-19 rRt-PCR positive patients, at least one neurological symptom was recorded in 95.5% of patients.[15] Again, researchers found the most common symptoms to be myalgia (48.5%), headache (39.6%), anosmia (34.8%), and dysgeusia (34%).[15] Interestingly, these symptoms manifested more commonly in ICU patients than those on regular inpatient floors.[15]

In the last edition of this chapter, as there was little to report on neurological manifestations in pediatric populations, no comments were made. In the time since, there still remains limited literature on pediatric cases. Perhaps because COVID-19 infections in children were perceived to be less severe, there are only a handful of studies that report neurological manifestations in children.[16] The existing literature suggests that while there may be some commonalities between the effects of COVID-19 in pediatric versus adult populations, the staggering difference in deceased and debilitated adults compared to children exemplifies that the disease does, in fact, affect children and adults differently.[16] Other than a generally milder course of pulmonary disease, children also tend to have fewer comorbidities.[16] Together, these components may contribute to the observed differences.

While there are differences in disease course between children and adults, the data holds that children, too, experience neurological manifestations of the virus. 28% of pediatric COVID-19 patients in the United Stats experienced headaches.[16] In 31–47% of those whose COVID-19 progressed to multisystem inflammatory syndrome in children (MIS-C), headache, altered mental status, and encephalopathy were observed.[16] A review study at Columbia University showed that out of 82 confirmed COVID-19 pediatric patients, 35 (43%) developed neurological symptoms. These were headache (34%), fatigue or malaise (25%), altered mental status (23%), weakness (14%), and seizure

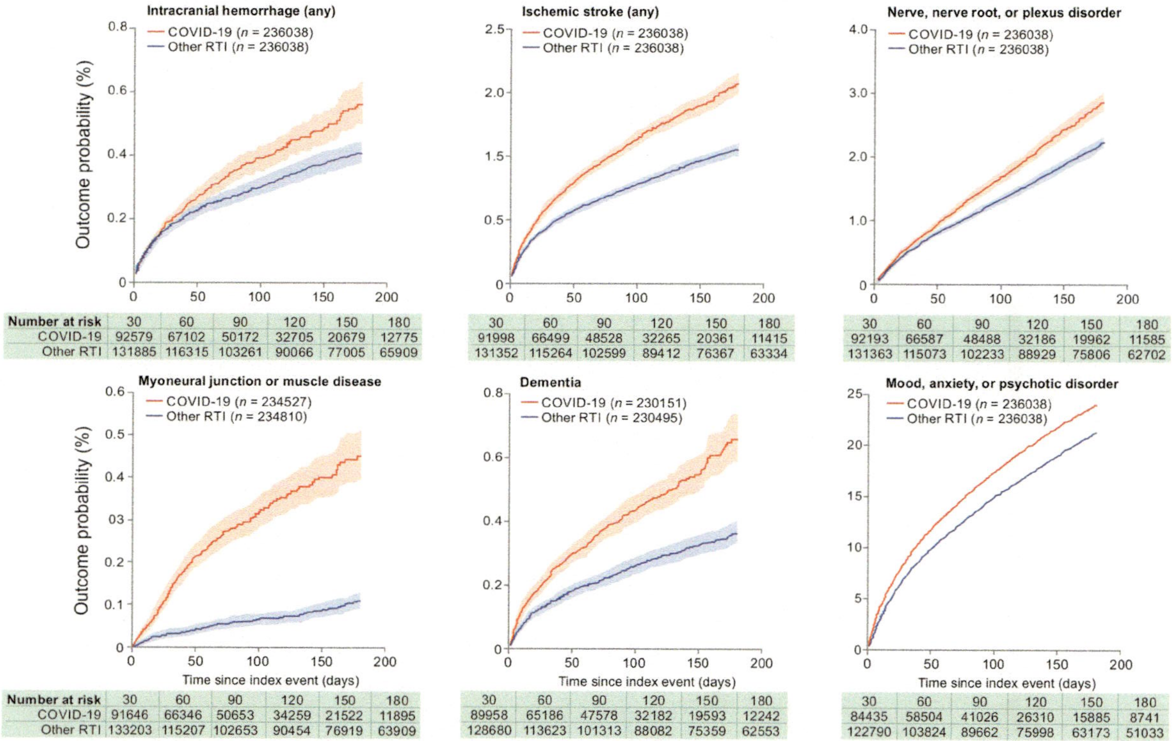

FIGURE 2: Kaplan–Meier estimates for major COVID-19 related neurological symptoms compared with other respiratory tract infections (RTI) based symptoms.[13]

(11%).[16] In this study, three patients presented with cranial nerve VI palsy, two with intracranial hypertension two with dysgeusia or ageusia, and one suffered a stroke.[16] No patients in this study had CSF positive for viral RNA tested via PCR.[16] Unfortunately, the long-term impact on neurodevelopment after COVID-19 infection is still largely unknown. Certainly, this is a field that warrants future study.

Though COVID-19 is incredibly complex, as mentioned above, it causes considerable comprehensive risk to the entire nervous system. The manifestations can, however, be categorized by CNS involvement or peripheral nervous system (PNS) involvement. Examples of COVID-19-related CNS disease include encephalopathy, acute disseminated encephalomyelitis, encephalitis, meningitis, ischemic and hemorrhagic stroke, venous sinus thrombosis, and endothelialitis.[17] Examples of COVID-19-related PNS disease are GBS, anosmia, chemosensory dysfunction, skeletal muscle damage, neuralgia, and epilepsy among others.[18]

NEUROLOGICAL MANIFESTATIONS OF LONG COVID

Long-COVID or post-COVID-19 syndrome initially garnered widespread recognition among social support groups and later among the scientific and medical communities.[5] Though the illness remains poorly understood, one study indicated that it occurs in at least 10% of those who were infected with SARS-CoV-2, albeit at varying degrees.[5,6] Another study, however, studying a cohort of 47,910 patients (age 17–81) estimated that long-term symptoms of COVID-19, defined as ranging from 14–110 days, developed in as many as 80% of the patient population.[19] Here, the most common symptoms were: fatigue (58%), headache (44%), attention disorder (27%), hair loss (25%), and dyspnea (24%).[19] This elucidates the need for a more robust conversation regarding defining terminology in the ever-evolving discussion surrounding COVID-19 **(Table 1)**.

Data suggest that more than 200 symptoms have been identified as potentially linked to long-COVID, impacting all organ systems, and at least 65 million individuals worldwide are estimated to have it.[6] Though there are several suggested mechanisms like long-term tissue damage and/or pathological inflammation from viral persistence or immune dysregulation, there remains a gap in the literature delineating the exact etiology.[6] Interestingly, studies indicate that there is no significant difference between long-COVID caused by the different strains of COVID-19.[25]

Though long-COVID is a multi-organ disorder that has an array of clinical manifestations, involvement in either the central or peripheral nervous system comprises almost one-third of patients who present with long-COVID.[20] The most common neurological manifestations of long-COVID are fatigue, "brain fog," headache, cognitive impairment, sleep/mood/smell/taste disorders, myalgias, sensorimotor deficits, and dysautonomia[20] **(Table 2)**. There is very little evidence in the literature that delineates an

TABLE 1: Various terminology often used to describe post-COVID syndrome.[20]

Nomenclature	Description
Long COVID[3,5]	Long-term COVID-19 symptoms characterized by cyclical, progressive, or multiphasic course
Long COVID[2]	Symptoms persisting for >2 months
Long COVID[4]	Signs and symptoms that persist for >4 weeks and can be attributed to COVID-19 infection
Long-haul COVID[10] Long-tail COVID	Symptoms persisting for >100 days
Long post-COVID symptoms[8]	Symptoms lasting for 12–24 weeks
Post-acute COVID syndrome (PACS)[21]	Persistent symptoms and/or delayed or long-term complications beyond 4 weeks from symptom onset
Post-acute sequelae of SARS-CoV-2 (PASC)[22,23]	Symptoms persisting for >1 month
Post-COVID-19[13]	Symptoms persisting for >2 months
Persistent post-COVID symptoms[8]	Symptoms lasting for >24 weeks
Post-COVID-19 syndrome[9,24]	Signs and symptoms that develop during or after an infection consistent with COVID-19, present for >12 weeks and are not attributable to alternative diagnoses

TABLE 2: Common neurological manifestations of long-COVID categorized by CNS or PNS findings.[20]

Localization in the nervous system	Neurological symptoms
Central nervous system	• Fatigue • "Brain fog" • Headache • Sleep disorders • Cognitive impairment • Emotional/Mood disorders • Dizziness • Dysautonomia
Peripheral nervous system	• Muscle weakness • Myalgias • Hyposmia • Hypogeusia • Hearing loss/tinnitus • Sensorimotor deficits (hypoesthesia, dysesthesia, tremor)

(CNS: central nervous system; PNS: peripheral nervous system)

exact pathophysiological mechanism in the neurological manifestations of long-COVID.[20] It is known that SARS-CoV-2 has a high affinity for ACE-2 receptors on type II pneumocytes.[26] As this receptor is also expressed on neurons and glial cells, some studies suggest that SARS-CoV-2 may also have a tropism for the nervous system, which may contribute to the widespread and long-lasting neurological manifestations.[26] One study suggests several potential mechanisms of long-COVID, including neuroinflammation increasing cytokines, chemokines, etc. and inducing a reactive state of resident microglia, the potential for SARS-CoV-2 to invoke an autoimmune response, the reactivation of previously latent viruses, like Epstein–Barr, or even that pulmonary and multiorgan dysfunction can cause hypoxemia, and metabolic disturbances that impact the brain.[27] Though these proposed mechanisms are not mutually exclusive, they remain theoretical as exact mechanism has been elucidated.

In one study of electronic health records analyzing 236,379 patients, researchers found that 34% of individuals in the 6 months following SARS-CoV-2 infection presented with a neurological or psychiatric diagnosis.[20] Importantly, when the researchers compared the probability of neurological outcomes in patients diagnosed with COVID-19 compared to matched controls with influenza or other respiratory infections, the patients who were previously diagnosed with COVID-19 were at a significantly higher risk to develop a neurologic manifestation.[20]

At present, neurologists are confronted with long-COVID on a daily basis, with ever increasing demand. But, because there is limited data on mechanisms and such varying presentations, diagnosis and treatment of long-COVID has proven to be a difficult feat. As a result, a multi-disciplinary approach should be employed, especially considering that long-COVID is a multi-system disease. After initial clinical assessment, tailored ancillary testing including neuroimaging, CSF and elctrophysiological studies, blood tests, cardiac and pulmonary function tests may be conducted, in addition to the standard neurological examination.[20] The decisions for appropriate, targeted treatment can be made next **(Flowchart 1)**.

CENTRAL NERVOUS SYSTEM MANIFESTATIONS

Encephalopathy and Neuroinflammatory Diseases (Encephalitis)

Among neurological manifestations of COVID-19, encephalopathy and encephalitis are considered to be serious.[28] Encephalopathy, collectively, is defined as alterations in mental status including disorientation, confusion, agitation, and somnolence or sleepiness.[29] Clinical manifestations can also include fever, headache, epilepsy, status epilepticus, and/or impaired consciousness,[28,30] and these manifestations can present before, after, or during respiratory symptoms.[30] Though altered mental status rarely impacts COVID-19 patients seeking care for respiratory illness, it impacts the majority

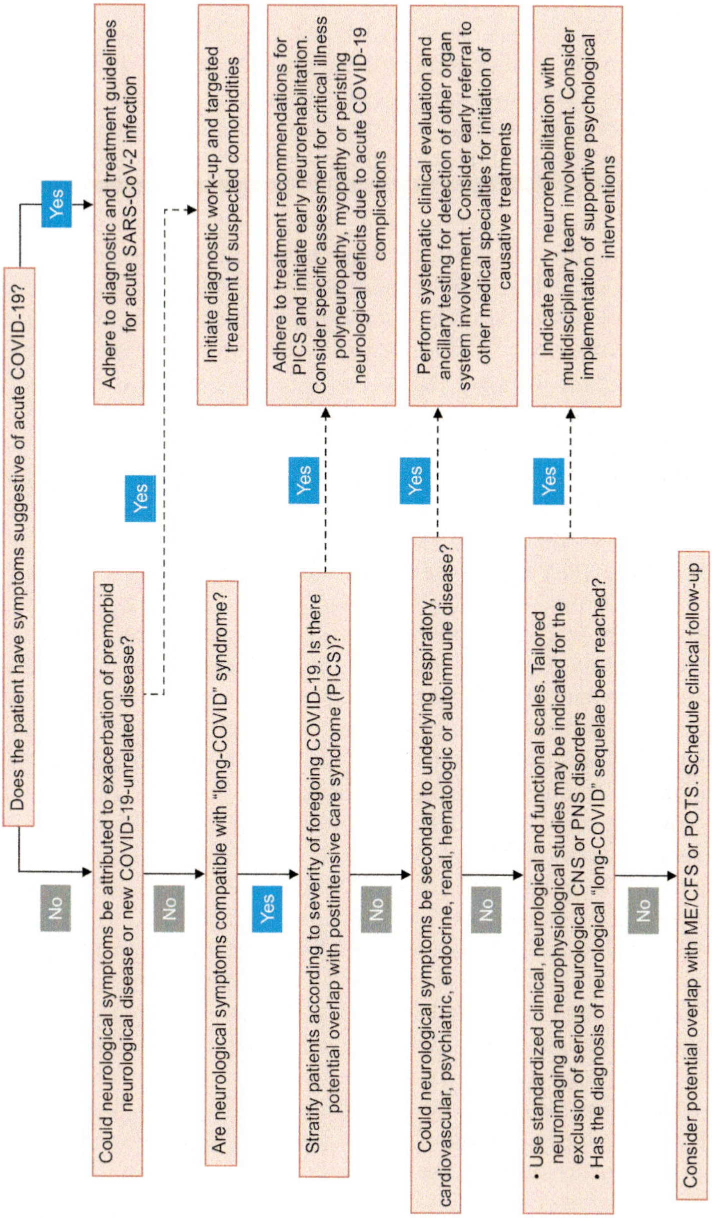

FLOWCHART 1: Proposed long-COVID diagnostic and treatment algorithm.[20]

of critically ill COVID-19 patients with ARDS or acute respiratory distress syndrome.[29] Importantly, the distinction between altered mental status as a result of encephalopathy caused by systemic illness or as a result of encephalitis directly caused by the SARS-CoV-2 virus itself must be made.

There are three broad classifications of COVID-related encephalitis/encephalopathy: (1) viral encephalitis which is caused by the direct viral infection of the CNS system, (2) encephalopathy caused by systemic inflammation (cytokine storm) precedes the neurological symptoms, and (3) autoimmune encephalitis that presents after a certain period of time after the COVID-19 infection and meets certain diagnostic criteria for "possible autoimmune encephalitis".[31] The classification of encephalitis and encephalopathy can be aided by the detection of certain cytokines and chemokines in the CSF in encephalitis and/or in the serum in encephalopathy, and a lumbar puncture can help in the diagnosis of encephalitis involvement.[30,31] The overproduction of inflammatory cytokines (IL-2R, IL-6, IL-8, IL-10, and TNF-α) appears to decrease the integrity of the blood–brain barrier (BBB), increasing the susceptibility of a COVID-19 infection. Additionally, higher levels of IL-6 were associated with auto-NMDA-R encephalitis.[32] Another paper reported that neuro-COVID patients presented with elevated levels of IL-6, IL-8, and IL-18 in both serum and CSF, MCP1 in CSF only, and IL-10, IL-1RA, IP-10, MIG, and NfL in serum only.[33]

Interestingly, SARS-CoV-2 can also promote post-infectious neurological complications. These delayed effects can impact both the CNS and the PNS. In the CNS, an example includes acute necrotizing hemorrhagic encephalopathy.[12] The first case of acute necrotizing hemorrhagic encephalopathy was reported in a 58-year-old woman with a 3-day history of cough, fever, and altered mental status.[34] Though the CSF fluid showed no evidence of SARS-CoV-2, evidence of the acute necrotizing hemorrhagic encephalopathy could be observed via MR imaging.[34]

The inflammatory mediated mechanism of the SARS-CoV-2 virus is postulated to play a crucial role in the pathogenesis of autoimmune encephalitis.[32] Although still not clear, there are proposed associations between certain autoantibodies (such as ones against VGKC, Caspr2, LGI1, and NMDA-R) and autoimmune encephalitis.[35] There has also been some evidence against anti-NDMA-R antibodies and autoimmune encephalitis.[32,36]

The MRI findings associated with COVID-related encephalitis include white matter changes with hyperintensities and hemorrhagic lesions, although there have also been reported cases of having normal brain MRI imaging **(Figs. 3A to D)**.[35] It is also visible in MRI as altered cortical and subcortical T2/FLAIR signals.[28] Additionally, IVIG therapy, plasma exchange, and corticosteroid were reported to be beneficial in the treatment of COVID-19-related encephalitis.[30]

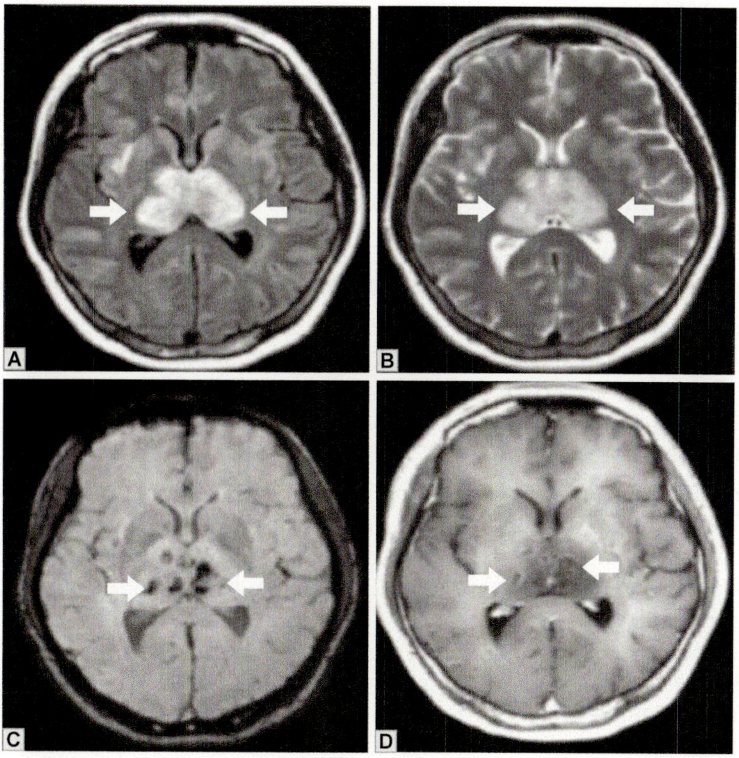

FIGURES 3A TO D: Magnetic resonance imaging (MRI) of COVID-19 positive 58-year-old female diagnosed with acute necrotizing hemorrhagic encephalopathy. (A) T2 FLAIR with bilateral thalamic hyperintensity. (B) T2 image depicting bilateral thalamic hyperintensity. (C) Evidence of bilateral thalamic hemorrhage. (D) T2 image with post contrast ring enhancement lesions.[12,34]

Cerebrovascular Disease or Stroke

Like other viruses, SARS-CoV-2 can also trigger acute cerebrovascular disease like acute and hemorrhagic stroke and cerebral venous sinus thrombosis.[37] The incidence of stroke ranges from 0.5 to 5% of hospitalized cases, with older age, comorbidities, and critical illness posing as risk factors.[38] A multinational observational study reported the risk to be slightly lower at 0.5% (pooled risk: 0.9%), with 79% ischemic stroke, 17% intracerebral/subarachnoid hemorrhage, and 4% cerebral sinus thrombosis.[39] Another study reported out of 1,916 patients who visited the emergency department or were hospitalized due to COVID-19, 1.6% of them experienced ischemic stroke. In comparison, only 0.2% of 1,486 patients with influenza developed ischemic stroke, emphasizing this considerable increase in risk associated with COVID-19.[40]

Although the exact mechanism remains unclear, critically-ill SARS-CoV-2 patients often show severe platelet reduction and elevated D-dimer levels which leave the patient more susceptible to acute cerebrovascular events.[41] SARS-CoV-2 can also promote cytokine storm syndromes, contributing to acute cerebrovascular disease.[41] SARS-CoV-2 can damage endothelial cells thus activating thrombotic pathways and leading to vascular complications in the brain.[11] The most common risk factors were hypertension, dyslipidemia, and diabetes mellitus. Ischemic stroke caused by COVID-19 was also reported to occur more in males.[42] Additionally, the average age of patients with COVID-19 who suffered from a stroke was slightly lower than those stroke patients who did not have COVID-19, although stroke was uncommon in patients <50 years, and was associated with a higher morbidity and mortality rate.[43]

Multiple Sclerosis

Multiple sclerosis (MS) is an autoimmune attack on the white matter of the central nervous system, which can be progressive in nature.[44] MS, like many other neurodegenerative disorders, often has a late presentation due to their slow progression, making it challenging to establish observable, causal relationships in epidemiological studies.[45] However, there may be an association between COVID-19 and neurodegenerative disorders, but further research is needed to understand this relationship.[15] A systematic review identified three cases of MS-like demyelination, aged 24, 28, and 29. In all three cases, the neurological symptoms followed 2–4 weeks after a mild COVID-19 infection. Two patients exhibited localized lesions in the brainstem, while the third presented primarily with unilateral optic neuritis. However, atypical patterns in all three cases pose challenges in classifying these as MS, as they could also indicate a post-viral demyelinating syndrome.[46] If an association does in fact exist between COVID-19 and MS, significant challenges may arise as treatments for MS typically involve immunotherapy, which may exacerbate the inflammatory damage of SARS-CoV-2.[47]

PERIPHERAL NERVOUS SYSTEM MANIFESTATIONS

Anosmia and Chemosensory Dysfunction

Anosmia and ageusia are increasingly common symptoms of COVID-19 and have become key diagnostic markers for COVID-19.[11] These symptoms are more prevalent among COVID-19 patients than for any cohort of influenza patients.[11] For instance, there have been reports that anosmia and hyposmia have a strong association with COVID-19 with risk ratio of 4.6 and other meta-analyses suggest that approximately 50% of patients who have COVID-19 develop symptoms of ageusia or dysgeusia in the acute phase.[48] Although symptoms of anosmia seem to recover in most patients, it is observed that this olfactory dysfunction persists longer than 12 months in approximately 7% of patients.[49] A systematic review and meta-analysis reported that older patients and symptoms of rhinorrhea and nasal congestion had a strong association with olfactory dysfunction, whereas sex, age, smoking, and comorbidity had no significant effect on chemosensory dysfunction.[50]

Although the exact mechanism of anosmia due to COVID-19 remains unclear, there have been proposed mechanisms such as the loss of conduction and delivery of odorants due to olfactory edema, injury to the olfactory epithelium, or injury to the olfactory bulb.[49] Additionally, the presence of ACE2 receptors in the tongue epithelial cells, buccal mucosa, and the oral cavity and its association in the regulation of taste perception, the oral cavity serves as a point of entry of the SARS-CoV-2 virus, leading to a localized infection and manifestation of dysgeusia.[51]

Guillain–Barré Syndrome

Guillain–Barré syndrome (GBS) is acute polyradiculopathy or immune attack on peripheral nerves characterized by rapidly progressive limb weakness, areflexia and can include facial weakness, as well. Though the incidence rate is not particularly high, there have been several patients who have been diagnosed with GBS and COVID-19.[11]

A cross-sectional study, which included 63 publications and represented all continents except Australia, reported 92 patients who presented with GBS and who tested positive for COVID-19.[52] The mean age of onset 55.2 ± 17.3 years and with a male preponderance with a M:F ratio of 1.6:1.[52] In all but three cases, GBS manifestations followed at a median time interval of 13 days after incidence of COVID-19 related respiratory and/or system symptoms, akin to the temporal pattern observed in other GBS cases following a viral infection, such as EBV, CMV, HEV, and influenza A.[52] The most common symptoms reported were lower limb weakness (57.6%), sensory symptoms (52.2%), and cranial nerve involvement (16.3%), which is similar to the general GBS population.[52] Respiratory failure related to the neuromuscular weakness as opposed to COVID-19 was observed in 32.1% of the reported patients in the study and 21.7% patients needed invasive ventilation.[52] Other factors such as frequent need for ICU stay and severity of disability outcomes suggest that COVID-19 could serve as a negative prognostic factor for GBS.[52]

Additionally, with the approval of 10 vaccines by the WHO, there have been 13.41 billion vaccine doses administered across the world with 70.1% of the world population having received at least one COVID-19 vaccine.[53] Inadvertently, there have been cases reporting the incidence of neurological manifestations as a result of the COVID-19 vaccine administration. A study, published in 2022, stated 51 individuals who developed neurological complications, with GBS being the most common PNS manifestation ($n = 14$, 27%). The majority of these occurred in males (71%) and aged 50 years or older (79%).[54]

OTHER COVID-19 RELATED NEUROLOGICAL MANIFESTATIONS

The overall presence of neurological symptoms is estimated to be 23%, and the high prevalence can contribute to the later recovery and longer hospital stays of COVID-19 patients.[55] In addition, there have been multiple neuropsychiatric issues such as depression, anxiety, delirium, paranoia, hallucination, suicidal trial, affect lability, and psychomotor agitation, with depression (41.5%) and anxiety (20.85%) being the most common symptoms of those reported cases.[55]

There have also been other neurodegenerative disorders, other than the aforementioned disorders. The prevalence of Parkinson's disease was reported to be around 5%, with an increased hospitalization and mortality rate at 49% and 12% respectively.[56] Moreover, COVID-19 appears to be attributed to a higher risk of Alzheimer's as well.[45,57] However, more research needs to be done to completely elucidate the relationship between COVID-19 and Parkinson's disease and Alzheimer's disease.

Long-term intensive care of critically-ill patients requiring mechanical ventilation, etc. can cause related neurological manifestations.[29] These symptoms are not necessarily directly induced by the disease, but instead are a byproduct of therapy. Some manifestations include an agitated confusional state (delirium) which occurs in >80% of patients on mechanical ventilators in ICUs.[29] Patients treated with heavy doses of sedatives and paralytic agents, like those with ARDS, are also at high risk of delirium.[29]

POTENTIAL SARS-CoV-2 MECHANISM OF NERVOUS SYSTEM INVASION

To date, including SARS-CoV-2, there have been seven known coronaviruses that have infected humans. Of these zoonotic viruses, three have caused severe widespread illness: severe acute respiratory syndrome coronavirus (SARS-CoV), Middle East respiratory syndrome coronavirus (MERS-CoV), and most recently SARS-CoV-2 or COVID-19.[21] Characterized as a beta coronavirus, SARS-CoV-2 shares almost 80% sequence identity with SARS-CoV and MERS-CoV.[8] Similar to SARS-CoV, it acts by binding to the enzymatic domain of the ACE-2 (angiotensin-converting enzyme 2) receptor on the surface of various cell types. Some include intestinal epithelial cells, alveolar cells, endothelial cells, kidney cells, neuroepithelial cells, and neurons.[8] Because of strong electrostatic differences between SARS-CoV-2 spike protein and the ACE-2 binding interface, there seems to be more powerful interactions between these two proteins than with SARS-CoV and ACE-2. This implies a potentially higher affinity for SARS-CoV-2.[8]

Importantly, since the onset of the pandemic, there have been several variants of concern (VOCs) that have differed in transmissibility, virulence, mechanism, and therapeutic/vaccine effectiveness.[58] The WHO has identified the following five VOCs: Alpha (B.1.1.7), reported in late December 2020,

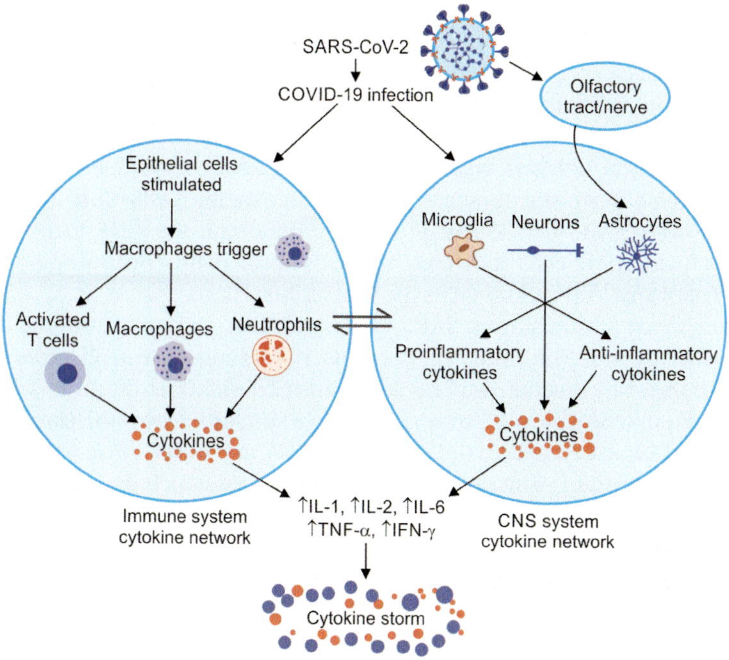

FIGURE 4: Potential modes of SARS-CoV-2 infection causing CNS damage. As seen above, coronavirus can (1) cause direct damage via infection through blood circulation and neuronal pathways, (2) attack the lung tissue promoting hypoxia, etc., and (3) enter through the olfactory nerve.

Source: Modified from Bhaskar S, Sinha A, Banach M, Mittoo S, Weissert R, Kass JS, et al. Cytokine storm in COVID-19-immunopathological mechanisms, clinical considerations, and therapeutic approaches: The REPROGRAM consortium position paper. Front Immunol. 2020;11:1648.[59] Creative Commons Attribution 4.0 International.

Beta (B.1.351), reported in December 2020, Gamma (P.1), reported in early January 2021, Delta (B.1.617.2), reported in December 2020, and Omicron (B.1.1.529), reported in November 2021.[58]

To date, there have been several theories for potential neuroinvasion of SARS-CoV-2. Despite the multiple barriers protecting the CNS, some viruses can still infiltrate the system **(Fig. 4)**. In most cases, viral infections begin with the peripheral tissues moving into the peripheral nerves and subsequently creeping into the central nervous system. In the case of SARS-CoV-2, the existence of olfactory dysfunction as a symptom also indicates potential involvement of the cranial nerves and olfactory system.[8] In one study analyzing autopsy materials from 33 patients with fatal cases of COVID-19, researchers mapped the viral infection through olfactory nervous tracts and CNS regions.[22] By measuring viral load using RT-qPCR in the olfactory mucosa, olfactory bulb, medulla oblongata, cerebellum, and other regions, scientists demonstrated that the greatest level of SARS-CoV-2 RNA was found in the olfactory mucosa beneath the cribriform plate.[22] Using this data, they concluded that one potential route of nervous system invasion is via the neuronal-mucosal interface in the olfactory mucosa.[22] After initial invasion and by taking advantage of close proximity to other relevant structures, SARS-CoV-2 can penetrate other neuroanatomical areas.[22]

Growing evidence indicates that among the peripheral nerves, the olfactory nerve is one of the strongest candidates for SARS-CoV-2 integration into the central nervous system.[8] Because olfactory endothelial cells have many ACE-2 receptors, they are great candidates for SARS-CoV-2 binding. In this case, SARS-CoV-2 can potentially penetrate the CNS through the olfactory receptor cells that pass the cribriform plate contacting second-order neurons.[8] This is known as the transcribial route.

In a study administering SARS-CoV and MERS-CoV to transgenic mice, viral CNS invasion was noted via the transcribial route via the olfactory bulb. Though the exact mechanism of access to the CNS was not fully understood, it suggested that SARS-CoV-2 may also behave similarly.[8] With the transcribial route and olfactory nerve, the virus may also use other forms of entry to the nervous system. One option is the vagus nerve which has lung and gut afferents reaching the brainstem. This theory is supported by the fact that SARS-CoV-2 was detected in COVID-19 patient feces, and in an in vitro study, SARS-CoV-2 demonstrated the ability to infect human intestinal epithelium.[8] Further research to support this hypothesis must still be conducted.

Another potential source of nervous system invasion is via what is known as the hematogenous route. In this mechanism, the virus, having entered the bloodstream, will go on to invade various organs including the brain. Release into the blood may increase permeability of the blood–brain barrier thus increasing the viral entry to the brain and viral encephalitis.[41] This theory, however, is considered secondary to the olfactory nerve hypothesis as there is not as much evidence supporting the hypothesis that SARS-CoV-2 acts in this way.[41]

Because COVID-19 neurological manifestations are classified based on CNS and PNS symptoms, one study organized these laboratory findings and clinical symptoms into mild, moderate, and severe categories: NeuroCovid stage I, NeuroCovid stage II, and NeuroCovid stage III.[60] According to the study, in NeuroCovid stage I, the binding of SARS-CoV-2 to ACE-2 receptors is largely related to nasal and gustatory epithelial cells, where the cytokine storm stimulated by the virus remains low. In these cases, patients who experience anosmia and ageusia are often spontaneously cured without intervention.[60] NeuroCovid stage II indicates a stronger immune response with higher levels of cytokines which increase ferritin, C-reactive protein, and D-dimer levels. These molecules trigger a hypercoagulable state wherein the patient is left at higher risk for blood clot, or venous thrombosis following stroke.[60] This immune response may also lead to vasculitis in muscles or nerve damage.[60] Finally, in NeuroCovid stage III, the cytokine storm damages the blood–brain barrier and may cause entry of viral particles to the CSF.[60] This may result in encephalopathy and/or seizures.[60] Patients in this category typically exhibit high total peripheral vascular resistance and hypertension, both of which increase risk for intracranial hemorrhage **(Table 3)**.[60]

TABLE 3: NeuroCovid stages, inflammatory response and mechanism of brain infection.[60]

Stages	Ways of brain infection	Inflammatory response	Symptoms	Cerebrospinal fluid test	Nasopharyngeal swab test
NeuroCovid Stage I Mild or neuroinvasion	Olfactory nerve bloodstream	The cytokine storm is low and controlled	• Smell or taste impairments (cure without any interventions) • Mild or no respiratory symptoms	Positive	Positive
NeuroCovid Stage II Moderate or CNS clearance	Brainstem respiratory brain center	High levels of cytokines	• Large or small strokes (formation of blood clots, arterial occlusion or venous thrombosis) • Vasculitis in muscles fatigue • Hemiplegia • Sensory loss • Double vision • Tetraplegia, aphasia ataxia • Respiratory symptoms	Negative	Positive
NeuroCovid Stage III Severe or immune response	• Brain • Lungs nerves connection with brain	Extreme cytokine storm	• Edema • Brain injury • Delirium • Encephalopathy • Seizures • Intracranial hemorrhage • Hypertension • Confusion • Coma • Loss of consciousness • Severe respiratory symptoms	Positive/ Negative	Positive

57. Zhang H, Zhou Z. COVID-19 and the risk of Alzheimer's disease, amyotrophic lateral sclerosis, and multiple sclerosis. Ann Clin Transl Neurol. 2022;9(12):1953-61.
58. Aleem A, Akbar Samad AB, Vaqar S. (2023). Emerging Variants of SARS-CoV-2 and Novel Therapeutics Against Coronavirus (COVID-19). [online] Available from http://www.ncbi.nlm.nih.gov/books/NBK570580/. [Last accessed February, 2024]
59. Bhaskar S, Sinha A, Banach M, Mittoo S, Weissert R, Kass JS, et al. Cytokine storm in COVID-19-immunopathological mechanisms, clinical considerations, and therapeutic approaches: The REPROGRAM consortium position paper. Front Immunol. 2020;11:1648.
60. Hosseini N, Nadjafi S, Ashtary B. Overview of COVID-19 and neurological complications. Rev Neurosci. 2021;32(6):671-91.
61. Centers for Disease Control and Prevention. (2020). COVID-19 and Your Health. [online] Available from https://www.cdc.gov/coronavirus/2019-ncov/your-health/treatments-for-severe-illness.html. [Last accessed February, 2024]
62. Tejada Meza H, Lambea Gil Á, Sancho Saldaña A, Martínez-Zabaleta M, Garmendia Lopetegui E, López-Cancio Martínez E, et al. Impact of COVID-19 outbreak in reperfusion therapies of acute ischaemic stroke in northwest Spain. Eur J Neurol. 2020;27(12):2491-8.
63. Zhang T, Chen C, Xu X, Xu J, Yang K, Xu Y, et al. Impact of the COVID-19 pandemic and post-epidemic periods on the process of endovascular treatment for acute anterior circulation ischaemic stroke. BMC Neurol. 2021;21(1):238.
64. Yamamoto V, Bolanos JF, Fiallos J, Strand SE, Morris K, Shahrokhinia S, et al. COVID-19: review of a 21st century pandemic from etiology to neuro-psychiatric implications. J Alzheimer's Dis. 2020;77(2):459-504.
65. Armocida D, Palmieri M, Frati A, Santoro A, Pesce A. How SARS-CoV-2 can involve the central nervous system. A systematic analysis of literature of the department of human neurosciences of Sapienza University, Italy. J Clin Neurosci. 2020;79:231-6.
66. Livingston EH. Necessity of 2 doses of the Pfizer and Moderna COVID-19 vaccines. JAMA. 2021;325(9):898.
67. Song E, Zhang C, Israelow B, Lu-Culligan A, Prado AV, Skriabine S, et al. Neuroinvasion of SARS-CoV-2 in human and mouse brain. J Exp Med. 2021;218(3):e20202135.
68. Reyes MSS, Medina PMB. Environmental pollutant exposure can exacerbate COVID-19 neurologic symptoms. Med Hypotheses. 2020;144:110136.
69. Yin R, Feng W, Wang T, Chen G, Wu T, Chen D, et al. Concomitant neurological symptoms observed in a patient diagnosed with coronavirus disease 2019. J Med Virol. 2020;92(10):1782-4.
70. Wong SH, Teoh JYC, Leung CH, Wu WKK, Yip BHK, Wong MCS, et al. COVID-19 and public interest in face mask use. Am J Respir Crit Care Med. 2020;202(3):453-5.
71. Mao L, Jin H, Wang M, Hu Y, Chen S, He Q, et al. Neurologic Manifestations of Hospitalized Patients with Coronavirus Disease 2019 in Wuhan, China. JAMA Neurol. 2020;77(6):683-90.

CHAPTER 30

Myocarditis: COVID-19 and COVID-19 Vaccines

Rajesh Mohan

INTRODUCTION

Myocarditis is an inflammatory disease of the myocardium that results from a variety of causes, including viral infections, autoimmune diseases, drug reactions, and toxic exposures.[1-3] Inflammation can lead to necrosis and dysfunction of cardiac myocytes, resulting in symptoms such as chest pain, shortness of breath, fatigue, palpitations, and heart failure.[1] According to the World Health Organization (WHO) classification, myocarditis is defined as "an inflammatory disease of the myocardium diagnosed by established histological, immunological, and immunohistochemical criteria, in the absence of a conventional cardiac disease."[2]

Several studies have investigated the definition and diagnostic criteria for myocarditis. In a review article by Cooper et al., they proposed a clinical definition of myocarditis as "inflammation of the heart muscle that results from an immune response to an offending agent, with or without associated myocyte necrosis."[1] They emphasized the importance of histopathological evaluation of endomyocardial biopsy (EMB) specimens for the diagnosis of myocarditis.

Another study by Kindermann et al. investigated the diagnostic criteria for myocarditis based on clinical, histological, and immunohistochemical findings.[4] They proposed the Dallas criteria, which define myocarditis as "an inflammatory infiltrate of the myocardium with necrosis and/or degeneration of adjacent myocytes not typical of acute ischemia." The criteria include histological, immunohistochemical, and clinical criteria for the diagnosis of myocarditis.

In summary, myocardial inflammation is commonly induced by a viral illness. Typical signs and symptoms range from chest pain, fever, life-threatening congestive heart failure, arrhythmias, or even death.[5] Acute pericarditis is the most prevalent form of pericardial disease and usually manifests as substernal chest pain.[6] The immune response to a viral insult may result in myocarditis and pericarditis.[7]

Cardiac complications, particularly myocarditis and pericarditis, have been associated with SARS-CoV-2 (the virus that causes COVID-19) infection and mRNA COVID-19 vaccination.[8-13]

EPIDEMIOLOGY OF MYOCARDITIS DUE TO COVID-19

Myocarditis is a heterogeneous disease with a variety of symptoms ranging from mild chest discomfort to cardiogenic shock. As it often mimics other common disorders, such as coronary artery disease (CAD), diagnosis may be challenging.[14,15] Evidence based medicine (EBM) is the gold standard for establishing the diagnosis of myocarditis.[16,17] Cardiac magnetic resonance (CMR) is a suitable noninvasive alternative in establishing the diagnosis in patients suspected of having myocarditis.[17-19] Advances in imaging such as CMR and other diagnostic tools have assisted in establishing the diagnosis of myocarditis indicating that in the past this entity may have been underdiagnosed. This is demonstrated in discrepancies within the published data regarding the prevalence of myocarditis.[20]

Determining the true incidence of myocarditis is challenging, as the inflammation has a patchy nature, and the infrequent use of EMB because of the invasiveness of the proceedure.[16,17] In the appropriate clinical setting, CMR is a reasonable noninvasive alternative to EMB.[21] Within the last decade, the "Lake Louise Criteria (LLC)" for CMR was established and revised to assist in the diagnosis of myocarditis. The initial LLC evaluate the severity of edema visualized on T2 weighted imaging as well as the timing of early and late gadolinium enhancement. This algorithm achieves 67% sensitivity and 91% specificity in the diagnosis of myocarditis.[22] CMR can also provide data to assist in prognosis and assist to objectify the degree of resolution and identify potentially fatal complications.[23] Multiple studies have demonstrated the utility of employing CMR in patients with myocardial infarction and nonobstructive coronary artery disease (MINOCA).[24,25] Concurrent myocarditis occurs in 15–75% of patients with MINOCA.[26-31] Pasupathy et al. employing CMR demonstrated that 33% of patients with MINOCA had myocarditis.[32] A study in a referring hospital in Switzerland demonstrated that employing CMR imaging in patients presenting with MINOCA increased the overall incidence of myocarditis up to 6.2-fold.[24,25]

Observations during the first wave of the COVID-19 pandemic reported cardiac injury, defined by increased levels of troponin, in up to 30% of patients.[33-35]

Richardson et al. and others have demonstrated that troponin elevation in patients hospitalized with COVID-19 infection, is associated with significant morbidity and mortality.[33-38] Previous experience with other Coronaviruses such as middle east respiratory syndrome (MERS) has demonstrated myocarditis is a potential complication, a link between COVID-19 and myocarditis seemed rational.[39,40]

EPIDEMIOLOGY OF MYOCARDITIS DUE TO COVID-19 VACCINE

Gao et al. performed systematic review and meta-analysis were in order to find the association between SARS-CoV-2 MRNA vaccination and myocarditis or pericarditis. The investigator included 11 studies and a total of 58,620,611 subjects. The study demonstrated a statistically significant association between COVID-19 vaccination and the development of myocarditis or pericarditis.[41] These findings suggest that there is a potential risk of developing cardiac injury following COVID-19 vaccination. However, further research is needed to comprehend the underlying mechanisms and to assess the overall risk–benefit ratio of vaccination. These findings have important implications for public health authorities and healthcare providers in monitoring and managing potential adverse events associated with COVID-19 vaccination.[41]

In comparison to unvaccinated subjects, myocarditis or pericarditis in those following COVID-19 vaccines was 2.13-fold higher. Gao et al. demonstrated a statistically significant association between COVID-19 vaccination and myocarditis.[41]

People who received their first dose of a COVID-19 vaccine had a higher risk of developing myocarditis or pericarditis compared to those who did not get vaccinated.[41] The risk escalates after receiving the second dose. Specifically, in comparison to unvaccinated subjects, the risk was 1.33 times higher after the first dose and 2.93 times higher after the second dose.[41] When both doses were considered, the overall risk was 4.06 times higher. Furthermore, when looking at different types of vaccines, there was a significant link between myocarditis and pericarditis and the BNT162b2 and mRNA-1273 vaccines, as opposed to viral vector vaccines.[41]

Cho et al. conducted an observational study in over 44 million subjects who received at least 1 COVID-19 MRNA dose of COVID-19 vaccination which demonstrated that vaccination related myocarditis (VRM) occurred in 480 subjects.[42] Chest pain was the most common presenting symptom occurring at a median time of 3 days after vaccination. VRM occurred more frequently in males in general and more frequently in those 12–17 years of age. Severe VRM occurred in 95 cases of which 17.7% required intensive care unit admission. Fulminant myocarditis developed in 7.5% of these patients.[42] In those with severe VRM, 4.4% required extracorporeal membrane oxygenation therapy, with 21 (4.4%) deaths.[42] All subjects who developed sudden cardiac death were under the age of 45.[42]

PATHOPHYSIOLOGY OF MYOCARDITIS DUE TO COVID-19

The SARS-CoV-2 virus uses its spike (S) protein to bind and enter host cells.[43] The S protein has two subunits—S1 and S2. S1 helps bind the virus to host cells.[43] S2 protein is responsible for the fusion between the membranes of the virus and host cell.[43] S protein binds to the angiotensin-converting enzyme (ACE)-2 receptor on the host cells.[44] The SARS-CoV-2 virus enters the host cell once the virus binds to the cell and is able to fuse its membrane with the host cell.[45] The cell surface protein type 2 transmembrane serine protease (TMPRSS2) cleaves ACE-2 and mediates the fusion of the virus and host cell membranes.[46] Once viral entry into the host cell occurs viral replication, and immune response follow, resulting in tissue damage and the clinical manifestations of COVID-19.[43] Early iterations of COVID-19 typically presented as pneumonia with symptoms of fever, cough, and dyspnea.[47] However, it is now known that COVID-19 can cause cardiovascular complications, including myocarditis. Myocarditis due to COVID-19 myocarditis can manifest itself in a broad range from mild to severe. Myocarditis if left untreated may progress to heart failure, arrythmias, and death making it important for COVID-19 myocarditis to be recognized and treated.[48-50]

Myocarditis has been described as inflammation of the heart muscle, resulting in myocardial injury in the absence of ischemia.[51,52] Various viruses have been shown to cause myocarditis.[52-55] SARS-CoV-2 virus is a new addition to the long list of viruses causing myocarditis. The pathophysiology of viral myocarditis has primarily been shown to be due to direct cell injury and immune-mediated cell death.[51]

In patients with COVID-19, SARS-CoV-2 virus binds to the ACE2 protein and enters human cells. ACE2 protein receptors, in addition to epithelial cells (type II alveolar cells) of the respiratory tract, are also found on cardiomyocytes.[56-58] SARS-CoV-2 viral particles were shown to be present in the myocardium of a patient with COVID-19 using EMB.[59] In another study that had autopsies of 20 human heart samples of patients infected with SARS-CoV, a virus related to SARS-CoV2, viral particles with macrophage infiltration were present in seven of them.[60] Therefore, SARS-CoV-2 virus can also infect cardiomyocytes leading to viral myocarditis.[61] SARSCoV-2 can also infect endothelial cells in the heart and cause myocardial damage.[62,63] Presence of SARS-CoV-2 in endothelial cells of numerous organs, including the heart, under histology substantiates the direct cell injury hypothesis.[64,65] Fox et al. found an increased number of diffusely distributed CD68+ cells in the myocardium of patients with COVID-19, compared to control groups and those with typical myocarditis.[66] The difference in immune cells on histology suggested that the inflammatory process of COVID-19 myocarditis is distinct from typical viral myocarditis.[66] The inflammatory process in COVID-19 can be described by essentially two mechanisms. Infection of endothelial cells within coronary vessels by SARS-CoV-2 can cause the migration of macrophages to these areas, resulting in the activation of complement and apoptosis.[66] In addition, thrombus formation in the coronary vessels as a consequence of inflammation can result in ischemic myocardial injury.[66]

The COVID-19 myocarditis can also be a result of systemic inflammation. Interleukin-6 (IL-6) is a cytokine that has been shown to recruit inflammatory cells to the myocardium and has been implicated in the pathophysiology of myocarditis.[67] Systemic inflammation has been shown to activate platelets and cause high levels of clotting factors (including factor V and VIII) leading to thrombus formation within coronary vessels.[62,68] Systemic inflammation induced cytokine storm may cause more myocardial injury by worsening established myocarditis.[61] Increased oxygen demands seen in patients with COVID-19 pneumonia with associated hypoxia of the myocardium worsen myocardial injury.[69]

Myocarditis was identified in 7.2% of 277 postmortem cases as opposed to less than 2% of cases identified as with clinically significant myocarditis in a study by Hauschka et al.[70] In a study by Puntmann et al. using CMR, cardiac involvement was seen in 78% of the 100 patients who had recovered from severe COVID-19 with 60% showing ongoing inflammation.[71] Such studies indicate that the actual incidence and prevalence of myocarditis due to COVID-19 may be underestimated. Mortality in patients hospitalized with COVID-19 has been shown to be increased with myocardial involvement.[37]

Myocarditis has been associated with sudden cardiac death in athletes.[72] In a study of 1,597 competitive athletes with CMR after COVID-19 infection by Daniel et al. for the presence of COVID19-induced myocarditis, 37 (2.3%) were diagnosed with COVID-19 myocarditis, 28 of whom had subclinical myocarditis.[73] The study noted that if cardiac testing was done based upon cardiac symptoms alone then only 5 cases (0.6%) of COVID-19 myocarditis would have been detected.[73] In another study of competitive athletes who tested positive for COVID-19, 15% were identified by CMR to have myocarditis and 30.8% had myocardial damage.[74] These athletes were either asymptomatic or had mild symptoms and none required hospitalization or received COVID-19 specific antiviral therapy.

Cardiac magnetic resonance imaging evidence of myocarditis has been associated with major adverse cardiac events (MACE) including death, heart failure decompensation requiring hospital admission, heart transplantation, documented sustained ventricular arrhythmia, and recurrent acute myocarditis.[23]

Studies such as these indicate that COVID-19 associated myocarditis and the associated sequalae and risks are likely underestimated.[23,74]

PATHOPHYSIOLOGY OF MYOCARDITIS DUE TO COVID-19 VACCINE

The precise mechanisms linking COVID-19 vaccination to the occurrence of myocarditis or pericarditis remain uncertain. A reasonable working hypothesis suggests potential connections to the vaccine's active component, the mRNA sequence responsible for encoding the spike protein of the severe acute respiratory syndrome coronavirus 2 (SARS-CoV-2), or the subsequent immune response generated by vaccination.[75] One proposed mechanism is molecular mimicry, wherein there is an interaction between vaccine components and the individual's immune predisposition.[76,77] The COVID-19 vaccine prompts the production of the SARS-CoV-2 viral spike glycoprotein and triggers an adaptive immune response aimed at recognizing and eliminating the virus expressing this spike protein, namely, the SARS-CoV-2 virus itself. However, because of the similarity between antibodies targeting SARS-CoV-2 spike glycoproteins and those targeting myocardial alpha-myosin heavy chain, there is a possibility of an immune cross-reaction occurring, potentially leading to autoimmune diseases **(Fig. 1)**.[76,77]

Similar to other investigators, Gao et al. demonstrated that both BNT162b2 vaccine and mRNA-1273 vaccines were associated with an increased risk of VRM and pericarditis.[41,79-81] No increased risks were found in other types of COVID-19 vaccines.[10,82] Studies have shown that the risk of myocarditis is greater after mRNA vaccination than viral vector vaccination.[10,82] A possible pathogenic mechanism of mRNA vaccine-induced myocarditis may related to increases in cytokine synthesis and release.[83] The reason for this lies in

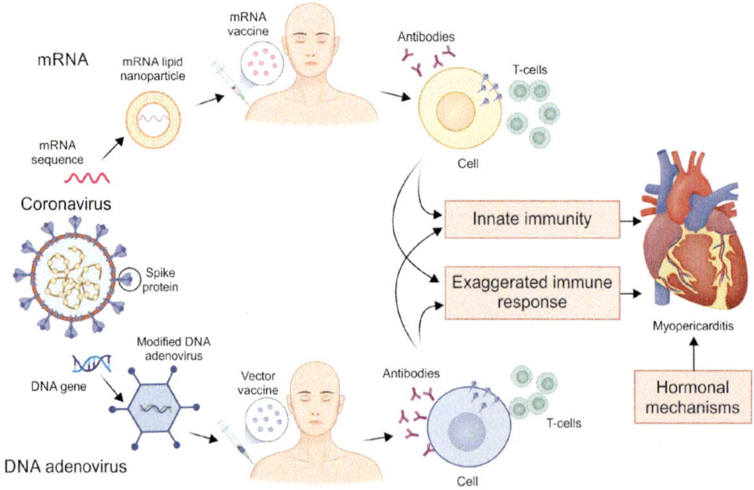

FIGURE 1: Potential mechanisms of COVID-19 vaccine induced myocarditis and pericarditis and activation of compliment cascade associated inflammatory response induced by lipid nanoparticles. Activation of adaptive immunity generating antispike protein antibodies which bind to myocardium either due to molecular mimicry or spike protein expressed on myocardium. Augmentation of the immune response by sex hormones or catecholamine release.[78]

Source:

1. Permission Creative Commons license 4.0.
2. Hromić-Jahjefendić A, Sezer A, Aljabali AAA, Serrano-Aroca Á, Tambuwala MM, Uversky VN, et al. COVID-19 Vaccines and Myocarditis: An Overview of Current Evidence. Biomedicines. 2023;11(5):1469.

the composition of mRNA vaccines, which incorporate an additive known as polyethylene glycol. This compound is primarily utilized to enhance the drug's water solubility but also has the capacity to trigger a more robust immune reaction.[84] While both the BNT162b2 and mRNA-1273 vaccines fall under the category of mRNA vaccines, they were assessed individually due to prior research indicating that mRNA-1273 was more commonly associated with myocarditis and pericarditis in younger individuals.[79,85] Gao et al. also showed a higher risk of myocarditis or pericarditis in those vaccinated with mRNA-1273 than in those vaccinated with BNT162b2.[41] Results from other studies corroborate this finding.[86,87] Younger patients particularly those <40 years of age seem to be more predisposed to VRM.[41] Previous studies have also suggested that myocarditis and pericarditis may be more likely to occur in younger people.[46,53]

A Canadian head-to-head study compared the two mRNA vaccines—BNT162b2 (Pfizer-BionTech Comirnaty) and mRNA-1273 (Moderna Spikevax). The study showed that in 18–29-year-old males who received a second dose of mRNA COVID-19 vaccine, attributable risk of myocarditis and/or pericarditis was found to be 5.69 times higher among mRNA-1273 recipients as compared to BNT162b2 recipients.[88] In the same group, Poisson regression modeling estimated that the risk of myocarditis and/or pericarditis was 4.72 times higher after mRNA-1723 compared to BNT162b2 vaccination.[88]

CLINICAL AND PATHOLOGICAL DIAGNOSIS OF VRM AND COVID-19 MYOCARDITIS

The clinical manifestations do not necessarily differ from VRM and COVID-19 and range from symptoms that are mild ranging from cough, fever, and dyspnea, although these symptoms may be due to acute COVID-19 rather than myocarditis.[48,49,89] Some patients may have additional symptoms of palpitations.[90-92] Patients may present with new-onset heart failure with no history of cardiovascular disease, hypotension, ECG changes with ST segment depression, bradyarrhythmias, and ventricular tachycardia which may lead to death as seen in fulminant myocarditis.[91-93]

Cardiac enzymes, troponin, and N-terminal pro-B-type natriuretic peptide (NT-pro-BNP) are known to be elevated in COVID-19 myocarditis.[94,95] Some patients with myocarditis may not have abnormal troponin. A normal troponin, therefore, does not rule out myocarditis.[89,96] The sensitivity for elevated troponin I levels in myocarditis is 34%.[97] Baseline levels of troponin I/T and NT-pro-BNP on admission of a patient with COVID-19 should be checked with subsequent tests to trend these tests.[61] Electrocardiogram (ECG) changes are nonspecific and are not diagnostic for myocarditis. They may include sinus tachycardia, which is most common, ST segment depression/elevation, tachyarrhythmia, bradyarrhythmia, and QT prolongation.[94,95] Cardiac magnetic resonance imaging is considered a noninvasive gold standard for diagnosing myocarditis (class I recommendation, level of evidence C in the 2012 ESC guidelines).[39,98] In 2018, consensus guidelines recommended the addition of T2-weighted cardiac MRI to the pre-existing LLC for the diagnosis of myocarditis.[99] The 2018 LLC showed better diagnostic performance than the original criteria owing to increased sensitivity.[100] Cardiac MRI continues to be underutilized in clinical practice due to in part difficulties in reimbursement of cardiac MRI associated costs, even though cost-effectiveness and value for the health-care system have been proven for various clinical indications.[101-103] It is also a prognostic marker for the increased risk of adverse cardiac outcomes in patients with myocarditis.[104]

Endomyocardial biopsy is considered the gold standard test to confirm the diagnosis of myocarditis since it can determine the nature of inflammation.[105] Samples from the biopsy sent for immunohistology and genomic analysis can confirm the diagnosis of COVID-19-induced myocarditis through the presence of SARS-CoV-2 RNA.[106] EMB samples have been interpreted using the Dallas criteria which described myocarditis as myocyte necrosis or damage associated with inflammatory infiltrates.[107]

The Dallas criteria have become more reliable with the addition of immunohistochemistry criteria.[62] Myocarditis using this criterion is defined as the presence of leukocytes ≥14/mm^2 with monocytes ≤4/mm^2 and CD3+ cells ≥7/mm^2 along with evidence of nonischemic necrosis under histology.[62]

CLINICAL AND PATHOLOGICAL DIAGNOSIS OF MYOCARDITIS DUE TO COVID-19 VACCINE

Successful clinical trials of mRNA-based vaccines demonstrating safety and efficacy led to their approval in December 2020 in the first year of the COVID-19 pandemic.[108,109] However, by March 2021, post-market safety surveillance systems in Israel, the United States, and other countries detected a disproportionate number of reports of myocarditis and/or pericarditis that had not been picked up during clinical trials.[110,111] The occurrence of myocarditis occurred rarely but the frequency was higher than expected during the week after mRNA vaccination, especially in younger age groups, in males, and after the second dose.[5,112-114] Reports from several countries also showed that mRNA-based COVID-19 vaccines may be associated with acute myocarditis.[12,75,112,114-116]

Although vaccination has been thought to possibly serve as a trigger for myocarditis, only the smallpox vaccine has previously been causally associated with myocarditis based on reports among US military personnel, with cases typically occurring 7–12 days after vaccination.[117]

In a study of mRNA-based COVID-19 vaccination in the US, symptom onset of myocarditis was within 7 days after vaccination for 947 reports of individuals who received the BNT162b2 vaccine and for 382 reports of individuals who received the mRNA-1273 vaccine.[13] In a Korean nationwide COVID-19 vaccination related myocarditis study, the median time from the vaccination to symptom onset was 3 days.[42] In both these studies, chest pain, pressure, or discomfort was the most common presenting symptom.[13,42] Troponin levels were elevated in 98% of the cases with myocarditis.[13] The electrocardiogram was abnormal in 72% of the cases with myocarditis.[13] In both the US and Korean studies, about 72% of the cases that received CMR had abnormal findings consistent with acute myocarditis.[42,112]

In the Korean study which was designed to mitigate underestimation despite which there were concerns of underreporting, VRM cases were identified, albeit rarely to have fulminant myocarditis, require intensive care unit admissions, extracorporeal membrane oxygenation (ECMO) and heart transplantation, and even lead to deaths.[42] In the same study, there were eight sudden cardiac deaths (SCDs) that were attributed to COVID-19 VRM in subjects aged under 45 years who received mRNA vaccination. In these SCD cases, VRM was not suspected as a clinical diagnosis or a cause of death before performing an autopsy.[42] In studies done in the US, there were no COVID-19 VRM associated deaths and appeared to have more favorable outcomes with less severity.[42,114] This was attributed to the use of Vaccine Adverse Event Reporting System (VAERS) in the US which is a passive reporting system that allows for underreporting or overreporting.[42,118]

Autopsies done on COVID-19 VRM cases by Schwab et al. showed patchy interstitial myocardial T-lymphocytic infiltration, predominantly of the CD4 positive subset, associated with mild myocyte damage. All cases showed a consisted phenotype that included focal interstitial lymphocytic myocardial infiltration, accompanied in some by demonstrable microfocal myocyte destruction; T-cell dominant infiltrate with CD4 positive T-cells outnumbering CD8 positive T cells; frequently associated with T-cell infiltration of epicardium and subepicardial fat tissue revealing a similar immune phenotype (CD4 >> CD8).[119] The authors concluded that autopsy findings in these cases indicated death due to acute arrhythmogenic cardiac failure.[119]

MANAGEMENT AND PROGNOSIS OF MYOCARDITIS DUE TO COVID-19 AND COVID-19 VACCINE

Cytokine storm as contributing pathway causing COVID-19 myocarditis has been shown to be mitigated by using steroids. The RECOVERY platform trial has shown that steroids help in reducing COVID-19 mortality.[120] Dexamethasone was found to decrease myocardial edema and improve systolic function in COVID-19 myocarditis.[121] Tocilizumab has been shown to reduce mortality in cases that have already been treated with steroids.[122-124] Hu et al. used a combination of glucocorticoid and intravenous immunoglobulin (IVIG) treatment to successfully treat COVID19 myocarditis.[125] IVIG showed a significant increase in survival rates in cases with life-threatening fulminant myocarditiis.[126] Nonsteroidal anti-inflammatory drugs (NSAIDs) have been shown to be potentially harmful and should be avoided in myocarditis.[127] NSAIDs neither affected all-cause mortality nor left ventricle function.[128] Moreover, none of the studies showed benefit of NSAIDs in myocarditis treatment.[3] Antibiotics in standard COVID care did not show any significant benefit and is unjustified.[129] Also, none of the antiviral agents used improved COVID survival.[130-132] Symptomatic treatment of COVID-19 patients with guideline directed medical therapy for heart failure, inotropic agents and mechanical support with intra-aortic balloon pump for cardiogenic shock may also be used in COVID-19 myocarditis patients.[3,96,105]

As per a study published in 2018 from the Multicenter Lombardy Registry, the overall incidence of combined in-hospital mortality and heart transplantations associated with myocarditis was 3.2%.[133] In a study published in 2022 of COVID-19 myocarditis cases, a higher mortality of 17% was reported.[134] A higher mortality ranging from 15.2 to 31.8% was reported in other COVID-19 myocarditis reviews.[94,135-137]

A recent study of COVID-19 VRM from October 2020 to January 2022 demonstrated that clinical course of mRNA related myocarditis appeared to be benign, although longer term follow-up data were limited.[138] In a study conducted between October 2020 and January 2022, Pillay et al. observed the clinical course of myocarditis related to mRNA COVID-19 vaccines appeared to be mild, although there was a lack of long-term follow-up data available.[138] Oster et al. evaluating the VAERS data found that the initial evaluation and treatment for COVID-19 vaccine-associated myocarditis were similar to typical myocarditis cases.[13] Treatment primarily involved supportive care, with additional cardiac or intensive care measures when necessary. Among those for whom treatment data was available, 87% received nonsteroidal anti-inflammatory drugs, while 12% received intravenous immunoglobulin and another 12% received glucocorticoids for myocarditis.[3,139-141]

According to guidelines from the American Heart Association and the American College of Cardiology, patients with myocarditis should avoid competitive sports for a period of 3–6 months. Before resuming sports, it is recommended to have documentation of a normal electrocardiogram result, ambulatory rhythm monitoring, and an exercise test. Cardiac magnetic resonance imaging (CMR) can be valuable in assessing the progression or resolution of myocarditis, particularly in individuals with baseline CMR abnormalities.[142]

The Centers for Disease Control and Prevention (CDC) advise deferring further doses of mRNA-based COVID-19 vaccines in most cases but considering them in specific circumstances.[143]

PERSPECTIVE

A higher risk of myocarditis and its sequalae is associated with COVID-19 mRNA vaccination compared to unvaccinated people. This risk is more pronounced in males younger than 40 years of age.[41] No such increase in risk was seen in viral vector vaccines for COVID-19.[41] However, there is some controversy that myocarditis or pericarditis due to vaccination has been shown to be less than in individuals infected with COVID-19.[144,145] Therefore, the quest for safer vaccines and properly controlled trials with inert placebos should be pursued to create better and safer vaccines including alternatives to mRNA.

Underreporting of myocarditis cases continues to be a challenge. As stated by Oster et al. in their study and others, VAERS is a passive reporting system subject to reporting bias and, given the high verification rate of reports of myocarditis to VAERS after mRNA based COVID-19 vaccination, underreporting is more likely. Actual rates of myocarditis per million doses of vaccine are likely higher than estimated.[13,42] Underreporting apparently may also be due to a high proportion of subclinical cases that would not normally be detected outside research studies.[73,146] Many cases of VRM myocarditis have likely been diagnosed in physician offices or not at all, and not captured in the data.[88] All SCDs in a Korean nationwide study were seen in subjects aged under 45 years within a week after receiving mRNA COVID-19 vaccine in whom VRM was not suspected as a clinical diagnosis or cause of death before performing an autopsy.[42] SCD has also been associated with mRNA based COVID-19 VRM on autopsy findings performed on individuals who died unexpectedly with 20 days of receiving mRNA COVID-19 vaccination.[119] SCD is likely a potential fatal complication mainly in males under 45 years of age who receive mRNA COVID-19 vaccine.[42]

Currently, long-term consequences of myocarditis due to COVID-19 and COVID-19 vaccines especially the mRNA-based vaccines are not clearly known. Cardiac MRI the gold standard should be the standard of care in places with availability in the diagnosis and follow-up of patients with myocarditis.[39]

REFERENCES

1. Cooper LT Jr, Keren A, Sliwa K, Matsumori A, Mensah GA. The Global Burden of Myocarditis: Part 1: A Systematic Literature Review for the Global Burden of Diseases, Injuries, and Risk Factors 2010 Study. Glob Heart. 2014;9(1):121-9.
2. World Health Organization. International Classification of Diseases (ICD), 11th revision. [online] Available from https://icd.who.int/browse11/l-m/en#/http://id.who.int/icd/entity/328460032. [Last accessed February, 2024]
3. Caforio ALP, Pankuweit S, Arbustini E, Basso C, Gimeno-Blanes J, Felix SB, et al. Current state of knowledge on aetiology, diagnosis, management, and therapy of myocarditis: a position statement of the European Society of Cardiology Working Group on Myocardial and Pericardial Diseases. Eur Heart J. 2013;34(33):2636-48.
4. Kindermann I, Barth C, Mahfoud F, Ukena C, Lenski M, Yilmaz A, et al. Update on myocarditis. J Am Coll Cardiol. 2012;59(9):779-92.
5. Rosner CM, Genovese L, Tehrani BN, Atkins M, Bakhshi H, Chaudhri S, et al. Myocarditis temporally associated with COVID-19 vaccination. Circulation. 2021;144(6):502-5.
6. Vecchie A, Chiabrando JG, Dell MS, Bonaventura A, Mauro AG, Wohlford G, et al. Clinical presentation and outcomes of acute pericarditis in a Large Urban Hospital in the United States of America. Chest. 2020;158(6):2556-67.

7. Brucato A, Valenti A, Maisch B. Acute and recurrent pericarditis: still idiopathic? J Am Coll Cardiol. 2017;69(22):2775.
8. Boehmer TK, Kompaniyets L, Lavery AM, Hsu J, Ko JY, Yusuf H, et al. Association between COVID-19 and myocarditis using hospital-based administrative data — United States, March 2020–January 2021. MMWR Morb Mortal Wkly Rep. 2021;70:1228-32.
9. Barda N, Dagan N, Ben-Shlomo Y, Kepten E, Waxman J, Ohana R, et al. Safety of the BNT162b2 mRNA Covid-19 vaccine in a nationwide setting. N Engl J Med. 2021;385:1078-90.
10. Patone M, Mei XW, Handunnetthi L, Dixon S, Zaccardi F, Shankar-Hari M, et al. Risks of myocarditis, pericarditis, and cardiac arrhythmias associated with COVID-19 vaccination or SARS-CoV-2 infection. Nat Med. 2022;28:410-22.
11. Block JP, Boehmer TK, Forrest CB, Carton TW, Lee GM, Ajani UA, et al. Cardiac Complications after SARS-CoV-2 Infection and mRNA COVID-19 Vaccination—PCORnet, United States, January 2021–January 2022. MMWR Morb Mortal Wkly Rep. 2022;71:517-23.
12. Witberg G, Barda N, Hoss S, Richter I, Wiessman M, Aviv Y, et al. Myocarditis after Covid-19 vaccination in a large health care organization. N Engl J Med. 2021;385: 2132-9.
13. Oster ME, Shay DK, Su JR, Gee J, Creech CB, Broder KR, et al. Myocarditis cases reported after mRNA-based COVID-19 vaccination in the US from December 2020 to August 2021. JAMA 2022;327:331-40.
14. Golpour A, Patriki D, Hanson PJ, McManus B, Heidecker B. Epidemiological Impact of Myocarditis. J Clin Med. 2021;10(4):603.
15. Sagar S, Liu PP, Cooper LT Jr. Myocarditis. Lancet. 2012;379:738-47.
16. Cooper LT, Baughman KL, Feldman AM, Frustaci A, Jessup M, Kuhl U, et al. The role of endomyocardial biopsy in the management of cardiovascular disease: A scientific statement from the American Heart Association, the American College of Cardiology, and the European Society of Cardiology Endorsed by the Heart Failure Society of America and the Heart Failure Association of the European Society of Cardiology. Eur Heart J. 2007;28:3076-93.
17. Bozkurt B, Colvin M, Cook J, Cooper LT, Deswal A, Fonarow GC, et al. Current diagnostic and treatment strategies for specific dilated cardiomyopathies: A scientific statement from the American Heart Association. Circulation. 2016;134:e579-e646.
18. Shanes J, Ghali J, Billingham M, Ferrans V, Fenoglio J, Edwards W, et al. Interobserver variability in the pathologic interpretation of endomyocardial biopsy results. Circulation. 1987;75:401-5.
19. Hauck AJ, Kearney DL, Edwards WD. Evaluation of Postmortem Endomyocardial Biopsy Specimens from 38 Patients with Lymphocytic Myocarditis: Implications for Role of Sampling Error. Mayo Clin Proc. 1989;64(10):1235-45.
20. Pollack A, Kontorovich AR, Fuster V, Dec GW. Viral myocarditis—diagnosis, treatment options, and current controversies. Nat Rev Cardiol. 2015;12:670.
21. Members WC, Hundley WG, Bluemke DA, Finn JP, Flamm SD, Fogel MA, et al. ACCF/ACR/AHA/NASCI/SCMR 2010 expert consensus document on cardiovascular magnetic resonance: A report of the American College of Cardiology Foundation Task Force on Expert Consensus Documents. Circulation. 2010;121:2462-508.
22. Friedrich MG, Sechtem U, Schulz-Menger J, Holmvang G, Alakija P, Cooper LT, et al. Cardiovascular magnetic resonance in myocarditis: A JACC White Paper. J Am Coll Cardiol. 2009;53:1475-87.
23. Gräni C, Eichhorn C, Bière L, Murthy VL, Agarwal V, Kaneko K, et al. Prognostic value of cardiac magnetic resonance tissue characterization in risk stratifying patients with suspected myocarditis. J Am Coll Cardiol. 2017;70:1964-76.

24. Heidecker B, Ruedi G, Baltensperger N, Gresser E, Kottwitz J, Berg J, et al. Systematic use of cardiac magnetic resonance imaging in MINOCA led to a five-fold increase in the detection rate of myocarditis: A retrospective study. Swiss Med Wkly. 2019;149:w20098.
25. Patriki D, Gresser E, Manka R, Emmert MY, Lüscher TF, Heidecker B. Approximation of the incidence of myocarditis by systematic screening with cardiac magnetic resonance imaging. JACC Heart Fail. 2018;6:573-9.
26. Gerbaud E, Harcaut E, Coste P, Erickson M, Lederlin M, Labèque JN, et al. Cardiac magnetic resonance imaging for the diagnosis of patients presenting with chest pain, raised troponin, and unobstructed coronary arteries. Int J Cardiovasc Imaging. 2012;28:783-94.
27. Mahmoudi M, Harden S, Abid N, Peebles C, Nicholas Z, Jones T, et al. Troponin-positive chest pain with unobstructed coronary arteries: Definitive differential diagnosis using cardiac MRI. Br J Radiol. 2012;85:e461-6.
28. Panovský R, Borová J, Pleva M, Feitová V, Novotný P, Kincl V, et al. The unique value of cardiovascular magnetic resonance in patients with suspected acute coronary syndrome and culprit-free coronary angiograms. BMC Cardiovasc Disord. 2017;17:170.
29. Assomull RG, Lyne JC, Keenan N, Gulati A, Bunce NH, Davies SW, et al. The role of cardiovascular magnetic resonance in patients presenting with chest pain, raised troponin, and unobstructed coronary arteries. Eur Heart J. 2007;28:1242-9.
30. Kawecki D, Morawiec B, Monney P, Pellaton C, Wojciechowska C, Jojko J, et al. Diagnostic contribution of cardiac magnetic resonance in patients with acute coronary syndrome and culprit-free angiograms. Med Sci Monit. 2015;21:171-80.
31. Leurent G, Langella B, Fougerou C, Lentz PA, Larralde A, Bedossa M, et al. Diagnostic contributions of cardiac magnetic resonance imaging in patients presenting with elevated troponin, acute chest pain syndrome and unobstructed coronary arteries. Arch Cardiovasc Dis. 2011;104:161-70.
32. Pasupathy S, Air T, Dreyer RP, Tavella R, Beltrame JF. Systematic review of patients presenting with suspected myocardial infarction and nonobstructive coronary arteries. Circulation. 2015;131:861-70.
33. Huang C, Wang Y, Li X, Ren L, Zhao J, Hu Y, et al. Clinical features of patients infected with 2019 novel coronavirus in Wuhan, China. Lancet. 2020;395:497-506.
34. Zhou F, Yu T, Du R, Fan G, Liu Y, Liu Z, et al. Clinical course and risk factors for mortality of adult inpatients with COVID-19 in Wuhan, China: A retrospective cohort study. Lancet. 2020;395:1054-62.
35. Wang D, Hu B, Hu C, Zhu F, Liu X, Zhang J, et al. Clinical characteristics of 138 hospitalized patients with 2019 novel coronavirus–infected pneumonia in Wuhan, China. JAMA. 2020;323:1061-9.
36. Richardson S, Hirsch JS, Narasimhan M, Crawford JM, McGinn T, Davidson KW. The Northwell COVID-19 Research Consortium. Presenting Characteristics, Comorbidities, and Outcomes among 5700 Patients Hospitalized with COVID-19 in the New York City Area. JAMA. 2020;323:2052-9.
37. Shi S, Qin M, Shen B, Cai Y, Liu T, Yang F, et al. Association of cardiac injury with mortality in hospitalized patients with COVID-19 in Wuhan, China. JAMA Cardiol. 2020;5:802-10.
38. Arentz M, Yim E, Klaff L, Lokhandwala S, Riedo FX, Chong M, et al. Characteristics and Outcomes of 21 Critically Ill Patients with COVID-19 in Washington State. JAMA. 2020;323:1612-4.
39. Tschöpe C, Ammirati E, Bozkurt B, Caforio AL, Cooper LT, Felix SB, et al. Myocarditis and inflammatory cardiomyopathy: Current evidence and future directions. Nat Rev Cardiol. 2021;18(3):169-93.
40. Alhogbani T. Acute myocarditis associated with novel Middle east respiratory syndrome coronavirus. Ann Saudi Med. 2016;36:78-80.

41. Gao J, Feng L, Li Y, Lowe S, Guo Z, Bentley R, et al. A Systematic Review and Meta-analysis of the Association between SARS-CoV-2 Vaccination and Myocarditis or Pericarditis. Am J Prev Med. 2023;64(2):275-84.
42. Cho JY, Kim KH, Lee N, Cho SH, Kim SY, Kim EK, et al. COVID-19 vaccination-related myocarditis: a Korean nationwide study. Eur Heart J. 2023;44(24):2234-43.
43. Parasher A. COVID-19: current understanding of its pathophysiology, clinical presentation and treatment. Postgrad Med J. 2021;97(1147):312-20.
44. Li W, Moore MJ, Vasilieva N, Sui J, Wong SK, Berne MA, et al. Angiotensin-converting enzyme 2 is a functional receptor for the SARS coronavirus. Nature. 2003;426(6965): 450-4.
45. Belouzard S, Millet JK, Licitra BN, Whittaker GR. Mechanisms of coronavirus cell entry mediated by the viral spike protein. Viruses. 2012;4(6):1011-33.
46. Wiersinga WJ, Rhodes A, Cheng AC, Peacock SJ, Prescott HC. Pathophysiology, transmission, diagnosis, and treatment of coronavirus disease 2019 (COVID-19): a review. JAMA. 2020;324(8):782-93.
47. Mele D, Flamigni F, Rapezzi C, Ferrari R. Myocarditis in COVID-19 patients: current problems. Intern Emerg Med. 2021;16(5):1123-9.
48. Marcinkiewicz K, Petryka-Mazurkiewicz J, Nowicki M, et al. Acute heart failure in the course of fulminant myocarditis requiring mechanical circulatory support in a healthy young patient after coronavirus disease 2019. Kardiol Pol. 2021;79(5):583-4.
49. Inciardi RM, Lupi L, Zaccone G, Italia L, Raffo M, Tomasoni D, et al. Cardiac involvement in a patient with coronavirus disease 2019 (COVID-19). JAMA Cardiol. 2020;5(7): 819-24.
50. Pascariello G, Cimino G, Calvi E, Bernardi N, Grigolato M, Garyfallidis P, et al. Cardiogenic shock due to COVID-19-related myocarditis in a 19-year-old autistic patient. J Med Cases. 2020;11(7):207-10.
51. Cooper LT Jr. Myocarditis. N Engl J Med. 2009;360(15):1526-38.
52. Baboonian C, Treasure T. Meta-analysis of the association of enteroviruses with human heart disease. Heart. 1997;78(6):539-43.
53. Caforio ALP, Calabrese F, Angelini A, Tona F, Vinci A, Bottaro S, et al. A prospective study of biopsy-proven myocarditis: prognostic relevance of clinical and aetiopathogenetic features at diagnosis. Eur Heart J. 2007;28(11):1326-33.
54. Agrawal AS, Garron T, Tao X, Peng BH, Wakamiya M, Chan TS, et al. Generation of a transgenic mouse model of Middle East respiratory syndrome coronavirus infection and disease. J Virol. 2015;89(7):3659-70.
55. Esfandiarei M, McManus BM. Molecular biology and pathogenesis of viral myocarditis. Annu Rev Pathol. 2008;3(1):127-55.
56. Qian Z, Travanty EA, Oko L, Edeen K, Berglund A, Wang J, et al. Innate immune response of human alveolar type II cells infected with severe acute respiratory syndrome-coronavirus. Am J Respir Cell Mol Biol. 2013;48(6):742-8.
57. Goulter AB, Goddard MJ, Allen JC, Clark KL. ACE2 gene expression is up-regulated in the human failing heart. BMC Med. 2004;2:19.
58. Sharma YP, Agstam S, Yadav A, Gupta A, Gupta A. Cardiovascular manifestations of COVID-19: an evidence-based narrative review. Indian J Med Res. 2021;153(1-2):7-16.
59. Tavazzi G, Pellegrini C, Maurelli M, Belliato M, Sciutti F, Bottazzi A, et al. Myocardial localization of coronavirus in COVID-19 cardiogenic shock. Eur J Heart Fail. 2020;22(5): 911-5.
60. Oudit GY, Kassiri Z, Jiang C, Liu PP, Poutanen SM, Penninger JM, et al. SARS-coronavirus modulation of myocardial ACE2 expression and inflammation in patients with SARS. Eur J Clin Invest. 2009;39(7):618-25.

61. Siripanthong B, Nazarian S, Muser D, Deo R, Santangeli P, Khanji MY, et al. Recognizing COVID19-related myocarditis: the possible pathophysiology and proposed guidelines for diagnosis and management. Heart Rhythm. 2020;17(9):1463-71.
62. Kawakami R, Sakamoto A, Kawai K, Gianatti A, Pellegrini D, Nasr A, et al. Pathological evidence for SARS-CoV-2 as a cause of myocarditis: JACC review topic of the week. J Am Coll Cardiol. 2021;77(3):314-25.
63. Ali M, Shiwani HA, Elfaki MY, Hamid M, Pharithi R, Kamgang R, et al. COVID-19 and myocarditis: a review of literature. Egypt Heart J. 2022;74(1):23.
64. Fox SE, Li G, Akmatbekov A, Harbert JL, Lameira FS, Brown JQ, et al. Unexpected features of cardiac pathology in COVID-19 infection. Circulation. 2020;142(11):1123-5.
65. Varga Z, Flammer AJ, Steiger P, Haberecker M, Andermatt R, Zinkernagel AS, et al. Endothelial cell infection and endotheliitis in COVID-19. Lancet. 2020;395(10234): 1417-8.
66. Fox SE, Falgout L, vandar Heide RS. COVID-19 myocarditis: quantitative analysis of the inflammatory infiltrate and a proposed mechanism. Cardiovasc Pathol. 2021;54: 107361.
67. Lee DW, Gardner R, Porter DL, Louis CU, Ahmed N, Jensen M, et al. Current concepts in the diagnosis and management of cytokine release syndrome. Blood. 2014;124(2): 188-95.
68. Talasaz AH, Sadeghipour P, Kakavand H, Aghakouchakzadeh M, Kordzadeh-Kermani E, Van Tassell BW, et al. Recent randomized trials of antithrombotic therapy for patients with COVID-19: JACC state-of-the-art review. J Am Coll Cardiol. 2021;77(15):1903-21.
69. Guzik TJ, Mohiddin SA, DiMarco A, Patel V, Savvatis K, Marelli-Berg FM, et al. COVID-19 and the cardiovascular system: implications for risk assessment, diagnosis, and treatment options. Cardiovasc Res. 2020;116(10):1666-87.
70. Hauschka MK, Vandar Heide RS. Myocarditis is rare in COVID-19 autopsies: cardiovascular findings across 277 postmortem examinations. Cardiovasc Pathol. 2021;50:107300.
71. Puntmann VO, Carerj ML, Wieters I, Fahim M, Arendt C, Hoffmann J, et al. Outcomes of cardiovascular nuclear magnetic resonance imaging in patients recently recovered from coronavirus disease 2019 (COVID-19). JAMA Cardiol. 2019;5(11):1265-73.
72. Maron BJ, Udelson JE, Bonow RO, Nishimura RA, Ackerman MJ, Estes NA 3rd, et al. Eligibility and disqualification recommendations for competitive athletes with cardiovascular abnormalities: task force 3: hypertrophic cardiomyopathy, arrhythmogenic right ventricular cardiomyopathy and other cardiomyopathies, and myocarditis: a scientific statement from the American Heart Association and American College of Cardiology. Circulation. 2015;132(22):e273-80.
73. Daniels CJ, Rajpal S, Greenshields JT, Rosenthal GL, Chung EH, Terrin M, et al. Prevalence of clinical and subclinical myocarditis in competitive athletes with recent SARS-CoV-2 infection. JAMA Cardiol. 2021;6(9):1078-87.
74. Rajpal S, Tong MS, Borchers J, Zareba KM, Obarski TP, Simonetti OP, et al. Cardiovascular magnetic resonance findings in competitive athletes recovering from COVID-19 infection. JAMA Cardiol. 2021;6(1):116-8.
75. Mevorach D, Anis E, Cedar N, Bromberg M, Haas EJ, Nadir E, et al. Myocarditis after BNT162b2 mRNA vaccine against Covid-19 in Israel. N Engl J Med. 2021;385(23):2140-9.
76. Fatima M, Ahmad Cheema H, Ahmed Khan MH, Shahid H, Saad Ali M, Hassan U, et al. Development of myocarditis and pericarditis after COVID-19 vaccination in adult population: a systematic review. Ann Med Surg (Lond). 2022;76:103486.
77. de Gregorio C, Calcaterra G, Kounis NG, Bassareo PP, Mehta JL. Cerebral venous thrombosis after COVID-19 vaccines: do we know the mechanism? Lancet Reg Health Eur. 2022;16:100387.

78. Hromić-Jahjefendić A, Sezer A, Aljabali AAA, Serrano-Aroca Á, Tambuwala MM, Uversky VN, et al. COVID-19 Vaccines and Myocarditis: An Overview of Current Evidence. Biomedicines. 2023;11(5):1469.
79. Yap J, Tham MY, Poh J, Toh D, Chan CL, Lim TW, et al. Pericarditis and myocarditis after COVID-19 mRNA vaccination in a nationwide setting. Ann Acad Med Singap. 2022;51(2):96-100.
80. Chelala L, Jeudy J, Hossain R, Rosenthal G, Pietris N, White CS. Cardiac MRI findings of myocarditis after COVID-19 mRNA vaccination in adolescents. Am J Roentgenol. 2022;218(4):651-7.
81. Chouchana L, Blet A, Al-Khalaf M, Kafil TS, Nair G, Robblee J, et al. Features of inflammatory heart reactions following mRNA COVID-19 vaccination at a global level. Clin Pharmacol Ther. 2022;111(3):605-13.
82. Gallo K, Goede A, Mura C, Abel R, Moahamed B, Preissner S, et al. A comparative analysis of COVID-19 vaccines based on over 580,000 cases from the vaccination adverse event reporting system. Vaccines. 2022;10(3):408.
83. Li C, Chen Y, Zhao Y, Lung DC, Ye Z, Song W, et al. Intravenous injection of coronavirus disease 2019 (COVID-19) mRNA vaccine can induce acute myopericarditis in mouse model [published correction appears in Clin Infect Dis.2021;73(12):2372-3]. Clin Infect Dis. 2022;74(11):1933-50.
84. Kounis NG, Koniari I, de Gregorio C, Velissaris D, Petalas K, Brinia A, et al. Allergic reactions to current available COVID-19 vaccinations: pathophysiology, causality, and therapeutic considerations. Vaccines (Basel). 2021;9(3):221.
85. Straus W, Urdaneta V, Esposito DB, Mansi JA, Sanz Rodriguez C, Burton P, et al. Analysis of myocarditis among 252 million mRNA-1273 recipients worldwide. Clin Infect Dis. 2023;76(3):e544-52.
86. Patone M, Mei XW, Handunnetthi L, Dixon S, Zaccardi F, Shankar-Hari M, et al. Risk of myocarditis following sequential COVID-19 vaccinations by age and sex. medRxiv. 2021; Preprint.
87. Husby A, Hansen JV, Fosbøl E, Thiesson EM, Madsen M, Thomsen RW, et al. SARS-CoV-2 vaccination and myocarditis or myopericarditis: population-based cohort study. BMJ. 2021;375:e068665.
88. Abraham N, Spruin S, Rossi T, Fireman B, Zafack J, Blaser C, et al. Myocarditis and/or pericarditis risk after mRNA COVID-19 vaccination: A Canadian head to head comparison of BNT162b2 and mRNA-1273 vaccines. Vaccine. 2022;40(32):4663-71.
89. Oleszak F, Maryniak A, Botti E, Abrahim C, Salifu MO, Youssef M, et al. Myocarditis associated with COVID-19. Am J Med Case Rep. 2020;8(12):498-502.
90. Das BB. SARS-CoV-2 myocarditis in a high school athlete after COVID-19 and its implications for clearance for sports. Children (Basel). 2021;8(6):427.
91. Gaine S, Devitt P, Coughlan JJ, Pearson I. COVID-19-associated myocarditis presenting as new-onset heart failure and atrial fibrillation. BMJ Case Rep. 2021;14(7):e244027.
92. Kociol RD, Cooper LT, Fang JC, et al. Recognition and initial management of fulminant myocarditis. Circulation. 2020;141(6):e69-e92.
93. Wang Z, Wang Y, Lin H, Wang S, Cai X, Gao D. Early characteristics of fulminant myocarditis vs non-fulminant myocarditis: a meta-analysis. Medicine. 2019;98(8):e14697.
94. Omidi F, Hajikhani B, Kazemi SN, Tajbakhsh A, Riazi S, Mirsaeidi M, et al. COVID-19 and cardiomyopathy: a systematic review. Front Cardiovasc Med. 2021;8:695206.
95. Ho JS, Sia CH, Chan MY, Lin W, Wong RC. Coronavirus-induced myocarditis: a meta-summary of cases. Heart Lung J Crit Care. 2020;49(6):681-5.
96. Schultz JC, Hilliard AA, Cooper LT Jr, Rihal CS. Diagnosis and treatment of viral myocarditis. Mayo Clin Proc. 2009;84(11):1001-9.

97. Smith SC, Ladenson JH, Mason JW, Jafe AS. Elevations of cardiac troponin I associated with myocarditis. Experimental and clinical correlates. Circulation. 1997;95(1):163-8.
98. McMurray JJ, Adamopoulos S, Anker SD, Auricchio A, Böhm M, Dickstein K, et al. ESC Guidelines for the diagnosis and treatment of acute and chronic heart failure 2012: The Task Force for the Diagnosis and Treatment of Acute and Chronic Heart Failure 2012 of the European Society of Cardiology. Developed in collaboration with the Heart Failure Association (HFA) of the ESC. Eur Heart J. 2012;33:1787-847.
99. Ferreira VM, Schulz-Menger J, Holmvang G, Kramer CM, Carbone I, Sechtem U, et al. Cardiovascular magnetic resonance in nonischemic myocardial inflammation: expert recommendations. J Am Coll Cardiol. 2018;72:3158-76.
100. Luetkens JA, Faron A, Isaak A, Dabir D, Kuetting D, Feisst A, et al. Comparison of original and 2018 Lake Louise criteria for diagnosis of acute myocarditis: results of a validation cohort. Radiol Cardiothorac Imaging. 2019;1(3):e190010.
101. Schneider JE, Stojanovic I. Economic evaluation of cardiac magnetic resonance with fast-SENC in the diagnosis and management of early heart failure. Health Econ Rev. 2019;9(1):13.
102. Ge Y, Pandya A, Steel K, Bingham S, Jerosch-Herold M, Chen YY, et al. Cost-effectiveness analysis of stress cardiovascular magnetic resonance imaging for stable chest pain syndromes. JACC Cardiovasc Imaging. 2020;13:1505-17.
103. Petrov G, Kelle S, Fleck E, Wellnhofer E. Incremental cost-effectiveness of dobutamine stress cardiac magnetic resonance imaging in patients at intermediate risk for coronary artery disease. Clin Res Cardiol. 2015;104:401-9.
104. Georgiopoulos G, Figliozzi S, Sanguineti F, Aquaro GD, di Bella G, Stamatelopoulos K, et al. Prognostic Impact of Late Gadolinium Enhancement by Cardiovascular Magnetic Resonance in Myocarditis: A Systematic Review and Meta-Analysis. Circ Cardiovasc Imaging. 2021;14:E011492.
105. Tschöpe C, Cooper LT, Torre-Amione G, van Linthout S. Management of myocarditis-related cardiomyopathy in adults. Circ Res. 2019;124(11):1568-83.
106. Leone O, Veinot JP, Angelini A, Baandrup UT, Basso C, Berry G, et al. 2011 Consensus statement on endomyocardial biopsy from the Association for European Cardiovascular Pathology and the Society for Cardiovascular Pathology. Cardiovasc Pathol. 2012;21(4):245-74.
107. Aretz HT. Myocarditis: the Dallas criteria. Human Pathol. 1987;18(6):619-24.
108. Health Canada. (2020). Pfizer-BioNTech Comirnaty COVID-19 vaccine. [online] Available from https://www.canada.ca/en/health-canada/services/drugs-health-products/covid19-industry/drugs-vaccines-treatments/vaccines/pfizer-biontech.html. [Last accessed February, 2024]
109. Health Canada; Government of Canada. (2020). Moderna Spikevax COVID-19 vaccine. [online] Available from https://www.canada.ca/en/health-canada/services/drugs-health-products/covid19-industry/drugs-vaccines-treatments/vaccines/moderna.html. [Last accessed February, 2024]
110. Polack FP, Thomas SJ, Kitchin N, Absalon J, Gurtman A, Lockhart S, et al. Safety and Efficacy of the BNT162b2 mRNA Covid-19 Vaccine. N Engl J Med. 2020;383(27):2603-15.
111. Baden LR, El Sahly HM, Essink B, Kotloff K, Frey S, Novak R, et al. Efficacy and Safety of the mRNA-1273 SARS-CoV-2 Vaccine. N Engl J Med. 2021;384(5):403-16.
112. Kim HW, Jenista ER, Wendell DC, Azevedo CF, Campbell MJ, Darty SN, et al. Patients with acute myocarditis following mRNA COVID-19 vaccination. JAMA Cardiol. 2021;6(10):1196-1201.
113. Bozkurt B, Kamat I, Hotez PJ. Myocarditis with COVID-19 mRNA Vaccines. Circulation. 2021;144(6):471-84.

114. Diaz GA, Parsons GT, Gering SK, Meier AR, Hutchinson IV, Robicsek A. Myocarditis and Pericarditis after Vaccination for COVID-19. JAMA. 2021;326(12):1210-2.
115. Marshall M, Ferguson ID, Lewis P, Jaggi P, Gagliardo C, Collins JS, et al. Symptomatic acute myocarditis in 7 adolescents after Pfizer-BioNTech COVID-19 vaccination. Pediatrics. 2021;148(3):e2021052478.
116. Montgomery J, Ryan M, Engler R, Hoffman D, McClenathan B, Collins L, et al. Myocarditis following immunization with mRNA COVID-19 vaccines in members of the US military. JAMA Cardiol. 2021;6(10):1202-6.
117. Halsell JS, Riddle JR, Atwood JE, Gardner P, Shope R, Poland GA, et al.; Department of Defense Smallpox Vaccination Clinical Evaluation Team. Myopericarditis following smallpox vaccination among vaccinia-naive US military personnel. JAMA. 2003;289(24):3283-9.
118. Shimabukuro TT, Nguyen M, Martin D, DeStefano F. Safety monitoring in the Vaccine Adverse Event Reporting System (VAERS). Vaccine. 2015;33:4398-405.
119. Schwab C, Domke LM, Hartmann L, Stenzinger A, Longerich T, Schirmacher P. Autopsy-based histopathological characterization of myocarditis after anti-SARS-CoV-2-vaccination. Clin Res Cardiol. 2023;112(3):431-40.
120. RECOVERY Collaborative Group, Horby P, Lim WS, Emberson JR, Mafham M, Bell JL, et al. Dexamethasone in Hospitalized Patients with COVID-19. N Engl J Med. 2021;384(8):693-704.
121. Rafiee MJ, Fard FB, Friedrich MG. COVID-19, myocardial edema and dexamethasone. Med Hypotheses. 2020;145:110307.
122. Ridker PM. Targeting cytokine storm in COVID-19: What have we learned? Eur Heart J Open. 2021;1:oeab005.
123. Gordon AC, Angus DC, Derde LPG. Interleukin-6 Receptor Antagonists in Critically Ill Patients with COVID-19. N Engl J Med. 2021;385:1147-9.
124. RECOVERY Collaborative Group. Tocilizumab in patients admitted to hospital with COVID-19 (RECOVERY): A randomized, controlled, open-label, platform trial. Lancet. 2021;397:1637-45.
125. Hu H, Ma F, Wei X, Fang Y. Coronavirus fulminant myocarditis treated with glucocorticoid and human immunoglobulin. Eur Heart J. 2021;42(2):206.
126. Huang X, Sun Y, Su G, Li Y, Shuai X. Intravenous immunoglobulin therapy for acute myocarditis in children and adults. Int Heart J. 2019;60(2):359-365.
127. Maisch B, Alter P. Treatment options in myocarditis and inflammatory cardiomyopathy: Focus on i. v. immunoglobulins. Herz. 2018;43:423-30.
128. Mirna M, Schmutzler L, Topf A, Boxhammer E, Sipos B, Hoppe UC, et al. Treatment with Non-steroidal Anti-inflammatory Drugs (NSAIDs) Does Not Affect Outcome in Patients with Acute Myocarditis or Myopericarditis. J Cardiovasc Dev Dis. 2022;9:32.
129. Chedid M, Waked R, Haddad E, Chetata N, Saliba G, Choucair J. Antibiotics in treatment of COVID-19 complications: A review of frequency, indications, and efficacy. J Infect Public Health. 2021;14:570-6.
130. Horby PW, Mafham M, Bell JL, Linsell L, Staplin N, Emberson J, et al. Lopinavir–ritonavir in patients admitted to hospital with COVID-19 (RECOVERY): A randomised, controlled, open-label, platform trial. Lancet. 2020;396:1345-52.
131. WHO Solidarity Trial Consortium. Repurposed Antiviral Drugs for COVID-19—Interim WHO Solidarity Trial Results. N Engl J Med. 2021;384:497-511.
132. Vegivinti CTR, Evanson KW, Lyons H, Akosman I, Barrett A, Hardy N, et al. Efficacy of antiviral therapies for COVID-19: A systematic review of randomized controlled trials. BMC Infect Dis. 2022;22:107.

133. Ammirati E, Cipriani M, Moro C, Raineri C, Pini D, Sormani P, et al. Clinical Presentation and Outcome in a Contemporary Cohort of Patients with Acute Myocarditis: Multicenter Lombardy Registry. Circulation. 2018;138:1088-99.
134. Urban S, Fułek M, Błaziak M, Iwanek G, Jura M, Fułek K, et al. COVID-19 Related Myocarditis in Adults: A Systematic Review of Case Reports. J Clin Med. 2022;11(19):5519.
135. Castiello T, Georgiopoulos G, Finocchiaro G, Claudia M, Gianatti A, Delialis D, et al. COVID-19 and myocarditis: A systematic review and overview of current challenges. Heart Fail Rev. 2022;27:251-61.
136. Jaiswal V, Sarfraz Z, Sarfraz A, Mukherjee D, Batra N, Hitawala G, et al. COVID-19 Infection and Myocarditis: A State-of-the-Art Systematic Review. J Prim Care Community Health. 2021;12:21501327211056800.
137. Rathore SS, Rojas GA, Sondhi M, Pothuru S, Pydi R, Kancherla N, et al. Myocarditis associated with COVID-19 disease: A systematic review of published case reports and case series. Int J Clin Pract. 2021;75:e14470.
138. Pillay J, Gaudet L, Wingert A, Bialy L, Mackie AS, Paterson DI, et al. Incidence, risk factors, natural history, and hypothesised mechanisms of myocarditis and pericarditis following covid-19 vaccination: living evidence syntheses and review. BMJ. 2022;378: e069445.
139. Yancy CW, Jessup M, Bozkurt B, Butler J, Casey DE Jr, Drazner MH, et al.; American College of Cardiology Foundation; American Heart Association Task Force on Practice Guidelines. 2013 ACCF/AHA guideline for the management of heart failure: a report of the American College of Cardiology Foundation/American Heart Association Task Force on Practice Guidelines. J Am Coll Cardiol. 2013;62(16):e147-239.
140. Law YM, Lal AK, Chen S, Čiháková D, Cooper LT Jr, Deshpande S, et al.; American Heart Association Pediatric Heart Failure and Transplantation Committee of the Council on Lifelong Congenital Heart Disease and Heart Health in the Young and Stroke Council. Diagnosis and management of myocarditis in children: a scientific statement from the American Heart Association. Circulation. 2021;144(6):e123-35.
141. US Centers for Disease Control and Prevention. Clinical considerations: myocarditis and pericarditis after receipt of mRNA COVID-19 vaccines among adolescents and young adults. [online] Available from https://www.cdc.gov/vaccines/covid-19/clinical-considerations/myocarditis.html. [Last accessed February, 2024]
142. Aquaro GD, Ghebru Habtemicael Y, Camastra G, Monti L, Dellegrottaglie S, Moro C, et al.; Cardiac Magnetic Resonance Working Group of the Italian Society of Cardiology. Prognostic value of repeating cardiac magnetic resonance in patients with acute myocarditis. J Am Coll Cardiol. 2019;74(20):2439-48.
143. US Centers for Disease Control and Prevention. Interim clinical considerations for use of COVID-19 vaccines currently authorized in the United States. [online] Available from https://www.cdc.gov/vaccines/covid-19/clinical-considerations/covid-19-vaccines-us.html. [Last accessed February, 2024]
144. Chou OHI, Zhou J, Lee TTL, Kot T, Lee S, Wai AKC, et al. Comparisons of the risk of myopericarditis between COVID-19 patients and individuals receiving COVID-19 vaccines: a population-based study. Clin Res Cardiol. 2022;111(10):1098-103.
145. Imazio M, Klingel K, Kindermann I, Brucato A, De Rosa FG, Adler Y, et al. COVID-19 pandemic and troponin: indirect myocardial injury, myocardial inflammation or myocarditis? Heart. 2020;106(15):1127-31.
146. Ling RR, Ramanathan K, Tan FL, Tai BC, Somani J, Fisher D, et al. Myopericarditis following COVID-19 vaccination and non-COVID-19 vaccination: a systematic review and meta-analysis. Lancet Respir Med. 2022;10(7):679-88.

CHAPTER 31

Injuries from the SARS CoV-2 Vaccines

Dan McDyer

INTRODUCTION

Review of the confidential Pfizer Clinical Trial documents[1] reveals the sad fact that this topic, "Injuries from the SARS CoV-2 Vaccines," should not even exist because a cursory review reveals that more participants died from all causes in the treatment arm of the study than in the control arm of the study. Historically, this has resulted in termination of a clinical trial with further detailed investigation into why the investigational drug resulted in more deaths than placebo administration. For unknown reasons, this was not the path undertaken by the regulatory agencies and the vaccine was cleared for emergency use authorization and rapid global deployment while ignoring the warning signals that became even more apparent in Pfizer's confidential post marketing analysis of the first 3 months of vaccine administration that identified over 1,220 deaths and over 42,000 serious adverse events in the first 90 days of global use.[2]

To understand how the SARS CoV-2 vaccines result in a multitude of injuries, it is necessary to review the components of the vaccines, what they do, how they work, their distribution pattern, how they differ from "traditional vaccines", and how they generally affect the body. These topics will be addressed in distinct sections for the purpose of organization. Thereafter, a review of the numerous SARS CoV-2 vaccine-related injuries and their underlying mechanisms, when understood, will be discussed. It is important to note that there has been difficulty getting vaccine injury-related reports accepted into the medical literature due to a global concerted effort to suppress information reporting on adverse effects from these vaccines. The vast majority of information in the literature consists of case reports of adverse effects. The narratives of these reports are typically prefaced by a comment about the safety and efficacy of the vaccines followed by a comment about the "rare nature" of the adverse events described. A representative example of these statements can be viewed in the first paragraph of an article by Cines and Bussel that appeared in the June 2021 issue of the New England Journal of Medicine.[3] This effort to conceal adverse effects to reduce "vaccine hesitancy" has not only hindered our knowledge of the extent of these injuries, but most importantly, our understanding of the mechanisms underlying the injuries so that treatment programs can be developed.

VACCINE ACTIVE INGREDIENTS[4]

The SARS CoV-2 vaccines available in the United States consist of two different transport models to deliver a payload of messenger RNA (mRNA) or DNA that encodes a message for the vaccine recipient to manufacture spike protein (the foreign substance, aka "antigen," recognized by the immune system). The two most administered vaccines in the US (Pfizer-BioNTech and Moderna) use a lipid nanoparticle (LNP) delivery system to provide an mRNA payload to the cells whereas the Johnson and Johnson/ Janssen vaccine utilizes a replication incompetent adenoviral vector (adenovirus type 26 that is not infectious in humans) to deliver a DNA segment to the cells. Once the payloads are transported to the cells by these two delivery systems, the actions of the mRNA and DNA are the production of SARS CoV-2 spike protein.

The mRNA contained in the Moderna and Pfizer-BioNTech vaccines is a modified genetic sequence that contains three regions. The first segment is a "nucleoside primer." It inhibits the degradation of the mRNA to prolong its activity of messaging for spike protein production. The second segment is the middle region that encodes for production of the SARS CoV-2 spike protein which elicits the immune response from the recipient's immune system. The third segment is a "membrane anchor." Its purpose is to capture the spike protein as it passes through the cell membrane and keep it on the surface of the cell so that the spike protein does not travel systemically throughout the body. In addition to the above components of the mRNA payload, the developers replaced one of the nucleotides, Uridine, with a synthetic nucleotide, Pseudouridine (P-uridine). P-uridine provides the same genetic message as Uracil, but is degraded at a slower rate than Uracil. The result of this creation is a synthetic mRNA molecule that instructs the recipient's cellular machinery to make SARS CoV-2 spike protein with an attached membrane anchor for a much longer time than a natural mRNA molecule due to the presence of the nucleoside primer and the P-uridine.

VACCINE BIODISTRIBUTION

The intention of the LNP vaccine development (Pfizer-BioNTech and Moderna) was to modify the chemical structure/electrical charge of the LNP's so that they would stay near the injection site in the deltoid (shoulder) muscle and enter the lymphatic system where the immune response to the spike protein would occur. Unfortunately, this is not what transpired and there is definitive evidence from Pfizer's confidential biodistribution studies that the LNPs invade every cell type and cross through every blood-tissue barrier, i.e., the blood-brain barrier, the blood-testis barrier, etc. **(Table 1)**. Pfizer's confidential rodent biodistribution study, obtained via a FOIA request of the Japanese government[5] (pages 6–7 of translated component), involved the administration of LNPs containing nucleoside modified mRNA to rats. This analysis demonstrated that these LNPs were detected in every tissue type within 15 minutes of injection, including the brain, testes, ovaries, heart, etc. This 48-hour duration study also revealed a progressive increase in the concentration of the LNPs in virtually every tissue type with the exception of blood and plasma **(Table 1)** which is expected as the LNPs are distributed to the bodily tissues.

The adenovirus vector vaccine (Johnson and Johnson/Janssen) is also injected into the deltoid (shoulder) muscle and transports its DNA cargo throughout the body, but it has a different biodistribution profile than the LNP-based vaccines. The adenovirus is unable to penetrate the blood-tissue barriers like the LNPs. Therefore, any tissue that is protected by one of these barriers is not exposed to the adenovirus and its DNA cargo.[6]

VACCINE MECHANISM OF ACTION[4]

After the vaccine is administered, the LNPs enter the bodily fluids and are electrically attracted to the cell membranes of the body's cells **(Figs. 1 and 2)**. The LNPs are absorbed into the cell membrane and then the mRNA is spilled into the cytoplasm (internal region) of the cell. Within the cytoplasm, there are ribosomes which are the structures that "read" the genetic messages encoded by mRNA. The vaccine's synthetic mRNA is read by the ribosome and the spike protein with the attached membrane anchor is produced. This protein is then delivered to the cell membrane by Golgi Bodies and then the spike protein sticks up from the cell membrane like a lollipop anchored into the cell membrane. This foreign spike protein is then recognized by the Humoral Immune System (B-cells and their antibodies) and a reaction occurs that results in the production of antibodies that specifically recognize the most immunogenic (elicit the greatest immune response) areas of the spike protein. Additionally, segmental portions of the produced spike protein are delivered by a different process to protein complexes on the surface of the cells called major histocompatibility complexes (MHCs). These MHCs are unique to each individual's body and are recognized by the cellular immune system (T-cells). These MHCs are part of the immune system's method of recognizing cells that are normal and that naturally belong to the body. Structural changes in the MHCs alert the cellular immune system (T-cells) to target and destroy cells with these structural changes, i.e., cancer cells and virally infected cells. So, the result is destruction of the cells that contain the altered MHCs.

TABLE 1: Pfizer confidential biodistribution of lipid nanoparticle, modRNA solution injection.

2.6.5.5B. Pharmacokinetics: Organ distribution continued	**Test Article: [^{3}H]-Labeled TNP-mRNA formulation containing ALC-0315 and ATC-0159 Report number: 185350**
Species (Strain)	Rat (Wistar Han)
Sex/Number of animals	Male and female/3 animals/sex time point (21 animals/sex total for the 50 µg dose)
Feeding condition	Fed ad libitum
Method of administration	Intramuscular injection
Dose	50 µg [3H]-08-A01-C0 (lot # NC-0552-1)
Number of doses	1
Detection	Radioactivity quantitation using liquid scintillation counting
Sampling time (hour):	0.25, 1, 2, 4, 8, 24, and 48 hours post-injection

Sample	Mean total lipid concentration (ug lipid equivalent/g (or mL) (males and females combined)							% of administered dose (males and females combined)						
	0.25 h	1 h	2 h	4 h	8 h	24 h	48 h	0.25 h	111	2 h	4 h	8 h	24 h	48 h
Adipose tissue	0.057	0.100	0.126	0.128	0.093	0.084	0.181	–	–	–	–	–	–	–
Adrenal glands	0.271	1.48	2.72	2.89	6.80	13.8	18.2	0.001	0.007	0.010	0.015	0.035	0.066	0.106
Bladder	0.041	0.130	0.146	0.167	0.148	0.247	0.365	0.000	0.001	0.001	0.001	0.001	0.002	0.002
Bone (femur)	0.091	0.195	0.266	0.276	0.340	0.342	0.687	–	–	–	–	–	–	–
Bone marrow (femur)	0.479	0.960	1.24	1.24	1.84	2.49	3.77	–	–	–	–	–	–	–
Brain	0.045	0.100	0.138	0.115	0.073	0.069	0.068	0.007	0.013	0.020	0.016	0.011	0.010	0.009
Eyes	0.010	0.035	0.052	0.067	0.059	0.091	0.112	0.000	0.001	0.001	0.002	0.002	0.002	0.003

Continued

Continued

2.6.5.5B. Pharmacokinetics: Organ distribution continued							**Test Article: [^{3}H]-Labeled TNP-mRNA formulation containing ALC-0315 and ATC-0159 Report number: 185350**							
Heart	0.282	1.03	1.40	0.987	0.790	0.451	0.546	0.018	0.056	0.084	0.060	0.042	0.027	0.030
Injection site	128	394	311	338	213	195	165	19.9	52.6	31.6	28.4	21.9	29.1	24.6
Kidneys	0.391	1.16	2.05	0.924	0.590	0.426	0.425	0.050	0.124	0.211	0.109	0.075	0.054	0.057
Large intestine	0.013	0.048	0.093	0.287	0.649	1.10	1.34	0.008	0.025	0.065	0.192	0.405	0.692	0.762
Liver	0.737	4.63	11.0	16.5	26.5	19.2	24.3	0.602	2.87	7.33	11.9	18.1	15.4	16.2
Lung	0.492	1.21	1.83	1.50	1.15	1.04	1.09	0.052	0.101	0.178	0.169	0.122	0.101	0.101

2.6.5.5B. Pharmacokinetics: Organ distribution continued							**Test Article: [^{3}H]-Labelled LNP-mRNA formulation containing ATC-0315 and ATC-0159 Report number: 185350**							
Sample	Total lipid concentration [μg lipid equivalent/g (or mL)] (males and females combined)							% of administered dose (males and females combined)						
	0.25 h	1 h	2 h	4 h	8 h	24 h	48 h	0.25 h	1 h	2 h	4 h	8 h	24 h	48 h
Lymph node (mandibular)	0.064	0.189	0.290	0.408	0.534	0.554	0.727	–	–	–	–	–	–	–
Lymph node (mesenteric)	0.050	0.146	0.530	0.489	0.689	0.985	1.37	–	–	–	–	–	–	–
Muscle	0.021	0.061	0.084	0.103	0.096	0.095	0.192	–	–	–	–	–	–	–
Ovaries (females)	0.104	1.34	1.64	2.34	3.09	5.24	12.3	0.001	0.009	0.008	0.016	0.025	0.037	0.095
Pancreas	0.081	0.207	0.414	0.380	0.294	0.358	0.599	0.003	0.007	0.014	0.015	0.015	0.011	0.019
Pituitary gland	0.339	0.645	0.868	0.854	0.405	0.478	0.694	0.000	0.001	0.001	0.001	0.000	0.000	0.001

Continued

Continued

2.6.5.5B. Pharmacokinetics: Organ distribution continued								Test Article: [^{3}H]-Labelled LNP-mRNA formulation containing ATC-0315 and ATC-0159 Report number: 185350						
Prostate (males)	0.061	0.091	0.128	0.157	0.150	0.183	0.170	0.001	0.001	0.002	0.003	0.003	0.004	0.003
Salivary glands	0.084	0.193	0.255	0.220	0.135	0.170	0.264	0.003	0.007	0.008	0.008	0.005	0.006	0.009
Skin	0.013	0.208	0.159	0.145	0.119	0.157	0.253	–	–	–	–	–	–	–
Small intestine	0.030	0.221	0.476	0.879	1.28	1.30	1.47	0.024	0.130	0.319	0.543	0,776	0.906	0.835
Spinal cord	0.043	0.097	0.169	0.250	0.106	0.085	0.112	0.001	0.002	0.002	0.003	0.001	0.001	0.001
Spleen	0.334	2.47	7.73	10.3	22.1	20.1	23.4	0.013	0.093	0.325	0.385	0.982	0.821	1.03
Stomach	0.017	0.065	0.115	0.144	0.268	0.152	0.215	0.006	0.019	0.034	0.030	0.040	0.037	0.039
Testes (males)	0.031	0.042	0.079	0.129	0.146	0.304	0.320	0.007	0.010	0.017	0.030	0.034	0.074	0.074
Thymus	0.088	0.243	0.340	0.335	0.196	0.207	0.331	0.004	0.007	0.010	0.012	0.008	0.007	0.008
Thyroid	0.155	0.536	0.842	0.851	0.544	0.578	1.00	0.000	0.001	0.001	0.001	0.001	0.001	0.001
Uterus (females)	0.043	0.203	0.305	0.140	0.287	0.289	0.456	0.002	0.011	0.015	0.008	0.016	0.018	0.022
Whole blood	1.97	4.37	5.40	3.05	1.31	0.909	0.420	–	–	–	–	–	–	–
Plasma	3.97	8.13	8.90	6.50	2.36	1.78	0.805							
Blood plasma ratio	0.815	0.515	0.550	0.510						–	–	–	–	–

Source: Pfizer report_Japanese government. SARS-CoV-2 mRNA Vaccine (BNT162, PF-07302048). [online] Available from https://www.docdroid.net/xq0Z8B0/pfizer-report-japanese-government-pdf, pages 6-7 of translated version. [Last accessed March, 2024].

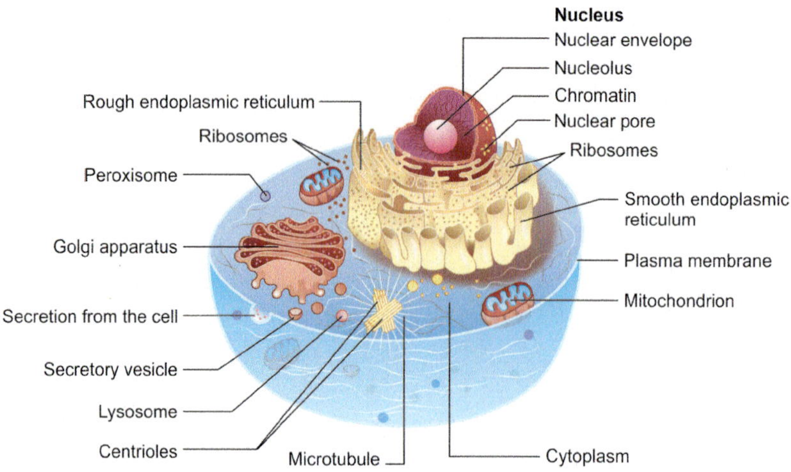

FIGURE 1: Anatomy of a cell.

Source: https://cdn.surfnetkids.com/resources/wp-content/uploads/2001/07/Cell-Structure.jpg

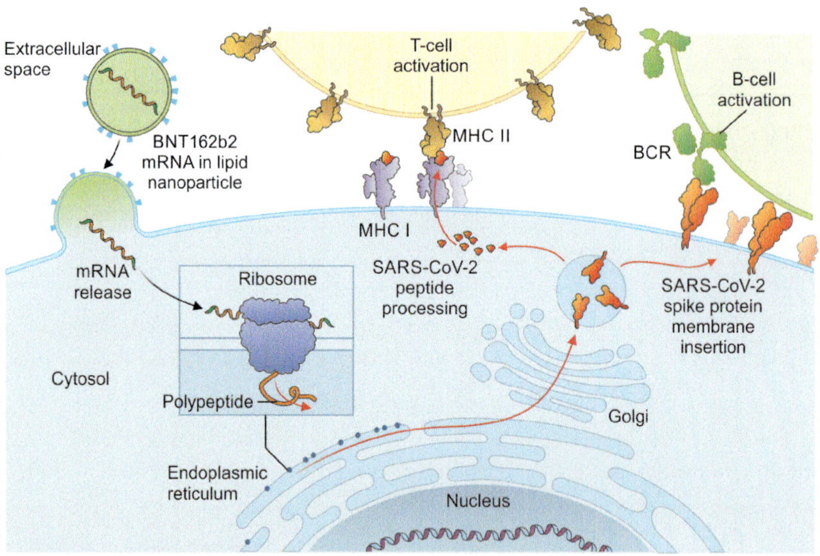

FIGURE 2: Cellular cycle of SARS CoV-2 vaccine activity.

The Johnson and Johnson/Janssen vaccine is slightly different in its actions in that an adenovirus is the delivery mechanism instead of an LNP. After injection, the adenovirus travels through the bodily fluids and binds to the coxsackie and adenovirus receptors on cell membranes and then delivers its DNA payload to the cell.[6] The DNA is then transferred to the nucleus where it is transcribed to mRNA that encodes for the same things described above, spike protein with a membrane anchor. The remaining succession of events is the same as described in the preceding paragraph.

PRIMARY DIFFERENCES FROM TRADITIONAL VACCINE TECHNOLOGIES

Prior to the introduction of these genetic vaccine platforms, vaccines consisted of an antigen (the component of an infectious organism to which an immune response is desired) contained in a solution with an adjuvant (a material that enhances immune responses). When the traditional vaccine is injected, an immune response to the antigen occurs and the antigen is rapidly cleared from the body by that immune response. In contrast, the SARS CoV-2 genetic vaccines deliver a genetic message that induces the cells of the recipient to become the antigen manufacturing systems, as described in the preceding section. Thus, the antigen sources differ—traditional vaccines consist of a limited antigen dose from an external source, whereas the SARS CoV-2 vaccines create the spike protein antigen from an internal source with an undetermined duration, and capacity, to produce it. Shockingly, none of these SARS CoV-2 vaccines underwent pharmacokinetic studies to determine how long the cells make the spike protein antigen. Heretofore, this was one of the basic requirements for a medication or vaccine to progress into clinical trials. Patient safety demands that we know how long a medication or vaccine is present in the body. Recent observational studies of vaccine recipients have provided some disturbing information in this regard. A study by Bansal et al.[7] discovered that the synthetic modifications to the vaccine mRNA result in prolonged production of spike protein for up to 4 months after the second injection (5 months after the first injection). Additionally, vaccine-derived mRNA has been detected in the blood of vaccine recipients for up to a month after vaccination.[8] So, unlike traditional vaccines that present a brief antigenic exposure, the SARS CoV-2 genetic vaccines create antigenic exposure to spike protein for several months.

SPIKE PROTEIN TOXICITY

The intention of the vaccine manufacturers was to expose the immune system to the highly immunogenic spike protein component of the coronavirus to elicit a powerful and durable immune response. This was planned to occur by two mechanisms **(Fig. 2)**. First was the creation of a humoral immune response (B cells and their antibodies) to the spike protein that was protruding from the cell membrane and anchored to it by the "membrane anchor" component of the protein complex. Second was the cellular immune response (T-cells) elicited by the spike protein fragments presented by the MHC complexes on the cell surface. This was expected to result in durable immunity to SARS CoV-2 with limited side effects. The flaw in this design is that any cell expressing spike protein on its surface or fragments of it in its

MHC complexes will not only elicit an immune response, but, importantly, that spike protein-laden cell will be destroyed by the triggered immune response. Thus, the process of developing immunity from this technique of immune exposure results in cytolysis (cell destruction) via the normal immune response.

Unfortunately, the membrane anchor failed to keep the spike proteins attached to the cell membrane resulting in the systemic release of spike protein into the extracellular spaces allowing it to exert its effects throughout the body.[9] The primary consequence of freely circulating spike protein is that it preferentially binds to cell membrane ACE-2 receptors. When this binding occurs, a cascade of events transpire that result in mitochondrial damage/dysfunction.[10] Mitochondria are the energy producing organelles within the cell. When the cell is unable to produce energy, the cell dies. Mitochondrial damage is a critical component of many of the SARS CoV-2 vaccine-related injuries.

LIPID NANOPARTICLE AND POLYETHYLENE GLYCOL TOXICITY

The lipid nanoparticles are another source of toxicity as are the polyethylene glycol molecules (PEG) that are bound to them to provide stabilization of the vaccine solution and to prevent them from aggregating. Studies in mice and rats have demonstrated significant inflammatory responses when LNPs are administered intramuscularly.[11] This inflammation may result in cell death via processes known as necroptosis and pyroptosis. Additionally, thousands of genes responsible for inflammatory responses are upregulated after administration of LNPs resulting in a significant inflammatory environment at the site of injection. This inflammatory response is most likely responsible for the common side effects experienced by vaccine recipients, such as pain, fever, swelling, and malaise.[11] Considering the fact that the above biodistribution studies **(Table 1)** indicate systemic delivery of the LNPs, one can extrapolate that these inflammatory responses are not isolated to the injection site as demonstrated in the above rodent study. Finally, PEG is highly immunogenic and can stimulate antibody formation that can result in deadly anaphylactic reactions to PEG after the first vaccine dose initiates exposure to PEG. Also, PEG is frequently used in many cosmetics and toothpaste, so individuals may have pre-existing PEG antibodies resulting in life-threatening allergic reactions to the first dose of the SARS CoV-2 vaccines.

RESULT OF SARS COV-2 VACCINE ADMINISTRATION—SUMMARY

Administration of SARS CoV-2 vaccines results in the systemic distribution of the mRNA or DNA encoding for SARS CoV-2 spike protein production by the cells that absorb the LNPs or those that are transfected by the adenovirus from the Johnson and Johnson/Janssen vaccine. The LNP containing vaccines initiate significant inflammatory changes that enhance immune responses (adjuvant effect) and result in significant generalized inflammatory responses along with those specifically initiated by the immune response to spike protein expressed on cell surfaces. This spike protein expression also results in humoral (B-cells and their antibody production) and cellular (T-cell) immune recognition which is the goal of the vaccination program. Unfortunately, this immune response also causes cell death mediated by the cellular immune response (T-cells) directed at these cells. The inflammatory response elicited by the LNPs may also result in localized cell death via processes known as necroptosis and pyroptosis.[11]

Thus, the final result of vaccine administration is a robust immune response to SARS CoV-2 spike protein with the associated cost of cellular death in addition to the production of significant inflammation as a result of the immune response and from that in response to the LNPs and PEG. There is also the unexpected release of spike proteins from the cell membranes allowing them to travel systemically. The effects of this systemic spike protein will be discussed in subsequent sections as it behaves like a toxin even when isolated from the SARS CoV-2 virus.

VASCULAR INJURIES

One of the first bodily systems that was recognized as a site of SARS CoV-2 vaccine injury was the vascular system. It is highly sensitive to the effects of spike protein and these effects have resulted in blood clots forming throughout the entire vascular system, hypertension, aneurysms (weakness of blood vessel walls predisposing to rupture), and vascular dissections (the lining of the blood vessel shears away from the underlying blood vessel structures resulting in vessel occlusion). Many of the vascular injuries result from damage to the endothelial cells that line the blood vessels **(Fig. 3)**. Injury to this tissue layer is caused by spike protein exposure, either from the virus or from the vaccine since it is released systemically, as previously noted. When spike protein binds to the ACE-2 receptors of the endothelial cells, a cascade of events, that are not completely understood, transpires resulting in malfunction of the mitochondria which are the energy producing organelles for our cells. When the mitochondria malfunction, there is no energy source for cellular activity and the affected cells die.[10]

This endothelial cell death results in changes that are interpreted as a vascular injury resulting in activation of the blood clotting mechanisms.[12] This injury along with spike protein-induced platelet activation results in blood clot formation throughout the circulatory system in the arteries, veins, and microcirculatory system.[13] These resultant clots can lead to serious morbidity and mortality including heart attacks, strokes, and tissue death from acutely obstructed arteries. Clots forming in the venous system can also

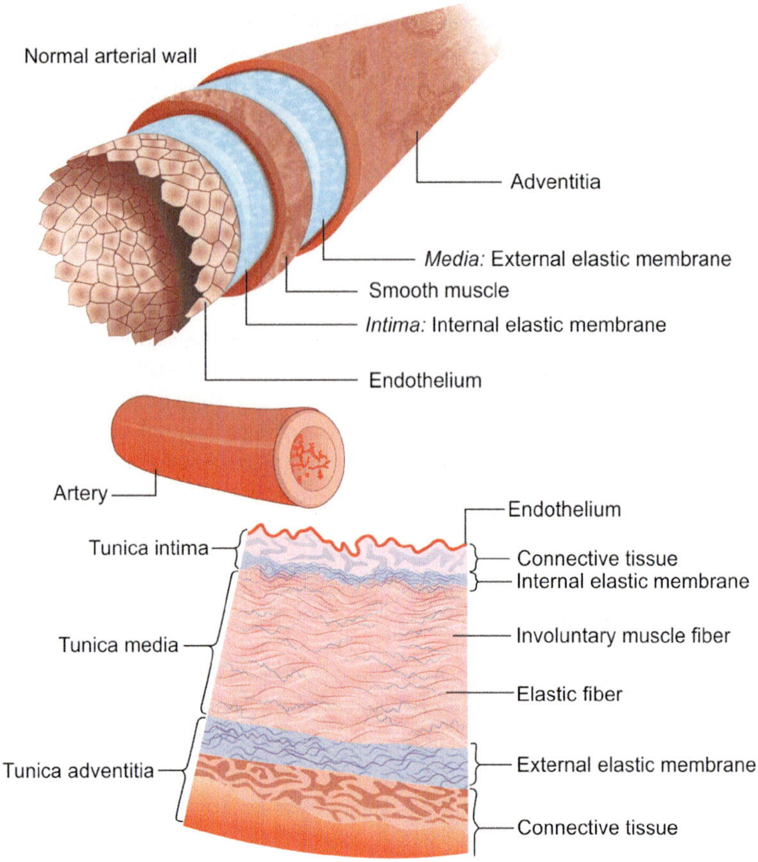

FIGURE 3: Structure of a normal arterial vessel.

Sources:

1. www.researchgate.net
2. www.humanbiologylab.pbworks.com

result in significant morbidity and mortality, especially if they fragment and travel to the lungs creating pulmonary emboli.

Another adverse event involving the vascular system is the development of hypertension (high blood pressure). A recent analysis has determined that 3.2% of SARS CoV-2 vaccine recipients develop hypertension.[14] The underlying cause is not yet understood, but there are numerous possibilities when considering the various types of injuries caused by the SARS CoV-2 vaccines with respect to the complex physiologic mechanisms of blood pressure control. Essentially, every contributing site or factor involved in blood pressure control is a candidate for alterations caused by these vaccines resulting in hypertension. Sites of vulnerability that deserve study include neurologic injury to baroreceptors or the nerves connecting them to the brain, direct brain injury, alterations in the availability of ACE2 enzyme, direct vascular injuries resulting in reduced elasticity of the arterial vessels,[15] alterations in various hormone secretions by their organs of origin, and alterations in various enzyme production involved in blood pressure regulation.

Another set of vascular injuries that have been reported in association with the SARS CoV-2 vaccines are arterial dissections[16] and aneurysms.[17] An arterial dissection occurs when the intima or media layers of the vessel wall **(Fig. 3)** separate and allow blood to collect in this new passageway. Accumulation of blood in this region can eventually occlude that vessel and result in injury to any tissue being supplied by the dissecting vessel.

Aneurysms are a ballooning effect of a vessel and result from a weakness or injury to the vessel wall. As these develop, they can cause blood clot formation which can block the blood vessel or the clots can fragment and block distant downstream vessels resulting in injury to the tissue supplied by that vessel. Additionally, as the aneurysm expands, it can rupture leading to significant bleeding. Common sites of aneurysms are in the brain vasculature or the aorta. When these aneurysms rupture, the resulting hemorrhage is often life threatening. The inflammatory response resulting from the endothelial damage induced by these vaccines[10] may be the cause of the vascular wall disruptions resulting in arterial dissections and aneurysms.

Finally, as mentioned above, the endothelial cell death induced by spike protein sets off a cascade of damaging events. In addition to activation of clotting, this cytotoxic outcome and immune response to spike-presenting endothelial cells results in the release of multitudes of inflammatory chemicals that create a toxic inflammatory environment resulting in the creation of tremendous oxidative stress via released reactive oxygen species and reactive nitrogen species. This inflammatory environment with the associated vascular injury is the same mechanism of action that initiates vascular plaque formation. If this plaque formation is occurring, it will eventually result in heart attacks, strokes, and peripheral vascular disease that will be seen many years after vaccine administration because these plaques evolve slowly. One study by Gundry using the protein unstable lesion signature (PULS) test, a laboratory test that predicts the risk of an acute coronary event, detected a 227% increased risk of an acute coronary event in the next 5 years post-vaccine supporting concern about the development of these delayed adverse outcomes.[18]

CARDIAC INJURIES

Another organ system that has received a great deal of attention for susceptibility to adverse events from the SARS CoV-2 vaccines is the heart. A detailed discussion of these adverse cardiac effects is covered in another chapter in this book. However, these injuries are important to note here in the chapter on injuries and include myocarditis (inflammation and associated dysfunction of the heart muscle cells), pericarditis (inflammation of the sac surrounding the heart), myocardial infarction ("heart attack"), and cardiac arrest.

NEUROLOGIC DISEASES AND INJURIES

The neurologic system is also particularly sensitive to adverse effects from the SARS CoV-2 vaccines. The most common adverse events seen include small fiber neuropathy, tinnitus, hearing loss, headaches, acute demyelinating polyneuropathy/Guillain–Barré syndrome, cerebral venous sinus thrombosis, Bell's palsy, acute disseminated encephalomyelitis, and transverse myelitis.[19,20] Other reported neurological disorders related to vaccine administration include prion disease, postural orthostatic tachycardia syndrome (POTS), strokes, and movement disorders. The vaccine-associated strokes typically result from previously described clot formation or aneurysmal rupture of the cerebral vasculature. They may also arise from dissection of the carotid or vertebral arteries. Cerebral venous sinus thrombosis results from clotting activation in the larger venous drainage tracts of the brain and may also result in stroke.

Acute disseminated encephalomyelitis, small fiber neuropathy, tinnitus, hearing loss, acute demyelinating polyneuropathy/Guillain–Barré syndrome, and transverse myelitis induced by the SARS CoV-2 vaccines appear to result from a phenomenon known as molecular mimicry in which the targeted agent for an immune response has a similar molecular appearance to a native substance in the human body resulting in an autoimmune attack of native tissue.[20-22] The molecular mimicry causing these neurodegenerative diseases is most likely an immune attack on myelin (the fatty insulating sheath coating nerve fibers). The resulting inflammation associated with this destructive process leads to these disorders whose effects range from temporary neurological deficits to death. Molecular mimicry is also hypothesized to be an underlying cause of POTS.[23]

There are also case reports of new-onset movement disorders or worsening of existing movement disorders, such as Parkinson's disease following SARS CoV-2 vaccination.[24] The underlying etiology is not understood, but several cases seem to have been amenable to treatment resulting in only temporary effects. Nevertheless, alterations in central nervous system function like this demand investigation to search for any permanent injury that may result from vaccine exposure.

Finally, there are several case reports of prion disease following SARS CoV-2 vaccination. The most common prion disease is Creutzfeldt Jacob Disease (CJD). This is generally a slow progressive neurodegenerative disorder of the brain that results in death. It is caused by misfolded prion proteins that create a cascading effect of protein misfolding of similar native proteins resulting in non-functional proteins that lead to degeneration of brain tissue and death. Prion-like domains have been identified in the SARS

CoV-2 spike protein.[25] These may serve as an initiator of protein misfolding. There is a pre-print report of 26 rapidly progressing cases of CJD with an average onset of 11.38 days post-vaccine. Twenty of the 26 patients died at an average of 4.76 months after the injection.[26] This is atypical behavior for CJD as it typically progresses slowly over several decades. There are also additional case reports of CJD following vaccination.[27]

IMMUNOLOGIC EFFECTS

The immune system is the ultimate target for responses to the SARS CoV-2 vaccines as with any other vaccine. Unfortunately, there are numerous reports of vaccine-induced adverse immune effects, including suppression of immune responses to infection with SARS CoV-2. There have also been numerous reports of the vaccine initiating autoimmune disorders. Upon exposure to the vaccination and subsequent boosters, the immune system is exposed to incredible and uncontrolled amounts of spike protein patterned after that of the Wuhan Strain. This results in a phenomenon known as immune imprinting in which exposure to future viral variants results in ineffective immune responses targeting the former variant.[28] Additionally, repeated exposure to the vaccines results in immune exhaustion leading to the inability to appropriately respond to SARS CoV-2 infection with the correct type of neutralizing antibodies.[29] These two anomalous immune responses induced by the vaccines are likely responsible for the observation of an increased risk of SARS CoV-2 infection being directly proportional to the number of vaccines received as demonstrated in a study performed by Cleveland Clinic involving 51,000 of their employees.[30]

There are also reports of the onset of autoimmune disorders of numerous organ systems after the vaccines are administered. The majority of available case reports involve the thyroid gland resulting in hyperthyroidism in addition to some of the neurological conditions previously mentioned that probably result from molecular mimicry, an autoimmune disorder.[20] The reported thyroid effects have involved hyperthyroidism (excessive thyroid hormone secretion).[31,32] There are also reports of diabetes developing post-vaccine.[33] There are no definitive underlying causes for these autoimmune disorders aside from molecular mimicry. However, with our understanding of how an immune response with associated cytolysis (cell destruction) is elicited by the spike protein presented on the surface of any cell type that is vaccine programmed to produce spike protein, it would appear that these cells would eventually be susceptible to continual immune targeting (autoimmunity) if the immune system transitions into a state where a particular cell type is no longer protected by being recognized as "self."

Finally, anaphylactic shock has been associated with the vaccines. These reactions often result in death and typically occur immediately after injection. They appear to result from an overwhelming inflammatory response to the highly immunogenic polyethylene glycol (PEG) component of the mRNA vaccines, as previously described.

GENETIC EFFECTS

There are concerning reports in the scientific literature that indicate the potential for significant genetic harms from the SARS CoV-2 vaccines. The mandatory genotoxicity studies that are normally performed on any new drug or vaccine to determine if it creates genetic damage to the recipient were not performed on the SARS CoV-2 vaccines. The observed damaging genetic effects from these vaccines include spike protein entering the cell nucleus and damaging DNA in addition to spike protein inhibiting the DNA repair mechanisms. The result of these adverse effects within cell nuclei is potential cancerous transformation of those affected cells or cell death.[34-36]

Also, spike protein has been observed to be reverse transcribed into DNA in human liver cells. This DNA was observed to enter the nuclei where it was integrated into the genome of the liver cells within 6 hours of exposure to the spike protein mRNA. If this is happening in any human cell line, those cells will produce spike protein in perpetuity. One can only imagine the harmful immune effects of this continual spike protein production. Worse yet, if the mRNA enters oogonia and/or spermatogonia and is reverse transcribed to DNA in those cells, this could result in the transfer of spike protein production to offspring.[37]

REPRODUCTIVE INJURIES

Since LNPs penetrate every tissue barrier and have been demonstrated to accumulate in the ovaries and, to a lesser extent, the testes, there is the potential for harm to the reproductive organs. A recent study by Gat et al. demonstrated reduced sperm motility and reduced sperm counts 3 months after the second vaccination followed by recovery to normality several months later.[38] Differing results were revealed in a study by Barda et al. which demonstrated increases in total sperm count and total motile sperm at 72 days post second vaccination.[39] These contradicting results may arise from the fact that the initial study by Gat et al. did not demonstrate alterations until 3 months after the second dose whereas the study by Barda et al. was completed an average of 72 days post vaccine. If the sperm are negatively affected, this delayed occurrence has yet to be explained.

A recent Vaccine Adverse Events Reporting System (VAERS) analysis by Thorp et al. comparing reported adverse events from the influenza vaccines to adverse events reported from the SARS CoV-2 vaccines revealed devastating impacts on women's reproductive outcomes.[40] Among their many findings, they discovered that menstrual disorders were reported 1,192 times more frequently from the SARS CoV-2 vaccines as compared to the flu vaccines. They also found miscarriage and stillbirth reports to be 57 times and 38 times more frequently from the SARS CoV-2 vaccines as compared to the flu vaccines, respectively. Other researchers have also found menstrual disturbances to be associated with the SARS CoV-2 vaccines.[41,42]

HEMATOLOGIC DISORDERS

The best known hematologic adverse event associated with the SARS CoV-2 vaccines is vaccine-induced immmune thrombotic thrombocytopenia (VITT) which is characterized by low platelet counts and clots forming in various locations within the vascular system.[3] An additional disorder with numerous case reports is autoimmune hemolytic anemia.[43,44] There are also case reports of dozens of other hematologic disorders. The underlying causes of these disorders have yet to be unraveled.

INFECTIOUS DISEASE EFFECTS

The SARS CoV-2 vaccines induce significant reactogenicity with broad effects on the delicate balance of the immune response. This disruption may result in susceptibility to adverse infectious outcomes. Case reports indicate concerns regarding reactivation of latent DNA viral infections, such as herpes simplex infections and Varicella Zoster reactivation (Shingles) following vaccination.[45-47] Although the exact mechanism underlying herpesvirus reactivation is unknown, it has been suggested that this may result from immunomodulation via attenuated T-cell activity particularly relating to functional impairment of CD4+ and CD8+ T-cells and Natural Killer cells along with a quantitative reduction of these T-cells, as seen in COVID-19 infection.[48]

An additional interesting finding is an increased susceptibility to SARS CoV-2 infection with each subsequent SARS CoV-2 vaccine.[30] This paradoxical outcome is discussed in detail in the "Immunologic Effects" section of this chapter.

PREGNANCY EFFECTS

Administration of experimental medications to pregnant women has never been an acceptable action due to the unknown risks to the developing fetus. For this reason, pregnant women are always excluded from vaccine and drug trials. However, on April 23, 2021, CDC Director Rachelle Walensky, MD announced that the CDC was recommending that all pregnant women receive the SARS CoV-2 vaccines. This unprecedented recommendation was merely 5 months after the initial vaccine release. This recommendation was followed by vaccine endorsement from the American College of OB/GYN's (ACOG) and the Society for Maternal Fetal Medicine (SMFM) on

July 30, 2021.[49] Given that the normal duration of pregnancy is 9 months, it is apparent that no evidence for vaccine-induced fetal effects could have been generated in that short interval of time. Thorp et al. analysis of the VAERS database for reported female reproductive vaccine effects reveals that this blatant disregard for adequate analyses of maternal and fetal vaccine effects has resulted in devastating consequences.[40] This comparison of flu vaccine versus SARS CoV-2 vaccine reported adverse events for each vaccine dose revealed that SARS CoV-2 vaccines in pregnancy have resulted in the following statistically significant findings:

- 57 times more miscarriage reports from SARS CoV-2 vaccines
- 38 times more stillbirth reports from SARS CoV-2 vaccines
- 20 times more fetal malformation reports from SARS CoV-2 vaccines
- 10 times more preterm delivery reports from SARS CoV-2 vaccines
- 33 times more preeclampsia (blood pressure disorder of pregnancy) reports from SARS CoV-2 vaccines
- 56 times more fetal growth anomalies reports from SARS CoV-2 vaccines
- 16 times more fetal cardiac anomaly reports from SARS CoV-2 vaccines
- 29 times more preterm premature rupture of membranes (premature rupture of the "sac of fluid") reports from SARS CoV-2 vaccines
- 16 times more low amniotic fluid reports from SARS CoV-2 vaccines
- A host of other pregnancy problems including fetal genetic anomaly reports from SARS CoV-2 vaccines that were never reported from flu vaccines

It is important to note that the CDC's standard operating procedures for COVID-19 indicate that a twofold increase of reported adverse events compared to those other vaccines represents a signal of safety concern.[50] However, the CDC uses a different analytic method known as Proportional Reporting Ratio which does not take sample size or uncertainty into account.[40] Thorp et al.'s study utilized statistical simulations to correct for sample size and uncertainty. The identified safety signals persist even if these statistical simulations are off by a factor of 5.

There are several unique aspects of the SARS CoV-2 vaccines that may influence these adverse pregnancy outcomes. The first is that the LNPs are less than 200 nm in size leading to their ability to cross the placenta and deliver the vaccine components to the developing fetus since nanoparticle studies have shown nanoparticles less than 240 nm cross the placenta.[51,52] This leads to the conclusion that all vaccine-related injuries seen in children and adults may also be experienced in the fetus and newborn if exposed to the vaccine in pregnancy. In addition to this concern, both the LNPs and the vaccine-induced immune response create a significant systemic inflammatory response in the host which is harmful to a developing pregnancy.[11,53-55] Finally, with a size of 180–200 kilodaltons, the spike protein may possess the ability to cross the placenta and interact with the fetus's developing immune system.

CONCLUSION

Significant evidence is accumulating regarding the adverse effects of the SARS CoV-2 vaccines. The evidence to support the causation of these effects is obtained by gaining an understanding of how these vaccines elicit the desired immune response due to the cascade of immune effects and cellular events that are triggered by this flawed vaccine platform. This flawed platform provides no control of the tissues penetrated by the LNP delivery system and no control of how much antigen (spike protein) is produced by the LNP-invaded cells that become spike protein production machines. Its design is also flawed in its inability to maintain the spike protein on the cell membranes leading to systemic release of the toxic spike protein and its associated adverse effects.[56]

In addition to the reviewed vaccine adverse effects appearing in the medical literature, there is significant evidence that the CDC, the agency legally responsible for vaccine safety surveillance, is derelict in their duties. Documents obtained via a FOIA request of the CDC by the Epoch Times revealed that CDC officials lied to federal officials and the public regarding when they started their safety analyses. The information obtained also revealed that the CDC has not reported to the public that their analyses have identified over 700 significant safety signals, 500 of which exceed the safety signals created by myocarditis, an acknowledged vaccine adverse effect.[57,58]

Additional concerning SARS CoV-2 vaccine data was reported in a recent study by Benn et al. that examined results from the randomized SARS CoV-2 vaccine clinical trials for nonspecific vaccine effects and found that in the short follow-up period in these studies, there was no difference in overall mortality for the Pfizer and Moderna mRNA vaccines.[59] They did find reduced overall mortality for the adenovirus vector vaccines from Johnson and Johnson/Janssen and from Astra Zeneca. However, since those initial trials concluded, significant warnings of other health issues, i.e., vascular thromboses (clots) have rendered limited public interest in adenovirus-vectored vaccine use in the United States. Additionally, on May 10, 2023, without any defined reason, the CDC announced that the Johnson and Johnson/Janssen SARS CoV-2 vaccine would no longer be available in the United States.[60]

When considering any medical intervention, it is critically important to perform its risk versus benefit analysis. This analysis assumes a much greater degree of importance when considering administering a vaccine to a population of healthy people. Given all of the above evidence, in addition to the death and adverse event reports available in Pfizer's confidential Post Marketing[2] with the fact that the vaccines do not prevent transmission or infection, it is uncertain as to how these vaccines are still available and why they are being promoted. The body of evidence indicates that the SARS CoV-2 vaccines produce substantial health risks with limited to no apparent benefit.

Historically, this outcome would result in this product being withdrawn from the market. For unknown reasons, the principle of "first do no harm" has been abandoned in the COVID era, placing healthy, low risk people in the crosshairs of a harmful intervention.

REFERENCES

1. Appendix 2.2 Cumulative and Interval Summary Tabulation of Serious and Non-serious Adverse Reactions From Post-marketing Data Sources (BNT162B2). Pfizer Inc., New York, NY; 2022. https://www.globalresearch.ca/wp-content/uploads/2023/05/pfizer-report.pdf.
2. Pfizer. (2021). 5.3.6 Cumulative Analysis of Post-authorization Adverse Event Reports received through 28-Feb-2021. [online] Available from https://www.onoway.ca/public/download/files/198030. [Last accessed March, 2024]
3. Cines DB, Bussel JB. SARS CoV-2 vaccine-induced immune thrombotic thrombocytopenia. N Engl J Med. 2021;384;2254-6.
4. Wilson B, Geetha KM. Lipid nanoparticles in the development of mRNA vaccines for COVID-19. J Drug Deliv Sci Technol. 2022;74:1-6.
5. Pfizer report_Japanese government.pdf. Pharmacokinetics overview Test article: BNT162b2. [online] Available from https://www.docdroid.net/xq0Z8B0/pfizer-report-japanese-government-pdf. [Last accessed March, 2024]
6. Bradshaw AC, Coughlan L, Denby L, McDonald RA, Waddington SN, Buckley SM, et al. Biodistribution and retargeting of FX-binding ablated adenovirus serotype 5 vectors. Blood. 2010;116(15):2656-64.
7. Bansal S, Perincheri S, Fleming T, Poulson C, Tiffany B, Bremner RM, et al. Cutting Edge: Circulating Exosomes with COVID Spike Protein are Induced by BNT162b2 (Pfizer-BioNTech) Vaccination prior to Development of Antibodies: A Novel Mechanism for Immune Activation by mRNA Vaccines. J Immunol. 2021;207:2405-10.
8. Castruita JAS, Schneider UV, Mollerup S, Leineweber TD, Weis N, Bukh J, et al. SARS CoV-2 spike mRNA vaccine sequences circulate in blood up to 28 days after COVID-19 vaccination. APMIS. 2023;131(3):128-32.
9. Ogata AF, Cheng C-A, Desjardins M, Senussi Y, Sherman AC, Powell M, et al. Circulating SARS-CoV-2 Vaccine Antigen Detected in the Plasma of mRNA-1273 Vaccine Recipients. Clin Infect Dis. 2022;74(4):715-8.
10. Yuyang L, Zhang J, Schiavon CR, He M, Chen L, Shen H, et al. SARS CoV-2 spike protein impairs endothelial function via downregulation of ACE 2. Circ Res. 2021;128(9): 1323-6.
11. Ndeupen S, Qin Z, Jacobsen S, Bouteau A, Estanbouli H, Igyártó BZ. The mRNA-LNP platform's lipid nanoparticle component used in preclinical studies is highly inflammatory. iScience. 2021;24(12):103479.
12. Moore KH, Murpy HA, George EM. The glycocalyx: a central regulator of vascular function. Am J Physiol RegulIntegr Comp Physiol. 2021;320(4):R508-18.
13. Kuhn CC, Basnet N, Bodakuntla S, Alvarez-Brecht P, Nichols S, Martinez-Sanchez A, et al. Direct cryo-ET observation of platelet deformation induced by SARS CoV-2 spike protein. Nat Commun. 2023;14(1):620.
14. Angeli F, Reboldi M, Santilli G, Trapasso M, Zappa M, Verdecchia P. Blood pressure increase following COVID-19 vaccination: A systematic overview and meta-analysis. J Cardiovasc Dev Dis. 2022;9(5):150.
15. Suzuki YJ, Gychka SG. SARS CoV-2 spike protein elicits cell signaling in human host cells: Implications for possible consequences of COVID-19 vaccines. Vaccines (Basel). 2021;9(1):36.

16. Takahashi M, Kondo T, Yamasaki G, Sugimoto M, Asano M, Ueno Y, et al. An autopsy case report of aortic dissection complicated with histiolymphocytic pericarditis and aortic inflammation after mRNA COVID-19 vaccination. Leg Med (Tokyo). 2022;59: 102154.
17. Oshida S, Akamatsu Y, Matsumoto Y, Suzuki T, Sasaki T, Kondo Y, et al. Intracranial aneurysm rupture within three days after receiving mRNA anti-COVID-19 vaccination: Three case reports. Surg Neurol Int. 2022;13:117.
18. Gundry SR. Abstract 10712: Observational findings of PULS test findings for inflammatory markers in patients receiving mRNA vaccines. Circulation. 2021;144:A10712.
19. Finsterer J. Neurological side effects of SARS CoV-2 vaccinations. Acta Neurol Scand. 2022;145(1):5-9.
20. Garg RK, Paliwal VK. Spectrum of Neurological complications following COVID-19 vaccination. Neurol Sci. 2022;43(1):3-40.
21. Ahmed SH, Waseem S, Shaikh TG, Qadir NA, Siddiqui SA, Ullah I, et al. SARS CoV-2 vaccine associated-tinnitus: A review. Ann Med Surg (Lond). 2022;75:103293.
22. Mastropaolo M, Hasbani MJ. Small fiber neuropathy triggered by COVID-19 vaccination: Association with FGFR3 Autoantibodies and improvement during intravenous immunoglobulin treatment. Case Rep Neurol. 2023;15(1):6-10.
23. Eldokla AM, Numan MT. Postural orthostatic tachycardia syndrome after mRNA COVID-19 vaccine. Clin Auton Res. 2022;32(4):307-11.
24. Imbalzano G, Ledda C, Artusi CA, Romagnolo A, Montanaro E, Rizzone MG, et al. SARS CoV-2 vaccination, Parkinson's disease, and other movement disorders: a case series and short review. Neurol Sci. 2022;43(9):5165-8.
25. Shahzad S, Wilcox M. The possible role of Prion-like viral protein domains on the emergence of novel viruses as SARS-CoV-2. J Mol Evol. 2022;90(3-4):227-30.
26. Perez JC, Moret-Chalmin C, Monatgnier L; Scienceopen.com. (2022). Towards the emergence of a new form of the neurodegenerative Creutzfeldt-Jakob disease. Twenty six cases declared a few days after a COVID-19 vaccine jab. [online] Available from https://www.scienceopen.com/document?vid=01340cc7-200a-40fc-8470-6b101f8ab39b. [Last accessed March, 2024]
27. Kuvanfik A, Serin S, Sungurtekin H, Özcan E. Creutzfeldt Jakob disease after the COVID-19 vaccination. Turk J Intensive Care. 2022;20(1):61-4.
28. Roitgen K, Nielsen SCA, Silva O, Younes SF, Zaslavsky M, Costales C, et al. Immune imprinting, breadth of variant recognition, and germinal center response in human SARS CoV-2 infection and vaccination. Cell. 2022;185(6):1025-40.
29. Irrgang P, Gerling J, Kocher K, Lapuente D, Steininger P, Habenicht K, et al. Class switch toward noninflammatory, spike-specific IgG4 antibodies after repeated SARS CoV-2 mRNA vaccination. Sci Immunol. 2023;8(79):eade2798.
30. Shrestha NK, Burke PC, Nowacki AS, Simon JF, Hagen A, Gordon SM. Effectiveness of the coronavirus disease 2019 (COVID 19) bivalent vaccine. Open Forum Infect Dis. 2023;10(6):ofad209.
31. Chee YJ, Liew H, Hoi WH, Lee Y, Lim B, Chin HX, et al. SARS CoV-2 mRNA vaccination and Graves' disease: A report of 12 cases and review of the literature. J Clin Endocrinol Metab. 2022;107(6):e2324-30.
32. Caron P. Autoimmune and inflammatory thyroid diseases following vaccination with SARS CoV-2 vaccine from etiopathogenesis to clinical management. Endocrine. 2022;78(3):406-17.
33. Yano M, Morioka T, Natsuki Y, Sasaki K, Kakutani Y, Ochi A, et al. New-onset Type 1 diabetes after COVID-19 mRNA vaccination. Intern Med. 2022;61(8):1197-200.
34. Jiang H, Me Y-F. SARS CoV-2 spike impairs DNA damage repair and inhibits V(d)J recombination in vitro. Viruses. 2021;13(10):2056.

35. Mirza-Aghazadeh-Attari M, Mohammadzadeh A, Yousefi B, Mihanfar A, Karimian A, Majidinia M. 53BP1: A key player of DNA damage response with critical functions in cancer. DNA Repair (Amst). 2019;73:110-9.
36. Mao Z, Bozzella M, Selkuanov A. Comparison of nonhomologous end joining and homologous recombination in human cells. DNA Repair (Amst). 2008;7(10):1765-71.
37. Aldén M, Olofsson Falla F, Yang D, Barghouth M, Luan C, Rasmussen M, et al. Intracellular Reverse Transcription of Pfizer BioNTech COVID-19 mRNA Vaccine BNT162b2 in Vitro in Human Liver Cell Line. Curr Issues Mol Biol. 2022;44(3):1115-26.
38. Gat I, Kedem A, Dviri M, Umanski A, Levi M, Hourvitz A, et al. Covid-19 vaccination BNT162b2 temporarily impairs semen concentration and total motile count among semen donors. Andrology. 2022;10:1016-22.
39. Barda S, Laskov I, Grisaru D, Lehavi O, Kleiman S, Wenkert A, et al. The impact of COVID-19 vaccine on sperm quality. Int J Gynaecol Obstet. 2022;158(1):116-20.
40. Thorp JA, Roger C, Deskevich MP, Tankersley S, Benavides A, Redshaw MD, et al. COVID-19 vaccines: The impact on pregnancy outcomes and menstrual function. J Am Phys Surg. 2022;28(1):28-43.
41. Wong KK, Heilig CM, Hause A, Myers TR, Olson CK, Gee J, et al. Menstrual irregularities and vaginal bleeding after COVID-19 vaccination reported to v-safe active surveillance, USA in December, 2020–January, 2022: an observational cohort study. Lancet Digit Health. 2022;4(9):e667-75.
42. Wang S, Mortazavi J, Hart JE, Hankins JA, Katuska LM, Farland LV, et al. A prospective study of the association between SARS-CoV-2 infection and COVID-19 vaccination with changes in usual menstrual cycle characteristics. Am J Obstet Gynecol. 2022;227(5):739.e1-739.e11.
43. Jackson EM, Harper S, Webb GJ, Thomas W. Severe refractory warm autoimmune haemolytic anaemia after the SARS-CoV-2 Pfizer-BioNTech vaccine (BNT162b2 mRNA) managed with emergency splenectomy and complement inhibition with eculizumab. BMJ Case Rep. 2022;15(8):e250774.
44. Okuno S, Hashimoto K, Shimizu R, Takagi E, Kajiguchi T. Development of autoimmune hemolytic anemia after BNT162b2 mRNA COVID-19 vaccination. Rinsho Ketsueki. 2021;62(10):1510-4.
45. Desai HD, Sharma K, Shah A, Patoliya J, Patil A, Hooshanginezhad Z, et al. Can SARS-CoV-2 vaccine increase the risk of reactivation of Varicella zoster? A systematic review. J Cosmet Dermatol. 2021;20(11):3350-61.
46. Furer V, Zisman D, Kibari A, Rimar D, Paran Y, Elkayam O. Herpes Zoster following BNT162b2 mRNA COVID-19 vaccination in patients with autoimmune inflammatory rheumatic diseases: a case series. Rheumatology. 2021;60(SI):SI90-5.
47. Fathy RA, McMahon DE, Lee C, Chamberlin GC, Rosenbach M, Lipoff JB, et al. Varicella-zoster and herpes simplex virus reactivation post-COVID-19 vaccination: a review of 40 cases in an International Dermatology Registry. J Eur Acad Dermatol Venereol. 2022;36(1):e6-e9.
48. Eid E, Abdullah L, Kurban M, Abbas O. Herpes zoster emergence following mRNA COVID-19 vaccine. J Med Virol. 2021;93(9):5231-2.
49. Thorp M, Thorp J. (2023) FOIA Reveals Troubling Relationship between HHS/CDC & the American College of Obstetricians and Gynecologists. [online] Available from https://www.americaoutloud.com/foia-reveals-troubling-relationship-between-hhs-cdc-the-american-college-of-obstetricians-and-gynecologists/. [Last accessed March, 2024]
50. Centers for Disease Control and Prevention; CDC VAERS Team. Vaccine Adverse Event Reporting System (VAERS) Standard Operating Procedures for COVID-19. [online] Available from https://www.cdc.gov/vaccinesafety/pdf/VAERS-v2-SOP.PDF. [Last accessed March, 2024]

51. Brohi RD, Wang L, Talpur HS, Wu D, Khan FA, Bhattarai D, et al. Toxicity of nanoparticles on the reproductive system in animal models: A review. Front Pharmacol. 2017;8:606.
52. Hassett KJ, Higgins J, Woods A, Levy B, Xia Y, Hsiao CJ, et al. Impact of lipid nanoparticle size on mRNA vaccine immunogenicity. J Control Release. 2021;335:237-46.
53. Han VX, Patel S, Jones HF, Nielsen TC, Mohammad SS, Hofer MJ, et al. Maternal acute and chronic inflammation in pregnancy is associated with neurodevelopmental disorders: a systematic review. Transl Psychiatry. 2021;11:71.
54. Shafiq M, Mathad JS, Naik S, Alexander M, Yadana S, Araújo-Pereira M, et al. Association of Maternal Inflammation during Pregnancy with Birth Outcomes and Infant Growth among Women with or without HIV in India. JAMA Netw Open. 2021;4(12):e2140584.
55. Rudolph MD, Graham AM, Feczko E, Miranda-Dominguez O, Rasmussen JM, Nardos R, et al. Maternal IL-6 during pregnancy can be estimated from newborn brain connectivity and predicts future working memory in offspring. Nat Neurosci. 2018;21:765-72.
56. Patterson BK, Francisco EB, Yogendra R, Long E, Pise A, Beaty C, et al. (2022). SARS-CoV-2 S1 Protein Persistence in SARS-CoV-2 Negative Post-Vaccination Individuals with Long COVID/PASC-Like Symptoms. [online] Available from https://assets.researchsquare.com/files/rs-1844677/v1/206f2ad5-a550-4359-a37e-18170828137a.pdf. [Last accessed March, 2024]
57. Stieber Z; Epoch Times. (2023). EXCLUSIVE: CDC Found COVID-19 Vaccine Safety Signals Months Earlier Than Previously Known, Files Show. [online] Available from https://www.theepochtimes.com/exclusive-cdc-found-covid-19-vaccine-safety-signals-months-earlier-than-previously-known-files-show_5151506.html?utm_source=open&utm_medium=search. [Last accessed March, 2024]
58. Stieber Z; Epoch Times. (2023). Exclusive: CDC finds hundreds of safety signals for Pfizer and Moderna COVID-19 vacines. [online] Available from https://www.theepochtimes.com/health/exclusive-cdc-finds-hundreds-of-safety-signals-for-pfizer-and-moderna-covid-19-vaccines_4956733.html. [Last accessed March, 2024]
59. Benn CS, Schaltz-Buchholzer F, Nielsen S, Netea MG, Aaby P. Randomized clinical trials of COVID-19 vaccines: Do adenovirus-vectored vaccines have beneficial non-specific effects? iScience. 2023;26(5):106733.
60. Centers for Disease Control and Prevention. Janssen (Johnson and Johnson) COVID-19 vaccine. [online] Available from https://www.cdc.gov/vaccines/covid-19/info-by-product/janssen/index.html. [Last accessed March, 2024].

CHAPTER 32

Tracheostomy during COVID-19 Pandemic; To Do or Not To Do

Christopher de Souza, Rosemarie de Souza

INTRODUCTION

Tracheostomy is a surgical procedure where the contents within the trachea could likely be aerosolized on opening the trachea. The prospect of a contaminated aerosol spray emanating from the tracheostomy site raised concerns about the safety of performing a tracheostomy to the hospital personnel performing it especially in the context of coronavirus disease-2019 (COVID-19). It was observed that during the first wave of COVID-19 in 2020 many frontline healthcare professionals advised deferral of the procedure. Their rationale was that healthcare workers (HCWs) would be exposed to the contaminated aerosol spray generated during the procedure and thus much more likely to contract the viral infection.

It was further reasoned that deferring the procedure would allow the patient to enter a phase where they would be less infectious and so lowered the possibility of transmission of the disease to those who were performing the procedure.

A review of these decisions and concerns led to the conclusion that such a course was solely from the perspective of the healthcare deliverers and not from how such a decision would affect the course of the disease in patients. These pertinent and extremely relevant questions needed answers that were based on sound, medically scientific data.

TRACHEOSTOMY IN COVID-19 SITUATIONS

Many papers were published on this subject. The long-term effects of these decisions can only be answered after rigorous scrutiny of accurate documentation and careful follow-up of these survivors on whom tracheostomy was performed during COVID.

Early experience[1] with severe acute respiratory syndrome coronavirus 2 (SARS-CoV-2) in China showed that HCWs involved in the tracheostomy were at greater risk (odds ratio 4.15) than those who were not. This led to guidelines that included correct donning a fully enhanced personnel protection equipment (PPE). This included protective surgical gown, N95 mask, helmet/face shields, gloves, and boots.

At the beginning of the COVID-19 pandemic, many treating HCWs were unsure about role and timing of tracheostomy and whether it would alter the course of the disease. This uncertainty led to deferral as a means to protect the HCWs involved in the performance of the tracheostomy.

They also postulated that while putting the patient in the prone position the tracheostomy tube would likely get blocked.

Early on in the pandemic during 2020, many thought it imperative to place patients on invasive mechanical ventilation (IMV). It soon became apparent that a majority of patients could be managed with noninvasive oxygenation (NIMV) and this caused the number of patients requiring IMV to drop significantly. This in turn caused the numbers of patients requiring tracheostomy to also decline.

Some reports point out that the N95 mask was the single most important piece of equipment needed when performing the tracheostomy procedure.

The N95 masks are effective at filtering 99.5% of particles >0.75 µm which travels within aerosol particles which are >1 µm. Thus, the N95 mask protects the wearer from the virus.

TIMING

A few recent studies clearly demonstrate that the performance of early tracheostomy in patients suffering from COVID-19 led to better outcomes in terms of survivorship as well as being weaned off IMV.[2]

Conversely delayed tracheostomy was associated with poorer survivorship and lengthy and costly delay in weaning off the ventilator.

Early tracheostomy was considered to be tracheostomy performed within the first 10 days of IMV and latest by day 10 of being placed on IMV.

Those studies advocating early tracheostomy demonstrated that it was significantly associated with the length of stay, 40 days for early tracheostomy (tracheostomy done within day 10 of being intubated) versus 49 days for late/deferred tracheostomy. Competing risks models with death as the competing risk demonstrated that late tracheostomies were 16% less likely to get off the ventilator.

Early tracheostomy led to early discharge from hospital. Full and complete PPEs for the operating surgeons were associated with low rates of transmission. More importantly, early tracheostomy was associated with diminished risk of mortality.[3]

Many papers[4-7] concede that there was no way of accurately determining the degree of infectivity and the viral load. It was thought that since the viral loads reduced substantially by day 8 the viral particles would also be very low. Thus, performance of tracheostomy by day 10 was considered not to pose as serious a possibility of disease transmission as was previously thought.[8,9]

All personnel who were involved in the procedure had to follow the protocol of donning a full and complete PPE when performing the tracheostomy.[10,11]

Recent data clearly demonstrates[12] that even after upper respiratory tract samples become negative, lower respiratory tract samples can remain positive for up to 39 days. The correlation between positive results by quantitative polymerase chain reaction (PCR) viral testing and infectivity is currently being investigated.[13]

Data also demonstrates that patients with the severe form of the disease present with a much higher viral load that decreases slowly.[14]

Another factor that was influential in decision-making was the presence of comorbidities. Patients with no comorbidities did much better than those with health issues.

Many studies conducted during the second wave clearly demonstrated that very few HCWs developed COVID-19 following tracheostomy.[15-17]

These studies focused on the following factors:[18] (1) Safety for HCWs, (2) timing of tracheostomy, and (3) were the outcomes influenced by tracheostomy?

Recommended protocols for tracheostomy in COVID-19 were the following:[19-21]

- Mandatory adequate PPE for the operating personnel. This included surgical gown, N95 mask, helmet/face shield, cap, gloves, and boots/appropriate footwear.
- Site to perform tracheostomy—bedside or operating room. Most preferred to perform it by the bedside. Transporting the patient to the operating room was considered to the risk of possible dissemination of disease.
- Precautions to reduce time of exposure to infected elements. Speed of performing tracheostomy is important, especially once the trachea is about to be opened. At that time the ventilator should be placed on standby. This is the period where aerosol spray of infected contents can be generated. At the time of opening the trachea the ventilator must be put on standby to prevent aerosolization. Once the trachea is opened the tracheostomy tube should be inserted correctly and swiftly.
- To avoid complications, delays, and confusion, a well-established tracheostomy team should be in place. Everyone in the team is expected to know their role and exactly how the procedure is to be conducted safely and efficiently.
- Open versus percutaneous tracheostomy is the team's choice and they should be familiar with both.

OUR PROTOCOL

Tracheostomy to be conducted at the earliest when it is apparent that the patient will need prolonged IMV support.

We have an established team of personnel familiar with open and percutaneous tracheostomies. At times we conducted hybrid procedures especially if the patient was obese. An incision was taken in the neck until the trachea was distinctly visible and palpable.

All tracheostomies were conducted by the bedside.

We favored the percutaneous tracheostomy procedure because it was quick and safe. As time went by expertise and confidence of performing it reliably, safely, and efficiently grew exponentially. Once the tracheostomy tube was correctly placed the ventilator was then connected to the tracheostomy tube. All parameters were checked to determine correct placement of the tracheostomy tube.

CONCLUSION

- Early tracheostomy is in general advocated for patients requiring IMV support.
- The benefits of early intervention include (1) shortened hospital stay, (2) early weaning off ventilator support, and (3) decreased mortality.
- Donning of recommended PPEs by HCW's performing the tracheostomy caused the risk of transmission of disease to be negligible.
- Percutaneous tracheostomy was found to be quick and devoid of complications when performing tracheostomies on COVID-19-affected patients.
- An established and experienced team should perform tracheostomy on COVID-19 patients. They should be familiar with both open and percutaneous methods. They should be able to perform this by the bedside.

REFERENCES

1. Chao TN, Harbison SP, Braslow BM, Hutchinson CT, Rajasekaran K, Go BC, et al. Outcomes after tracheostomy in COVID-19 patients. Ann Surg. 2020;272(3):e181-6.
2. Cazzador D, Franchella S, Navalesi P. Tracheostomy During COVID-19 Pandemic—In Search of Lost Timing. JAMA Otolaryngol Head Neck Surg. 2020;146(10):981-2.
3. Bertroche JT, Pipkorn P, Zolkind P, Buchman CA, Zevallos JP. Negative pressure aerosol cover for COVID 19 tracheostomy. JAMA Otolaryngol Head Neck Surg. 2020;146(7): 672-4.
4. Rosano A, Martinelli E, Fusina F, Albani F, Caserta R, Morandi A, et al. Early percutaneous tracheostomy in coronavirus disease 2019. Associated with hospital mortality and factors associated with removal of tracheostomy tube at ICU discharge. A cohort study of 121 patients. Crit Care Med. 2021;49:261-70.
5. Tay JK, Khoo ML, Loh WS. Surgical considerations for tracheostomy during the COVID-19 pandemic: Lessons learned from the severe acute respiratory syndrome outbreak. JAMA Otolaryngol Head Neck Surg. 2020;146(6):517-8.
6. Goldman RA, Swendseid B, Cognetti DM. Comment on "Tracheostomy in COVID-19 Patients: Why Delay or Avoid?" Otolaryngol Head Neck Surg. 2021;164(3):684.

7. McGrath BA, Brenner MJ, Warrillow SJ, Pandian V, Arora A, Cameron TS, et al. Tracheostomy in the COVID-19 era: global and multidisciplinary guidance. Lancet Respir Med. 2020;8(7):717-25.
8. Kwak PE, Connors JR, Benedict PA, Timen MR, Wang B, Zhang Y, et al. Early outcomes from early tracheostomy for patients with COVID-19. JAMA Otolaryngol Head Neck Surg. 2021;147(3):239-44.
9. Kwak PE, Persky MJ, Angel L, Rafeq S, Amin MR. Tracheostomy in COVID-19 patients Why delay or avoid? Otolaryngol Head Neck Surg. 2021;164(3):683-4.
10. Givi B, Schiff BA, Chinn SB, Clayburgh D, Iyer NG, Jalisi S, et al. Safety recommendations for evaluation and surgery of the head and neck during the COVID-19 pandemic. JAMA Otolaryngol Head Neck Surg. 2020;146(6):579-84.
11. Heyd CP, Desiato VM, Nguyen SA, O'Rourke AK, Clemmens CS, Awad MI, et al. Tracheostomy protocols during COVID-19 pandemic. Head Neck. 2020;42(6):1297-302.
12. Avilés-Jurado FX, Prieto-Alhambra D, González-Sánchez N, de Ossó J, Arancibia C, Rojas-Lechuga MJ, et al. Timing, complications and safety of tracheotomy in critically ill patients with COVID-19. JAMA Otolaryngol Head Neck Surg. 2020;147(1):1-8.
13. Aviles Jurado FX, Vilaseca I. Measuring Tracheotomy Risk in Patients With COVID-19-Time to Look Beyond Surgery and Surgeons-Reply. JAMA Otolaryngol Head Neck Surg. 2021;147(7):679-80.
14. Andriolo BN, Andriolo RB, Saconato H, Atallah AN, Valente O. Early versus late tracheostomy for critically ill patients. Cochrane Database Syst Rev. 2015;1:CD007271.
15. Chiesa-Estomba CM, Lechien JR, Calvo-Henríquez C, Fakhry N, Karkos PD, Peer S, et al. Systematic review of international guidelines for tracheostomy in COVID-19 patients. Oral Oncol. 2020;108:104844.
16. Staibano P, Levin M, McHugh T, Gupta M, Sommer DD. Association of tracheostomy with outcomes in patients with Covid-19 and SARS-COV2 transmission among health care professional. A systematic review and meta-analysis. JAMA Otolaryngol Head Neck Surg. 2021;147(7):646-55.
17. Thal AG, Schiff BA, Ahmed Y, Cao A, Mo A, Mehta V, et al. Tracheotomy in a high volume center during the COVID-19 pandemic: Evaluating the surgeon's risk. Otolaryngol Head Neck Surg. 2021;164(3):522-7.
18. Fiacchini G, Tricò D, Ribechini A, Forfori F, Brogi E, Lucchi M, et al. Evaluation of the incidence and potential mechanisms of tracheal complications in patients with COVID-19. JAMA Otolaryngol Head Neck Surg. 2021;147(1):70-6.
19. Schultz MJ, Teng MS, Brenner MJ. Timing of tracheostomy for patients with COVID-19 in the ICU-setting precedent in unprecedented times. JAMA Otolaryngol Head Neck Surg. 2020;146(10):887-8.
20. Sommer DD, Engels PT, Weitzel EK, Khalili S, Corsten M, Tewfik MA, et al. Recommendations from the CSO-HNS taskforce on performance of tracheotomy during the COVID-19 pandemic. J Otolaryngol Head Neck Surg. 2020;49(1):23.
21. Takhar A, Walker A, Tricklebank S, Wyncoll D, Hart N, Jacob T, et al. Recommendation of a practical guideline for safe tracheostomy during the COVID-19 pandemic. Eur Arch Otorhinolaryngol. 2020;277(8):2173-84.

CHAPTER 33

Telemedicine for Medical Students—Lessons Learnt from the Pandemic

Anish Patil

BACKGROUND

In simple terms, telemedicine refers to the remote provision of healthcare services that would traditionally be performed in person. Wallace, Wyatt, and Taylor (1998) described it more specifically as *"combining computer and telecommunications technology with medical expertise to enable health professionals to send and receive information and provide medical diagnostic and consulting services from locations distant from patients and their attending doctors".*[1] It has been taking an increasing foothold in various clinical settings for a long time now. While the coronavirus pandemic has accelerated this process, it by no means started. Even since before coronavirus disease 2019 (COVID-19), telemedicine was becoming hugely popular around the world.[2] In fact, the telephone was even used to diagnose childhood croup before the 1900s.[1]

There are many patient factors and logistical advantages which can explain why telemedicine is becoming more of a mainstay in healthcare services, leaving aside the obvious reasons presented by COVID-19. Even before the pandemic, there were many data showing that clinical outcomes and patient satisfaction are similar or even better with telemedicine compared to face-to-face services.[3-6] Patients find significantly more convenience in the lack of travel to appointments. Reduced costs to the patient as well as the ability for clinicians to triage more effectively have also been reported.[7,8]

The evidence for telemedicine is not all positive, however. Some studies have shown increased readmission rates[9] and slower processing times,[10] though the latter did not affect clinical outcomes in the cited study. Technical issues sometimes interfere with consultations.[11] However, telemedicine can be of great benefit when it comes to serving patients who are frail or in more remote geographic locations and can widen access to care.

Irrespective of the pros and cons of telemedicine, it seems like it is here to stay and will become part of the professional duties of many more clinicians. It was predicted that telemedicine would grow by 30% between 2017 and 2022.[12,13] Therefore, in order to educate and develop future clinicians that are sufficiently equipped to handle the ever-expanding influence of telemedicine, it is also clear that medical education will need to adapt. A key method to achieve this would be to integrate telemedicine into medical school curricula. Telemedicine requires a brand-new set of clinical skills and acumen, some of which are completely different to traditional bedside skills. For example, a traditional history-taking face-to-face does not only require asking the relevant questions to drill down on a diagnosis, but also involves picking up on nonverbal patient cues. These include patient expression and emotion, bedside clues, or reaction from relatives.

There are global efforts aimed at developing a set of curriculum learning objectives to teach remote history taking and basic virtual examination skills, as well as some underlying principles of telehealth, to medical students. There is already some precedent for telemedicine teaching in medical schools and postgraduate curricula.[14,15]

CURRENT TELEMEDICINE EDUCATION

A review of PubMed using the following inclusion criteria—papers that (1) study a teaching initiative aimed at training learners in telehealth skills, (2) include a clear method of program evaluation for effectiveness, (3) clearly define their learning goals, (4) publish their teaching methods, and (5) have their full-text available—and the following search terms returned over 10,000 results:

[(Telemedicine) or (telehealth) or (remote clinics) or (virtual consultations)] and [(education) or (training) or (teaching) or (medical students) or (curriculum)]

However, most of the returned results were related to educating patients on how to remotely engage with their clinical teams to monitor their conditions, rather than teaching telemedicine skills to prospective or current clinicians. Many papers put forward a framework for education in telemedicine, while some provided tips and guidance for telemedicine teaching.

A 2021 review performed in Turkey included seven journal articles.[16] A common educational strategy across these articles was to first start with a series of didactic lectures to provide a foundation for students in the application and intricacies of telehealth, followed by practical sessions such as mock patient encounters and hands-on exposure to telehealth equipment. In this context, "hands-on exposure" commonly referred to simulation, mock virtual encounters, or remote consultations with real patients. A review from New Zealand found that while lecture-based teaching was important in achieving learning outcomes, students were more satisfied with experiential learning alongside it.[14] Other literature reviews have shown similar trends with didactic teaching and a hands-on component appearing to be the mainstream method of telemedicine education.[12,13] Jonas, Durning, Zebrowski, and Cimino (2019) implemented a multidisciplinary, multi-institutional telemedicine course for third year medical students using Kern's Six Step Approach.[17] They started by administering a precourse multiple choice question (MCQ) to ascertain baseline knowledge. They then enlisted a number of telehealth experts from a variety of academic disciplines to deliver asynchronous teaching that they saw as essential for conducting a telehealth encounter. The knowledge was then put into practice during mock patient encounters, in which participants performed a history and a physical examination via video conference. Students were then scored on a checklist by faculty observers to assess achievement of learning objectives.

Liu, Lim, McCabe, Taylor, and Calvo (2016) focused on communication skills, verbal, and nonverbal. Communication is one of the most essential attributes to a good clinician, and can tremendously aid in appropriately diagnosing and managing a patient.[18] Liu and team used a computer-based communication training platform called EQClinic to improve skills,[18] and found this to be effective. Bulik and Shokar (2010) offered telemedicine as an elective for fourth year medical students.[19] This started off with online introductory courses on telemedicine, with learning objectives which were very clearly defined, followed by site visits to telemedicine operators. The aim of this was to provide technology provider perspectives to students. The University of Zürich has integrated a telemedicine and e-health module into their curriculum in response to the rapid digitization of healthcare services worldwide. The main aim of the module is to teach internet and telephone consultation, as well as the basics of telemonitoring. It has been shown to be very well received by students who highly rate their new skills learned in the module.[20]

Bramstedt et al. (2014) took a completely different approach to introducing telemedicine into their curriculum.[21] They instead opted to use telemedicine to teach their ethics curriculum in nephrology. Using videoconferencing, they set up a session for medical students to have in-depth discussions with chronic kidney disease patients about their disease and the impact on their lives that comes with it. The advantage of using this technology was that the students and patients could be anywhere, and they could still have a conversation with each other. Based on feedback from students, they were able to determine that telehealth can be a useful tool to teach other curricula such as ethics, without compromising the vital patient contact component. Students said that telemedicine technology aided them in understanding the psychosocial burden and human suffering associated with chronic kidney diseases. However, this curriculum approach did not actually focus on teaching telehealth skills to students, but rather using telehealth as a vehicle to teach other subjects.

There is currently no accepted best practice guideline for teaching telehealth. However, there is quite a lot of evidence-based guidance on practicing telemedicine as a clinician.[22,23] Stovel, Gabarin, Cavalcanti, and Abrams (2020) have performed an excellent scoping review of the literature in search of telemedicine learning objectives.[12] In order to determine the best practice in telemedicine education, they searched for curricula meeting the requirements set by CanMEDS, the framework for professional competencies for physicians in Canada. To do this, they looked for existing telemedicine curricula which follow competency-based medical education (CBME). 43 articles were included in their review. They found that the most commonly covered curriculum topics (in order) were technology, clinical skills, communication, medical expert topics, professionalism, business and administration, and legal issues among many others. 65% of included studies covered all CanMEDS competencies. The review found that curricula that included a clinical rotation component were the most successful in achieving this. This was the most common method of hands-on training. Lum, van Galen, and Car (2020) presented a good example of how a telemedicine curriculum, designed as an entrustable professional activity (EPA),[24] can be clearly matched to ACGME and CanMEDS core competencies.

One of the most fundamental telemedicine learning outcomes would be communication. Communication is paramount to a good clinical relationship with a patient and no effort should be spared to ensure that this is not lost during a virtual encounter. The Cleveland Clinic has introduced a very handy tool in their telemedicine curriculum in order to strive for good communication. The *Cleveland Clinic Communication Tips for Virtual Visits* is based on the Relationship: Establishment, Development, and Engagement (REDE) model which is a well-known, validated instrument for teaching effective healthcare communication. The Cleveland guide features 10 tips for optimizing the experience including setting the agenda, reflective listening and asking the patient to repeat back what they understand.[25] Hovaguimian, Joshi, Onorato, Schwartz, and Frankl (2021) have used educational literature to create 12 tips for clinical teachers training medical students in telemedicine.[26,27] They advocate aiding good communication by allowing students and patients to engage and interact prior to the telemedicine encounter. This allows students to confirm that patients are set up on the platform, and if they have any questions about it, ensure patients know how to use vital signs monitoring in preparation for the consultation, assess need for an interpreter if necessary, or confirm medication lists.

A common learning objective identified from existing papers was to focus on ensuring that the technology aspect has been optimized. This includes ensuring that students are taught how to use the technology, as students have varying levels of computer literacy, so any potential curriculum should include a component that covers this competency.[28] It should be made clear whom to contact in the event of a technical difficulty. Jonas, Durning, Zebrowski, and Cimino (2019) took a robust approach here.[17] They created a comprehensive checklist of learning outcomes including ensuring security and privacy, ensuring microphone and camera is working, explaining to the patient what to do in the event of a technical difficulty, and obtaining contact details for the patient in case the connection is lost. Privacy is a common theme in the literature with the curriculum of Asprey, Zollo, and Kienzle (2001) dedicating a large part of its content to security and confidentiality.[29] This is, understandably, a key concern for patients using these modalities and this needs to be reinforced in potential clinicians. It is also important to know some of the legal guidance surrounding telemedicine in the country or territory in which it is being practiced.[30]

Perhaps the most essential learning objective that we need to carefully consider is the clinical competencies. Specifically, this refers to how we will ensure that the virtual interaction can obtain a safe clinical assessment of the patient. A thorough review of the literature identifies a few ways in which one can achieve this. A pediatrics telemedicine curriculum implemented at a large New York hospital focused on delineating the main conditions that residents are expected to know, and specifically created learning standards and competencies for each of these conditions against which residents could be assessed. For example, residents are asked to describe an effective musculoskeletal virtual examination, use a telemedical abdominal examination to identify which patients need admitting to hospital, and assess hydration status.[31] The framework for these virtual physical examinations can be extremely easily obtained from the vast array of literature available on the topic. For example, Laskowski et al. (2020) have presented an extremely detailed paper on the remote musculoskeletal examination.[32] While it is not mentioned in the aforementioned Costich et al.'s paper where they sourced their virtual examination teaching material from, it is quite likely that they used this large swathe of published guidance. The key to an effective telemedicine physical examination is that it is a clinician-directed patient self-examination. Benziger, Huffman, Sweis, and Stone (2021) have created a very useful 10-step system-by-system approach to carrying out a virtual examination,[33] and it puts a strong emphasis on using patient environmental cues and a judicious self-performed physical examination. Such literature is very practical for developing a telemedicine curriculum. In fact, certain physical examination tools can be adapted for the purpose of virtual patient consultations. For example, Tanaka, Oh, Martin, and Berkson (2020) have developed an extremely thorough virtual orthopedic examination guide, including guidance on body and camera position in order to best assess joint function and stability.[34] This includes making use of tools that are commonly available on telemedicine software portals, such as the virtual goniometer. One must be mindful of the patient and clinician implications of telehealth that could impact on clinical assessment. For example, some patients are uncomfortable with undergoing a telemedicine consultation by a doctor with whom they are unfamiliar, but are happy to have one with a doctor that they have met before in person. This suggests that meeting a doctor for the first time virtually is not conducive to the formation of a strong doctor-patient relationship.[11]

Hovaguimian, Joshi, Onorato, Schwartz, and Frankl (2021) also astutely mentioned that we should clearly define which conditions are suitable for telemedicine assessment, because there are clearly many that are not (e.g., a suspected traumatic brain injury).[26] The GMC has released some guidance on this (General Medical Council, n.d.),[27] as has the Royal College of Physicians.[35] One key Royal College recommendation is that remote consultation should only be used if one can provide the patient with all of the treatment that they want or need without the need to see them in person. One should also have access to the patient's medical records. It would be logical to call on guidance from major healthcare stakeholders such as the Royal Colleges when designing a telemedicine curriculum for medical students. Patients are obviously the most important stakeholder in the process, and need to be happy engaging in a virtual encounter instead of an in-person one. The need to ensure patient's satisfaction has to be reflected in a telemedicine curriculum.[30]

DISCUSSION

Telemedicine is a rapidly emerging, evolving medium for clinical assessment. Even before the unique role it took during the pandemic, it has widened access to healthcare for those who traditionally struggle to access it, such as those in remote locations and frail patients. In much of the literature, overall patient's satisfaction with telemedicine is markedly high; a 2019 systematic review of 36 studies found >70% patient's satisfaction with telehealth across most of the papers (Orlando, Beard, and Kumar, 2019).[36] It will continue to be part of the healthcare world postpandemic. We urgently need to train future healthcare professionals in this important skill from an early stage so that they can adapt to the changing nature of how healthcare services are being delivered. This creates a pressing need for the best practice guideline for teaching telehealth, however, this will likely require more evidence from program evaluation initiatives in order to determine the most effective curriculum strategy. As improved patient care is the main motivation to develop better medical education, we believe that evaluating the impact of a telehealth course on student's behavior and patient's outcomes would be the most ideal way to build an evidence base for the best practice in telehealth education.

A detailed literature review finds numerous existing examples of telemedicine curricula across the world, covering a vast range of different learner audiences. There is some consistency in the content and learning objectives in many of the courses. It is also noted that that there is a broad agreement with using didactic lectures to teach a solid foundation in underlying theory and concepts, followed by a clinical or practical component for experiential learning. This goes to demonstrate that a unanimous guideline for telemedicine education could be closer to becoming a reality than we think. And this, ultimately, will have a beneficial knock-on effect for patient's care. It is essential that students appreciate telemedicine from the patients' perspective, and take their possible reservations into account. Ultimately, their experience is the most important thing. It is also vital to get across the human nuances of virtual assessment in telemedicine teaching. The patient's experience and satisfaction with a specific encounter is very multifactorial, and each of these different factors forms a small portion to the way in which the patient perceives the encounter. Therefore, we need to be holistic in the way we teach how to approach a telemedicine encounter, keeping these various factors in mind. A good way to achieve this is to take advantage of the fact that these patients' factors and perceptions have been extensively researched in the literature. For example, it is very understandable that patients do not necessarily want to discuss very serious or personal issues such as breaking bad news over a virtual medium, and would prefer a face-to-face interaction for matters that could be potentially upsetting.[11] Patient's considerations such as these absolutely must be included in a curriculum on telemedicine.

CONCLUSION

There is desire within the medical education world to implement telehealth teaching as a core skill. As remote consultation continues to take a center-stage position in clinical triage and assessment, there will be an increased demand for education in telehealth in order to train the future clinicians who will subsequently engage in it. Even though there is currently no consensus on the best way to teach telemedicine, the preexisting literature on the telemedicine curriculum, as well as the available guidance on how to best practice telemedicine as a clinician, can be consolidated to form a simple evidence-based curriculum for medical students that is relatively easy to implement.

REFERENCES

1. Wallace S, Wyatt J, Taylor P. Telemedicine in the NHS for the millennium and beyond. Postgrad Med J. 1998;74(878):721-8.
2. Bashshur R, Howell J, Krupinski E, Harms K, Bashshur N, Doarn C. The Empirical Foundations of Telemedicine Interventions in Primary Care. Telemed E-Health. 2016;22(5):342-75.
3. Flodgren G, Rachas A, Farmer A, Inzitari M, Shepperd S. Interactive telemedicine: effects on professional practice and health care outcomes. Cochrane Database Syst Rev. 2015;2015(9):CD002098.
4. Kruse C, Krowski N, Rodriguez B, Tran L, Vela J, Brooks M. Telehealth and patient satisfaction: a systematic review and narrative analysis. BMJ Open. 2017;7(8):e016242.
5. Luo C, Sanger N, Singhal N, Pattrick K, Shams I, Shahid H, et al. A comparison of electronically-delivered and face to face cognitive behavioural therapies in depressive disorders: A systematic review and meta-analysis. EClinicalMedicine. 2020;24:100442.

6. Robb J, Hyland M, Goodman A. Comparison of telemedicine versus in-person visits for persons with multiple sclerosis: A randomized crossover study of feasibility, cost, and satisfaction. Multiple Scler Related Disord. 2019;36:101258.
7. Cui S, Sedney C, Daffner S, Large M, Davis S, Crossley L, et al. Effects of telemedicine triage on efficiency and cost-effectiveness in spinal care. Spine J. 2021;21(5):779-84.
8. Lin C, Tseng W, Wu J, Tay J, Cheng M, Ong H, et al. A Double Triage and Telemedicine Protocol to Optimize Infection Control in an Emergency Department in Taiwan during the COVID-19 Pandemic: Retrospective Feasibility Study. J Med Internet Res. 2020;22(6):e20586.
9. Li J, Thomas A, Kilduff C, Logeswaran A, Ramessur R, Jaselsky A, et al. Safety of video-based telemedicine compared to in-person triage in emergency ophthalmology during COVID-19. EClinicalMedicine. 2021;34:100818.
10. Chowdhury M, Birns J, Rudd A, Bhalla A. Telemedicine versus face-to-face evaluation in the delivery of thrombolysis for acute ischaemic stroke: a single centre experience. Postgrad Med J. 2012;88(1037):134-7.
11. Donaghy E, Atherton H, Hammersley V, McNeilly H, Bikker A, Robbins L, et al. Acceptability, benefits, and challenges of video consulting: a qualitative study in primary care. Br J Gen Pract. 2019;69(686):e586-94.
12. Stovel R, Gabarin N, Cavalcanti R, Abrams H. Curricular needs for training telemedicine physicians: A scoping review. Med Teacher. 2020;42(11):1234-42.
13. Waseh S, Dicker A. Telemedicine Training in Undergraduate Medical Education: Mixed-Methods Review. JMIR Med Edu. 2019;5(1):e12515.
14. Basu A, Seaton P, Kirk R, Hanley E, Sheehan D, O'Steen B, et al. Review of the effectiveness of educational tools for teaching Telehealth care. Canterbury. 2010.
15. Di Cerbo A, Morales-Medina JC, Palmieri B, Iannitti T. Narrative review of telemedicine consultation in medical practice. Patient Prefer Adherence. 2015;9:65-75.
16. Budakoğlu Iİ, Sayılır MÜ, Kıyak YS, Coşkun Ö, Kula S. Telemedicine curriculum in undergraduate medical education: a systematic search and review. Health Technol (Berl). 2021;11(4):773-81.
17. Jonas C, Durning S, Zebrowski C, Cimino F. An Interdisciplinary, Multi-Institution Telehealth Course for Third-Year Medical Students. Acad Med. 2019;94(6):833-7.
18. Liu C, Lim R, McCabe K, Taylor S, Calvo R. A Web-based Telehealth Training Platform Incorporating Automated Nonverbal Behavior Feedback for Teaching Communication Skills to Medical Students: A Randomized Crossover Study. J Med Internet Res. 2016;18(9):e246.
19. Bulik R, Shokar G. Integrating telemedicine instruction into the curriculum: expanding student perspectives of the scope of clinical practice. J Telemed Telecare. 2010;16(7):355-8.
20. Brockes C, Wirth F, Schmidt-Weitmann S, Battegay E, Gerke W. Implementation of the module "Clinical Telemedicine/E-Health" in the University of Zurich Medical Curriculum [Implementierung des Moduls "Klinische Telemedizin/E-Health" in das Medizinstudium der Universität Zürich]. GMS J Med Edu [Gesellschaft für Medizinische Ausbildung]. 2010;27(1):doc14.
21. Bramstedt K, Prang M, Dave S, Shin P, Savy A, Fatica R. Telemedicine as an Ethics Teaching Tool for Medical Students within the Nephrology Curriculum. Prog Transplant. 2014;24(3):294-7.
22. Car J, Freeman G, Partridge M, Sheikh A. Improving quality and safety of telephone-based delivery of care: teaching telephone consultation skills. Qual Safe Health Care. 2004;13(1):2-3.
23. Derkx H, Rethans J, Maiburg B, Winkens R, Muijtjens A, van Rooij H, et al. Quality of communication during telephone triage at Dutch out-of-hours centres. Patient Edu Counsel. 2009;74(2):174-8.

24. Lum E, van Galen L, Car J. Competency-Based Training for Entrustment in Telehealth Consultations. Pediatr Clin North Am. 2020;67(4):735-57.
25. Savage D, Gutierrez O, Montané B, Singh A, Yudelevich E, Mahar J, et al. Implementing a telemedicine curriculum for internal medicine residents during a pandemic: the Cleveland Clinic experience. Postgrad Med J. 2022;98(1161):487-91.
26. Hovaguimian A, Joshi A, Onorato S, Schwartz A, Frankl S. Twelve tips for clinical teaching with telemedicine visits. Med Teacher. 2021;1-7.
27. General Medical Council. (2024). Remote consultations. General Medical Council. [online] Available from https://www.gmc-uk.org/ethical-guidance/ethical-hub/remote-consultations [Last accessed Feb., 2024].
28. Atack L, Luke R, Sanderson D. Development of an online, team-based programme in telecare. J Telemed Telecare. 2004;10(6):355-60.
29. Asprey D, Zollo S, Kienzle M. Implementation and Evaluation of a Telemedicine Course for Physician Assistants. Acad Med. 2001;76(6):652-5.
30. Seifert C, Veronin M, Kretschmer T, McBeath D, Stanford S, Turner D, et al. The Training of a Telepharmacist: Addressing the Needs of Rural West Texas. Am J Pharmaceut Edu. 2004;68(3):60.
31. Costich M, Robbins-Milne L, Bracho-Sanchez E, Lane M, Friedman S. Design and implementation of an interactive, competency-based pilot pediatric telemedicine curriculum. Med Edu Online. 2021;26(1):1911019.
32. Laskowski E, Johnson S, Shelerud R, Lee J, Rabatin A, Driscoll S, et al. The Telemedicine Musculoskeletal Examination. Mayo Clin Proceed. 2020;95(8):1715-31.
33. Benziger C, Huffman M, Sweis R, Stone N. The Telehealth Ten: A Guide for a Patient-Assisted Virtual Physical Examination. Am J Med. 2021;134(1):48-51.
34. Tanaka M, Oh L, Martin S, Berkson E. Telemedicine in the Era of COVID-19. J Bone Joint Surg. 2020;102(12):e57.
35. Lee P, Koo S, Panter S. The value of physical examination in the era of telemedicine. J Royal Coll Phys Edinburgh. 2021;51(1):85-90.
36. Orlando J, Beard M, Kumar S. Systematic review of patient and caregivers' satisfaction with telehealth videoconferencing as a mode of service delivery in managing patients' health. PLoS One. 2019;14(8):e0221848.

CHAPTER 34

Censorship of the Biomedical Literature during the COVID-19 Era

Ronald Neil Kostoff

INTRODUCTION

The published biomedical literature has been the gold standard for—(1) setting toxic substance exposure limits, (2) identifying efficacious and safe treatments for myriad diseases, and (3) copious other applications that contribute to human health. Central to these functions is the integrity of the literature's contents. The coronavirus disease 2019 (COVID-19) pandemic was accompanied by massive contributions to the biomedical literature. Many questions have been raised about the integrity of some of the additions to, and retractions from, this literature during the COVID-19 era.

This chapter will examine distortions in the biomedical literature, mainly (but not limited to) those made during the COVID-19 era. Retractions of published articles for nontechnical (e.g., political) reasons are probably the most well-known because they are the most tangible examples of deliberate distortions. However, retractions for political purposes are but one example of the larger literature censorship issue, where high-quality biomedical articles are not only removed, but also prevented from being published at all. Censorship, in turn, is one component of the larger distortion issue, which also includes politically motivated publication of low-quality biomedical articles that are not removed.

This chapter will draw heavily on the concepts presented in a 2023 Op-ed in Trial Site News (TSN),[1] and will present some real-world examples to put a human face to these concepts. The Op-ed's initial focus was article retractions from the biomedical literature, but that was expanded to include the censorship that prevented publication from occurring. The present chapter will provide censorship examples and will add a few examples of the literature distortion resulting from the addition of politically motivated articles.

The literature survey for the Op-ed identified many academic treatises on retraction. Those published before the COVID-19 era focused exclusively on retractions for technical reasons (e.g., plagiarism, fabrication of data, other forms of fraud, etc.).[2-10] Those published during the COVID-19 era focused on the technical reasons for retraction, but had a secondary focus on what they termed "misinformation".[11-20] Almost none focused on the politically driven motivations for retraction, with few exceptions.[12,13] None addressed the full extent of the censorship issues and the distortions from adding politically driven articles with the help of compliant Editors, Editorial Boards, and Publishers. Were these gaps in coverage themselves a result of Editor and/or Publisher censorship, or were they due to lack of topical interest on the part of performers? The present chapter will address these coverage gaps to some degree.

There are three major components of censorship: (1) the motives for censorship; (2) the mechanics of censorship; (3) the consequences from censorship. The motives for the highest level COVID-19 era censorship will not be addressed in this chapter, and the motives for the lower level executioners of the censorship (e.g., journal Editors and Publishers) will be addressed obliquely. What the public hears about the highest level censorship are the *stated* motives, which may or may not be the *actual* motives. Since the latter are difficult to ascertain, substantial speculation would be involved in addressing them. Most of the effort in this chapter will be devoted to the mechanics of censorship, covering both conceptual issues and examples. Finally, because of the enormity of the consequences that (1) have resulted, (2) are resulting, and (3) are projected to result from the COVID-era censorship of the biomedical literature, a very short section at the end will address the potential magnitude of these consequences.

BACKGROUND

"Retraction of a published paper from a journal is its removal from the journal. It is typically done after findings of malfeasance, such as fabrication of data and substantial plagiarism. However, in the era of COVID-19, retractions have taken on a new (or perhaps previously hidden) politically driven dimension. Papers of high technical quality have been retracted if they question the government-industry approach to the treatment of COVID-19, and especially adverse effects resulting from the COVID-19 vaccines."[1] [*Note*: These injectants being marketed as COVID-19 vaccines are not vaccines in the classical sense. They prevent neither infection nor transmission].

The Website Retraction Watch[21] has been tracking retracted COVID-19 papers, and has identified 405 as of this writing (March 2024). COVID-19 paper retractions have been addressed in substack articles,[22] journal articles,[12] and many other forums. The retraction of the author's paper on vaccinating children against COVID-19 was described in detail in an online newsletter.[23]

However, it is important that retractions do not become distractions. A paper's retraction is the tail end of a long multi-step process, where culling and blatant censorships are applied at each step. The remainder of this chapter will describe mainly the larger process of journal paper censorship (with some examples of additions or retention of politically driven articles in the biomedical literature), and will examine each of these steps that precedes the actual retraction.[1]

MECHANICS OF CENSORSHIP AND DISTORTION OF THE BIOMEDICAL LITERATURE

Step 1: Funding of Research

For research to be published, it must be performed. To be performed, in most (not all) cases, research will require some external funding support, especially laboratory-based or field study-based research. In the USA today, there are three major sources of funding for biomedical research support: the Federal Government (mainly NIH), Industry, and Foundations. All three were strong promoters of (1) the measures taken to control the COVID-19 pandemic and (2) the COVID-19 vaccines.

For funds to be allocated to studies on adverse effects of COVID-19 vaccines, two conditions must be met: (1) the potential sponsor's Program Manager must be willing to fund such proposals and (2) there need to be potential performers willing to conduct such studies. Unfortunately, in the COVID-19 era, sponsoring and performing such studies is not a career-enhancing move for either the sponsor's Program Manager or the potential performer.

The sponsor's Program Manager would gain little, and potentially lose much, by funding research whose results would run counter to the agenda of the sponsoring organization's upper management. The potential performer would also gain little in producing such results. Performers' careers are enhanced by publishing many papers, garnering high citations and awards, and receiving continuing grants. For a study that would show the extensive damage from the COVID-19 vaccines, much time would be required to find a journal willing to publish such results, with the potential of additional time required to prevent a retraction. Further, such publications would act as disincentives for potential sponsors to provide grant money to the performer for future research. Finally, as has happened repeatedly during the COVID-19 era, performers who have published negative results on government measures taken during the pandemic, such as type and timing of treatments for COVID-19 or adverse effects from the COVID-19 vaccines, have lost their jobs, lost medical certifications, and have been subjected to continual attacks and harassment from their colleagues and the media. The last section of this chapter provides examples of retractions based on nontechnical reasons, nonretractions based on nontechnical reasons, harassment for views opposing the mainstream narrative, and censorship of concepts/products that preclude the possibility of literature publication. In summary, the incentives are not in place for such studies to be funded or performed.[1]

Step 2: Submission of Results for Publication

For those few cases where funds are made available for research that challenges the government–industry–media narrative, or even where the research was done without external funding, the next step in the publication process is to submit the paper to a journal. At this point, the journal Editor has three main choices: (1) reject the paper outright; (2) accept the submission, and send out for peer-review to reviewers who will most probably recommend rejection; (3) accept the submission, and send out for peer-review to reviewers who will most probably be unbiased.

Before proceeding further on the Editor's choices, the Editor's perspectives need to be discussed. There are myriad stakeholders for any journal, and they will influence the selection of the Editor. First is the Publisher of the journal, and the Publisher will want an Editor who advances the interests of the Publisher. For those journals that are sponsored by a professional society, the society will want an Editor who advances the society's interests, especially the interests of (1) the main donors to the society and (2) the members of the society (who will typically be employed in the discipline represented by the journal). Because of the strong role played by government and industry in funding (1) many of the Publishers, (2) many of the professional societies, and (3) many of those employed in the area of the journal's discipline, the interests of government and industry will play a strong role in the selection of any journal Editor. In the case of COVID-19 (given the strong support of government and industry for the measures taken to combat the pandemic and the development and distribution of the COVID-19 vaccines), the person selected (and maintained) for the Editor position will most likely be a strong supporter of the measures and vaccines as well (at least outwardly).[1]

Step 3: Response of Editor

3A—Reject Submission Outright

Detailed data on article submission acceptances and rejections (such as comments of peer-reviewers) is not advertised and would be extremely difficult to obtain. In the COVID-19 era, outright submission rejection is probably the most frequent action taken by the Editors who reject an article for political reasons. There are standard reasons they can give for rejection (e.g., out of scope, poor research merit, poor research approach, etc.). Given the subjectivity of the acceptance/rejection process under any circumstances, it is difficult to counter such subjective reasons. Outright rejection minimizes wasting the time required by a peer-review (whose ending the Editor can control and predict by selection of appropriate peer-reviewers), and it minimizes the problems and unwanted notoriety the Editor would face from a potential retraction.

3B—Send for Peer-review to Selected Opponents of the Paper's Results

This action would compete with 3A in terms of occurrence frequency. Many Editors want to give the appearance of objectivity, if not the substance, and therefore are willing to spend the time and effort on a peer-review whose results they can predict beforehand. Most journal Editors know many of the experts in the field, and know quite well on whom they can rely for acceptance or rejection of papers to be reviewed.

3C—Send for Objective Peer-review

For those few paper submissions that are sent for an objective peer-review based on the merits, some will be recommended for rejection and some for publication. Because of the incentives that are in place presently, it is difficult to see how any Editor would be incentivized materially to have such a paper published. The only incentives would be higher order, such as ethical and moral.

Step 4: Retraction

For those few papers that have survived Steps 1–3 to get published, they now face the hurdle of avoiding retraction. At this point, those motivated to retract the article for political reasons surface. Much of the underlying collusion is unknown, since it is not something the perpetrators would want to advertise. Typically, it is the academics at the bottom of the chain who form the public face of the opposition, supported by the media (including the captive Publishers), while the industry and their government proxies remain hidden in the background. As will be seen in many reported cases of retraction, the Publishers/Editors will use the misinformation provided by the lowest level detractors to justify retraction.[1]

EXAMPLES OF CENSORSHIP AND DISTORTION OF THE BIOMEDICAL LITERATURE

Retractions

This section will provide four examples of COVID-19 era retractions that appear to have been based on nontechnical reasons.

Rose–McCullough Paper

An article titled "A Report on Myocarditis Adverse Events in the US Vaccine Adverse Events Reporting System (VAERS) in Association with COVID-19 Injectable Biological Products" was published in Current Problems in Cardiology on October 1, 2021. The paper showed "that myocarditis cases spiked after teenagers began receiving COVID-19 vaccines".[24] In mid-October 2021, the article was withdrawn by the Publisher, Elsevier. The only explanation provided by Elsevier's spokesperson (in an email to Dr Peter McCullough dated October 21, 2021) was "I am afraid the journal is not willing to publish the paper."[25] The Retraction Watch articles[24,25] emphasized both Dr Rose's and Dr McCullough's associations with organizations Retraction Watch characterized as critical of vaccines.

Is this how science is being conducted today? What kind of objective publication criterion is "the journal is not willing to publish the paper"? Why go through the time and expense of a peer-review if the review's results can be ignored and the paper arbitrarily withdrawn by the Publisher Editor?

Obviously, no one involved in the retraction process was willing to give the real reason for the retraction. As will be shown by other examples in this section, expression of opposition to the COVID-19 vaccines was cause for paper retractions and other forms of censorship and harassment. That appears to be the main driving force in the Rose-McCullough retraction.

Equally important are the responses, or lack thereof, from other principals involved with the retraction process, directly or indirectly. Why did the Editor agree to publish the article, and then retract it a few weeks later? One assumes the Editor approved of the article's contents by agreeing to publish. Why did not the Editor resign, rather than reverse position (obviously due to external pressures)? And what about the Editorial Board? Why did they not resign en masse after such a blatant politically motivated decision?

A quote commonly attributed to Edmund Burke states: "The only thing necessary for the triumph of evil is for good men to do nothing". Unfortunately, if men or women do nothing in the face of evil, *they are not "good" by any measure*! The compliance shown above by those associated with the retraction process, directly or indirectly, mirrors the societal compliance that occurred with all the extreme measures that were imposed by government and the private sector during the pandemic. Because of this compliance, millions were maimed or crippled and hundreds of thousands were killed in the USA alone.[26]

Lyons-Weiler-Thomas Paper

An article titled "Relative Incidence of Office Visits and Cumulative Rates of Billed Diagnoses Along the Axis of Vaccination" was published in the International Journal of Environmental Research and Public Health on November 22, 2020. Based on the anonymous comments of one reader, the article was retracted on July 22, 2021. Retraction Watch[27] summarized the retraction process, and again remarked on the authors' past writings on the problem with vaccinations.

During the retraction process, the authors "asked the Editor-in-Chief and the Editorial Board of the journal to publish the readers' comments, and our reply. They did not respond to that request. Instead, they decided to retract it without further discussion of our reply."[28] The authors then reproduced the comments of the anonymous reader and their responses.[28] According to Retraction Watch, "Thomas' efforts to discourage vaccinations in his patients prompted the state medical board to suspend his license last December—a move the authors have alleged was in retaliation for the publication of their study".[27]

Again, the pattern of retraction associated with the authors' critical views on vaccinations is repeated, accompanied by medical board harassment of one of the authors (as will be shown later, harassment by medical boards through license suspension and other drastic measures was/is commonplace for those who expressed views about the dangers from COVID-19 vaccines). It is also disconcerting that the Editor did not publish the authors' responses to the anonymous reviewers' comments. This would have allowed the readership to judge for themselves the merit for each side of the argument, and the merit for retracting the article.

Kostoff et al. Paper

An article titled "Why are we vaccinating children against COVID-19?" was published in Toxicology Reports (TR) on September 14, 2021, as part of a TR Special Issue titled "COVID-19 Pandemic: Health impact and Novel research". The article was retracted by the Publisher (Elsevier)/replacement Editor on April 30, 2022. The retraction process was documented in detail by the paper's first author in a Trial Site News Op-ed.[23] As in the other three retracted papers described in this section, this retracted paper was critical of the reported efficacy and safety of the COVID-19 vaccines, and showed that even under a best case scenario, the vaccines had a very unfavorable cost–benefit ratio.

Three points from the detailed review of the retraction process[23] will be emphasized here, but it is strongly recommended the reader examine the full Op-ed to get both the verbatim technical exchanges and the politically motivated aspects.

The first two points are technical, and the third is completely nontechnical. Elsevier had initiated a re-review of this referenced peer-reviewed and published article (and of all the nine articles in the TR Special Issue), and comments from the Elsevier review were sent to the authors for a response. The first two comments on the Kostoff et al. paper (which one assumes were the highest priority concerns for the reviewers) are as follows.

First, "The lead technical comment from each reviewer in the Appendix was that our paper was not within the scope of TR."[23] This comment was extremely strange for the following reasons. The theme of TR is toxicology, and the theme of the Special Issue of TR in which the paper was published was the COVID-19 pandemic. The main thrust of the Kostoff et al. paper was the toxic effects of the COVID-19 vaccine. This was a perfect match with the theme of the Special Issue of TR, yet was deemed out-of-scope by the two reviewers of the paper. Interestingly, the lead reviewer is a toxicologist, yet had no comments on any toxicology issues in the paper.

Second, "The Elsevier reviewers objected to our use of the term 'inoculation' instead of 'vaccination'. We used the term 'inoculation' rather than 'vaccine' in the TR paper because the substance does not meet the legal definition of a vaccine, nor does it function as a vaccine (prevent infection, prevent viral transmission)... The reviewers state that our use of the terms 'diverges from common use and are incorrect'. That is an opinion, not a technical argument. Nowhere do they offer technical reasons showing why the statement is incorrect and why this substance should be called a vaccine.

That is not a mystery; credible evidence of the injected substance acting as a COVID-19 'vaccine' does not exist!"[23]

It was surprising that Elsevier would approve, and release, a review of such low technical caliber. What was even more disturbing was the third nontechnical point. The Editor-in-Chief (EIC) of TR during the re-review was Dr Tsatsakis. The person who managed the review for Elsevier (and also served as a reviewer) was Dr Lash (founder of TR and an *in-house Elsevier contractor* who was the Editor of another Elsevier journal). "On 21 March 2022, the TR EIC (Dr Tsatsakis) resigned as EIC for personal reasons, and later that same day, Dr Lash was appointed the permanent EIC for TR. I cannot emphasize this last point too strongly. *Dr Lash, an Elsevier contractor, conducted the re-review at Elsevier's request, and then was rewarded with the permanent TR EIC position on the same day that the TR EIC resigned.*"[23]

Mead et al. Paper

An article titled "COVID-19 mRNA Vaccines: Lessons Learned from the Registrational Trials and Global Vaccination Campaign" was published on 24 January 2024 in the journal Cureus, after having passed a rigorous peer-review that included *eight* reviewers. The article concluded, in part: "Reanalysis of the Pfizer trial data identified statistically significant increases in serious adverse events (SAEs) in the vaccine group. Numerous SAEs were identified following the Emergency Use Authorization (EUA), including death, cancer, cardiac events, and various autoimmune, hematological, reproductive, and neurological disorders. Furthermore, these products never underwent adequate safety and toxicological testing in accordance with previously established scientific standards. Among the other major topics addressed in this narrative review are the published analyses of serious harms to humans, quality control issues and process-related impurities, mechanisms underlying adverse events (AEs), the immunologic basis for vaccine inefficacy, and concerning mortality trends based on the registrational trial data. The risk–benefit imbalance substantiated by the evidence to date contraindicates further booster injections and suggests that, at a minimum, the mRNA injections should be removed from the childhood immunization program until proper safety and toxicological studies are conducted."[29]

On 26 February 2024, the article was retracted. The retraction letter, signed by Mr Tim Kersjes (Head of Research Integrity, Resolutions, Springer Nature Research Integrity Group), raised the following eight points of concern:

1. We find that the article is misrepresenting all-cause mortality data.
2. We find that the article appears to be misrepresenting VAERS data.
3. The article states that the Pfizer COVID-19 vaccine saved two lives and caused 27 deaths per 100,000 vaccinations, and the Moderna vaccine saved 3.9 lives and caused 10.8 deaths per 100,000 vaccinations, though there does not appear to be convincing evidence for this claim.
4. *Incorrect claim*: Vaccines are gene therapy products.

5. The article states that vaccines are contaminated with high levels of DNA. Upon review, we found that the cited references are not sufficient to support these claims.
6. The article states that SV40 promoter can cause cancer because SV40 virus can cause cancer in some organisms and inconclusively in humans. However, we find that this is misrepresenting the cited study (Li S, MacLaughlin F, Fewell J, et al. Muscle-specific enhancement of gene expression by incorporation of SV40 enhancer in the expression plasmid. Gene Ther. 2001;8:494-7. https://doi.org/10.1038/sj.gt.3301419).
7. The article states that mRNA COVID-19 vaccines did not undergo adequate safety and efficacy testing, which the journal considers to be incorrect.
8. The article incorrectly states that spike proteins produced by COVID-19 vaccination linger in the body and cause adverse effects.

The first author of the retracted paper, M Nathaniel Mead, addressed each of the eight points raised by Mr Kersjes. Based on analyses and publications I have done on (1) COVID-19 and (2) the side effects from its vaccines, I can state unequivocally that Mead's rebuttal demolished the credibility and validity of each of these points. The eight points raised by Mr Kersjes and the detailed rebuttal can be found on the substack of Dr Peter McCullough, one of the retracted paper's co-authors.[30] However, as in all the other retractions shown in this section, rebuttals are irrelevant to the final retraction decision. Mead's excellent rebuttal had no impact on the retraction.

To show how deep the tentacles of the censorship industry have penetrated, consider the journal that retracted the paper, Cureus. This journal has an impact factor of ~1.2, which puts it at the very low end of journals indexed in Web of Science. A study by two Emory university librarians assessing where the Emory faculty are publishing[31] concluded the following: "Our findings highlight two journals that represented 50% of the controversial or predatory publications among our faculty: Cureus and Oncotarget. These use nontraditional publishing practices, and there have been arguments for and against considering each legitimate... We would like to communicate with the authors of papers that were published in these journals to understand their level of awareness of the controversy surrounding these titles. We are not able to determine from our analysis if faculty have fallen prey to controversial or predatory tactics or if they have made strategic, fully informed choices when disseminating their work".

It is not clear to me why the authors would choose such a low-tier journal for their publication venue of this extremely important paper. Further, the fact that even such a low-tier journal was targeted by the vaccine promoters shows the depths that they will go to ensure that the truth about the COVID-19 vaccines never sees the light of day. Most disturbing to me, however, is the fact that the Editors-in-Chief of Cureus and their Editorial Board allowed this retraction to happen without a mass resignation. It is this widespread compliance with the censorship of the vaccine promoters that will (1) destroy the credibility of the biomedical literature and (2) enable widespread harm among the COVID-19 vaccine recipients because they were deliberately denied knowledge of this suppressed information.

To summarize this section, different approaches were used to retract the papers in the four examples. Technical feedback from the authors was either not requested or not taken into consideration. However, the real victims of these politically driven retractions are not the authors of the retracted article. The real victims are those who will make decisions on COVID-19 vaccination without having access to all the information showing the vaccine's potential dangers, and will then have to bear the health and financial consequences.

Distortions

This section contains examples of two articles that have remained in the literature despite questionable findings and conclusions. The first occurred in the pre-COVID-19 era, and the second occurred at a crucial point in the early COVID-19 era.

CDC Study on MMR Vaccine-Autism Link

Dr William W Thompson is a senior researcher/epidemiologist with the Centers for Disease Control and Prevention (CDC). Among other accomplishments, he was first author of two journal papers that received over 1,000 citations apiece. The following excerpts summarize his allegations that the CDC removed critical data from a study exploring the link between the MMR (measles, mumps, and rubella) vaccine and autism, thereby altering the results.

"On August 27, 2014, the following excerpted statement by Dr William Thompson (a CDC Senior Researcher) appeared on the website of Morgan Verkamp, LLC, a legal organization representing Dr Thompson."

"I regret that my co-authors and I omitted statistically significant information in our 2004 article published in the journal Pediatrics. The omitted data suggested that African American males who received the MMR vaccine before age 36 months were at increased risk for autism. Decisions were made regarding which findings to report after the data were collected, and I believe that the final study protocol was not followed... My concern has been the decision to omit relevant findings in a particular study for a particular subgroup for a particular vaccine. There have always been recognized risks for vaccination and I believe it is the responsibility of the CDC to properly convey the risks associated with receipt of those vaccines."

According to taped phone conversations between Dr Brian Hooker and Dr Thompson, not only were the African-American children who received the MMR vaccine at substantially greater risk for autism (as alleged by Dr Thompson), but according to Dr Hooker, Dr Thompson mentioned that children of all races were shown to have an increased risk of "Isolated Autism" [young children, regardless of race, who had (1) received the MMR vaccine on schedule, as recommended by the CDC, and (2) had no other factors sometimes observed to accompany autism, such as cerebral palsy, mental retardation, and birth defects].

The MMR vaccine-autism study to which Dr Thompson referred had been performed shortly after the turn of the new millennium, and the stated results (no link between MMR vaccine and autism) had been published in the journal Pediatrics... As of September 1, 2016, the article has not been retracted by Pediatrics, despite the serious allegations of intentional omission of critical data by one of its co-authors.

Thus, according to Dr Thompson's allegations of August 27, 2014, CDC had known for at least a decade that these two groups of children were at increased risk for autism from the MMR vaccine, and did not disclose this information to the public. Internal CDC memos also showed the highest levels of CDC management had been informed of these problems with the MMR vaccine since the early 21st century.[32]

What more credible evidence of wrongdoing is there than one of the authors of the Pediatrics paper alleging in public that data were deliberately omitted to alter the results? But even that was insufficient for retraction. Again, the real victims of this nonretraction (assuming Thompson's allegations are correct) are (1) the children who developed autism and might not have if the correct information had been available, (2) the parents/caretakers of these children who will spend inordinate amounts of time and money in having to care for them, and (3) the American taxpayer, who will finance the government aid provided for these children and the added insurance premiums that will result.

Further, why would we believe this situation with vaccine (and other) studies is unique? Given the motivations of the principals, what excludes similar alterations of data in other studies to achieve the desired results? We only know about the alleged data manipulations in the MMR vaccine-autism study because one of the participants in the alteration admitted/alleged these alterations in public. How many participants in other such alleged data alterations would be willing to risk their careers and follow in Dr Thompson's footsteps?

RECOVERY Trials Paper

Because of the rapid development and testing of the COVID-19 vaccines, they could not be granted full FDA approval before mass distribution. In order to be released before clinical trials were complete, they had to be granted Emergency Use Authorization (EUA). What is EUA? Yale Medicine defines EUA as follows: "an emergency use authorization (EUA) is a tool the Food and Drug Administration (FDA) can use to expedite the availability of medical products, including drugs and vaccines, during a public health emergency. An EUA can only be granted when no adequate, approved, available alternatives exist, and when the known and potential benefits outweigh the potential risks."[33]

Therefore, in order to qualify the potential COVID-19 vaccines for EUA, there had to be evidence that no credible treatment alternatives existed. While much evidence of effectiveness and safety of alternative treatments for COVID-19 (including hydroxychloroquine, azithromycin, zinc, vitamin D3, intravenous vitamin C, and other alternatives) was being gathered and demonstrated from the earliest days of the pandemic,[34,35] it was being ignored by health policy bureaucrats and the mainstream media. Actions were taken by many bureaucrats and politicians to suppress recommendations of these alternatives. Studies were being commissioned and published showing ineffectiveness and potential dangers from these alternatives.

One study that had substantial influence on COVID-19 treatment policy was published in NEJM in late 2020.[36] It was based on the RECOVERY study, a large, randomized, multi-center clinical trial. The RECOVERY study and similar large-scale studies Solidarity and REMAP were analyzed in detail and criticized severely by Dr Meryl Nass, Board-Certified in Internal Medicine.[37] As stated in the latter reference: "It is remarkable that a large series of events taking place over the past 3 months produced a unified message about hydroxychloroquine, and produced similar policies about the drug in the US, Canada, Australia, New Zealand, and western Europe. The message is that generic, inexpensive hydroxychloroquine is dangerous and should not be used to treat a potentially fatal disease, COVID-19, for which there are no (other) reliable treatments.

Hydroxychloroquine has been used safely for 65 years in many millions of patients. And so the message was crafted that the drug is safe for its other uses, but dangerous when used for COVID-19. It does not make sense, but it seems to have worked."

Dr Nass summarized what happened in these three trials in the format of a to do list:

"1. You stop doctors from using the drug in ways it is most likely to be effective (in outpatients at onset of illness). You prohibit use outside of situations you can control.
   Situations that were controlled to show no benefit included three large, randomized, multi-center clinical trials (RECOVERY, Solidarity, and REMAP-COVID), the kind of trials that are generally believed to yield the most reliable evidence. However, *each of them used excessive hydroxychloroquine doses that were known to be toxic and may have been fatal in some cases*; and a fourth Chinese study that also used excessive doses (3.6 g HCQ in the first 3 days and 800 mg/day thereafter, comparable to the above studies) also found no benefit from HCQ.
2. You play up the danger of the drug, emphasizing side effects that are very rare when the drug is used correctly. You make sure everyone has heard about the man who died after consuming hydroxychloroquine in the form of fish tank cleaner. Yet its toxicity at approved doses is minimal. Chloroquine was added to table salt in some regions in the 1950s as a

malaria preventive, according to Professor Nicholas White in his study for the RECOVERY trial.

3. You limit clinical trials to hospitalized patients, instead of testing the drug in outpatients, early in the illness, when it is predicted to be most effective.
4. You design clinical trials to give much too high a dose, ensuring the drug will cause harm in some subjects, sufficient to mask any possible beneficial effect. You make sure that trials in 400 hospitals in 35 countries (Solidarity) plus most hospitals in the UK (RECOVERY) use these dangerous doses, as well as additional sites in 13 countries (REMAP-COVID trial)."[37]

Based on the results of these three questionable clinical trials and other similar trials, decisions were made to severely restrict access to hydroxychloroquine by politicians, clinicians, pharmacists, etc., and deny the public the benefits of a treatment proven to be safe and effective on thousands of patients by some hands-on physicians. Why was a paper that contained this disinformation about the benefits of hydroxychloroquine not withdrawn or retracted?

The two examples in this section (and many others like them) show that papers known to contain disinformation can remain published if the disinformation supports the agenda of government and industry.

Censorship

Two of the essential elements of literature censorship are (1) creation of disincentives for potential authors to work on, or promote, alternatives to mainstream interests, and (2) creation of incentives for the media and licensing bodies to disparage such people and their activities. This section will provide examples of how the CDC/FDA/NIH and other government entities effectively censored alternative treatments for COVID-19 and promoted the vaccines by sending large sums of money to censoring organizations. Additionally, this section will show how alternative treatments for chronic diseases were censored by government actions against the developers of these alternative treatments, using the same playbook that was used in the COVID-19 era for censoring alternative COVID-19 treatments.

CDC/FDA/NIH Censorship of Alternative Treatments for COVID-19

Hospital and drug manufacturer subsidies: The Federal agencies responsible for healthcare, in concert with other non-healthcare Federal agencies, actively (1) suppressed alternative treatments for COVID-19 using a combination of bribery, coercion, and regulations, (2) promoted mainstream treatments using the same tactics, and (3) promoted the use of vaccines using all these measures. All the funds provided came directly from the American taxpayers.

For example, "According to section 3710 of the Cares Act, hospitals are reimbursed by the government an extra 20% for each hospitalized Medicare patient. The only criteria for that extra money? A positive COVID test."[38] The COVID-19 tests were performed using polymerase chain reaction (PCR), even though the scientist responsible for the PCR test "was the first to say that

PCR technology could not be used for diagnostic purposes."[39] Assessments have been done showing that PCR tests give false positives anywhere from 90–97% of the time (at the amplification cycle levels that were used in the tests).[40]

Further, "More than 1,000 hospitals in high-impact areas will get a share of $10 billion in new federal assistance. The new payments will be $50,000 per COVID-19 admission, less than the $77,000 in an earlier round."[41] Additionally, "Hospitals were paid $13,000 per person who was admitted as a COVID case, and another $39,000 for every patient put on a ventilator."[42]

Incentives were provided to hospitals that used specific drugs in the treatment of COVID-19: "CMS issued an Interim Final Rule with Comment Period that established the New COVID-19 Treatments Add-on Payment (NCTAP) under the Medicare Inpatient Prospective Payment System (IPPS). The NCTAP, designed to mitigate potential financial disincentives for hospitals to provide new COVID-19 treatments, is effective from November 2, 2020, until September 30, 2023.

Through the NCTAP, Medicare will provide an enhanced payment through September 30, 2023, for eligible inpatient cases that use certain new products with current FDA approval or emergency use authorization (EUA) to treat COVID-19, including the following: VEKLURY (remdesivir)".[43] The use of remdesivir, and the additional Federal subsidy for its use, were discussed in the following: "The antiviral drug remdesivir, brand name Veklury, is approved for use against COVID-19 despite research showing it lacks effectiveness and can cause high rates of organ failure.

John Beaudoin is calling for a criminal investigation into remdesivir, citing data that it may have killed 100,000 people in the US.

Beaudoin received all the death certificates in Massachusetts from 2015 to 2022, finding 1,840 excess deaths from acute renal failure from January 1, 2021, to November 30, 2022, which he believes may be due to remdesivir.

A study published in the Lancet found 'no clinical benefit' from the use of remdesivir in hospitalized patients.

The US government pays hospitals a 20% upcharge on the entire hospital bill when remdesivir is used."[44]

For patients whose death was attributed to COVID-19, FEMA will cover up to $9,000 in funeral expenses.[45]

To summarize the above, once a person was tagged as having COVID-19, based mainly on the results of PCR tests that gave anywhere from 90–97% false positives, they were given special treatment protocols when hospitalized, and the hospitals received substantial subsidies for following these government-authorized protocols. If these patients died, their funeral costs were subsidized by the government if they were tagged as COVID-19. In effect, the American taxpayer subsidized hospitals and drug manufacturers for treatment of patients who most likely did not have COVID-19 based on flawed PCR diagnostic tests. The purpose of subsidizing protocols that followed the mainstream narrative was to reinforce the concept that COVID-19 was a pandemic, no alternative treatments were available, and only the COVID-19 vaccines could control COVID-19 globally.

There were additional subsidies for administering the vaccines. For example, Blue Cross Blue Shield announced the following in 2021: "the Blue Cross and Blue Shield (BCBS) Government-wide Service Benefit Plan, also known as the Federal Employee Program® (FEP®) announced it will launch a COVID-19 Vaccination Incentive Program starting Friday, June 11, 2021, to encourage members to get vaccinated against COVID-19. Eligible members—those over the age of 18 with an FEP MyBlue® account—will receive $50 on their MyBlue Wellness Card when they provide official documentation of their COVID-19 vaccination record."[46]

Vaccine providers were also given BCBS financial incentives. The following referenced URL (containing an announcement from the Kentucky BCBS) shows the magnitude of the incentives.[47] States, cities, and businesses also offered incentives to vaccine recipients, ranging from lotteries for financial rewards and scholarships to smaller cash bonuses and prizes.[48] In summary, providers and recipients of the COVID-19 vaccines were rewarded financially for administering and receiving the vaccines.

Subsidies of other organizations: Many other organizations were provided subsidies/bribes (depending on one's perspective) for promoting the government treatment and prevention protocols for COVID-19. Some of these organizations disparaged those who opposed the protocols.

For example, "According to FOIA documents obtained by the Blaze, the current administration paid the whole of corporate media, including the so-called 'conservative' outlets, a billion of your tax dollars to carry out a massive campaign to push positive information about the COVID-19 vaccines. The Department of Health and Human Services admitted that it spent hundreds of millions of dollars on the purchasing of advertising from major news networks including ABC, CBS, and NBC, as well as cable TV news stations Fox News, CNN, and MSNBC, legacy media publications including the New York Post, the Los Angeles Times, and the Washington Post, digital media companies like BuzzFeed News and Newsmax, and hundreds of local newspapers and TV stations. These outlets were collectively responsible for publishing countless articles and video segments regarding the vaccine that were nearly uniformly positive about the vaccine in terms of both its efficacy and safety."[49]

Many of these media organizations also published disparaging articles about researchers who showed the dangers of the vaccines. These articles served not only the purpose of disinforming the public about the vaccines, but served to set an example for other researchers of what can happen if they choose to oppose the mainstream approach to COVID-19 treatments and vaccines. This is the human side of the censorship that has occurred and is occurring with respect to COVID-19.

Each State has various physician societies that can regulate the certification and licensing of physicians. As stated by Sonia Elijah in an online newsletter "By March 2021, as part of the Biden administration's emergency countermeasure efforts involving COVID-19 vaccines, the administration handed out nearly $10 billion in money to influential groups across American society such as physician societies to advocate and aggressively promote the vaccines across low-income and underserved communities as part of the COVID-19 response. The safety data was not well understood, and in fact, still remains unclear, especially when it comes to pregnant women and their gestating babies, lactation, and very young children per the to date Food and Drug Administration package inserts.

Part of Biden administration's nearly $10 billion COVID-19 vaccine promotional campaign included the launching of 'COVID-19 Community Corps,' a nationwide grassroots network of local voices people know and trust to encourage Americans to get vaccinated. A total of $6,113,504,125 was injected into 1,377 health centers, hence the intense push to promote the vaccine and unfortunately, suppression of any critical information. A founding member was the American College of Obstetricians and Gynecologists (ACOG)—the group received money, and as it happens, was literally the very first organization to declare that the COVID-19 vaccines were safe for pregnant women and gestating babies."[50]

At approximately 10.5 minutes into the following video interview of Dr James A Thorp (a Board-Certified Obstetrician/Gynecologist), Dr Thorp presents a vugraph titled "COVID-19 Community Corps", with the subtitle "$13 Billion to 298 Sectors of USA Society".[51] The vugraph contains a list of twelve categories of recipients (who can be characterized as influencers, such as public health and medical organizations, business leaders, union leaders, faith leaders, etc.), and the percentage of funds each category received. The purpose was to have trusted community leaders encourage vaccinations. Depending on one's perspective, this could be interpreted as (1) supporting an important life-enhancing measure or (2) bribing willing officials to push an essentially untested and unsafe product. Given all the other rewards and incentives described previously, it is quite apparent which interpretation of the $13 Billion handout is correct!

Censorship of Alternatives to Mainstream Chronic Disease Treatments

Dr Dale Bredesen, a long-time neurologist/researcher/clinician who specialized in Alzheimer's disease (AD), made a profound observation (in the journal Aging, 2014) with respect to AD: "In the case of Alzheimer's disease, there is not a single therapeutic that exerts anything beyond a marginal, unsustained symptomatic effect, with little or no effect on disease progression. Furthermore, in the past decade alone, hundreds of clinical trials have been conducted for AD, at an aggregate cost of billions of dollars, without success. This has led some to question whether the approach taken to drug development for AD is an optimal one".[52]

This statement by Dr Bredesen is applicable well beyond AD to perhaps all chronic diseases and many infectious diseases as well. Perhaps the most widely discussed suppression of alternative treatments, including both active suppression and exclusion from clinical trials, is for cancer. Therefore, this section will summarize the cancer alternative treatments suppression. The remainder is excerpted from a 2023 Trial Site News Op-ed on cancer alternative treatments.[53]

Alternative cancer therapies have been propounded for over a century. A 1995 study summarized the concepts underlying some of these alternative cancer therapies.[54] The concepts were divided into the following classes: Diet Therapy (e.g., Gerson Method, Macrobiotic Diet, Shark Cartilage, etc.); Megavitamins (e.g., High-dose Vitamins A, B, C, D, E, etc.); Metabolic Therapy (e.g., Laetrile, Dimethyl Sulfoxide, etc.); Herbal Remedies (e.g., Essiac, Barley Green, Blue-Green Algae, etc.); Electronic Devices (e.g., Galvanic Therapy, Magnetic Field Therapy, Negative Ion Therapy, Color and Light Therapy, etc.); and Immune Therapy (e.g., Autologous and fetal vaccines, Burton Treatment, etc.). The names associated with some of these therapies include the following: Gerson, Rife, Hoxsey, Budwig, and many others. Other more recent cancer therapy alternatives include antineoplaston therapy (Burzynski) and bioresonance ultrasound healing therapy (Venter).[53]

These alternative cancer therapies appear to be far less invasive, painful, disfiguring, and expensive compared to the mainstream cancer therapies (costs of these mainstream cancer therapies are estimated in the following references: 55, 56). Whether these alternative cancer therapies are safe and effective is another story. None of these alternative therapies have been approved by the FDA for cancer treatment. Many of the proponents of these alternative cancer therapies have been attacked in various ways by the government. Many/most practitioners had their practices closed, and some had to establish practices in foreign countries to continue patient treatment.[53]

However, the pandemic-related events of the last 4 years, and the role of the FDA and other healthcare agencies in the pandemic responses, have radically changed the public image of (1) the FDA and the associated Federal healthcare agencies (CDC, NIH, etc.), as well as (2) their grantees in academia. The FDA and the CDC have become completely untrustworthy and corrupted, with the upper levels of the NIH not far behind [while the FDA and CDC are singled out for criticism here because they were the public face of Federal government response to the pandemic, it should be remembered that they are two tentacles of the octopus that is the Federal government. The octopus controls the tentacles. The highest levels of all branches of the Federal government (executive, legislative, and judicial) abdicated their responsibilities during the pandemic].[53]

It is questionable whether the COVID-19-era level of collusion (among the healthcare and all other Federal agencies, the healthcare industry, the media, the governing Boards of the medical profession, and much of academia) started with COVID-19. Such widespread collusion must have taken decades to develop. Therefore, some of the FDA's past decisions on alternative cancer (and other chronic disease) therapies, and the media's compliant blackout about the potentially positive effects of such therapies, should be re-examined.

For the pandemic, the safe, effective (when given early), and inexpensive COVID-19 treatments (e.g., hydroxychloroquine, ivermectin, etc.) were not approved by the Federal agencies for treating patients diagnosed as COVID-19. Rather, they were actively opposed and outlawed. More expensive and ineffective treatments (applied late) were promoted by these healthcare agencies. Most egregiously, essentially untested "vaccines" were promoted by the healthcare agencies for all demographics, even those that did not suffer any serious side effects from COVID-19. These Federal dictates were parroted by the popular and biomedical media, which suppressed essentially all discussion of adverse effects from the COVID-19 vaccines and only published papers purportedly showing benefits from the vaccines. When papers were published in the mainstream biomedical literature on COVID-19 vaccine adverse events, they typically portrayed the adverse event as extremely rare and/or mild and transient.

How does this concerted Government–Industry–Media approach for COVID-19 differ from that taken for the alternative cancer therapy approaches? In the latter case, the alternative cancer treatments did not receive FDA approval. The media only published negative results from these treatments, and did not publish positive results. Thus, *the playbook to advance mainstream cancer therapies (chemotherapy, surgery, radiation) and suppress alternative cancer therapies is almost identical to the playbook used to advance the vaccines and mainstream expensive (and ineffective) treatments for COVID-19 and suppress the alternative safe, effective, and inexpensive approaches.*[53]

The above should not be interpreted as support for the alternative cancer therapies that were proposed and tested in the past. Their validity is open to question, and the FDA may have been correct in not approving them. Unfortunately, because of the COVID-19 fiasco, the recommendations of (1) the Federal healthcare agencies whose job it is to provide credible healthcare information to the American public and (2) their parroting State and local counterparts can no longer be trusted. Thus, the FDA's disapproval of these alternative cancer therapies, and the media's parroting of the FDA-industry position, are not adequate proof that none of the alternative cancer therapies have worked or could work. An independent objective evaluation (by nonconflicted experts) of some of these alternative cancer therapies would need to be conducted before one could conclude (1) they have not worked, (2) they do not, and (3) could not work.[53]

Harassment

This section continues the theme of previous section "Censorship", showing some harsh measures that were used to dissuade people from promoting alternatives to the mainstream approaches. Four brief examples are shown, with three of them occurring prior to the COVID-19 era. For the COVID-19 era alone, tens (if not hundreds) of such examples could be presented.

David Lewis

In 1993, Environmental Protection Agency (EPA) generated a sludge rule that allows very toxic biosolids, or treated sewage sludge, to be used for farms, forests, playgrounds, and parks. Dr David Lewis (ex-EPA senior researcher) exposed how EPA, in coordination with other Federal Agencies, research institutions, and advisory groups, suppressed public knowledge of potential biosludge adverse health effects for years.

He did this exposure through published research articles; testimony and depositions before Congress; testimony and depositions before Department of Labor hearings; and lawsuits that revealed (under oath) the detailed participation of EPA officials and others in the science distortions. Dr Lewis was forced to retire and, in 2014, published a book (recounting his experiences) entitled Science for Sale. He implied that EPA-sponsored research had to support EPA policy; implied that there was selective funding of scientists who supported EPA's sludge rule; showed myriad ways the science was distorted to present biosludge as safe; and showed collusion among EPA and other agencies.

The book is unique in its portrayal of collusion among the diverse groups mentioned in its subtitle: "How the US Government uses Powerful Corporations and Leading Universities to Support Government Policies, Silence Top Scientists, Jeopardize Our Health, and Protect Corporate Profits". One can draw a straight line from the harassment of Dr Lewis and the suppression of his findings to the harassment and suppression that was the norm in the COVID-19 pandemic. The examples of harassment and suppression presented in this chapter provide strong evidence that what we have in practice (for these commercially, militarily, and politically sensitive issues) is a Government–Industrial–Media–Academia–Complex that monopolizes the discourse and exerts strong influence on what the public knows and believes about these topics.[32]

William Marcus

Dr William Marcus was a toxicologist and Senior Science Advisor at EPA. He reported potential cover-up of cancers (by the National Toxicology Program)...resulting from fluoride ingestion... and was fired in 1992. He challenged this decision in court, and was re-instated. While there is substantial credible evidence in the published literature that water fluoridation carries high health risks, the literature remains infested with voluminous "manufactured" research on the safety of fluoride, sowing confusion on appropriate limits of fluoride concentrations in water. The EPA maximum contaminant level goals (MCLG) limit of 4 milligrams per liter for fluoride remains in effect, even though the Public Health Service recommends 1/6 that concentration as a limit.

Interestingly, EPA's risk control methodology, the Reference Dose (daily dose that a person can receive over the long term with reasonable assurance of safety from adverse effects), when applied to neurotoxicity data, led to a Reference Dose for fluoride of 0.000007 mg/kg per day. Persons who drink about one quart of fluoridated water per day from the public drinking water supply of the District of Columbia while at work receive about 0.01 mg/kg per day from that source alone. This amount of fluoride is more than 100 times the Reference Dose.[32]

This level of discrepancy between doses yielding adverse health effects shown in the literature and regulatory agency guidelines is not unique to either fluoridation or the EPA. A 2018 study on the Permissible Exposure Limits (PELs) established by OSHA to ostensibly protect workers showed "the PELs are orders of magnitude higher than what the premier biomedical literature would suggest is protective".[57]

Rather than reward Dr Marcus for his valuable contribution in exposing the dangers of fluoride, the EPA chose to harass and punish him, and suppress his valuable findings. Again, a straight line can be drawn from Dr Marcus to the suppressions and harassments that occurred during the COVID-19 era.

Tyrone Hayes

Dr Tyrone Hayes was a researcher and member of the biology faculty at the University of California, Berkely. In 1998, "Syngenta, one of the largest agribusinesses in the world, had asked Hayes to conduct experiments on the herbicide atrazine, which is applied to more than half the corn in the United States. Hayes was thirty-one, and he had already published twenty papers on the endocrinology of amphibians. David Wake, a professor in Hayes's department, said that Hayes 'may have had the greatest potential of anyone in the field.' But, when Hayes discovered that atrazine might impede the sexual development of frogs, his dealings with Syngenta became strained, and, in November, 2000, he ended his relationship with the company."[58]

Rachael Aviv, a reporter with the New Yorker Magazine, chronicled how Syngenta harassed Dr Hayes over the next few years to discredit his findings and reputation.[58] It is a must-read for anyone who wants to understand the lengths to which organizations will go to discredit anyone whose findings can adversely impact their bottom line, and was repeated in different forms throughout the COVID-19 era. Collusion between industry, the media, some members of academia, and the EPA was also described in Ms Aviv's article, although this collusion was much less than occurred during the COVID-19 era.

Meryl Nass

Dr Meryl Nass is Board-Certified in Internal Medicine, and is a practicing physician in Maine. She has criticized the suppression of alternative treatments for COVID-19 since early in the pandemic, and gained special notoriety for an article she wrote exposing the use of known toxic dose of hydroxychloroquine in a supposedly objective clinical trial of its efficacy and safety.[59] As a result of this article, and many others on alternative COVID-19 treatments and the dangers of the COVID-19 vaccines, The Board of Licensure in Medicine (BOLIM), a state agency that regulates medical licensing in Maine, suspended Dr Meryl Nass's medical license on January 12, 2022 following an investigation that started with an activist's complaint that she was spreading misinformation in media interviews and on the Internet.[60] There have been multiple hearings by the Board, and they have had to retract multiple allegations of spreading misinformation. But the harassment continues, and neither most of the physicians in the State of Maine nor most of the residents have taken appropriate actions to end the harassment.

In summary, what all these examples have shown generally, and what the last group of examples has shown specifically, is that (1) suppression of information that is counter to commercial, political, and military interests and (2) harassment and punishment of those who supply such information have been occurring for many decades. What is new for the COVID-19 era is (1) the scale of the suppression and harassment, and (2) the potential scale of the damage caused by the denial of appropriate treatments for COVID-19, and (3) deployment of the vaccines.

CONSEQUENCES OF CENSORSHIP AND DISTORTION

This final section will address the consequences of the mRNA-based COVID-19 vaccines, since they were the vaccines used most frequently in the USA. These mRNA vaccines (while labeled as vaccines) are not vaccines in any traditional sense. They prevent neither infection nor viral transmission. In fact, they could not prevent infection or transmission because of their fundamental mode of operation.[61] Given the damage that results from their fundamental mode of operation, *it is difficult to see how anyone who has received doses of a functional mRNA vaccine can avoid having their lifespan reduced*. If the worst comes to pass, and these shots result in producing vastly increased sterility and infertility, then future generations will be greatly impacted as well.

Even more disturbing, a 2023 interview (with the eminent microbiologist Dr Sucharit Bhakdi) shows that the fundamental mode of operation of *any* of the myriad mRNA vaccines being studied for many different diseases will end up producing similar damage to that from the COVID-19 mRNA shots that encoded the spike protein.[62]

Dr Bhakdi (and many others) have stated that, even though these mRNA vaccines are injected into the deltoid muscle, most of the vaccine will end up in the bloodstream, directly or indirectly. The central mechanism for the COVID-19 mRNA shots involves the lipid-nanoparticle (LNP)-encased mRNA coalescing with cells on the inside of blood vessels (endothelial cells). These cells then express the spike protein produced on their surface. To the bloodstream immune cells in the area, the cells with spike protein on their surface are foreign bodies, and the immune cells attack and destroy them as nature intended. This destruction of the vessel wall by the immune cells allows the remaining LNP-encased mRNA packages to enter the organs and tissues adjacent to the degraded blood vessel, and produce destruction of the organ and tissue cells by the same process.

Dr Bhakdi's main point is that this pseudo-autoimmunity-generating process will occur for the mRNA of *any* protein, not just the spike protein. Any cell in the body with foreign protein expressed on the surface is viewed by the immune system as foreign, and will be attacked and killed. Thus, if these new mRNA vaccines are approved, there will be multiple opportunities for cell, tissue, and organ destruction for people who allow themselves to be injected with such toxic substances. Not informing the public of these actual and potential dangers is the real downside of this biomedical literature censorship!

CONCLUSION

Retractions are important and (for those researchers/clinicians at the beginning or mid-point of their careers) can be career-threatening. However, the retractions are at the tail end of a long culling process, where most culling and censorship occur well before the retraction process. The real culling probably occurs at Step 1 (research funding), especially for the potential performers. If they do not see studies on COVID-19 vaccines adverse effects as career-enhancing, but rather as career-stagnation at best, they will not propose such studies, and eventually will not even think about ideas for such studies. More effort needs to be expended exposing the dangers of Steps 1–3 (not funding potential research, not publishing results of studies opposing official government narrative), because focusing on retractions will shift attention away from where the bulk of actual censorship is occurring.

As some of the examples of censorship and distortion have shown, censorship and distortion of the biomedical literature are not new phenomenon. Censorship and distortion have been in effect for many decades. What is new for the COVID-19 era level of censorship is the magnitude of the potential consequences. The actual numbers of people who were killed and maimed because censorship denied them (or their caretakers) the ability to give informed consent to government-imposed measures, especially vaccination, is a subject for debate. However, these numbers of necessity will be large for two main reasons: (1) the fundamental mode of operation of the COVID-19 vaccines will result in tissue and organ destruction throughout the body of the recipient, and (2) tracking databases such as VAERS, V-Safe, and the European Medicines Agency tracking database (EudraVigilance) have all shown that the numbers of injured and killed post-COVID-19 vaccination are enormous. The challenge for society is identifying and implementing required actions to ensure that the probability of future manipulations of the literature (with devastating consequences) can be reduced substantially.

REFERENCES

1. Kostoff RN; Trial Site News. (2023). Retractions are the tip of the censorship iceberg. [online] Available from https://www.trialsitenews.com/a/retractions-are-the-tip-of-the-censorship-iceberg-d16ae28b. [Last accessed April, 2024]
2. Budd JM, Sievert M, Schultz TR. Phenomena of retraction: reasons for retraction and citations to the publications. JAMA. 1998;280(3):296-7.
3. Campos-Varela I, Ruano-Ravina A. Misconduct as the main cause for retraction. A descriptive study of retracted publications and their authors. Gac Sanit. 2019;33(4): 356-60.
4. Faggion CM Jr., Ware RS, Bakas N, Wasiak J. An analysis of retractions of dental publications. J Dent. 2018;79:19-23.
5. Katavic V. Retractions of scientific publications: responsibility and accountability. Biochem Med. 2014;24(2):217-22.
6. Moylan EC, Kowalczuk MK. Why articles are retracted: a retrospective cross-sectional study of retraction notices at BioMed Central. BMJ Open. 2016;6(11):e012047.
7. Nath SB, Marcus SC, Druss BG. Retractions in the research literature: misconduct or mistakes? Med J Aust. 2006;185(3):152-4.
8. Wager E, Williams P. Why and how do journals retract articles? An analysis of Medline retractions 1988-2008. J Med Ethics. 2011;37(9):567-70.
9. Steen RG. Retractions in the scientific literature: do authors deliberately commit research fraud? J Med Ethics. 2011;37(2):113-7.
10. Steen RG. Retractions in the scientific literature: is the incidence of research fraud increasing? J Med Ethics. 2011;37(4):249-53.
11. Kohl CBS, Faggion CM Jr. A comprehensive overview of studies that assessed article retractions within the biomedical sciences. Account Res. 2023:1-19. Online ahead of print.
12. Shir-Raz Y, Elisha E, Martin B, Ronel N, Guetzkow J. Censorship and Suppression of COVID-19 Heterodoxy: Tactics and Counter-Tactics. Minerva. 2022:1-27. Epub ahead of print.
13. Walach H, Klement RJ, Aukema W. The risk-benefit ratio of Covid-19 vaccines: Publication policy by retraction does nothing to improve it. Clin Transl Discov. 2022;2(1):e35.
14. Anderson C, Nugent K, Peterson C. Academic Journal Retractions and the COVID-19 Pandemic. J Prim Care Community Health. 2021;12:21501327211015592.
15. Audisio K, Robinson NB, Soletti GJ, Cancelli G, Dimagli A, Spadaccio C, et al. A survey of retractions in the cardiovascular literature. Int J Cardiol. 2022;349:109-14.
16. Campos-Varela I, Villaverde-Castaneda R, Ruano-Ravina A. Retraction of publications: a study of biomedical journals retracting publications based on impact factor and journal category. Gac Sanit. 2020;34(5):430-4.
17. Valencise FE, Palamim CVC, Marson FAL. Retraction of Clinical Trials about the SARS-CoV-2 Infection: An Unaddressed Problem and its Possible Impact on Coronavirus Disease (COVID)-19 Treatment. Int J Environ Res Public Health. 2023;20(3):1835.
18. Yeo-Teh NSL, Tang BL. An alarming retraction rate for scientific publications on Coronavirus Disease 2019 (COVID-19). Account Res. 2021;28(1):47-53.

19. Schonhaut L, Costa-Roldan I, Oppenheimer I, Pizarro V, Han D, Diaz F. Scientific publication speed and retractions of COVID-19 pandemic original articles. Rev Panam Salud Publica. 2022;46:e25.
20. Frampton G, Woods L, Scott DA. Inconsistent and incomplete retraction of published research: A cross-sectional study on COVID-19 retractions and recommendations to mitigate risks for research, policy and practice. PloS One. 2021;16(10):e0258935.
21. Retraction Watch. Retracted coronavirus (COVID-19) papers. [online] Available from https://retractionwatch.com/retracted-coronavirus-covid-19-papers/. [Last accessed April, 2024]
22. McCullough PA; Courageous Discourse. (2023). Retracted COVID-19 Articles: Significantly More Cited than Others. [online] Available from https://petermcculloughmd.substack.com/p/retracted-covid-19-articles-significantly. [Last accessed April, 2024]
23. Kostoff RN; Trial Site News. (2022). Anatomy of a Retraction. [online] Available from https://www.trialsitenews.com/a/anatomy-of-a-retraction-ea3c16b1. [Last accessed April, 2024]
24. Retraction Watch. Paper linking COVID-19 vaccines to myocarditis is temporarily removed without explanation. [online] Available from https://retractionwatch.com/2021/10/17/paper-linking-covid-19-vaccines-to-myocarditis-is-temporarily-removed-without-explanation/. [Last accessed April, 2024]
25. Retraction Watch. COVID-19 vaccine-myocarditis paper to be permanently removed: Elsevier. [online] Available from https://retractionwatch.com/2021/10/25/covid-19-vaccine-myocarditis-paper-to-be-permanently-removed-elsevier/. [Last accessed April, 2024]
26. Rancourt DG, Baudin M, Hickey J, Mercier J; CORRELATION Research in the Public Interest. (2023). COVID-19 vaccine-associated mortality in the Southern Hemisphere. [online] Available from https://correlation-canada.org/covid-19-vaccine-associated-mortality-in-the-Southern-Hemisphere/. [Last accessed April, 2024]
27. Retraction Watch. Authors blame a "ghoul" for retraction of paper claiming vaccines lead to health and behavioral issues. [online] Available from https://retractionwatch.com/2021/08/11/authors-blame-a-ghoul-for-retraction-of-paper-claiming-vaccines-lead-to-health-and-behavioral-issues/. [Last accessed April, 2024]
28. Lyons-Weiler J. MDPI'S "The International Journal of Environmental Research and Public Health" Does Not Publish Unbiased Research or Advances in Methodology. [online] Available from https://jameslyonsweiler.com/2021/07/25/mdpis-the-international-journal-of-environmental-research-and-public-health-does-not-publish-unbiased-research-or-advances-in-methodology/. [Last accessed April, 2024]
29. Mead M, Seneff S, Wolfinger R, Rose J, Denhaerynck K, Kirsch S, et al. COVID-19 mRNA Vaccines: Lessons Learned from the Registrational Trials and Global Vaccination Campaign. Cureus. 2024;16(1):e52876.
30. McCullough PA; Courageous Discourse. (2024). BREAKING--Springer Nature Cureus Journal of Medical Science Violates Committee on Publication Ethics (COPE) Guidelines. [online] Available from https://petermcculloughmd.substack.com/p/breaking-springer-nature-cureus-journal?r=14jb45&utm_campaign=post&utm_medium=web&open=false. [Last accessed April, 2024]
31. Sparks K, Powell KR. (2022). Assessing Predatory Journal Publishing within Health Sciences. [online] Available from https://www.sla.org/wp-content/uploads/2022/08/Predatory-Journal-Publishing.pdf. [Last accessed April, 2024]
32. Kostoff RN. Under-reporting of Adverse Events in the Biomedical Literature. J Data Inform Sci. 2016;1(4):10-32.
33. MacMillan C; Yale Medicine. (2022). Emergency Use Authorization vs. Full FDA Approval: What's the Difference? [online] Available from https://www.yalemedicine.org/news/what-does-eua-mean. [Last accessed April, 2024]

34. Ried K, BinJemain T, Sali A. Therapies to Prevent Progression of COVID-19, Including Hydroxychloroquine, Azithromycin, Zinc, and Vitamin D3 with or without Intravenous Vitamin C: An International, Multicenter, Randomized Trial. Cureus. 2021;13(11):e19902.
35. Alexander PE, Armstrong R, Fareed G, Lotus J, Oskoui R, Prodromos C, et al. Early multidrug treatment of SARS-CoV-2 infection (COVID-19) and reduced mortality among nursing home (or outpatient/ambulatory) residents. Med Hypotheses. 2021;153:110622.
36. Horby P, Mafham M, Linsell L, Bell JL, Staplin N, Emberson JR, et al. Effect of hydroxychloroquine in hospitalized patients with COVID-19. N Engl J Med. 2020;383(21):2030-40.
37. Jalsevac S; LifeSiteNews. (2020). How a false hydroxychloroquine narrative was created, and more. [online] Available from https://www.lifesitenews.com/blogs/how-a-false-hydroxychloroquine-narrative-was-created-and-more/. [Last accessed April, 2024]
38. Casso M; KGNS. (2022). Government pays hospitals more money for Covid-19 patients than non-Covid patients. [online] Available from https://www.kgns.tv/2022/03/28/government-pays-hospitals-more-money-covid-19-patients-than-non-covid-patients/. [Last accessed April, 2024]
39. Young RO. (2022). The Father of the PCR Test - Kary Mullis. [online] Available from https://www.drrobertyoung.com/post/the-father-of-the-pcr-test-kary-mullis. [Last accessed April, 2024]
40. ELMS. Research LLC. (2021). PCR Testing Report. [online] Available from https://www.brlax.net/wp-content/uploads/2021/04/PCR-Test.pdf. [Last accessed April, 2024]
41. Daly R; HFMA. (2020). Hospitals in COVID-19 hotspots to receive $10 billion more in federal aid \ HFMA. [online] Available from https://www.hfma.org/payment-reimbursement-and-managed-care/the-new-round-will-pay-50-000-per-covid-19-admission-compared/. [Last accessed April, 2024].
42. Edwards S; Organic Lifestyle Magazine. (2020). CDC admits financial hospital incentives drove up COVID-19 death rates. [online] Available from https://www.organiclifestylemagazine.com/cdc-admits-finacial-hospital-incentives-drove-up-covid-19-death-rates. [Last accessed April, 2024]
43. CMS.gov. New COVID-19 Treatments Add-On Payment (NCTAP). [online] Available from https://www.cms.gov/medicare/covid-19/new-covid-19-treatments-add-payment-nctap. [Last accessed April, 2024]
44. Mercola J; The Defender. (2023). Lawsuits Pile Up Alleging Remdesivir Killed COVID Patients. [online] Available from https://childrenshealthdefense.org/defender/lawsuits-remdesivir-covid-cola/. [Last accessed April, 2024]
45. FEMA. COVID-19 Funeral Assistance. [online] Available from https://www.fema.gov/disaster/historic/coronavirus/economic/funeral-assistance. [Last accessed April, 2024]
46. BlueCross BlueShield. (2021). Blue Cross and Blue Shield Federal Employee Program (FEP) Joins White House Effort to Achieve National Vaccination Goal. [online] Available from https://www.bcbs.com/press-releases/blue-cross-and-blue-shield-federal-employee-program-fep-joins-white-house-effort. [Last accessed April, 2024]
47. Anthem Medicaid. COVID-19 Vaccine Provider Incentive program. [online] Available from https://providers.anthem.com/docs/gpp/KY_CAID_PU_COVID19VaccineProviderIncentiveProgram.pdf?v=202110121818. [Last accessed April, 2024]
48. Delfino D; GoodRX Health. (2021). Incentives for COVID-19 Vaccination: Food, Cash, & Other Perks. [online] Available from https://www.goodrx.com/health-topic/vaccines/covid-19-vaccination-incentives. [Last accessed April, 2024]
49. Agorist M; Truth Unmuted. FOIA Request Reveals Biden Admin Paid $1 Billion to Corporate Media Outlets to Push Covid Vaccines. [online] Available from https://truthunmuted.org/foia-request-reveals-biden-admin-paid-1-billion-to-corporate-media-outlets-to-push-covid-vaccines/. [Last accessed April, 2024]

50. Elijah S; Trial Site News. (2023). Did Biden Administration Pay Physician Networks to Push COVID-19 Vaccine Prematurely?. [online] Available from https://www.trialsitenews.com/a/did-biden-administration-pay-physician-networks-to-push-covid-19-vaccine-prematurely-bcf50597. [Last accessed April, 2024]
51. Thorpe J, Macko G. TakeDownPfizer Campaign—Dr. James Thorp and Glen Macko extensively review the corruption in progress with CDC, HHS, Pfizer and much, much more. Humanity Coalition. [online] Available from https://rumble.com/v2logp0-dr.-james-thorp-with-glen-mackow.html. [Last accessed April, 2024]
52. Bredesen DE. Reversal of cognitive decline: a novel therapeutic program. Aging (Albany NY). 2014;6(9):707-17.
53. Kostoff RN; Trial Site News. Where are Clinical Trials for Alternative Cancer Therapies? [online] Available from https://www.trialsitenews.com/a/where-are-clinical-trials-for-alternative-cancer-therapies-d0b3365e. [Last accessed April, 2024]
54. Brigden ML. Unproven (questionable) cancer therapies. West J Med. 1995;163(5):463-9.
55. Asbestos.com. High cost of cancer treatment. [online] Available from https://www.asbestos.com/featured-stories/high-cost-of-cancer-treatment/. [Last accessed April, 2024]
56. Levey N; NPR.org. (2022). She was already battling cancer. Then she had to fight the bill collectors. [online] Available from https://www.npr.org/sections/health-shots/2022/07/09/1110370391/cost-cancer-treatment-medical-debt#:~:text=The%20National%20Cancer%20Institute%20calculated,Usually%2C%20most%20costs%20are%20covered. [Last accessed April, 2024]
57. Kostoff RN; Repository.gatech.edu. (2018). OSHA Permissible Exposure Limits (PELs) are too Permissive. [online] Available from https://repository.gatech.edu/entities/publication/d01f9c2e-4bb6-4f96-9c9f-699e4c150039. [Last accessed April, 2024]
58. Aviv R; New Yorker Magazine. (2014). A valuable reputation. [online] Available from https://www.newyorker.com/magazine/2014/02/10/a-valuable-reputation. [Last accessed April, 2024]
59. Nass M. (2020). WHO and UK trials use potentially lethal hydroxychloroquine dose—according to WHO consultant. Anthrax Vaccine—Posts by Meryl Nass, M.D. [online] Available from https://anthraxvaccine.blogspot.com/2020/06/who-trial-using-potentially-fatal.html. [Last accessed April, 2024]
60. Robinson S. (2023). The Dr. Meryl Nass Interview—Maine Wire TV. [online] Available from https://www.themainewire.com/2023/04/the-dr-meryl-nass-interview-maine-wire-tv/. [Last accessed April, 2024]
61. Kostoff RN; Trial Site News. (2021). COVID-19 "vaccines": the wrong bomb over the wrong target at the wrong time. [online] Available from https://www.trialsitenews.com/a/covid-19-vaccines-the-wrong-bomb-over-the-wrong-target-at-the-wrong-time. [Last accessed April, 2024]
62. CHD.TV. (2023). Dr. Sucharit Bhakdi's Warning to the World. [online] Available from https://live.childrenshealthdefense.org/chd-tv/shows/good-morning-chd/dr-sucharit-bhakdis-warning-to-the-world/?utm_source=luminate&utm_medium=email&utm_campaign=chdtv. [Last accessed April, 2024]

Index

Page numbers followed by *b* refer to box, *f* refer to figure, *fc* refer to flowchart, and *t* refer to table.

A

B

D

E

H

I

J

K

L

M

N

T

U

V

W

Y

Z